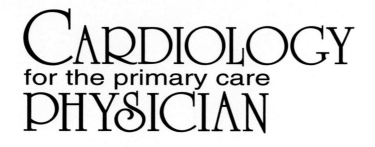

CARDIOLOGY
for the primary care
PHYSICIAN

2nd edition

Edited by:

Joseph S. Alpert

Professor and Chairman
Department of Medicine
University of Arizona
Health Sciences Center
Tucson, Arizona

with 70 contributors

From the Series:
CURRENT PRACTICE OF MEDICINE 2nd edition
Roger C. Bone and Faith Fitzgerald, Editors

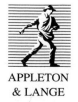

APPLETON
& LANGE

Developed by Current Medicine, Inc., Philadelphia

Current Medicine, Inc.

MANAGING EDITOR . . . . Lori J. Bainbridge

DEVELOPMENTAL EDITORS . . . . Crystal G. Norris, Elizabeth Rexon

EDITORIAL ASSISTANT . . . . Daniel J. McCue

ART DIRECTOR . . . . Paul Fennessy

COVER DESIGN . . . . Lisa Caro

LAYOUT . . . . Jerilyn Bockorick and Patrick Whelan

ILLUSTRATION DIRECTOR . . . . Ann Saydlowski

ILLUSTRATOR . . . . Gary Welch, Lisa Weischedel

PRODUCTION MANAGER . . . . Lori Holland

ASSISTANT PRODUCTION MANAGER . . . . Sally Nicholson

TYPESETTER . . . . Ryan Walsh

Cardiology for the primary care physician/Edited by Joseph S. Alpert; with
  69 contributors. — 2nd ed.
    p. cm.
    "From the series: Current practive of medicine, 2nd edition, Roger C. Bone
and Faith Fitzgerald, editors"
  - Includes bibliographical references and index.
    ISBN 0-8385-1563-0 (hardcover)
    1. Cardiology 2. Primary care (Medicine) 3. Cardiovascular system —
Diseases.   I. Alpert, Joseph S. II. Current practice of medicine.
    [DNLM: 1. Heart Diseases.   WG 210 C2677 1997]
RC667.C3834 1997
616.1'2—dc21
DNLM/DLC   97-41983
for Library of Congress   CIP

Library of Congress Cataloging-in-Publication Data

Printed and bound in Singapore by Imago
10 9 8 7 6 5 4 3 2 1

ISBN: 0-8385-1563-0

Although every effort has been made to ensure that drug doses and other information are presented accurately in this publication, the ultimate responsibility rests with the prescribing physician. Neither the publishers nor the author can be held responsible for errors or for any consequences arising from the use of the information contained therein. Any product mentioned in this publication should be used in accordance with the prescribing information prepared by the manufacturers. No claims or endorsements are made for any drug or compound at present under clinical investigation.

Contributors

JOSEPH S. ALPERT, MD
Professor and Chairman
Department of Medicine
University of Arizona
Health Sciences Center
Tucson, Arizona

JACK E. ANSELL, MD
Professor and Vice Chair
Department of Medicine
Boston University School of Medicine
Boston, Massachusetts

MOHAMMAD ASIF, MD
Cardiology Fellow
Department of Cardiology
University of Medicine and Dentistry of
   New Jersey
Newark, New Jersey

RICHARD C. BECKER, MD
Associate Professor of Medicine
University of Massachusetts Medical School
Director, Coronary Care Unit
Director, Thrombosis Research Center
University of Massachusetts Medical Center
Worcester, Massachusetts

DALE BERG, MD
Assistant Professor of Medicine
Department of Medicine
Medical College of Wisconsin
Milwaukee, Wisconsin

CHARLES M. BLATT, MD
Instructor in Medicine
Harvard Medical School
Associate Physician
Brigham and Women's Hospital
Boston, Massachusetts

BRAD S. BURLEW, MD
Associate Professor
University of Tennessee School of Medicine
Director, Cardiac Catheterization Laboratory
University of Tennessee Bowld Hospital
Memphis, Tennessee

SEEMANT CHATURVEDI, MD
Assistant Professor
Department of Neurology
Wayne State University
Staff Neurologist
Detroit Medical Center
Detroit, Michigan

MELVIN D. CHEITLIN, MD
Professor of Medicine
Division of Cardiology
Department of Medicine
University of California, San Francisco,
   School of Medicine
San Francisco General Hospital
San Francisco, California

JOHN S. CHILD, MD, FACC
Co-Chief for Clinical Cardiology
Adult and Congenital Heart Disease Center
UCLA School of Medicine
Department of Medicine
Division of Cardiology
Los Angeles, California

JULIUS J. CHOSY, MD
Professor of Medicine
University of Wisconsin
Associate Chief of Staff for
   Ambulatory Care
William S. Middleton Memorial
   Veteran's Hospital
Madison, Wisconsin

JACK W. COBURN, MD
Professor
Department of Medicine
University of California, Los Angeles,
   School of Medicine
Staff Physician
West Los Angeles VA Medical Center
Los Angeles, California

PETER F. COHN, MD
Professor of Medicine
Division of Cardiology
Department of Medicine
State University of New York at
   Stony Brook
Stony Brook, New York

DEBORAH M. DeMARCO, MD
Associate Professor of Medicine
Division of Rheumatology
Department of Medicine
University of Massachusetts Medical School
Worcester, Massachusetts

VINCENT DeQUATTRO, MD
Professor of Medicine
Department of Medicine
University of Southern California
   School of Medicine

Chief, Hypertension Service
Los Angeles County University of Southern
   California Medical Center
Los Angeles, California

RICHARD B. DEVEREUX, MD
Professor of Medicine
Cornell University Medical College
Director, Echocardiography Laboratory
The New York Hospital
New York, New York

GORDON A. EWY, MD
Professor and Chief of Cardiology
Department of Medicine
University of Arizona College of Medicine
Director, Department of Cardiology
University of Arizona Medical Center
Tucson, Arizona

MARK N. FIENGO, DO
Eastern Connecticut Cardiology Group, PC
New London, Connecticut;
Clinical Instructor of Medicine
Allegheny University Hospital,
   Hahnemann Campus
Philadelphia, Pennsylvania

MICHAEL A. FIFER, MD
Associate Professor of Medicine
Harvard University
Director, Coronary Care Unit
Massachusetts General Hospital
Boston, Massachusetts

EDWARD A. FISHER, MD
Clinical Associate Professor
Department of Medicine
Assistant Director of Echocardiography
Mt. Sinai Hospital
New York, New York

MARC FISHER, MD
Professor of Neurology and Radiology
Department of Medicine
University of Massachusetts
   School of Medicine
Chief of Neurology
Medical Center of Central Massachusetts
Worcester, Massachusetts

GERALD F. FLETCHER, MD
Professor of Medicine
Mayo Medical School

Senior Associate Consultant
Mayo Clinic Jacksonville
Jacksonville, Florida

BARRY A. FRANKLIN, PHD
Director, Cardiac Rehabilitation and
    Exercise Laboratories
William Beaumont Hospital
Professor of Physiology
Wayne State University School of Medicine
Detroit, Michigan

JOÃO M. FRAZÃO, MD
Visiting Assistant Professor
Department of Medicine
University of California, Los Angeles
Research Fellow
West Los Angeles VA Medical Center
Los Angeles, California

DAVID F. GIANSIRACUSA, MD
Professor of Medicine
Associate Chair
Department of Medicine
University of Massachusetts Medical Center
Worcester, Massachusetts

MARTIN E. GOLDMAN, MD
Associate Professor
Department of Medicine
Mt. Sinai Medical School
Director, Non-Invasive Cardiology
Mt. Sinai Hospital
New York, New York

THOMAS B. GRABOYS, MD
Associate Clinical Professor of Medicine
Harvard Medical School
Director, Lown Cardiovascular Center
Physician, Brigham and Women's Hospital
Boston, Massachusetts

HAIM HAMMERMAN, MD
Director, Coronary Care Unit
Department of Cardiology
Rambam Medical Center
Haifa, Israel

ROBERT C. HENDEL, MD
Associate Professor of Medicine
Division of Cardiology
Department of Medicine
Northwestern University Medical School
Chicago, Illinois

L. DAVID HILLIS, MD
Professor
Department of Internal Medicine
University of Texas Southwestern
    Medical Center
Dallas, Texas

THOMAS A. HOLLY, MD
Fellow in Cardiovascular Medicine
Department of Medicine
University of Massachusetts Medical Center
Worcester, Massachusetts

HOWARD R. HORN, MD
The LW Diggs Alumni Professor of
    Medicine and Chair of Excellence in
    Medical Education
Department of Medicine
University of Tennessee at Memphis
    School of Medicine
Senior Physician
University of Tennessee Bowld Hospital
Memphis, Tennessee

**RUSSELL D. HULL, MSC, FRCP(C),
FACP, FCCP**
Professor of Medicine
Department of Medicine
University of Calgary
Calgary, Alberta, Canada

MICHAEL H. HUMPHREYS, MD
Chief, Division of Nephrology
University of California, San Francisco
San Francisco, California

**WILLIAM B. KANNEL, MD, MPH,
FACC**
Professor of Medicine and Public Health
Department of Medicine
Boston University School of Medicine
Boston, Massachusetts

ROBERT A. KLONER, MD, PHD
Professor of Medicine
University of Southern California
Director of Research
Heart Institute
Good Samaritan Hospital
Los Angeles, California

DEPING LEE, MD
Assistant Professor
Department of Research Medicine
Associate Director
Hypertension Diagnostic Laboratory
University of Southern California
    School of Medicine
Los Angeles, California

CARL V. LEIER, MD
Overstreet Professor of Medicine
    and Pharmacology
Director of Cardiology
The Ohio State University
    College of Medicine
Columbus, Ohio

MARTIN M. LEWINTER, MD
Director of Cardiology
Professor of Medicine
University of Vermont College of Medicine
Burlington, Vermont

A. JAMES LIEDTKE, MD
Professor of Medicine
Department of Medicine
University of Wisconsin Medical School
Madison, Wisconsin

ROBERT G. LUKE, MD
Taylor Professor of Medicine
Director, Department of Internal Medicine
University of Cincinnati
    College of Medicine
Cincinnati, Ohio

ERIC L. MICHELSON, MD
Professor of Medicine
Allegheny University of the Health Sciences
Philadelphia, Pennsylvania;
Director, Cardiovascular Research
Astra Merck
Wayne, Pennsylvania

CHARLES K. MOORE, MD
Assistant Professor of Medicine
Department of Medicine
University of Mississippi Medical Center
Jackson, Mississippi

NAVIN C. NANDA, MD
Professor of Medicine
Division of Cardiology
Department of Medicine
University of Alabama School of Medicine
Birmingham, Alabama

J.V. NIXON, MD
Professor of Medicine
Medical College of Virginia
Virginia Commonwealth University
Richmond, Virginia

IRA S. OCKENE, MD
Associate Professor of Cardiology
Department of Medicine
University of Massachusetts Medical Center
Worcester, Massachusetts

JOHN B. O'CONNELL, MD
Professor and Chairman
Department of Medicine
University of Mississippi Medical School
Jackson, Mississippi

ELIZABETH O. OFILI, MD, MPH
Chief, Section of Cardiology
Associate Professor of Medicine

Department of Internal Medicine
Morehouse School of Medicine
Atlanta, Georgia

JOHN A. PARASKOS, MD
Professor of Medicine
Department of Cardiovascular Medicine
University of Massachusetts Medical School
Worcester, Massachusetts

THOMAS G. PICKERING, MD, DPHIL
Professor of Medicine
Department of Medicine
The Cornell University Medical College
New York, New York

WILLIAM R. PITTS, MD
Senior Fellow
Internal Medicine
University of Texas Southwestern
   Medical Center
Dallas, Texas

ERIC N. PRYSTOWSKY, MD
Consulting Professor of Medicine
Department of Medicine
Duke University Medical Center
Durham, North Carolina;
Director, Clinical Electrophysiology
   Laboratory
St. Vincent Hospital
Indianapolis, Indiana

TIMOTHY J. REGAN, MD
Professor of Medicine
Department of Medicine
University of Medicine and Dentistry of
   New Jersey
Newark, New Jersey

STUART RICH, MD
Professor of Medicine
Department of Medicine
Rush Medical College
Rush Heart Institute
Center for Pulmonary Heart Disease
Chicago, Illinois

CLIFFORD J. ROSEN, MD
St. Joseph Hospital
Maine Center for Osteoporosis Research
   and Education
Bangor, Maine

JOHN SPEER SCHROEDER, MD
Professor of Medicine
Department of Medicine
Stanford University School of Medicine
Stanford, California

ERNST R. SCHWARZ, MD
Research Fellow
Division of Cardiology
University of Southern California
Heart Institute
Good Samaritan Hospital
Los Angeles, California

JAMES SEBASTIAN, MD
Associate Professor of Medicine
Department of Medicine
Medical College of Wisconsin
Milwaukee, Wisconsin

SUSAN SIMANDL, MD
Assistant Professor of Medicine
Division of Cardiology
Department of Medicine
State University of New York at
   Stony Brook
Stony Brook, New York

SIDNEY C. SMITH, JR., MD
Chief, Division of Cardiology
Professor of Medicine
University of North Carolina at Chapel Hill
Chapel Hill, North Carolina

JOHN A. SPITTELL, JR., MD, MACP, FACC
Professor (Emeritus) of Medicine
Cardiovascular Department
Mayo Medical School
Consultant, Cardiovascular Disease
Mayo Clinic
Rochester, Minnesota

PETER C. SPITTELL, MD, FACC
Assistant Professor of Medicine
Division of Cardiovascular Diseases
Department of Internal Medicine
Mayo Medical School
Rochester, Minnesota

KELLY ANNE SPRATT, DO
Assistant Professor of Medicine
Division of Cardiology
University of Pennsylvania
Director, Women's Cardiovascular Health
Philadelphia, Pennsylvania

PAUL D. STEIN, MD
Henry Ford Professor of Medicine
Case Western Reserve University
   School of Medicine
Cleveland, Ohio;
Medical Director, Cardiac Wellness Center
Henry Ford Hospital
Detroit, Michigan

NEIL J. STONE, MD
Professor of Clinical Medicine
Division of Cardiology
Department of Medicine
Northwestern University Medical School
Chicago, Illinois

JAY M. SULLIVAN, MD
Chief, Division of Cardiology
Professor of Medicine
Department of Medicine
University of Tennessee, Memphis,
   College of Medicine
Senior Physician
University of Tennessee Bowld Hospital
Memphis, Tennessee

PAUL T. VAITKUS, MD
Professor
Case Western Reserve University
   School of Medicine
Cardiology Division
University Hospitals of Cleveland
Cleveland, Ohio

PANTEL S. VOKONAS, MD
Professor of Medicine and Public Health
Department of Medicine
Boston University School of Medicine
Director, Department of Veteran's Affairs
Normative Aging Study
Boston, Massachusetts

PARK W. WILLIS IV, MD
Associate Professor
Division of Cardiology
Department of Medicine
University of North Carolina at Chapel Hill
School of Medicine
Chapel Hill, North Carolina

GREGG M. YAMADA, MD
Instructor
Department of Medicine
University of Arizona College of Medicine
Tucson, Arizona

Preface

The response to the first edition of this book was remarkable. More physicians called, wrote, and spoke to me concerning this text than with any previous book I have written or edited. The book reached a wide audience of primary care physicians; it was also positively reviewed. Consequently, a second edition seemed warranted. Much of the material contained in *Cardiology for the Primary Care Physician* was also printed as part of Current Medicine's large internal medicine text, *Current Practice of Medicine*. This second edition of *Cardiology for the Primary Care Physician* contains the latest diagnostic and therapeutic concepts in cardiovascular medicine. Most of the authors from the first edition have updated their chapters for the second edition.

I would like to acknowledge the untiring efforts of my academic administrative staff, Mrs. Barbara Raney and Mrs. Charlene Sass, who have helped me in innumerable ways with both editions of this text. I would also like to thank the editors of Current Medicine whose efforts have been essential to the success of *Current Practice of Medicine* and *Cardiology for the Primary Care Physician*.

Joseph S. Alpert, MD
Tucson, Arizona

Contents

Physical Diagnosis in Medicine

Dale Berg
James Sebastian

> ### Key Points
>
> - Physical diagnosis plays a central role in making diagnostic and management decisions in the everyday practice of medicine.
>
> - Physical diagnostic techniques are most useful when the clinician approaches them with knowledge of the techniques, outcomes, and scientific characteristics (*ie*, knowledge of sensitivity and specificity of the tests).
>
> - With a thorough but succinct examination of various musculoskeletal structures (*eg*, shoulder, knees, back or hands), the clinician will be able to define the underlying diagnosis.
>
> - Knowledge of the techniques of cardiac palpation and auscultation provides the clinician tools for evaluating cardiac extrasounds, especially murmurs.
>
> - Knowledge of the techniques of percussion, tactile fremitus, and auscultation afford the clinician tools for evaluating pulmonary problems.

The past several decades have seen increasing use of the technologic aspects of medicine for making diagnostic and therapeutic decisions. These methods, which include computed tomography and magnetic resonance imaging, echocardiography, cardiac catheterization, and a veritable potpourri of laboratory tests, have provided new and exciting modalities to assist physicians in providing quality medical care. These techniques, via their emphasis in medical school and postgraduate training, have taken over as the central features of medical diagnosis and management at the expense of the techniques of physical examination and history taking.

Objective evidence that medical students and house staff are deficient in physical examination skills is provided in a 1992 study by St. Clair and coworkers [1], in which internal medicine house staff were asked to auscult classic cardiac findings under optimal auscultatory conditions. Only 37% of the house staff at this institution could detect incontrovertible mitral stenosis. Only a slight majority (52% and 54%, respectively) detected mitral regurgitation or aortic insufficiency.

Yet physical examination is indeed a first-line, pivotal, basic foundation on which the remainder of the evaluative and management schemes are based. This is self-evident to general internists and other primary care providers, and has been demonstrated by several studies, *eg*, Peterson and coworkers [2]. When the examination is performed correctly and the result interpreted using scientific parameters of sensitivity, specificity, positive predictive values, negative predictive values, and likelihood ratios, as eloquently described by Sackett and coworkers [3], it becomes integral to effective, appropriate, efficient, and economical patient care, thus often precluding the need for expensive and invasive examinations. Even when a specific diagnosis cannot be established on the basis of the bedside history and physical examination, clinicians can construct a weighted differential diagnosis on which a logical and diagnostic approach can be formulated.

This chapter provides a brief overview of some of the most commonly used physical examination techniques for seven discrete and common medical problem areas.

Hand Pain, Stiffness, or Dysfunction

It is exceedingly common for patients to present with pain, stiffness, or dysfunction of one or both hands. The primary care physician can evaluate and diagnose most of these problems by performing a basic physical examination of the hands (Table 1).

Felon

A felon is an exquisitely tender, swollen, erythematous nodule at the tip of a digit. This lesion is a type of "collar button abscess" that forms in the terminal pulp cavity of the distal phalanx, usually as the result of an antecedent puncture wound.

Heberden's and Bouchard's Nodes

Heberden's and Bouchard's nodes are nontender nodules on the distal interphalangeal (Heberden's) or proximal interphalangeal (Bouchard's) joints of the digits. They usually occur on the digits of the hands, the feet, or both in middle-aged or older patients and are consistent with degenerative joint disease.

Sclerodactyly

Sclerodactyly is characterized by a diffuse and quite painless decreased range of motion of the digits resulting from a palpable thickening of the skin and underlying connective tissue about the digits. The differential diagnosis of etiologies includes the autoimmune and rheumatologic disorders of mixed connective tissue disease, CREST syndrome (calcinosis, Raynaud's disease, esophageal dysmotility, sclerodactyly, and telangiectasia), rheumatoid arthritis, scleroderma, Buerger's disease, and diabetes.

Swan Neck and Boutonnière Signs

Swan neck deformity is hyperextension contracture of the proximal interphalangeal and joint flexion contracture of the distal interphalangeal joint; the boutonnière deformity is the converse, in that the proximal interphalangeal joint has a significant flexion contracture and the distal interphalangeal joint has a contracture of hyperextension. These signs are found in severe chronic polyarticular arthritides in patients who have sustained previous trauma to the interphalangeal joint.

Boxer's Fracture

The presence of tenderness and swelling over the ulnar aspect of the hand that occurs after the patient forcibly hits an object with a closed fist is a simple fracture of the diaphysis of the fifth metacarpal bone.

Trigger Finger and Locked Finger

Triggering is the snapping sensation of the digit on flexion, extension, or both. Locking is the reversible inability to extend the affected finger or fingers, usually at the proximal interphalangeal joint. These conditions result from inflammation at the site where the long flexor tendons pass through the metacarpophalangeal joint pulley.

Ganglion

Ganglions are soft, fluctuant, nontender lesions that occur on the palmar or dorsal side of the hands, wrists, or both, each adjacent to a tendon or tendon sheath. They are well-defined benign cystic structures and have nothing to do with the nervous system in spite of the name.

Dupuytren's Disease

Dupuytren's disease is the presence of a flexion contracture, usually in the fourth and fifth digits, which cannot be actively or passively extended. Palpable nodules are often present in the palmar fascia of the affected digits. The presence of this disease is correlated with ethanol abuse and chronic hepatic diseases, trauma, and use of anticonvulsants.

de Quervain's Disease

The presence of tenderness in and about the tendons that comprise the anatomic "snuff box" at the dorsal aspect of the base of the thumb characterizes de Quervain's disease. In this entity, there is inflammation of the tendons of the abductor pollcis longus muscle, the extensor pollicis longus muscle, and the extensor pollicis brevis muscle. Examination reveals Finklestein's sign (pain is reproduced when the patient is instructed to grasp the thumb with adjacent digits while passively flexing the wrist ulnarly and palmarly).

Radial Nerve Dysfunction

If any evidence of radial nerve dysfunction is present, a screening examination should be performed (Table 2).

TABLE 1 OVERALL PHYSICAL EXAMINATION OF THE HANDS

Perform active and then passive range-of-motion assessment of the wrist, metacarpophalangeal, proximal interphalangeal, and distal interphalangeal joints

Wrist joints
  Flexion: 80°
  Extension (dorsiflexion): 70°
  Abduction: 30°
  Adduction: 30°
Metacarpophalangeal joints
  Flexion: 90°
  Extension: 30°
Proximal interphalangeal joints
  Flexion: 120°
  Extension: 0°
Distal interphalangeal joints
  Flexion: 80°
  Extension: 0°
Immobilize the joint or joints if a fracture is suspected
Visually inspect and palpate the digits and hands
Screen for the function of the three nerves that innervate the hands: the ulnar, median, and radial nerves (*see* Table 2).

TABLE 2 OVERALL SCREENING EXAMINATION OF NERVES IN THE HANDS	
Procedure	**Nerve**
Fine touch on the palmar skin of digits 1, 2, and 3	Median
Fine touch on the dorsal skin of digits 1, 2, and 3	Radial
Fine touch on the ulnar aspect of the hand	Ulnar
Active flexion (apposition) of the thumb	Median
Active abduction of the digits	Ulnar
Active dorsiflexion of the hand at the wrist	Radial

TABLE 3 OVERALL PHYSICAL EXAMINATION OF THE BACK
Perform passive and active range-of-motion assessment of the lower back
Extension: 30°
Flexion: 75° to 90°
Lateral bending: 30°, left and right
Rotation: 30°, left and right
Palpate the spinous processes of the back
Palpate the paraspinous musculature
Perform a screening neurologic examination of the S-1, L-5, and L-4 roots of the lower extremities (*see* Table 4)
Perform a rectal examination to determine sphincter tone
Perform the straight-leg-raising examination by placing the patient in a supine position and passively flexing each leg at the hip

Wristdrop

Wristdrop is the development of significant weakness in dorsiflexion at the wrist joint. The patient has a "limp" wrist that can be passively but not actively extended. This may be the result of damage to the radial nerve, possibly secondary to a Colles fracture of the radius or a spiral fracture of the humeral shaft.

Median Nerve Dysfunction

If any evidence of median nerve dysfunction is present, a screening examination should be performed (Table 2).

Carpal tunnel syndrome

The sensory manifestations of carpal tunnel syndrome, which is a very common entity, include the development of paresthesias and numbness of the volar (palmar) side of digits 1, 2, and 3. A further manifestation is the presence of thenar (thumb) muscular atrophy. In addition, Tinel's sign may be present. This is the development of paresthesias and dysthesias in the distribution of the median nerve when the examiner percusses over the midpoint of a line transversely placed at the base of the thenar and hypothenar eminences for more than 30 seconds. The site for percussing should be adjacent to the palmaris longus tendon immediately on the radial side. In Phalen's sign, the patient is directed to flex both hands at the wrist passively (reverse prayer position) for 60 seconds. The development of paresthesias and dysthesias in the distribution of the median nerve is consistent with carpal tunnel syndrome. In their review of carpal tunnel syndrome, Katz and coworkers [4] reported the sensitivity of Tinel's and Phalen's signs to be in the range of 25% to 75%, whereas the specificity of these signs was 70% to 90%.

LOW BACK PAIN OR STIFFNESS

Physical examination plays a central role [5] in the evaluation of back pain and dysfunction and effectively supersedes all other techniques (Table 3).

Acute Musculoskeletal or Ligamentous Strain

With acute musculoskeletal or ligamentous strain, there is often spasm and tenderness of the involved back musculature but no radicular findings or neurologic deficits. The underlying pathology is the tearing of muscle and ligamentous structures from the lifting of a heavy object, with resultant pain and inflammation.

Herniated Disk

With sciatica or herniated disk [6], weakness of the muscles innervated by the L-5 and S-1 nerve roots is manifest by weakness of great toe dorsiflexion and an inability to perform a heel walk for L-5 deficit and by weakness of great toe plantarflexion, an inability to perform a tiptoe walk, and a decreased ankle jerk (Achille's reflex) for S-1 deficit (Table 4). Concurrent posterolateral thigh and leg pain, paresthesias, and sensory deficits are invariably present. The underlying pathology is often the posterior herniation of the disk annulus, the soft connective tissue bridge between two vertebral bodies. This herniation may result in entrapment or impingement of the nerve root (*ie*, the manifestations of sciata, unilaterally).

Compression Fracture

With compression fracture, there is significant tenderness over the affected vertebra, which is quite localized and can be severe. Concurrent findings are usually due to the underlying process. For example, dowager's hump, which is an accentuated thoracic kyphosis in patients with past compression fractures, occurs in osteoporosis. The compression can be trauma related or result from a loss of bone substance, thus weakening the individual vertebral body. Disorders predisposing to compression fractures include osteoporosis, neoplastic disease, and infectious diseases, *eg*, osteomyelitis.

Ankylosing Spondylitis

Ankylosing spondylitis is characterized by a marked abnormal straightening of the back, manifested specifically with a loss of the normal thoracic kyphosis and lumber lordosis. Further-more, palpable tenderness exists over the sacroiliac joints, and the normal range of motion of the back is significantly decreased. The underlying pathogenesis is inflammatory arthritis affecting the central (*ie*, appendicular) skeleton.

Epidural Disease

On examination, the patient with epidural disease (includ-ing cauda equina and cord compression syndromes) may have fever and quite often has pain over the affected verte-bra. There can be weakness of the musculature innervated by L-4, L-5, and the sacral nerves (*see* Table 4). This weak-ness is manifest as great toe weakness; weakness of foot dorsiflexion and foot plantar flexion; and an inability to walk on the toes, the heels, or both. Furthermore, a weak-ened anal sphincter and the presence of an enlarged, fluid-filled urinary bladder are often demonstrable. This condi-tion is a result of disease from an infectious source, either endocarditis or an adjacent osteomyelitis, or from a malig-nant neoplastic source.

KNEE PAIN OR DYSFUNCTION

As the members of our society become more active, more injuries of and problems with the knees occur. Therefore, the primary care physician must know the physical examination of the knee. This is especially true given the fact that the vast majority of knee problems can be diagnosed by a thorough, site-specific physical examination [7,8•] (Table 5). A number of specific entities are diagnosed by physical examination.

Prepatellar Bursitis

Prepatellar bursitis is characterized by tender swelling and fluc-tuance over the anterior and superior aspects of the patella. This results from an inflammation of the prepatellar bursa, a bursa that is located immediately anterior (superficial) to the patella.

Infrapatellar Bursitis

Infrapatellar bursitis is characterized by moderately tender swelling on one side or both sides of the inferior aspect of the patellar ligament. The most marked manifestations are located immediately deep and inferior to the patella. This results from an inflammation of the infrapatellar bursa, a bursa that is located immediately deep and inferior to the patella itself.

TABLE 4 NEUROLOGIC SCREENING EXAMINATION OF THE LOWER EXTREMITIES	
Procedure	**Nerve**
Instruct the patient to walk on tiptoes, *ie*, actively plantar flex at the ankle	S-1
Instruct the patient to walk on the heels, *ie*, actively dorsiflex at the ankle	L-5
Instruct the patient to actively extend the leg at the knee	L-4

Semimembranous Bursitis

Semimembranous bursitis is marked by a moderately tender fullness in the superior medial aspect of the popliteal fossa. The mass becomes more palpable on extension, whereas it relaxes on knee flexion and thus becomes nonpalpable. This is the result of an inflammation of the semimembranous bursa, a bursa that is located deep in the superior medial popliteal fossa and immediately adjacent to the head of the gastrocnemius and the insertion of the semimembranous muscle.

Anterior Cruciate Ligament Tear

The presence of a moderate to large effusion and a marked decrease in range of motion characterize an anterior cruciate ligament tear. On further examination there are positive anterior drawer sign and positive Lachman's sign findings. These two signs can be difficult to demonstrate if the injury is acute because of the pain and swelling. The underlying pathogenesis is a partial or complete tear of the anterior cruciate ligament, usually resulting from a force applied to the tibia anteriorly (recall that this ligament connects the anterior tibia with the femur).

Posterior Cruciate Ligament Tear

The presence of a tender effusion in the affected knee and decreased range of motion characterize a posterior cruciate ligament tear. On further examination, there is a positive posterior drawer sign finding. The underlying pathogenesis is a partial or complete tear of the posterior cruciate liga-ment. As one can recall, the posterior cruciate ligament attaches the posterior tibia to the femur. The tear is usually the result of a direct blow to the proximal tibia when the knee is flexed.

Medial Meniscus Tear

With a medial meniscus tear, minimal joint instability or effu-sion is present. On further examination, there is a positive McMurray's test finding. The results of Childress' test (*ie*, the "duck waddle test," in which the patient is unable to fully flex the affected knee while instructed to move in the duck waddle position) may also be positive. Positive results are indicative of a rupture of the posterior horn of the medial meniscus. The underlying pathogenesis is one of damage to the cartilage (meniscus) in the medial compartment of the knee. The damage occurs when the knee is twisted medially and flexed, with concurrent bearing of weight.

Lateral Meniscus Tear

With a lateral meniscus tear, minimal joint instability or effu-sion is present. On further examination, McMurray's test findings are positive. The underlying pathogenesis is one of damage to the cartilage (meniscus) in the lateral compartment of the knee. The damage occurs when the knee is twisted laterally and flexed, with concurrent bearing of weight.

Medial Collateral Ligament Tear

The knee with a medial collateral ligament tear often has mild to moderate medial mobility, which is even more prominent if there has been concurrent damage to the anterior cruciate ligament. Valgus stress test results are positive. The underlying pathogenesis is partial or complete tear of the medial collateral ligament, usually a result of excessive valgus bending of the knee during activity.

Lateral Collateral Ligament Tear

On examination, the knee with a lateral collateral ligament tear often has mild to moderate lateral mobility, which is even more prominent if there has been concurrent damage to the anterior cruciate ligament. Valgus stress test results are positive. The underlying pathogenesis of this is the partial or complete tear of the lateral collateral ligament, usually as a result of excessive varus bending of the knee during activity.

Degenerative Joint Disease

In degenerative joint disease, crepitus is quite often present in the affected knee or knees, as is decreased range of motion. Furthermore, a small effusion in the involved knee

may be present. Often, a valgus or varus deformity exists, the lateral or medial compartments, respectively, are more significantly involved.

SHOULDER PROBLEMS

Physical examination is extremely important in the evaluation of the shoulder. Clearly the vast majority of problems can by diagnosed by a site-specific, thorough physical examination [9] (Table 6). The specific entities that can be diagnosed by physical examination are described in the following sections.

Anterior Glenohumeral Dislocation

In anterior glenohumeral dislocation, the acromion is inappropriately prominent and the head of the humerus is anteriorly and medially displaced to a position beneath the coracoid process. The patient positions and holds the arm close to the body, with the elbow flexed. Finally, there is a complete loss of passive or active range of motion of the arm at the shoulder. This disloca-

---

TABLE 5 OVERALL EXAMINATION OF THE KNEE

Perform active and passive range-of-motion assessment of the knee:
  Flexion: 130°
  Extension: 5°
  Adduction and abduction: Minimal
  Internal and external rotation: Minimal

Ballot the patellas. With the patient in a supine position and the knee extended, gently press on the suprapatellar area with one hand and on the patella with the other hand, attempting to press the patella against the tibial condyles

Palpate the structures around the knee for areas of fluctuance, swelling, or both

With the patient in a supine position and the knee extended, gently press on the lateral side of the knee 1 cm inferior to the patella, visually inspecting the medial side of the knee. Repeat the procedure on the medial side, visually inspecting the lateral side, if there is a concavity before that remains concave after applying pressure. If a loss of the concavity or even a convex appearance to the side of the knee (a bulge), an effusion is present

Instruct the patient to assume and maintain a neutral anatomic stance. If the tibia is abnormally adducted on the femur, the patient has a varus deformity (ie, is bowlegged). If the tibia is abnormally abducted on the femur, the patient has a valgus deformity (ie, is knock-kneed)

Perform Lachman's maneuver: With the patient in a supine position and the knee held by examiner and flexed at 30°, gently yet firmly pull on the tibia in an anterior direction so as to sublux it anteriorly. Perform with the knee in internal and external rotation positions to increase the sensitivity of the examination. If the tibia slides anteriorly over the femur (positive Lachman's sign) it is consistent with an anterior cruciate ligament tear.

Examine the patient for the perform posterior drawer sign. With the patient in a supine position and the knee held by the examiner and flexed at 90°, gently yet firmly push on the tibia in a posterior direction so as to sublux it posteriorly; use the contralateral knee as a control. If the tibia slides posteriorly under the femur (positive posterior drawer sign) it is consistent with a posterior cruciate ligament tear.

Perform McMurray's test. With the patient in a supine position, flex the hip and the knee until the heel touches the buttock. Steady the knee with one hand and grasp the heel with the other hand rotating the foot as far lateral (external rotation) as possible and the extend the knee to 90°. Return to the beginning and rotate the foot as far medial (internal rotation) as possible, and then passively extend the knee to 90°. Concurrently palpate the knee being tested. Repeat in the contralateral knee as a control. The presence of a click over the lateral aspect of the knee (a lateral McMurray sign) is consistent with a lateral meniscal tear, whereas, the presence of a click over the medial aspect of the knee (a medial McMurray sign) is consistent with a medial meniscal tear

Perform varus and valgus stress tests on affected knee. With the patient in a surpine position and the knee held by the examiner at 30°, gently yet firmly pull on the tibia with varus intent, palpating the lateral condyles. Pain or laxity over the condyles is consistent with lateral collateral ligament sprain. Repeat test with valgus intent, palpating over the medial condyle. Pain or laxity is consistent with medial collateral sprain.

From Daniel [7] and Rothenberg and Graf [8•]; with permission.

tion usually results from arm hyperextension (*eg*, while pitching a baseball overhand or serving a tennis ball overhand).

Acromioclavicular Separation

In acromioclavicular separation, the distal clavicle is superiorly displaced from the acromion. Furthermore, the patient is unable to abduct or flex the ipsilateral arm actively. In most cases, the separation of the clavicle from the acromion can be detected via visual and tactile inspection. This separation is the result of trauma, specifically force being placed on the shoulder with an inferoposterior thrust.

Clavicular Fracture

The patient with a clavicular fracture is unable to abduct or elevate the entire upper extremity. On visual inspection and palpation, the fracture is quite evident. The underlying pathogenesis is one of direct trauma to the shoulder, the anterosuperior chest wall, or both, usually as the result of a fall.

Bicipital Tendinitis

The patient with bicipital tendinitis has tenderness over the anterior shoulder and positive findings for Yergason's sign (*ie*, reproduction of the pain on flexion of the elbow against force) and Speed's sign (*ie*, reproduction of the pain on curling the shoulders actively inward). This is the result of inflammation of the long head of the biceps in the bicipital groove.

Subacromial Bursitis

With subacromial bursitis, there is significant tenderness over the anterior and inferior aspects of the acromion and the development of signs of impingement, including both the presence of positive impingement test findings (*ie*, pain over the anterior acromion when the patient's arm is maximally passively flexed and the examiner presses on the shoulder girdle).

Supraspinatus Tendinitis

With supraspinatus tendinitis, there is significant tenderness over and adjacent to the greater tuberosity of the humerus and the acromion process and a marked decrease in active and passive abduction of the humerus at the glenohumeral joint over 90°. The underlying pathogenesis of this entity is the noninfectious inflammation of the rotator cuff tendons, of the supraspinatus tendon specifically.

Rotator Cuff Tears

Rotator cuff tears are characterized by tenderness over the greater tuberosity of the humerus and weakness of the motions of abduction and external rotation of the arm at the shoulder. The passive range of motion of the arm is normal, but active motion, especially abduction, is significantly limited. Furthermore, there is a marked limitation to active abduction from 0° to 30°. This is the result of a tear in the supraspinatus muscle or tendon. If there is a marked decrease in active external rotation the infraspinatus and/or teres minor are involved.

MURMURS

Cardiac murmurs are frequently noted during routine physical examination [10] (Table 7). Although many murmurs are benign (innocent), others require further definition because they may be correlated with a malignant natural history. Furthermore, some lesions that these murmurs represent can be markers for other disease processes or may need antibiotic prophylaxis to prevent procedure-induced endocarditis (Table 8).

On the basis of the initial physical examination findings and the preliminary differential diagnosis, the examiner can then use other bedside maneuvers to assist in defining the underlying lesion. These specific maneuvers should not be performed blindly without having first defined the basic attributes of the murmur. Specific maneuvers are discussed in the following sections.

Systolic Murmurs Loudest at the Base

An attempt should be made to differentiate between aortic stenosis, a pathologic lesion that can result in malignant outcomes (including heart failure, left ventricular hypertrophy, syncope and sudden cardiac death) and that sometimes requires antibiotic prophylaxis; idiopathic hypertrophic subaortic stenosis (IHSS) another malignant lesion; and the benign entity aortic sclerosis, which does not require antibiotic prophylaxis.

To differentiate an aortic lesion from a subaortic lesion, such as IHSS, refer to Table 9. With the patient supine and breathing at baseline, auscultate using the diaphragm over the base, and then repeat the examination at this location 30 seconds after the patient has assumed a standing position [11]. If the murmur intensity decreases or is unchanged after standing, it is aortic stenosis or sclerosis, whereas an increase on standing is consistent with IHSS. Furthermore, if the murmur increases in intensity or stays the same with squatting, it is aortic stenosis or sclerosis, whereas if it decreases with squatting, it is IHSS. Finally, if the carotid pulse

TABLE 7 DIAGNOSTIC FEATURES OF A MURMUR

Place the patient in a supine position and auscult over the base and apex using the diaphragm with the patient breathing at baseline; note the following features of the murmur:

Timing—when the murmur occurs in the cardiac cycle
Systolic—between S_1 and S_2
Diastolic—between S_2 and S_1

Location—the location that is is easiest to auscult and/or palpate
Base—deep to the manubrium sternum
Apex—deep to the left fourth interspace

Intensity [10]
Heard, but not immediately
Faintest murmur is heard immediately after placing the stethoscope on the chest
Loud, without a thrill
Loud, with a thrill (*ie*, a palpable vibratory component to the murmur)
Can be heard with the stethoscope at an angle
Heard even with the stethoscope not touching the chest wall

Radiation—locations where the murmur can be heard distant from the loudest point

Associated manifestations—the company that the murmur keeps. Examples include the fixed split S_2 of atrial septal defect, the decreased intensity of S_2 in aortic stenosis, and the systolic click of mitral valve prolapse. Specifics are described in the text

S_1—first heart sound; S_2—second heart sound.

TABLE 8 DIFFERENTIAL DIAGNOSIS OF LESIONS FOR VARIOUS MURMURS

If systolic murmur is loudest at the base
Aortic sclerosis
Aortic stenosis
Idiopathic hypertrophic subaortic stenosis
Pulmonic stenosis, organic or functional

If diastolic murmur is loudest at the base
Aortic insufficiency
Pulmonic insufficiency

If diastolic murmur is loudest at the apex
Austin Flint murmur of aortic insufficiency
Mitral stenosis

If systolic murmur is loudest at the apex
Mitral insufficiency
Tricuspid insufficiency
Mitral valve prolapse
Ventricular septal defect

Procedure	Outcome
Change in the intensity of the murmur after attaining a standing from a supine position	Increased IHSS Decreased aortic valve
Change in the intensity of the murmur after attaining a squatting from a supine position	Decreased IHSS Increased aortic valve

IHSS—idiopathic hypertrophic subaortic stenosis.

decreases in intensity after an extrasystole, it is IHSS.

Severe aortic stenosis, unlike aortic sclerosis, results in a loss in the intensity of the second heart sound, a paradoxical splitting of the second heart tone (*ie*, P_2A_2 with inspiration, rather than the normal splitting of A_2P_2 with inspiration), or both; and has a decrease in the pulse pressure, with carotid upstrokes that are low and slow (*ie*, pulsus parvus et tardus) [12] (Table 10).

Systolic Murmurs Loudest at the Apex

The four most common lesions that manifest with systolic murmurs best heard at the apex are tricuspid regurgitation, mitral regurgitation, mitral valve prolapse, and ventricular septal defect. Maneuvers to differentiate these lesions are extremely useful.

The first step is to differentiate tricuspid regurgitation from the other lesions. This is accomplished by several specific maneuvers. The first is the Rivero-Carvallo maneuver, which consists of auscultating over the apex with the diaphragm at the end of expiration and then during a deep, held inspiration. If the intensity of the murmur is increased with inspiration, it is tricuspid regurgitation. There have been reports of 100% sensitivity and 88% specificity [13]. Furthermore, if the examiner auscultates over the apex with the diaphragm before and during the placement of manual pressure on the liver for 15 to 20 seconds and the intensity of the murmur increases (Vitums' sign), it is consistent with tricuspid

regurgitation. This sign has been reported to be 56% sensitive and virtually 100% specific [14]. Finally, if the examiner visually inspects the patient for jugular venous pulsations, these pulsations are often elevated, with large V waves and great Y descents (Lancisi's sign), in tricuspid regurgitation [14].

Once tricuspid regurgitation has been diagnosed, no further maneuvers are necessary. However, if tricuspid regurgitation is unlikely based on these maneuvers, the next step is to differentiate mitral valve prolapse from mitral regurgitation. Mitral valve prolapse has a concurrent click before the murmur in systole, whereas none of the other lesions have a systolic click. Furthermore, the murmur and click of mitral valve prolapse increase in intensity after the patient assumes a standing position; if the murmur does not change, it is consistent with mitral regurgitation or another lesion.

ABDOMINAL PAIN

One of the most common problems with which patients present to physicians, and to primary care physicians specifi-

Procedure	Aortic stenosis	Aortic sclerosis
Radiation of the murmur	Into the right carotid and right midclavicular areas	Minimal
Brachioradial delay [12]: with the patient supine or sitting, palpate the brachial and radial pulses simultaneously in one arm	The pulse in the radial site is delayed Sensitivity: 100% in severe aortic stenosis and 25% in mild aortic stenosis Specificity: 100%	Pulses are simultaneous
Second heart tone	Decreased intensity Paradoxical splitting (P_2A_2) with inspiration)	Discrete S_2 Physiological splitting (A_2P_2) with inspiration
Point of maximal impulse	Laterally displaced	Normal
Pulse wave contour	Pulsus parvus et tardus (low and slow)	Normal
Pulse pressure	<40 mm Hg	>40 mm Hg

S_2—second heart sound.

cally, is abdominal pain. Physical examination of the abdomen is pivotal in the evaluation of abdominal pain (Tables 11, 12, and 13). It will assist not only in making a diagnosis, but in an emergency (*ie*, an acute abdomen).

High-pitched bowel sounds heard on auscultation of the abdomen are called tinkles and are consistent with small bowel obstruction. Periods of markedly increased bowel sounds that are intermittent and few in nature are rushes; they are consistent with either normal findings, or early small bowel obstruction. Periods of markedly increased bowel sounds that are recurrent and heard without the assistance of a stethoscope are referred to as borborygmi and are consistent with a hyperdynamic small bowel. Finally, decreased or absent bowel sounds are consistent with ileus (*ie*, hypofunctioning of the small intestine).

To assess the liver, place the patient in a supine position and auscultate using the diaphragm of the stethoscope over the area inferior to the xiphoid process. Concurrently, scratch the skin lightly in the right midclavicular line, starting at the right nipple and moving inferiorly. This is used as a screening test to estimate the size and location of the liver. The scratching sound is accentuated over the liver itself. A scratching sound 10 to 12 cm in the right midclavicular line indicates a normal sized liver; if the hepar is greater than 12 cm, hepatomegaly is indicated; and, if it is less than 8 cm, a small liver is indicated. The upper border of the liver can be confirmed by percussion in the right midclavicular line, whereas the inferior border can be confirmed and described in further detail via palpation. If the edge is smooth and nontender, it is normal; if nodules or masses are present, it is consistent with cirrhosis, primary hepatocellular carcinoma, or metastatic disease; and if the liver is diffusely tender and enlarged, it is consistent with hepatitis.

To discover any direct tenderness, instruct the patient to assume a supine position with the knees and hips flexed. Directly palpate, the abdomen in all four quadrants and about the umbilicus using the dominant hand with the palm adjacent to the skin. Always palpate the painful area last. If there is tenderness to deep palpation (*ie*, pain produced by direct pressure), it is quite nonspecific, except to localize the tenderness to a specific quadrant. Voluntary guarding (*ie*, the patient voluntarily contracts muscles to prevent palpation) is nonspecific, whereas in involuntary guarding the abdominal wall is rigid to palpation, which is indicative of peritoneal irritation. Although this is not specific for a diagnosis, it is a marker for an emergent or acute abdomen.

With the patient in a supine relaxed position, auscultate the abdomen using the diaphragm for 30 to 40 seconds. Perform this procedure before any other abdominal examination

Determine liver size and consistency by performing the scratch test and by performing percussion and palpation

Perform direct palpation using the dominant hand in the abdomen in all four quadrants and about the umbilicus. Always palpate the painful area last

Perform rebound palpation, using the dominant hand in the abdomen in all four quadrants and about the umbilicus. Always palpate the painful area last

Visually inspect the skin of the adbomen, with attention given to the periumbilical and flank areas

Attempt to localize the tenderness to one quadrant of the abdomen, and then perform quadrant-specific manuevers to assist in divining the diagnosis (see Table 12)

If the abdomen appears to be distended, perform specific maneuvers to differentiate between adipose, gas, a gravid uterus, and ascites (*see* Table 13) [15•,16]

Perform a rectal examination

Perform a genitourinary examination in men and women. Palpate the penis and scrotum in men, and perform a pelvic examination in women

TABLE 12 MANEUVERS TO EVALUATE ABDOMINAL PAIN

Quadrant	Maneuver or procedure	Outcome and diagnosis
Right upper quadrant	With the patient supine and with the hips and knees flexed, deeply palpate the right upper quadrant as the patient is instructed to inhale deeply	If inspiration is inhibited by pain: Cholecystitis Ascending cholangitis
Right upper quadrant	Directly palpate the liver	If the liver is diffusely enlarged and tender: Hepatitis Distention from acute congestive failure
Right or left upper quadrant	With the patient sitting upright, percuss, using the second digit, over the right costophrenic angle, using the contralateral side as a control; a variant is to punch the costophrenic angle gently with the ulnar aspect of a closed fist	If tenderness is present over the costophrenic angle: Pyelonephritis Psoas abscess
Right lower quadrant	With the patient in supine and with the hips and knees flexed, perform deep and rebound palpation at McBurney's point (one third of the distance medial to the anterosuperior iliac spine on a line drawn from the anterosuperior iliac spine to the umbilicus)	If tenderness is present: Appendicitis
Right lower quadrant	With the patient supine and with the hips and knees flexed, perform deep and rebound palpation in the left lower quadrant	If rebound and deep tenderness are present in the right lower quadrant (Rovsing's sign): Appendicitis
Left or right lower quadrant (in women)	Perform a bimanual pelvic examination	If adnexal tenderness or an adnexal mass is present: Ectopic pregnancy Pelvic inflammatory disease Ovarian cyst

TABLE 13 MANEUVERS TO DIFFERENTIATE THE ETIOLOGY OF ABDOMINAL DISTENTION

Procedure	Outcome	Sensitivity and specificity
With the patient supine, percuss the abdomen in an arc from the umbilicus inferolaterally; note the location of a change in percussion note from resonant to dull	Dull throughout: Adipose Dull in flanks only: Ascites	Sensitivity: 80% [15,16] Specificity: 69% [15,16] Sensitivity: 94% [15] Specificity: 29% [15]
Examine the patient for shifting dullness: If there is a level of dullness perceived by percussion, note and mark that level, then roll the patient over 90° and repercuss in the same arc; note and mark the level of dullness	If no change in the level occurs: Adipose No significant ascites If a change in the level occurs: Ascites Severe mesenteric adiposity	Sensitivity: 60% [15,16] Specificity: 90% [15,16]
With the patient in a supine position, percuss with a sharp staccato motion over a specific spot in the left or right inferolateral abdomen; concurrently, place the contralateral hand, palm to abdominal skin, on the contralateral side of the abdomen; if possible instruct an assistant to gently place the ulnar aspect of the hand longitudinally over the midline of the abdomen	If there is a wave, fast and seen in the skin: Adipose If the presence of a wave sensation felt by the contralateral hand occurs after the adipose wave: Fluid wave of ascites	Sensitivity: 50% [15] Specificity: 82% [15] Sensitivity: 80% [15,16] Specificity: 92% [15,16] Sensitivity: 53% [15] Specificity: 90% [15]

To discover any rebound tenderness, palpate the abdomen and rapidly withdraw the hand from the point of maximal deep palpation. Always palpate the painful area last. If no pain is present on withdrawal of the hand, there is no rebound tenderness, whereas if pain is present, this is rebound tenderness and indicates local or diffuse peritoneal irritation. If the rebound tenderness is localized, it is an aid in developing a quadrant-specific differential diagnosis and is a marker for an emergent or acute abdomen.

TABLE 14 OVERALL EXAMINATION OF A PATIENT WITH SHORTNESS OF BREATH

Percuss the lung fields with the third digit of the dominant hand on the third digit of the nondominant hand applied to specific sites in the thorax. A tympanic note (*ie*, hyperresonance) is consistent with decreased lung tissue emphysema or pneumothorax. A dull note is consistent with a pleural effusion or consolidation

Instruct the patient to state the word "coin," "toy," or "boy" repetitively. Each time feel for the transmission of the sound using the palms of both hands as the sensor (tactile fremitus)

With the patient sitting up and leaning forward, auscult using the diaphragm and the lung fields

Visually inspect the mucous membranes and nail beds; use your own mucous membranes as a control

Auscultate the heart for any gallops or evidence of heart failure. S_3 is quite specific for systolic heart failure, whereas S_4 may indicate diastolic heart failure

Perform a sputum examination if the patient has a productive cough. Yellow-green (*ie*, purulent) sputa is correlated with an inflammatory (asthma) or infectious etiology. Pink frothy sputa is consistent with pulmonary edema, and hemoptysis may result from bronchitis, cancer, or mycobacterial diseases

S_3—third heart sound; S_4—fourth heart sound.

SHORTNESS OF BREATH

Another quite common problem with which patients present to primary care physicians is shortness of breath, with or without a cough. The many causes of this problem, including bronchitis, pneumonia, asthma, chronic obstructive pulmonary disease, pneumothorax, pleural effusions, and heart failure, can all be diagnosed via the techniques of physical diagnosis (Table 14).

Breath sounds are quite helpful in assessing the underlying etiology of shortness of breath. If the peripheral breath sounds have an expiratory phase that is longer than the inspiratory phase and are louder than those in control areas (*ie*, if they sound similar to those over the trachea [bronchial breath sounds]), they are consistent with consolidation or atelectasis. Table 15 provides information on differentiating pleural effusion from consolidation.

Adventitious sounds [17] include wheezes and rales. Wheezes indicate partial airway obstruction. Predominantly inspiratory wheezes suggest rigid stenosis of an airway, whereas predominantly expiratory wheezes suggest reversible airway disease. A high-pitched wheeze (*ie*, stridor) is consistent with high-grade stenosis of an airway, an emergent condition. If the stridor is predominantly inspiratory, it is consistent with upper airway obstruction, whereas if it is predominantly expiratory, it is consistent with lower airway obstruction. Crackles and rales will sound like the rubbing of hairs next to the ears, and may indicate interstitial inflammation, fibrosis, or fluid in the pulmonary parenchyma itself. Sounds that sound like secretions in tubes or something that needs to be coughed up, are rhonchi, which are suggestive of fluid or secretions in the airways themselves.

During the inspection of the mucous membranes and nail beds, the examiner can assess certain features of the severity and chronicity of the pulmonary dysfunction. The color of the mucous membranes and nail beds is important to note: pink is normal; a bright red discoloration is suggestive of carbon monoxide inhalation or ingestion of cyanide; a diffuse blue discoloration is consistent with cyanosis; and a pallor or white discoloration is consistent with anemia.

The nails should be carefully examined for clubbing through visual inspection of the nail plate, and attention given to the angle made by the nail plate and the proximal nail fold. This angle is normally 160°; an angle of greater than 160° is one criterion for clubbing. If this first criterion for clubbing is present, press on the proximal nail plate with finger, attempting to move the plate from the bed. If the plate cannot be moved on the bed, this is normal, whereas if the plate can be moved on the bed (*ie*, if there is sponginess at the base), this is consistent with clubbing. Clubbing is a marker for chronic hypoxemia or a chronic neoplastic or inflammatory condition.

The specifics regarding examination for the diagnoses of pleural effusion, typical pneumonia, atypical pneumonia, bronchitis, asthma, chronic obstructive pulmonary disease, heart failure, and pneumothorax are listed in Table 16.

CONCLUSION

This brief overview of physical examination has hopefully served to reinforce the tools we as physicians have virtually at the tips of our fingers, at the focal point of our vision, at our threshold of hearing, and within the range of our olfactory senses. These techniques, when used and interpreted effectively are a time- and cost-effective set of tools for providing quality medical care. In addition, we hope that this overview has piqued interest in further developing skills in physical examination.

TABLE 15 MANEUVERS TO DIFFERENTIATE CONSOLIDATION FROM PLEURAL EFFUSION

Procedure	Consolidation	Pleural effusion
Percussion	Dull over site	Dull over site
Examination for tactile fremitus	Increased usually	Decreased
Auscultation	Increased breath sounds	Decreased breath sounds

TABLE 16 PHYSICAL EXAMINATION FINDINGS OF COMMON ETIOLOGIES OF SHORTNESS OF BREATH

Etiology	Percussion	Auscultation Breath sounds	Adventitous sounds	Tactile fremitus	Heart	Sputum
Pleural effusion	Dull over effusion	Decreased over effusion	Minimal	Decreased over effusion	Tachycardia	Scant
Typical pneumonia	Dull over pneumonia	Increased over pneumonia	Diffuse rhonchi; crackles over pneumonia	Increased over pneumonia	Tachycardia	Green-yellow
Atypical pneumonia	Normal	Normal	Diffuse crackles	Normal	Tachycardia	Scant
Bronchitis	Normal	Normal	Diffuse wheezes; diffuse rhonchi	Normal	Tachycardia	Yellow-white
Asthma	Normal	Normal	Diffuse wheezes	Normal	Tachycardia	Yellow-white
Chronic bronchitis	Normal	Normal	Diffuse wheezes; diffuse rhonchi	Normal	Tachycardia; increased P_2; wide split S_2	Yellow-white
Emphysema	Tympanic	Diffusely decreased	A few wheezes	Normal	Tachycardia; increased P_2; wide split S_2	Scant
Heart failure	Normal, unless an effusion is present	Normal	Diffuse crackles	Normal	Tachycardia; S_3	Frothy, pink
Pneumothorax	Unilateral tympany	Unilateral decrease	Minimal	Unilateral decrease	Tachycardia	Scant

S_2—second heart sound; S_3—third heart sound (ventricular gallop).

REFERENCES

1. St. Clair EW, Oddone EZ, Waugh RA: Assessing housestaff diagnostic skills using a cardiology patient simulator. *Ann Intern Med* 1992, 117:751–756.

2. Peterson MC, Holbrook JH, Von Hales D, *et al.*: Contributions of the history, physical examination, and laboratory investigation in making a medical diagnosis. *West J Med* 1992, 156:163–165.

3. Sackett DL: The science and art of the clinical examination. *JAMA* 1992, 267:2650–2657.

4. Katz JN: The carpal tunnel syndrome: diagnostic utility of the history and physical examination findings. *Ann Intern Med* 1990, 112:321–327.

5. Deyo RA, Rainville J, Kent DL: What can the history and physical examination tell us about low back pain? *JAMA* 1992, 268:760–766.

6. Deyo RA, Loeser JD, Bigos SJ: Herniated lumber intervertebral disk. *Ann Intern Med* 1990, 112:598–603.

7. Daniel DM: Diagnosis of a ligament injury. In *Knee Ligaments: Structure, Function, Injury, and Repair.* Edited by Daniel DM, *et al.* New York: Raven Press; 1990:3–10.

8. Rothenberg MH, Graf BK: Evaluation of acute knee injuries. *Postgrad Med* 1993, 93:75–86.

9. Smith DL, Campbell SM: The painful shoulder. *J Gen Intern Med* 1992, 7:328–339.

10. Freeman AR, Levine SA: Clinical significance of systolic murmurs. *Ann Intern Med* 1933, 6:1371–1379.

11. Rothman A, Goldberger AL: Aids to cardiac auscultation. *Ann Intern Med* 1983, 99:346–353.

12. Leach RM, McBrien RM: Brachioradial delay in severe aortic stenosis. *Lancet* 1990, 335:1199–1201.

13. Lembo NJ, Dell'Italia LJ, Crawford MH, O'Rourke RA: Bedside diagnosis of systolic murmurs. *N Engl J Med* 1988, 318:1572–1578.

14. Cha SD, Gooch AS: Diagnosis of tricuspid regurgitation. *Arch Intern Med* 1983, 143:1763–1764.

15. Williams JW, Simel DL: Does this patient have ascites? *JAMA* 1992, 267:2645–2648.

16. Simel DL: Quantitating bedside diagnosis: clinical evaluation of ascites. *J Gen Intern Med* 1988, 3:423–428.

17. Bohadana AB: Breath sounds in the clinical assessment of airflow obstruction. *Thorax* 1978, 33:345–351.

SELECT BIBLIOGRAPHY

Berg D, Worzala K, Pachner R, Sebastian J: *Advanced Physical Diagnosis.* Boston: Blackwell Science; 1997.

Sapira JD: *The Art and Science of Bedside Diagnosis.* Baltimore: Urban and Schwarzenberg; 1990.

Schneiderman H, Wilms J, eds: *Physical Diagnosis.* Baltimore: Williams and Wilkins; 1994.

Schneiderman H: *Bedside Diagnosis.* Philadelphia: American College of Physicians; 1992.

Referrals 2
Julius J. Chosy

Key Points

- Proper referral and consultation are important for optimum health care delivery, control of costs, and quality of care.
- Accurate communication is essential; referring physicians should state clearly what it is they want to know and what they want the consultant to do.
- Consultants must define the task, address the referring physician's concerns, and know what responsibility for care is to be assumed.
- Consultants should use problem lists, make recommendations that are succinct, to the point, and specific, and then follow up if possible.
- Consultants should transmit what is important to both the patient and the referring physician.

Referral and consultation among physicians and other health care providers facilitates optimum health care delivery. The primary physician as care coordinator matches patients' needs and preferences with the judicious use of medical services. Doing so protects patients from the possible adverse effects of unnecessary care and ensures the appropriate use of health care services [1]. In this era of explosive growth in biomedical knowledge, technology, subspecialized care, and costs, referral and consultation decisions greatly affect the cost and quality of care [2].

Physicians in training are exposed to a variety of consultation services, but few training programs offer formal instruction in the principles and the art of referral and consultation (seven leading medical textbooks do not cover the subject at all). In this chapter the principles of referral and consultation and the rules of behavior involved are discussed.

REFERRAL

Referrals may involve requests for a wide range of services, from a limited consultation (for example, to a nutrition service for diet assessment) to a complete transfer of patient care responsibility. The outcome of these arrangements among the primary physician, the patient, and the consultant is generally improved care for the patient; however, poor communication between the participants can lead to misunderstanding, duplication of care, delayed or missed diagnoses, or even lapses in care [1,3••,4].

Consultation and referral patterns, their variability, and the clinical decision processes that govern them are not well understood. Patient characteristics, physician specialty, length of training experience, and reimbursement plan appear to be important [2,5,6]. The results of two recent studies suggest that the greater a practitioner's diagnostic certainty or knowledge in a specialty area, the higher the referral rate to that specialty [7,8].

TABLE 1 REASONS FOR REFERRAL

Diagnosis or confirmation of diagnosis
Recommendations for therapy or management
Implementation of therapy or management
Performance of a specialty procedure
Routine specialty examination
Prior care by subspecialty consultant
Reassurance for patient, relative, or physician
Request by patient
Education of patient or physician
Medical-legal reasons
Transfer of patient care

TABLE 2 THE FIVE STEPS OF REFERRAL AND CONSULTATION

1. Referring physician and patient recognize need for consultation
2. Referring physician communicates reason for consultation and clinical information about patient to consultant
3. Consultant evaluates patient's condition
4. Consultant communicates findings and recommendations to referring physician
5. Patient, referring physician, and consultant decide about continuing care

The reasons for referral and consultation are varied and complex (Table 1) [2,9–11]. They mainly involve seeking advice or help in diagnosis or patient management, performing a procedure, reassurance, pleasing someone, patient education, and divestiture of responsibility for care.

The literature includes many articles regarding when to refer patients with a particular problem or disease. The chief plea of consultants is that patients be referred "soon enough." "Soon enough" depends on the problem in question, the condition of the patient, and the skills of the primary physician and consultant. Certainly, when a physician is feeling a certain level of discomfort, it is time to refer. When the patient's condition is at a plateau or getting worse and further improvement might be possible, it is time to refer. A physician should not wait until the patient has become resentful or is compelled to ask for a referral. Patients often know when they are being held back from a second opinion. Enough medical information is available through the media for patients to be familiar with their options. Physicians should not be afraid to seek a second opinion: to do so will either validate their care and thereby their reputation, or it will lead to patients' getting the care they need, or both.

A somewhat sensitive reason for referral is the wish to be free of a particularly troublesome or hypochondriacal patient. It is an appropriate reason to refer when the physician can no longer provide the attentive listening and objective responses good medical care requires. In fairness to both the patient and the consultant, it should be made clear to the consultant.

What should be done when a patient asks for a referral that is not indicated or a second opinion that is believed unnecessary? Unless the patient can be readily convinced otherwise, it is probably best to arrange it. What if the patient asks to see a specific consultant whom the physician believes to be a poor one? Always, the physician's obligation is to do right by the patient so that the issue must be handled tactfully but honestly and an alternate consultant suggested.

Steps in Referral

The process of referral and consultation involves five essential steps (Table 2) [2,10,12•]. Problems may occur at any point, usually because of failures in communication or discordant expectations [1,3••,4,9,10,12•,13–15]. The most

important step is formulating the question being asked. The consultant can't provide what is wanted if physicians themselves don't know or have not asked for it clearly. The physician must ask, "What is it I want to know, and what is it I want the consultant to do?"

For example, in requesting a neurology consultation, rather than saying, "Diabetic patient with progressive lower extremity weakness," say, "Insulin-dependent diabetic with steroid-dependent chronic obstructive pulmonary disease and three-month history of progressive lower extremity weakness. Considering diabetic plexopathy versus steroid myopathy. Would appreciate your opinion and suggestions for evaluating the cause of this problem."

In requesting a rehabilitation medicine consultation, it is less helpful to say, "Admitted for pneumonia, needs rehab" than to say "76-yo patient admitted for treatment of pneumonia who is now deconditioned because of extended bedrest. Wishes to be discharged home. Lives alone. Please evaluate for self care and mobility and intervene as necessary."

When choosing a consultant, the primary physician's responsibility is to ensure the best possible outcome for the patient. In these days of managed care, capitation, gatekeepers, and pressure to generate revenue and contain costs, there may be limitations on referral choices. In a system with referral limitations, the physician remains obliged to get the right consultant for the patient when needed, even if it means requesting approval from a medical director to go outside.

Physicians choose consultants based on reputation, the recommendations of colleagues, and their own personal experience. Consultants are sought who will give a skilled and thoughtful response, whose personality fits the patient well, and who will keep the referring physician informed.

The mode of contact with the consultant varies with circumstances and personal style. Commonly, contact is by telephone, which has the advantage of speed and the opportunity to clarify questions and expectations. In other instances formal letters or consultation forms are used. Some physicians use verbal instructions to their patients to convey the purpose of a consultation, but this carries a great risk for miscommunication.

It is important to provide the consultant with all relevant clinical information (Table 3), including results of diagnostic tests and procedures to avoid unnecessary duplication [12•,16]. It is helpful for the consultant to know of any previous therapy that has failed so that the same therapy is not recommended again. Consultants must know what responsibility for care they are to assume. It is courting disaster, for example, for the consulting physician to write aminoglycoside orders while thinking, incorrectly, that the primary physician will monitor blood levels and renal function. The consultant needs to know if a request is an emergency, urgent, or routine, as emergency consults must be seen immediately and urgent ones urgently. It is helpful for the consultant to know what the referring physician has told the patient about the referral so that the patient's expectations can be anticipated. Similarly, it is helpful for the consultant to know about any preferences or special attitudes of the patient, such as inordinate fear, fixed opinions of tests or treatments, or unreasonable expectations of outcome.

CONSULTATION

Now we turn to the consultant's role and the rules of effective consultation (Table 4) [3••,8–10,13–16]. The consultant's first task is to define what the referring physician wants. That is not always evident in the written consultation request or referral letter. A quick phone call to the referring physician may be needed to ascertain what the questions are and what specifically the consultant is being asked to do and when.

Next, consultants should look for themselves. It may be that they will have more time for interviewing and examining the patient, reviewing old records, or tracking down information than did a time-pressured referring physician. Because of their expertise and special perspective they may recognize the significance of information overlooked by others. They can also give the patient another chance to provide answers. The problem of one patient referred to find the cause of chronic postcholecystectomy right upper quadrant pain was illuminated when the consultant, after listening to the patient, confirmed the presence of a tender mass just where the patient said it was; at laparotomy, a stitch abscess was removed. And a telephone call to another hospital's record room may easily answer the question of whether a lung nodule was there 2 years ago. Consultants who look at the radiographs themselves may see something important that the radiologist didn't see or report.

Recommendations should be succinct and directed to the questions that generated the consultation. Compliance with recommendations increases when recommendations are fewer than six [14], are specific, and are focused on issues central to current patient care, when drug doses are specific and when frequent follow-up visits are made by the consultant [9,13–15]. Use problem lists in consultation note or letter. A group of British general practitioners overwhelmingly preferred a letter with a problem list over one containing the same information in the conventional narrative format (Fig. 1) [7]. Unless it is certain that the referring physician will see the consultant's note in the chart in suitable time, the referring physician should be telephoned. There is no substitute for direct contact to discuss recommendations and plans [13].

Secondary referrals or major interventions should not be undertaken that have not been mutually agreed upon beforehand [12•]. It is extremely disconcerting for a referring physician to learn that a patient referred for evaluation of an abnormal mammogram has had a radical mastectomy.

Finally, it is important to communicate with the patient as well as the referring physician. Most consultants report their conclusions and recommendations verbally to the patient. Others think the results of the consultation should be conveyed to the patient by the referring physician, who knows the patient better, particularly if there is bad news. A more controversial approach is to provide the patient with an individualized letter with a copy to the referring physician. This method was heavily favored by a group of Australian cancer consultants who believed that for initial cancer consultations, doctor–patient and doctor–doctor communications would be improved by this technique [18].

AWKWARD ISSUES

In the process of referral and consultation several awkward issues can be counted upon to arise. One is the problem of the referring physician or the consultant concluding that poor medical care has been given by the other. In this situation, as always, the patient's best interests come first, and an appropriate care plan should be recommended to the patient as gently and tactfully as possible.

A more serious problem is that of disagreement between a referring and a consulting physician over an important matter

TABLE 3 INFORMATION CONSULTANTS NEED FROM REFERRING PHYSICIAN
Specific reason for consultation
Current medical problems
Current medications
Diagnostic test and procedure results
Previous therapeutic failures
Specific responsibility for care consultant is to assume
How soon consultant needs to see patient
What patient has been told about referral
Any special patient attitude about the problem

TABLE 4 RULES FOR EFFECTIVE CONSULTATION
Define what referring physician wants
Establish urgency
Look for yourself
Address referring physician's concerns
Make specific and succinct recommendations
Limit number of recommendations to fewer than six, if possible
Include problem list
Call referring physician
Make follow-up visits

A	B

Re John Jones, Date of birth: 1/1/1985
456 Any Street, London N17 33X
 	
Dear Dr Smith,
 	
    Thank you for referring this boy with frequent attacks of cough and wheeze. He misses a lot of school, sleeps badly, and is short of breath on exertion. I think he has poorly controlled asthma. I note that both his parents smoke and that their housing conditions are very poor. As you know, his younger brother has Down's syndrome.
 	
    I was very generally optimistic but emphasized the potential for serious attacks and the need for close family involvement in the management.
 	
    I prescribed sodium cromoglycate 10 mg (two puffs) three times a day. His relief drug is terbutaline 1 mg (four puffs) four hourly. Both are to be taken via a nebuhaler (he has excellent technique). I have advised his parents to stop smoking.
 	
    His peak flow was 180 today. I have issued a peak flow meter, and the parents will establish what his best peak flow is. I have given them a danger peak flow value of 100—if his peak flow falls to less than this they will bring him to casualty.
 	
    Review 1 month.
	Re John Jones, Date of birth: 1/1/1985
	456 Any Street, London N17 33X
	
	Dear Dr Smith,
	
	Problems:
	  Poorly controlled asthma
	  Passive smoker
	  Poor housing
	  Younger brother has Down's syndrome
	
	    Thank you for referring this boy with frequent attacks of cough and wheeze. He misses a lot of school, sleeps badly, and is short of breath on exertion.
	
	    I was generally optimistic but emphasized the potential for serious attacks and the need for close family involvement in the management.
	
	    I prescribed sodium cromoglycate 10 mg (two puffs) three times a day. His relief drug is terbutaline 1 mg (four puffs) four hourly. Both are to be taken via a nebuhaler (he has excellent technique). I have advised his parents to stop smoking.
	
	    His peak flow was 180 today. I have issued a peak flow meter, and the parents will establish what his best peak flow is. I have given them a danger peak flow value of 100—if his peak flow falls to less than this they will bring him to casualty.
	
	    Review 1 month.

FIGURE 1 Referral letters without (**A**) and with (**B**) a problem list. (*From* Lloyd and Barnett [17]; with permission.)

of management. Resolution of the conflict will most often be achieved by discussion between the two physicians [13,19•]. But what if it cannot? The literature offers little guidance for this dilemma involving the primacy of the patient's referring physician and the obligation of the consulting physician to the care of the patient. The consulting physician should document any recommendations in the chart and has the right to discuss the recommendations with the patient, preferably with the permission of or in the presence of the referring physician. A second opinion should be sought [19•].

Last is the situation in which the patient wants the consultant to become the primary physician or to completely take over care when such was not intended by the referring physician. A sure way for a consulting physician's practice to suffer is to develop a reputation for "stealing" patients [12•,13]. The referral-consultant relationship should be explained to the patient, who should be urged to discuss concerns with the referring physician. Should the patient be unwilling to do so, however, it is not unethical to accept the patient in this circumstance.

It would be proper for the consultant to inform the referring physician of the patient's wishes and the reasons for them, along with a description of the consultant's attempts to return the patient to the referring physician.

To be a good consultant, make communication a priority, establish what the consultant's task is, be specific and to the point, follow up, and transmit what is important to the patient and to the referring physician.

KEY REFERENCES

Recently published papers of outstanding interest, as identified in *References and Recommended Reading*, have been annotated.

•• Epstein R: Communication between primary care physicians and consultants. *Arch Fam Med* 1995, 4:403–409.
A comprehensive review of the topic. Discussed are the context of the relationship between primary care physicians and consultants, communication barriers, the reasons for communication difficulties, consequences of poor communication, and possible solutions. Excellent tables of the communication problems, the reasons, and possible solutions are provided.

REFERENCES AND RECOMMENDED READING

Recently published papers of particular interest have been highlighted as:
• Of interest
•• Of outstanding interest

1. Franks P, Clancy C, Nutting P: Gatekeeping revisited—protecting patients from overtreatment. *N Engl J Med* 1992, 327:424–429.

2. Nutting P, Franks P, Clancy C: Referral and consultation in primary care: do we understand what we're doing? *J Fam Pract* 1992, 35:21–23.

3.•• Epstein R: Communication between primary care physicians and consultants. *Arch Fam Med* 1995, 4:403–409.

4. Wu CH, Kao JC, Chang CJ: Analysis of outpatient referral failures. *J Fam Pract* 1996, 42:498–502.

5. Salem-Schatz S, Moore G, Rucker M, Pearson S: The case for case-mix adjustment in practice profiling. *JAMA* 1994, 272:871–874.

6. Vehvilainen A, Kumpusalo E, Voutilainen S, Takala J: Does the doctors' professional experience reduce referral rates: evidence from the Finnish referral study. *Scand J Prim Health Care* 1996, 14:13–20.

7. Reynolds G, Chitnis J, Roland M: General practitioner outpatient referrals: do good doctors refer more patients to hospital? *BMJ* 1991, 302:1250–1252.

8. Calman N, Hyman R, Licht W: Variability in consultation rates and practitioner level of diagnostic certainty. *J Fam Pract* 1992, 35:31–38.

9. Lee T, Pappius E, Goldman L: Impact of inter-physician communication on the effectiveness of medical consultations. *Am J Med* 1983, 74:106–112.

10. McPhee S, Lo B, Saika G, Meltzer R: How good is communication between primary care physicians and subspecialty consultants(?) *Arch Intern Med* 1984, 144:1265–1268.

11. Armstrong D, Fry J, Armstrong P: Doctors' perceptions of pressure from patients for referral. *BMJ* 1991, 302:1186–1188.

12.• Williams PT, Peet G: Differences in the value of clinical information: referring physicians versus consulting specialists. *J Am Board Fam Pract* 1994, 7:292–302.

13. Goldman L, Lee T, Rudd P: Ten commandments for effective consultations. *Arch Intern Med* 1983, 143:1753–1755.

14. Sears C, Charlson M: The effectiveness of a consultation: compliance with initial recommendations. *Am J Med* 1983, 74:870–876.

15. Pupa L, Coventry J, Hanley J, Carpenter J: Factors affecting compliance for general medicine consultations to non-internists. *Am J Med* 1986, 81:508–514.

16. Newton J, Eccles M, Hutchinson A: Communication between general practicioners and consultants: what should their letters contain? *BMJ* 1992, 304:821–824.

17. Lloyd B, Barnett P: Use of problem lists in letters between hospital doctors and general practitioners. *BMJ* 1993, 306:247.

18. Stockler M, Butow P, Tattersall M: The take-home message: doctors' views on letters and tapes after a cancer consultation. *Ann Oncol* 1993, 4:549–552.

19.• Stinson M: Conflicts in consultation. *J S C Med Assoc* 1996, Jan:14–17.

Preoperative Consultation   3

Thomas A. Holly
Ira S. Ockene

> ### Key Points
> - Consideration of the risk of the surgical procedure is the first step in preoperative risk assessment.
> - Clinical history, including functional capacity, is an important component of the evaluation.
> - Noninvasive and invasive testing where appropriate can help to risk-stratify patients and guide possible therapy to reduce the perioperative risk.
> - Preoperative consultation should also give an assessment of long-term prognosis, because this may affect decisions regarding type of surgery and possible preoperative interventions.

More than 25 million patients undergo noncardiac surgery in the United States each year. One million of these patients have known coronary artery disease (CAD), another 2 to 3 million have multiple risk factors for CAD, and another 4 million are at risk because they are over 65 years of age. Surgery imposes many stresses on the cardiovascular system (Table 1), and can tip the myocardial supply/demand balance over the line that separates tolerable function from ischemia. Thus, it is not surprising that the occurrence of perioperative cardiac events is the leading cause of death after noncardiac surgery [1].

Risk stratification is therefore an important part of the preoperative evaluation of patients. It requires knowledge of the planned procedure and anesthesia and the stresses they impose on the cardiovascular system, the general medical condition of the patient, and the specific degree of CAD, myocardial dysfunction, and risk of ischemia that the patient brings to the procedure. Evaluation requires a good history and physical examination, and where appropriate, further noninvasive and/or invasive testing and medical stabilization. A thorough evaluation also provides an assessment of long-term prognosis.

TYPE OF SURGERY

To stratify patients appropriately by risk, one must consider the risk of the specific procedure. Thoracic, intraperitoneal, vascular, major orthopedic, and emergency surgical procedures are generally considered high risk for cardiac complications. Vascular surgery carries many potential stresses including blood loss, intraoperative hypotension, and large fluid shifts. The same holds true for thoracic surgery, which also may be associated with prolonged mechanical ventilation. Orthopedic surgery often involves prolonged operative time with considerable blood loss and large fluid shifts, and is often performed on elderly patients. Conversely, head and neck, prostate, and ophthalmologic procedures are generally believed to carry a lower risk. Procedures performed under local anesthesia and uncomplicated endoscopies fall into this category, as well.

TABLE 1 SURGICAL STRESSES

Preoperative

Anxiety—increases BP, heart rate, catecholamine levels

Sedation—may impair ventilation

Intraoperative

Anesthesia—can cause myocardial depression

Impaired ventilation—decreases oxygenation and causes acid-base disturbances

Blood pressure fluctuations—may cause myocardial ischemia due to decreased coronary blood flow (hypotension) or increased myocardial oxygen demand (hypertension)

Blood loss—decreases myocardial oxygen delivery

Compromised function of vital organs, especially secondary to hypotension

Acid-base disturbances

Reactions to drugs, blood products

Volume overload—increases preload; decreases oxygenation secondary to pulmonary congestion

Hypovolemia—decreases cardiac output; decreases flow to myocardium and other vital organs

Hyper- or hypothermia, shivering—increases myocardial oxygen demand

Postoperative

Hypovolemia related to blood loss, vomiting, diaphoresis, poor intake, excessive diuresis

Anemia secondary to blood loss—decreases myocardial oxygen delivery

Volume overload from excessive transfusion, fluid infusions

Sepsis—markedly increases myocardial oxygen demands

Venous or arterial thrombosis related to postoperative clotting factor changes and immobility

Endocarditis—can directly affect cardiac valvular function, as well as increasing metabolic demands

Reactions to drugs, blood products

Anxiety

BP—blood pressure.
From Ockene and Holly [28]; with permission.

ANESTHESIA

Consideration of the risk of surgery necessitates some comment regarding the choice of anesthesia. There is limited evidence that spinal or epidural anesthetic techniques are safer for the cardiac patient [2,3]. Both spinal and epidural anesthesia can cause hypotension secondary to sympathetic blockade; furthermore, these techniques are not as easily reversible as is general anesthesia. However, Goldman and colleagues [4] found that patients with a history of congestive heart failure (CHF) or severe left ventricular dysfunction were less likely to develop postoperative CHF when spinal or epidural anesthesia was used.

CLINICAL ASSESSMENT

Dripps and colleagues developed one of the first strategies for assessing preoperative risk (Dripps–American Society of Anesthesiologists Index) [5]. Although still in use, the Dripps classification has been shown to be poorly reproducible and is of limited value in developing specific patient management strategies [6].

Perhaps the most comprehensive study of cardiac risk for patients undergoing noncardiac surgical procedures was reported by Goldman and colleagues in 1977 [3]. In this prospective study, 1001 patients older than 40 years of age who underwent general surgery were studied. Minor surgical procedures performed under local anesthesia, uncomplicated endoscopic studies, and transurethral resections of the prostate were excluded from the analysis. A multivariate discriminant analysis identified nine factors that had statistically independent correlations with cardiac outcome; these are listed in Table 2. The discriminant analysis was used to develop a point system that could be used to predict risk. Based on point totals, patients were separated into four risk categories (Table 3). Progression from class I to class IV was associated with an incremental increase in the percentage of patients suffering cardiac complications or cardiac death.

Subsequently Detsky and colleagues [7] carried out a validation study using Goldman's index and found that modifying it by adding categories for angina and for history of pulmonary edema improved its predictive power. The Detsky study also differed from Goldman's in that it applied the score obtained on the multifactorial index (patient characteristics) to the pretest probability of a cardiac complication to yield a final, posttest probability. The pretest probability is based on the average risk of a cardiac complication, and is dependent on the

TABLE 2 COMPUTATION OF THE CARDIAC RISK INDEX

Criteria	Points
History	
Age >70 yr	5
MI in previous 6 mo	10
Physical examination	
S_3 gallop or JVD	11
Important VAS	3
Electrocardiogram	
Rhythm other than sinus or PAC's on last preoperative ECG	7
>5 PVCs/min documented at any time before operation	7
General status	
PO_2 < 60 or PCO_2 > 50 mm Hg, K < 3.0 or HCO_3 < 20 meq/liter, BUN > 50 or Cr > 3.0 mg/dl, abnormal SGOT, signs of chronic liver disease or patient bed ridden from noncardiac causes	3
Operations	
Intraperitoneal, intrathoracic, or aortic operation	3
Emergency operation	4
Total possible	53

MI—myocardial infarction; JVD—jugular-vein distention; VAS—valvular aortic stenosis; PAC—premature atrial contractions; ECG—electrocardiogram; PVC—premature ventricular contractions; PO_2—partial pressure of oxygen; PCO_2—partial pressure of carbon dioxide; K—potassium; HCO_3—bicarbonate; BUN—blood urea nitrogen; Cr—creatinine; and SGOT—serum glutamic oxalacetic transaminase.
From Goldman *et al.* [3]; with permission.

TABLE 3 CARDIAC RISK INDEX

Class	Point total	No or only minor complication	Life-threatening complication (N = 39)	Cardiac deaths (N = 19)
I (N =537)	0–5	532 (99)†	4 (0.7)	1 (0.2)
II (N =316)	6–12	295 (93)	16 (5)	5 (2)
III (N = 130)	13–25	112 (86)	15 (11)	3 (2)
IV (N =18)	≥26	4 (22)	4 (22)	10 (56)

*Documented intraoperative or postoperative myocardial infarction, pulmonary edema, or ventricular tachycardia without progression to cardiac death.
†Figures in parentheses denote %.
From Goldman [3]; with permission.

procedure, the institution, and referral bias, among other factors (Tables 4 and 5; Fig. 1).

A number of studies have examined the relationship between CAD, especially antecedent myocardial infarction (MI), and the risk of surgery. Steen and colleagues reviewed the records of 73,321 patients who underwent anesthesia and noncardiac surgery at the Mayo Clinic; 587 of these patients had suffered previous MIs [2]. Thirty-six patients (6.1%) had a reinfarction, and 25 of the 36 patients (69%) died. The relationship of morbidity and mortality to the length of time between infarction and surgery in this study is shown in Table 6. The explanation for the higher morbidity and mortality in these patients is probably related to residual ischemia, as well as left ventricular dysfunction.

If at all possible, major surgery should be delayed for 6 months after an MI, although risk stratification with noninvasive testing may permit the identification of a low-risk subset that may safely undergo surgery earlier.

Patients with peripheral vascular disease (PVD) present a particularly interesting problem. These patients have a high incidence of associated CAD, but because their ability to exercise may be limited by claudication, they may have little or no angina. Routine coronary arteriography in patients with PVD has shown that the incidence of significant (but often asymptomatic) CAD may be more than 30%. In a study of 1000 patients from the Cleveland Clinic, Hertzer and colleagues [8] found that 34% of patients undergoing peripheral vascular surgery and clinically suspected of having CAD as well as 14%

TABLE 4 MODIFIED MULTIFACTORIAL INDEX

Condition	Points
Coronary artery disease	
Myocardial infarction within 6 months	10
Myocardial infarction more than 6 months	5
Canadian Cardiovascular Society angina	
Class III	10
Class IV	20
Unstable angina within 6 months	10
Alveolar pulmonary edema	
Within 1 week	10
Ever	5
Valvular disease	
Suspected critical aortic stenosis	20
Arrhythmias	
Rhythm other than sinus or sinus plus APBs on last preoperative electrocardiogram	5
More than five premature ventricular contractions at any time before surgery	5
Poor general medical status*	5
Age over 70 y	5
Emergency operation	10

*As defined in original multifactorial index (see Table 2).
APB—atrial premature beat.
From Detsky et al. [7]

TABLE 5 PRETEST PROBABILITIES FOR TYPES OF SURGERY

Types of surgery	Severe cardiac complications*
Major surgery	
Vascular	10/76 (13.2%)
Orthopedic	9/66 (13.6%)
Intrathoracic/intraperitoneal	7/88 (8.0%)
Head and neck	1/38 (2.6%)
Minor surgery	
(eg, TURP, cataracts)	3/187 (1.6%)

*Cardiac death, myocardial infarction, alveolar pulmonary edema.
TURP—transurethral resection of the prostate.
From Detsky et al. [7]; with permission.

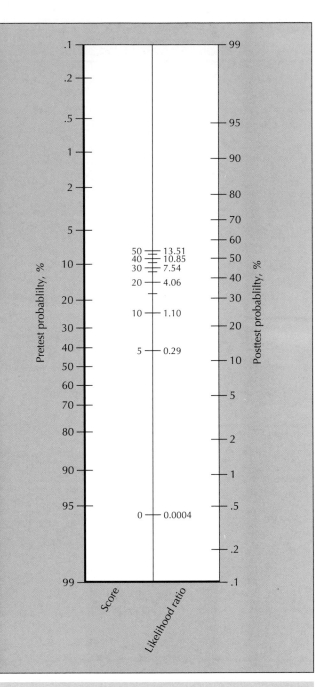

FIGURE 1 Likelihood ratio nomogram. Anchor a straight edge at the value on the pretest side of the nomogram determined by the surgical procedure. Direct the straight edge through the point in the center column reflecting the patient's index score and associated likelihood ratio. The point where the straight edge meets the right-hand column denotes the posttest probability for the patient, ie, his risk of perioperative cardiac complication. (From Detsky et al. [7]; with permission.)

of those without clinical evidence for CAD had "severe, correctable" CAD documented by catheterization.

NONINVASIVE TESTING

The value of exercise testing and, in particular, the determination of functional capacity in preoperative evaluation, has been known for some time. In 1981, Cutler and colleagues [9] showed that electrocardiographic stress testing was especially valuable in the preoperative assessment of patients with PVD. Patients who achieved >75% of maximum predicted heart rate (MPHR) and had no ischemic electrocardiographic (ECG) changes (35 of 105 patients) had no postoperative cardiac complications. In contrast, in the highest risk group (26 patients with an ischemic ECG response at <75% of maximum predicted heart rate), there were ten postoperative cardiac complications (38%), including seven MIs (27%), five of which were fatal. Other studies have shown

TABLE 6 MYOCARDIAL REINFARCTION AND MORTALITY*

Time of surgery after infarct, *mo*	No. of patients	No. (%) postoperative reinfarctions	Deaths, No. (%)
0–3	15	4 (27)	4 (100)
4–6	17	2 (11)	1 (50)
7–12	31	2 (6)	2 (100)
13–18	30	1 (3)	0 (0)
19–24	17	1 (6)	1 (100)
>25	383	15 (4)	8 (53)
Unknown	93	11 (12)	9 (82)
Total	587	36 (6.1)	25 (69)

*Relation to interval from previous myocardial infarction.
From Steen *et al.* [2]; with permission.

that failure to achieve 85% MPHR, 5 metabolic equivalents (METs), or a heart rate of 100 are predictors of a poor outcome [10–13]. ECG evidence of ischemia is less predictive than poor functional capacity, but when added to it, indicates even greater risk.

Dipyridamole-thallium testing has become an established noninvasive alternative to conventional stress testing for patients at high risk for CAD who cannot exercise because of PVD or orthopedic problems. Several studies have demonstrated the utility of dipyridamole-thallium imaging in the preoperative assessment of cardiac risk. Thallium redistribution, indicating ischemia, is a significant predictor of perioperative cardiac events.

Although its sensitivity for detecting patients at increased risk is excellent, dipyridamole-thallium imaging for preoperative screening carries a relatively low specificity for clinical events. To improve the specificity and positive predictive value, some investigators have tried combining clinical markers with noninvasive testing, whereas others have demon-

strated that quantifying the amount of myocardium at risk can better define those patients at risk for perioperative cardiac events.

Eagle and colleagues [14] performed preoperative dipyridamole-thallium testing and clinical evaluation in 254 patients before major vascular procedures. Surgery was subsequently performed in 200 patients. Of these 200 patients, 30 (15%) had early postoperative ischemic events; 9 (4.5%) had nonfatal MIs; and 6 (3%) died. Thallium redistribution was highly predictive of subsequent events, as were five clinical variables (Q waves on ECG, history of ventricular ectopic activity, diabetes, age >70 years, and angina). Use of both the clinical and thallium data yielded significantly higher specificity with no loss of sensitivity. The authors noted that for nearly half of the patients, very low or very high operative risk could be predicted on the basis of clinical variables alone, making dipyridamole-thallium imaging unnecessary (Fig. 2).

A number of other studies have demonstrated a strong correlation between the extent of reversible thallium defects

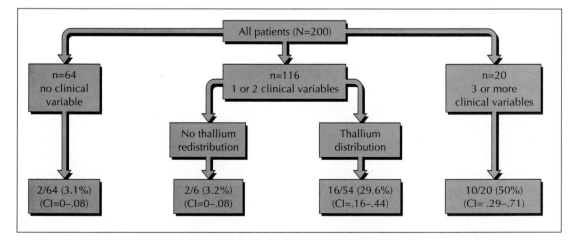

FIGURE 2 Algorithm for using clinical variables and results of dipyridamole-thallium imaging to stratify cardiac risk as applied to this group of 200 patients. Event refers to postoperative cardiac ischemic events including unstable angina, ischemic pulmonary edema, myocardial infarction, or cardiac death. Clinical variables are presence of Q wave on electrocardiogram, age > 70 years, history of angina, history of ventricular ectopic activity requiring treatment, and diabetes mellitus requiring treatment. CI—confidence interval. (*From* Eagle *et al.* [14]; with permission.)

and the risk of cardiac death or MI. Recently, Brown and Rowen [15] developed a method to stratify perioperative risk based on the number of segments with transient thallium defects and a history of diabetes mellitus. The impact of combining these methods with clinical indices such as those described by Eagle has not yet been tested.

Ambulatory electrocardiographic monitoring also has been shown to identify ischemia in symptomatic patients with normal 12-lead ECGs and negative exercise tolerance tests [16] and in patients with silent ischemia [17]. Raby and colleagues [18] prospectively studied 176 patients undergoing elective vascular surgery. Thirty-two patients had S-T segment depression on preoperative ambulatory electrocardiographic monitoring. Of these 32 patients, 12 had postoperative ischemic events (MI, unstable angina, or ischemic pulmonary edema) compared with only 1 of 144 patients who did not have preoperative ischemia on ambulatory monitoring. The sensitivity of S-T depression on ambulatory monitoring was 92%, specificity was 88%, positive predictive value was 38%, and negative predictive value was 99%.

Dobutamine stress echocardiography (DSE) has been used recently to identify patients at risk for cardiac complications of surgery. Several studies have described the usefulness of DSE in diagnosing CAD. A recent study by Poldermans and colleagues [19] demonstrated the ability of DSE to identify patients at high and low risk for vascular surgery. All 15 patients with perioperative cardiac events had positive tests (new or worsened wall-motion abnormality), and no one with a negative DSE had an event. DSE had a positive predictive value of 42% and a negative predictive value of 100%. These results are similar to data presented by Lalka and colleagues [20] with a smaller group of patients undergoing aortic surgery (positive predictive value = 29%, negative predictive value = 95%). DSE is a promising new tool that deserves further investigation.

In summary, clinical information combined with appropriate noninvasive testing can select a subset of patients who are at high risk for a perioperative cardiac event. These patients, if appropriate, should undergo invasive testing for possible revascularization before their noncardiac surgery.

LONG-TERM PROGNOSIS

Although the immediate purpose of preoperative examination is to assess the patient's perioperative risk, determination of long-term prognosis is an important part of the evaluation, since long-term prognosis affects the risk/benefit ratio of the contemplated procedure. This topic has been most extensively studied in patients undergoing vascular surgery. Hendel and colleagues demonstrated the value of thallium scanning for this purpose [21]. While reversible defects are associated with perioperative cardiac events, fixed defects are associated with late events. A poor long-term outlook may lead to the conclusion that the planned surgery is inappropriate, and such knowledge may help the patient and physician make decisions regarding the necessity of high-risk surgery or the benefit of major preoperative interventions (*eg*, coronary artery bypass surgery [CABG] or percutaneous transluminal coronary angioplasty [PTCA]).

MANAGEMENT

The place of CABG and PTCA in the preoperative management of the patient with CAD undergoing noncoronary surgery is unsettled, although many physicians believe that under appropriate circumstances, mechanical revascularization prevents ischemic morbidity and mortality during subsequent noncardiac surgery.

Foster and colleagues [22] examined this issue in an analysis of data from the Coronary Artery Surgery Study (CASS). Patients without significant CAD had an operative mortality of 0.5%, similar to that of patients with significant CAD who underwent CABG before noncardiac surgery (0.9%). For patients with significant CAD undergoing noncardiac surgery without prior CABG, the operative mortality was 2.4%, significantly higher than in the other two groups. The incidence of perioperative MI and arrhythmia was similar in the three groups. Of note, the perioperative mortality associated with CABG itself was 1.4%.

Two recent studies have examined the use of PTCA before noncardiac surgery. Huber and colleagues [23] looked at the incidence of perioperative MI and death in a group of 50 high-risk patients undergoing 54 procedures a median of 9 days after angioplasty. The overall frequency of perioperative MI was 5.6%, and the mortality was 1.9%. Although there was no control group, they concluded that patients who have had successful PTCA for severe CAD have a low risk of major cardiac complications associated with noncardiac surgery.

Another study from the Mayo Clinic compared the cardiac morbidity, mortality, and survival of patients who underwent PTCA (n = 14) or CABG (n = 86) before abdominal aortic aneurysm repair [24]. The rate of perioperative MI was 0% for the PTCA group and 5.8% for the CABG group, and no hospital deaths occurred in either group. However, the 3-year survival was not statistically different between groups.

The studies cited above are weakened in that they are not randomized, prospective trials, and in many the number of patients in each treatment arm is inadequate for statistical power. However, the available data suggest that antecedent mechanical intervention may be indicated in selected, high-risk patients who are scheduled to undergo a major noncardiac surgical procedure, bearing in mind the morbidity and mortality of the myocardial revascularization procedure itself.

The management of drug therapy deserves special comment. Many surgical patients are receiving antihypertensive drugs, β-blocking agents for ischemia, or digoxin. Almost all cardiac medications should be continued up to the time of surgery and resumed as soon as possible after surgery. β-blockers or nitrates may be given intravenously or topically (nitroglycerin paste) during periods when the patient is unable to take oral medications.

The prophylactic use of β-blockers may actually decrease the occurrence of perioperative ischemia. Only a few studies have been published, but some have indicated a decrease in intraoperative ischemic episodes [25–27], and one demonstrated a decrease in perioperative MI [27]. Even fewer data exist regarding the use of other antianginal agents during surgery, and no clear consensus has been reached regarding the use of these agents.

Preoperative assessment of the patient is generally easily carried out; only history, physical examination, and ECG are necessary in the large majority of patients. Using some form of risk assessment criteria such as those described by Goldman, Detsky, and Eagle is helpful and may select out patients in whom further functional or anatomic information is needed. Exercise testing (ECG monitored or thallium), dipyridamole-thallium imaging, echocardiography, dobutamine stress echocardiography, ambulatory electrocardiographic monitoring, and cardiac catheterization provide additional information in those situations where the expense and risk (in the case of catheterization) can be justified.

REFERENCES

1. Mangano DT: Perioperative cardiac morbidity. *Anesthesiology* 1990, 72:153–184.

2. Steen PA, Tinker JH, Tarhan S: Myocardial reinfarction after anesthesia and surgery. *JAMA* 1978, 239:2566–2570.

3. Goldman L, Caldera DL, Nussbaum SR, *et al.*: Multifactorial index of cardiac risk in noncardiac surgical procedures. *N Engl J Med* 1977, 297:845–850.

4. Goldman L, Caldera DL, Southwick FS, *et al.*: Cardiac risk factors and complications in non-cardiac surgery. *Medicine* 1978, 57:357–370.

5. Dripps RD, Lamont A, Eckenhoff JE: The role of anesthesia in surgical mortality. *JAMA* 1961, 178:261–266.

6. Owens WD, Felts JA, Spitznagel EL: ASA physical status classifications: A study of consistency of ratings. *Anesthesiology* 1978, 49:239–243.

7. Detsky AS, Abrams HB, McLaughlin JR, *et al*: Predicting cardiac complications in patients undergoing non-cardiac surgery. *J Gen Intern Med* 1986, 1:211–219.

8. Hertzer NR, Beven EG, Young JR, *et al*: Coronary artery disease in peripheral vascular patients. *Ann Surg* 1984, 199:223–233.

9. Cutler BS, Wheeler HB, Paraskos JA, *et al.*: Applicability and interpretation of electrocardiographic stress testing in patients with peripheral vascular disease. *Am J Surg* 1981, 141:501–506.

10. Carliner NH, Fisher ML, Plotnick GD, *et al.*: Routine preoperative exercise testing in patients undergoing major noncardiac surgery. *Am J Cardiol* 1985, 56:51–58.

11. McPhail N, Calvin JE, Shariatmader A, *et al.*: The use of preoperative exercise testing to predict cardiac complications after arterial reconstruction. *J Vasc Surg* 1988, 7:60–68.

12. Gerson MC, Hurst JM, Hertzberg VS, *et al.*: Cardiac prognosis in noncardiac geriatric surgery. *Ann Intern Med* 1985, 103:832–837.

13. Kopecky SL, Gibbons RJ, Hollier LH: Preoperative supine exercise radionuclide angiogram predicts perioperative cardiovascular events in vascular surgery. *J Am Coll Cardiol* 1986, 7:226A.

14. Eagle KA, Coley CM, Newell JB: Combining clinical and thallium data optimizes preoperative assessment of cardiac risk before major vascular surgery. *Ann Intern Med* 1989, 110:859–866.

15. Brown KA, Rowen M: Extent of jeopardized viable myocardium determined by myocardial perfusion imaging predicts perioperative cardiac events in patients undergoing noncardiac surgery. *J Am Coll Cardiol* 1993, 21:325–330.

16. Stern S, Tzivoni D: Early detection of silent ischemic heart disease by 24-hour electrocardiographic monitoring of active subjects. *Br Heart J* 1974, 36:481–486.

17. Cohn PF: Silent myocardial ischemia: Classification, prevalence, and prognosis. *Am J Med* 1985, 79(suppl. 3A):2–6.

18. Raby KE, Goldman L, Creager MA, *et al.*: Correlation between preoperative ischemia and major cardiac events after peripheral vascular surgery. *N Engl J Med* 1989, 321:1296–1300.

19. Poldermans D, Fioretti PM, Forster T, *et al.*: Dobutamine stress echocardiography for assessment of perioperative cardiac risk in patients undergoing major vascular surgery. *Circulation* 1993, 87:1506–1512.

20. Lalka SG, Sawada SG, Dalsing MC, *et al.*: Dobutamine stress echocardiography as a predictor of cardiac events associated with aortic surgery. *J Vasc Surg* 1992, 15:831–842.

21. Hendel RC, Whitfield SS, Villegas BJ, *et al.*: Prediction of late cardiac events by dipyridamole thallium imaging in patients undergoing elective vascular surgery. *Am J Cardiol* 1992, 70:1243–1249.

22. Foster ED, Davis KB, Carpenter JA, *et al.*: Risk of noncardiac operation in patients with defined coronary disease: The coronary artery surgery study (CASS) registry experience. *Ann Thorac Surg* 1986, 41:42–50.

23. Huber KC, Evans MA, Bresnahan JF, *et al.*: Outcome of noncardiac operations in patients with severe coronary artery disease successfully treated preoperatively with coronary angioplasty. *Mayo Clin Proc* 1992, 67:15–21.

24. Elmore JR, Hallett JW, Gibbons RJ, *et al.*: Myocardial revascularization before abdominal aortic aneurysmorrhaphy: effect of coronary angioplasty. *Mayo Clin Proc* 1993, 68:637–641.

25. Stone JG, Foex P, Sear JW, *et al.*: Myocardial ischemia in untreated hypertensive patients: effect of a single small oral dose of a β-adrenergic blocking agent. *Anesthesiology* 1988, 68:495–500.

26. Pasternack PF, Grossi EA, Baumann FG, *et al.*: β blockade to decrease silent myocardial ischemia during peripheral vascular surgery. *Am J Surg* 1989, 158:113–116.

27. Pasternack PF, Imparato AM, Baumann FG, *et al.*: The hemodynamics of a-blockade in patients undergoing abdominal aortic aneurysm repair. *Circulation* 1987, 76(suppl 3):1–7.

28. Ockene IS, Holly TA: Noncardiac surgery in the cardiac patient. In *Intensive Care Medicine*, 3rd edn. Edited by Rippe J, *et al.* Boston: Little, Brown and Co.; 1995:1369.

SELECT BIBLIOGRAPHY

Abraham SA, Coles NA, Coles CM: Coronary risk of noncardiac surgery. *Prog Cardiovasc Dis* 1991, 34:205–234.

Fleisher LA, Eagle KA: Screening for cardiac disease in patients having noncardiac surgery. *Ann Intern Med* 1996, 124:767–772.

Shaw LJ, Eagle KA, Gersh BJ, *et al.*: Meta-analysis of intravenous dipyridamole-thallium-201 imaging (1985 to 1994) and dobutamine echocardiography (1991 to 1994) for risk stratification before vascular surgery. *J Am Coll Cardiol* 1996, 27:787–798.

Eagle KA, Brundage BH, Chaitman BR, *et al.*: Guidelines for perioperative cardiovascular evaluation for noncardiac surgery- American Collage of Cardiology/American Heart Association Task Force on Practice Guidelines. *J Am Coll Cardiol* 1996, 27:910–948.

Interpreting Noninvasive Cardiac Tests

Robert C. Hendel

4

> ### Key Points
> - The clinician must use his or her clinical judgment in deciding how to interpret diagnostic tests, because no test is 100% accurate.
> - Electrocardiograms can help to diagnose myocardial ischemia and arrhythmias, and suggest other conditions such as drug overdoses and electrolyte disturbances.
> - Exercise or pharmacologic stress testing is used to diagnose coronary artery disease, offer prognostic information, and assess the need for or adequacy of revascularization.
> - Echocardiography is used to assess systolic and diastolic function, evaluate valve function and pathology, and assess pericardial and myocardial pathology; alone and in conjunction with exercise and pharmacologic stress testing.
> - Nuclear cardiology is used to diagnose coronary artery disease, offer prognostic information after myocardial infarction and before noncardiac surgery, and in patients with known or suspected coronary disease.
> - New technetium-99m–based radionuclides allow the physician to obtain information regarding ventricular function and myocardial perfusion from the same test.
> - Newer uses of noninvasive tests include imaging in the emergency department in patients with nondiagnostic electrocardiograms and early imaging after myocardial infarction to assess the degree of myocardium damage and myocardial salvage.

Noninvasive cardiac testing is playing an increasingly prominent role in the diagnosis and treatment of patients with known or suspected heart disease. This trend is likely to continue given the current economic climate and the high expense and potential risk associated with invasive procedures. Recent technological advances in nuclear cardiology, echocardiography, and electrocardiography now allow for enhanced diagnostic capabilities, and ample research supports the prognostic value of these methods. New myocardial perfusion agents and improved instrumentation in nuclear cardiology have significantly improved the diagnostic accuracy for detection of coronary artery disease (CAD). Echocardiography has undergone rapid development; transesophageal probes are now able to detect thrombi or tumors as small as 1 mm. In addition, stress echocardiography is being used with increasing frequency and in a variety of patient populations.

This chapter reviews the different noninvasive cardiac modalities currently available and their applications as related to evaluation of coronary artery disease, valvular abnormalities, pericardial disorders, and arrhythmia evaluations.

ELECTROCARDIOGRAPHY

The electrocardiogram (ECG) is the most commonly used diagnostic test in cardiology, providing a definitive diagnosis or helpful clues for many disorders. The ECG is predominantly used to diagnose myocardial ischemia or infarction and arrhythmias, but also reveals clues to electrolyte imbalances, medication-induced abnormalities, and metabolic derangements.

Ischemia/Infarction

There are many possible electrocardiographic manifestations of myocardial ischemia including ST segment elevation, horizontal or downsloping ST segment depressions, symmetric T-wave inversion, normalization of a previously abnormal T wave (also called "pseudonormalization"), or QT prolongation. The location of myocardial injury may be ascertained by the ECG, as shown in Table 1. While a single ECG may provide a diagnosis, often a series of ECGs showing evolving changes or

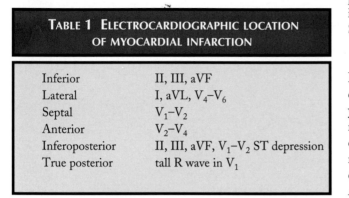

TABLE 1 ELECTROCARDIOGRAPHIC LOCATION OF MYOCARDIAL INFARCTION	
Inferior	II, III, aVF
Lateral	I, aVL, V_4–V_6
Septal	V_1–V_2
Anterior	V_2–V_4
Inferoposterior	II, III, aVF, V_1–V_2 ST depression
True posterior	tall R wave in V_1

patterns is crucial. The classic sequence of ECG changes in the setting of an acute myocardial infarction (MI) begins with tall and peaked T waves (hyperacute) followed by convex ST segment elevations with ≥1 mm ST elevation in two or more contiguous leads (Fig. 1). The next step is the inversion of the T waves and the formation of Q waves. Other causes of ST segment elevations that may be confused with an acute MI are pericarditis (Fig. 2), electrolyte abnormalities, and a normal juvenile (variant) pattern. The presence of reciprocal changes with ST segment depression in leads other than those with ST segment elevation is a helpful clue for the diagnosis of acute infarction. Resting ST segment depression portends a poorer prognosis after MI than its absence [1,2]. Right ventricular involvement may be accurately diagnosed by the presence of ST elevation in the 4th right precordial lead [3].

Arrhythmias

In addition to diagnosing myocardial ischemia, the ECG may document and diagnose arrhythmias. Supraventricular tachyarrhythmias (SVT), which are usually narrow QRS complex rhythms, include atrial fibrillation, atrial flutter, atrial tachycardia, AV nodal reentrant tachycardia (AVNRT), and atrial reentrant tachycardia (also referred to as a bypass tract tachycardia, preexcitation, Wolff-Parkinson-White syndrome). AVNRT is the most common SVT and is characterized by an

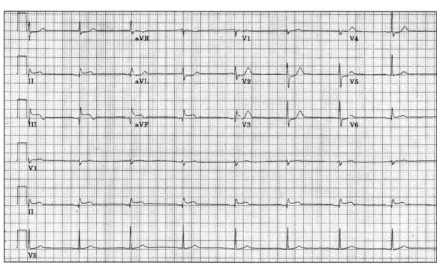

FIGURE 1 Evolutionary electrocardiographic changes associated with an acute myocardial infarction. Notice the ST segment elevations and small Q waves in the inferior leads, and the reciprocal ST segment depressions in the lateral leads. The ST depressions in leads V_1 and V_2 indicate posterior involvement as well. A cardiac catheterization revealed an occluded proximal right coronary artery. Temporal factors for these patterns are highly variable and may be influenced by acute interventions, such as thrombolytic therapy or angioplasty. See text for further details.

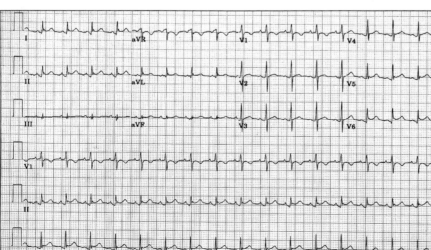

FIGURE 2 Electrocardiogram recording. The patient had a history of breast cancer and developed shortness of breath and severe, sharp chest pain worsened by motion and a supine position. Concave ST segment elevation is noted in virtually all leads, with prominent PR depression. The patient was diagnosed with pericarditis, and a moderate-sized pericardial effusion was noted on echocardiography.

abrupt onset and abrupt termination. ECG manifestations feature an absence of a P wave or an inverted P wave just after the QRS. Preexcitation syndrome is characterized by delta waves on the ECG and a short P-R cycle. Adenosine may be used with the ECG to differentiate among several arrhythmias. If the SVT terminates abruptly, the rhythm was likely AVNRT. The transient AV block induced by adenosine also may uncover the "F" waves produced in atrial flutter. When a history of preexcitation is present, adenosine must be used with caution, because it may induce ventricular fibrillation.

When a wide QRS complex is present, it is often difficult to differentiate between ventricular tachycardia and SVT with aberrant conduction. However, criteria have been defined to improve the accuracy of the ECG diagnosis for wide complex tachycardias (Table 2) [4].

Chamber Enlargement/ Left Ventricular Hypertrophy

Although there are established criteria for diagnosing chamber enlargement, the anatomic correlation tends to be poor. While characterization of ECG abnormalities associated with enlargement or hypertropy of the cardiac chambers is beyond the scope of this text, left ventricular hypertrophy (LVH) is a common and often-discussed entity [5]. Numerous diagnostic criteria have been proposed for the diagnosis of LVH (Table 3). The sensitivity of most criteria is in the range of 30% to 50%. In addition to prominent QRS voltage, the ST-segment and T-wave abnormalities seen reflect a shift of subendocardial to subepicardial repolarization. ECG evidence of LVH in hypertensive patients is associated with a threefold increase in overt CAD and an increased risk of death [6].

Bundle Branch Block

A bundle branch block is characterized by a prolonged (> 0.12 sec) QRS complex (Tables 4 and 5). A right bundle branch block (RBBB) is more common than left bundle branch block (LBBB) and is usually benign. In contrast, the most common cause of a LBBB is CAD. In contrast to RBBB, a LBBB may confound the determination of myocardial infarction. In fact, a new LBBB when associated with classic symptomatology should be taken as evidence of an acute MI. Although difficult, it may be possible to diagnose myocardial ischemia with a LBBB: inferior ST elevation may represent an acute infarction, and T-wave deflections in the same direction as the primary QRS forces represent primary T-wave changes and are consistent with ischemia.

EXERCISE STRESS TESTING

Exercise stress testing is often indicated to establish the diagnosis of CAD, using graded exercise treadmill or bicycle ergometry with a variety of exercise protocols (Table 6). For example, the Bruce protocol employs 3-minute stages with gradual increases in speed and grade. Patients who have recently had an MI or patients that may have difficulty keeping up can exercise with a modified Bruce protocol, which has no incline for the first two stages of exercise.

TABLE 2 CRITERIA FOR VENTRICULAR TACHYCARDIA

Classic criteria suggesting ventricular tachycardia

QRS duration > 0.14 sec

Superior QRS axis

Fusion beats

Atrioventricular dissociation

Brugada criteria for diagnosis of ventricular tachycardia

1. Absence of an RS complex in all precordial leads
   If present, VT
   If absent, continue algorithm
2. R-to-S interval >100 ms (0.1 sec) in one precordial lead
   If present, VT
   If absent, continue algorithm
3. AV dissociation
   If present, VT
   If absent, continue algorithm
4. Morphology criteria (see below) for VT present in V_1, V_2, and V_6
   If present, VT
   If absent, then SVT with aberrant conduction

Morphology criteria

LBB type

R>0.3 sec in lead V_1 or V_2

Onset of R to nadir of

S>0.7 sec in V_1

No S wave in V_6

RBB type

R/S ratio in V_6<1

RSR*, QR, or monophasic R in V_1

LBB—left bundle branch; RBB—right bundle branch.

A positive ECG test is usually defined as ≥ 1 mm of horizontal or downsloping ST segment depression 0.08 sec after the J point of the QRS (Figure 3). Upsloping ST segment depression of ≥ 1.5 mm in magnitude 0.08 sec after the QRS also indicates a positive test. The sensitivity and specificity of the test is approximately 75%. In addition to the ECG response, much clinical information is obtained from an exercise test, including the assessment of functional capacity, blood pressure changes, and the production of symptoms. Severe or multivessel CAD may be suggested by a marked reduction in exercise capacity (less than 6 min of exercise), a decrease in blood pressure during exercise, or severe and prolonged symptoms or ECG changes.

As with any test, the pretest probability strongly influences the outcome as well as what to do with the information. Patients with a high pretest likelihood of coronary disease and a negative test may still have CAD. Patients with an intermediate likelihood of CAD are the best candidates for exercise stress testing. Women and patients who are receiving digoxin, who have LVH, or who have resting ECG abnormalities have a higher incidence of false-posi-

TABLE 3 CRITERIA FOR LEFT VENTRICULAR HYPERTROPHY

Estes criteria*

1. Amplitude	3 points
Largest R or S in limb leads >20 mm	
S wave in V_1 or $V_2 \geq 30$ or R wave in V_5 or $V_6 \geq 30$ mm	
2. ST-T wave shifts (LV strain pattern) in the opposite direction of mean QRS	
Without digoxin	3 points
With digoxin	1 point
3. Left atrial involvement	3 points
4. Left axis deviation > 30°	2 points
5. QRS duration ≥ 0.09	1 point
6. Intrinsicoid deflection in leads V_5 or $V_6 \geq 0.05$	1 point

Cornell Voltage criteria

S wave in V_3 plus R wave in aVL ≥ 28 in men, ≥ 20 in women

Sokolow and Lyons criteria

S wave in V_1 plus R wave in V_5 or $V_6 \geq 35$ mm

LVH in the presence of a LBBB

S wave in V_2 plus R in $V_6 \geq 45$ mm

Left atrial enlargement

QRS duration greater than 0.16 s

*Point scoring system: 5 points = LVH, 4 points probable LVH.
LBBB—left bundle branch block; LVH—left ventricular hypertrophy.

tive ECG stress tests and may require adjunctive noninvasive imaging for the accurate assessment of CAD. Additional applications of exercise testing beyond the detection of coronary disease include risk stratification after MI, evaluation of arrhythmias, assessment of therapy, and determination of long-term prognosis. For example, patients who exercise to the end of stage III of a Bruce protocol have an excellent 5-year survival, irrespective of the degree of CAD. A comprehensive review of the indications, performance, and interpretation of exercise testing is presented in a recent series of practice guidelines [7•].

NUCLEAR CARDIOLOGY

Myocardial Perfusion Imaging

Myocardial perfusion imaging is used in conjunction with exercise electrocardiography or pharmacologic stress testing and can be performed using planar or single photon emission computed tomography (SPECT) imaging. Planar images are acquired in three primary views, while SPECT imaging collects a series of planar projections acquired as a camera rotates in an arc around the patient. SPECT images are then reconstructed three dimensionally and are typically displayed in three orientations: 1) short axis, 2) horizontal long axis, and 3) vertical long axis. SPECT allows for better localization of perfusion abnormalities and enhanced diagnostic sensitivity (≈ 85%).

There are two classes of agents used for perfusion imaging. Thallium-201 has been used for more than 20 years for perfusion imaging. More recently, technetium-99m (Tc-99m) compounds have been used such as Tc-99m sestamibi (Cardiolite, DuPont Pharma, N. Billerica, MA), Tc-99m tetrofosmin (Myoview, Amersham Healthcare, Arlington Heights, IL) and Tc-99m teboroxime (Cardiotec, Bracco Diagnostic, Princeton, NJ). Within the normal physiologic range, myocardial uptake of tracer is proportional to coro-

TABLE 4 ELECTROCARDIOGRAPHIC DIAGNOSIS OF A LEFT BUNDLE BRANCH BLOCK

Diagnostic findings

QRS duration > 0.12 ms

Broad R wave in leads I, V_5, and V_6

Absence of Q waves in same leads

Delay in intrinsicoid deflection in V_5 and V_6

ST and T waves in the opposite direction of *major* QRS deflection

Clues to diagnosis

Poor R-wave progression

Broad S wave in the right precordial leads

Left axis deviation

QS pattern in the inferior leads

nary blood flow. Therefore, regional differences in myocardial blood flow caused by CAD will manifest regional differences in tracer uptake, resulting in defects on the initial scan. A second set of images obtained at rest after a second injection of a Tc-99m tracer will provide the comparison necessary to determine if the perfusion defect is permanent, such as after MI, or if it is reversible and consistent with ischemia (Fig. 4). Usually only one injection of thallium is used, but relative changes of tracer distribution occur with time. Ischemic myocardium is characterized by a slower washout of thallium, so that a second set of images acquired at a later time may show normalization or redistribution. Some myocardium may improve further if a third image is acquired as much as 24 hours later or if a second injection of thallium is administered immediately after the second image (viable myocardium). Several laboratories now perform dual isotope imaging with rest thallium/stress sestamibi in an attempt to decrease the amount of time required for each study and maximize the detection of myocardial viability, while optimizing image quality [8].

Although the Tc-99m-based agents are better suited for gamma camera imaging because of their physical properties, the extensive literature supports the diagnostic and prognostic value of thallium [9,10]. The Tc-99m agents now appear to have similar utility, and the newer tracers provide images of superior quality, and importantly, permit the assessment of ventricular function in addition to myocardial perfusion.

Using techniques such as gated SPECT imaging [11], viable myocardium is found to thicken and brighten, and the global left ventricular ejection fraction may be quantitated with accuracy. Functional information also may be obtained using first-pass techniques with Tc-99m sestamibi, whereby data regarding right and left ventricular function are gathered as the isotope passes through the cardiac chambers in addition to perfusion information.

In addition to the identification of CAD, perfusion imaging provides geographic localization of stenosis and extent of perfusion abnormality. The number of segments with abnormal perfusion is not only related to the severity of CAD, but also to prognosis. Transient cavity dilatation or an increased lung uptake of thallium with a lung:heart ratio of greater than 0.5 are markers of multivessel disease, left ventricular dysfunction, and a worse prognosis.

Myocardial perfusion imaging has been demonstrated in many studies to provide incremental prognostic value after

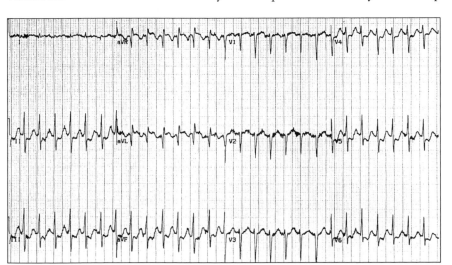

FIGURE 3 Electrocardiographic tracing at peak exercise (5 minutes) demonstrating 2 to 3 mm of downsloping ST segment depression in the inferolateral leads. The patient developed chest pain after 3 minutes of exercise and stopped soon thereafter. The patient is a 50-year-old male smoker who denied any history of angina. These changes persisted long into recovery, and at cardiac catheterization, the patient was found to have severe three-vessel coronary disease.

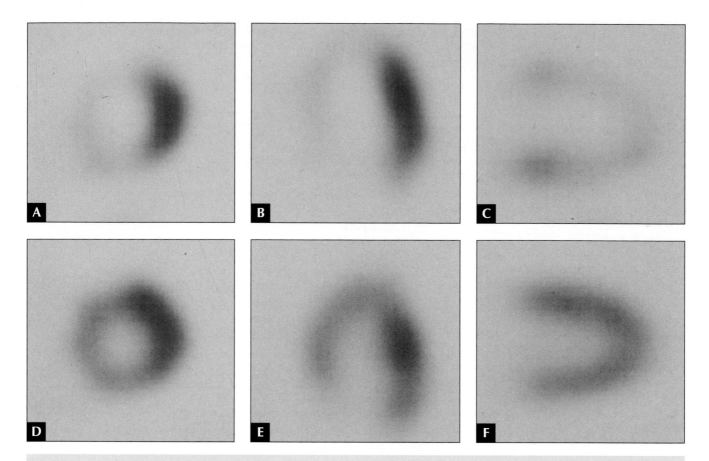

FIGURE 4 Single proton emission computed tomographic (SPECT) myocardial perfusion images obtained 10 minutes after an injection of thallium-201 at peak exercise (**A–C**) and approximately 3 hours later (**D–F**). The patient is a 61-year-old woman with hypertension and exertional chest pain. She developed exercise-induced ST changes and became dizzy and nauseated after 5 minutes of exercise. The perfusion images reveal reversible perfusion defects in the septum (short axis [**A** and **D**] and horizontal long axis [**B** and **E**]), anterior (short axis [**A** and **D**] and vertical long axis [**C** and **F**]), and apex (long axes [**B,C,E,** and **F**]). Subsequent evaluation revealed single-vessel coronary artery disease with a 90% diameter narrowing of the proximal left anterior descending coronary artery.

infarction, revascularization or catheterization, as well as in patients without previously known coronary artery disease [12•]. A very low risk (< 1%) for sustaining a cardiac event within the next year is associated with a normal perfusion study.

Left ventricular dysfunction may improve after revascularization in patients who demonstrate myocardial viability. Although there is no true gold standard for the noninvasive identification of viability, positron emission tomography (PET) is currently the most effective modality used. Thallium imaging, however, may be an inexpensive and simple alternative to PET and has been correlated with postoperative outcome and PET imaging [13]. There are two protocols for detecting viability: 1) a small dose of thallium is injected immediately after the second set of images is acquired of a regular stress test and a third image is acquired; and 2) thallium is injected at rest and then two sets of images are taken. Quantitation of sestamibi activity also may allow for the accurate detection of viable myocardium.

In patients who are unable, unwilling, or should not undergo exercise, pharmacologic stress testing is a valuable alternative (Table 7). Two categories of pharmacologic stress agents are available: 1) vasodilators, including dipyridamole and adenosine, and 2) catecholamines, including dobutamine and arbutamine. The intravenous vasodilators cause regional disparities in blood flow when a coronary stenosis is present, causing a perfusion defect. These actions may be reversed by aminophylline; consequently caffeine and theophylline should be withheld before testing. Because of the direct bronchoconstriction produced by adenosine and dipyridamole, patients with severe lung disease or active wheezing should not undergo pharmacologic stress testing with the vasodilators. Vasodilator stress testing is recommended for patients with LBBB, because exercise testing may produce false-positive perfusion defects, wall-motion abnormalities, or ECG changes. Unlike adenosine and dypridamole, dobutamine and arbutamine cause an increase in myocardial oxygen consumption and produce ischemia and subsequent perfusion abnormalities and regional wall-motion disturbances. The catecholamines are most useful in conjunction with perfusion imaging in patients unable to receive dipyridamole or adenosine.

In addition to the detection of coronary artery disease, myocardial perfusion imaging has a variety of prognostic applications including preoperative risk assessment, stratification after a myocardial infarction, determination of therapeutic efficacy, evaluation of the functional significance of angio-

TABLE 7 INDICATIONS FOR PHARMACOLOGIC STRESS TEST
Inability to exercise
Vascular, neurologic, or orthopedic patients
Limited exercise capacity
High risk from exercise
Aortic aneurysm, aortic stenosis, severe hypertension
Left bundle branch block

graphically determined stenoses, and assessment for the presence of myocardial viability.

PET is a relatively new technique that can be used in the detection of CAD, the estimation of its severity, and for the assessment of myocardial viability in patients with left ventricular dysfunction. PET is considered the gold standard in the noninvasive assessment of viability, as this method can directly measure and quantitate markers of myocardial metabolism, such as fatty acid or glucose utilization. The most commonly used agent for detection of viability is fluorodeoxyglucose (FDG). FDG is a marker of regional exogenous glucose uptake. Areas that have reduced perfusion but normal or increased glucose uptake indicate viable tissue. Because of the limited availability of cyclotrons for production of tracers and the cost of PET equipment, it is unlikely that PET scanning will become a widespread and standard technique for the evaluation of CAD. However, it is now feasible to image FDG with a modified SPECT camera, making metabolic imaging more available for clinical use [14].

Radionuclide Angiography

Radionuclide angiography is a highly reproducible and accurate method for the determination of ventricular function. One technique is first-pass angiography, which involves analysis of counts during the first 15 to 20 seconds after an intravenous injection of a tracer. More frequently, gated equilibrium radionuclide angiography, is performed, where the R wave of the ECG is used as a "gate" for serial static images in relation to the cardiac cycle. Several hundred beats are collected and summed to allow for adequate counts. Both first-pass and equilibrium studies may be performed at rest or in conjunction with exercise, obtaining measurements of left ventricular ejection fraction at each stage of exercise. Abnormal exercise ejection fraction response or absolute value less than 50% have been shown to be powerful prognostic indicators [15,16].

Besides being able to measure left ventricular function, radionuclide angiography can evaluate left ventricular volumes, right ventricular function and volume, regurgitant fraction in patients with valvular incompetence, and left ventricular diastolic function. Because many patients who present with heart failure may in fact have diastolic dysfunction, it is often important to distinguish systolic from diastolic dysfunction, since the treatment of each process is dramatically different.

ECHOCARDIOGRAPHY

M-Mode, Two-Dimensional, and Doppler Echocardiography

Echocardiography uses high-frequency ultrasonic waves for the real-time imaging of cardiac structures and blood cells as they transit the heart. A transducer applied to the chest wall emits and receives acoustic data, which then may be displayed in a variety of formats. M-mode echocardiography has largely been replaced by two-dimensional information, but may still be useful in measuring dimensions and wall thickness of cardiac chambers. Two-dimensional echocardiography provides an accurate representation of cardiac structures and reveals the anatomic relationships of various structures. Wall motion can be visualized and classified as normal, hypokinetic, akinetic, or dyskinetic. Although true quantitation is not yet a reality, this semiquantitative analysis, in conjunction with a segmental model, provides useful diagnostic and prognostic information. Doppler echocardiography provides physiologic information regarding valvular function and the patterns of blood flow through the heart. The signal is reflected off the moving erythrocytes and produces a slight shift in frequency, permitting determination of the direction and velocity of flow. There are three forms of Doppler imaging: 1) pulse wave, 2) continuous wave, and 3) color flow. Color-flow Doppler imaging permits visualization of this information superimposed on the two-dimensional echocardiogram. Doppler imaging is frequently used to detect valve regurgitation and quantitate the degree of valvular and subvalvular stenosis. The echocardiographically derived valve areas in the setting of mitral or aortic stenosis correlate well with data obtained from cardiac catheterization. Additionally, Doppler flows can be used to assess diastolic left ventricular function and estimate right ventricular and pulmonary artery pressures.

Echocardiography has a variety of applications including the evaluation of global and regional left ventricular function, determination of left ventricular mass and volume, detection of thrombi or tumors in cardiac chambers, assessment for the presence and degree of pericardial effusion, and the initial evaluation of valve pathology (stenosis, prolapse, flail, incompetence). Echocardiography is useful for the evaluation of complications after acute MI such as mitral regurgitation, papillary muscle dysfunction, rupture of the ventricular septum or papillary muscle (Fig. 5), or apical thrombus. Echocardiography is often used in critical care settings because of its portability.

Transesophageal Echocardiography

Transesophageal echocardiography (TEE) is performed in the same manner as an upper endoscopic procedure. Because of the invasive nature of the procedure, certain precautions are necessary during the test. For example, oxygen saturation and blood pressure monitoring should be performed during and after the test, especially if the patient has received sedation. The risk of bacterial endocarditis is low, and in general, antibiotic prophylaxis is not indicated. However, patients with prosthetic valves or

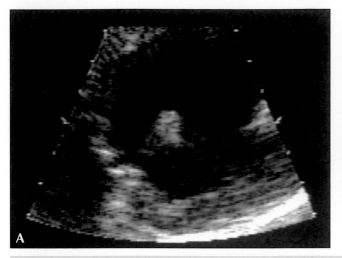

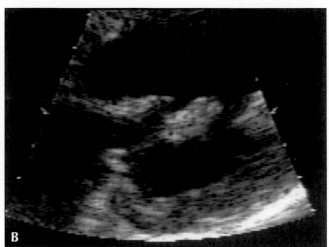

FIGURE 5 A, Systolic and B, diastolic images from a two-dimensional echocardiogram. Subcostal view demonstrates a ruptured papillary muscle from a patient who suffered a myocardial infarction 2 days before the echocardiogram was obtained.

those in high-risk groups should receive antibiotics before and after the procedure. The only real contraindication to TEE is esophageal pathology, although patients who have difficulty swallowing represent a challenging group. All probes are now equipped with biplane technology; anatomic relationships and pathology can be seen in multiple views and with less uncertainty. The newer TEE probes allow investigation in multiple planes, further enhancing diagnostic abilities. Doppler imaging also can be performed with the TEE probes (Fig. 6).

The indications for transesophageal echocardiography (TEE) are expanding rapidly (Table 8) [17]. Because of the anatomic relationship of the heart and the esophagus, many structures can be visualized in great detail. The most common use of TEE is to evaluate the heart as a source of embolism or to rule out endocarditis. The left atrium is the most posterior structure, and therefore is uniquely suited to examination by TEE. Most thrombi are located within the left atrial appendage, which is rarely seen on standard transthoracic echocardiography. Clinicians are using TEE with increasing frequency to help monitor early cardioversion in patients with new onset atrial fibrillation. TEE is ideal for examination of the intraatrial septum for atrial septal defects, a patent foramen ovale, and intraatrial septal aneurysms. TEE also is useful in the setting of suspected infective endocarditis, because it may reveal vegetations as small as 1 to 2 mm. This method may also detect complications of endocarditis, such as ring abscesses, valve dehiscence, or leaflet perforation. Intraoperatively, TEE may be employed as a means of assessing for myocardial ischemia during surgery, as well as assisting in the determination of whether a valve needs replacement during coronary bypass surgery.

Stress Echocardiography

Stress echocardiography is a recently developed modality, permitting the assessment of coronary artery disease by means

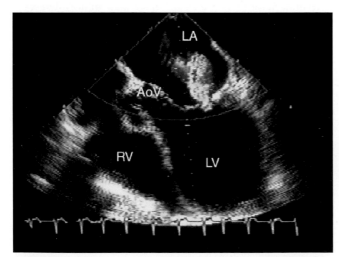

FIGURE 6 Color flow Doppler image from a transesophageal echocardiogram. The image reveals a normal left ventricle, a large left atrium, and a single broad turbulent jet of mitral regurgitation extending far back into the left atrium during systole. (See Color Plate.)

TABLE 8 INDICATIONS FOR TRANSESOPHAGEAL ECHOCARDIOGRAPHY
Potential source of embolism
Evaluate left atrium and left atrial appendage
Rule out left ventricle thrombus
Assess aorta for atheroma
Rule out atrial septal defect or patent foramen ovale
Complications of infective endocarditis
Evaluate LV and LV outflow tract
Rule out atrial septal defect or ventricular septal defect
Intraoperative monitoring
Evaluating congenital heart disease
Evaluating aorta for possible dissection, atheroma, or aneurysm
LV—left ventricle.

of regional wall-motion analysis [18]. Despite its potential advantages regarding cost and time efficiency, stress echocardiography has significant limitations: up to 30% of patients do not have adequate acoustic windows, and image interpretation is highly observer dependent.

Exercise echocardiography has a sensitivity and specificity similar to that of nuclear stress testing, with a concordance between the techniques of approximately 82% [19]. Unfortunately, limited outcome data are available regarding exercise echocardiography because of the recent origin of the method. In addition to exercise, pharmacologic stress echocardiography also may be performed, primarily using a dobutamine infusion. This catecholamine is delivered in increasing doses to allow for identification of new wall-motion abnormalities. Dobutamine stress echocardiograms have been used for a variety of scenarios including risk stratification before surgery, ischemia evaluation, and in patients who have recently undergone angioplasty [20•]. Additionally, in patients with left ventricular dysfunction, low-dose dobutamine echocardiography can detect myocardial viability by demonstration of improved contractility. Its ability to detect viability is comparable to thallium studies and has been confirmed by outcomes and postoperative evaluation of LV function [21•].

ELECTROPHYSIOLOGY

The field of cardiac electrophysiology has grown dramatically in the past 10 years. In addition to invasive electrophysiologic studies, several noninvasive techniques are currently available. Twenty-four hour ambulatory or Holter monitoring is used for the evaluation of patients with bradycardia or tachycardia, detecting prolonged pauses or episodes of tachycardia. The presence of significant ventricular ectopy increases a patient's risk of sudden death [22]. An alternative method for patients with less frequent symptoms or arrhythmia is the use of an event monitor, a recorder that the patient wears and can activate whenever he or she experiences symptoms. These data can then be transmitted telephonically and interpreted by a physician.

Tilt-table testing is used to evaluate the patient whose history suggests vasodepressor syncope (simple faint). The bed is gradually tilted to an angle of approximately 70° while the patient's heart rate and blood pressure are monitored. If this does not provoke symptoms, then isoproterenol is infused and the bed is again tilted until the test is over or the patient develops symptoms. Currently, most patients are treated with β-adrenergic blockers and then are retested to ascertain efficacy of drug therapy. If unsuccessful, other drugs can be assessed.

The role of signal average electrocardiograms (SAECG) in the prediction of sudden death is unclear. In post-MI patients with a narrow QRS complex on their ECG, the SAECG appears valuable in identifying a high-risk group. Although this technique may also be useful in patients with hypertrophic cardiomyopathy or nonischemic dilated cardiomyopathy, the predictive value of SAECG is not as powerful [23]. The presence of late potentials in the terminal portion of the QRS conveys an increased risk of sudden death. Another measure of increased risk is loss of heart rate variability (HRV). HRV is determined by having the patient lie flat with a standard ECG recording the heart rate. HRV is usually performed just before electrophysiology studies and has yet to demonstrate enough independent prognostic value to be of clinical use.

MAGNETIC RESONANCE IMAGING/COMPUTED TOMOGRAPHY

Magnetic resonance imaging (MRI) has experienced explosive growth, but currently has limited clinical uses in cardiology. It is chiefly employed in evaluating cardiac tumors and masses, pericardial disease, and in the assessment of possible aortic dissection. The following potential applications for MRI are still being investigated and are not widely used clinically: assessment of ventricular volumes, severity of diastolic dysfunction, perfusion imaging, assessment of valvular regurgitation, and myocardial viability.

Computed tomography (CT) is employed primarily for the diagnosis of aortic dissection. Some authors suggest that TEE may be superior to CT in diagnosing acute dissection. Cine CT or "ultrafast" CT reveals coronary calcification, a marker of atherosclerosis. Therefore, this method has been suggested as a screening tool for the presence of CAD. However, an American Heart Association advisory board has recommended that the electron beam CT not be used as a screening tool for CAD detection [24]. Overall, it does appear that the assessment of coronary calcification with electron beam CT has diagnostic value [25•].

CLINICAL APPLICATIONS

Diagnosis of Myocardial Infarction

ST segment elevation is the hallmark of acute infarction, permitting triage and rapid intervention with thrombolytic therapy or angioplasty. However, the initial electrocardiogram is diagnostic of an acute MI in only 50% to 60% of patients, with serial ECGs identifying an additional 10%. Right ventricular involvement is an important clinical entity and may be detected using right-sided ECG leads and confirmed by the presence of ≥ 1 mm ST elevation in V_{3R} or V_{4R} in the setting of an inferior infarction [3].

The current gold standard for the diagnosis of an acute MI is the measurement of serum creatine kinase (CK)–MB isoenzymes. The typical pattern consists of an increase in CK-MB within 4 to 8 hours of an acute MI and peak activity at 12 to 24 hours. Recently, additional serologic tests have become available for the early detection of acute injury such as CK-MB isoforms, troponin-T, and serum myoglobin [26,27].

Imaging also may be performed to visualize a wall-motion abnormality with echocardiography or a scintigraphic perfusion defect after administration of sestamibi, both of which confirm an acute ischemic syndrome in the absence of prior infarction [28•]. Echocardiography also may allow for the diagnosis of infarct-related complications, such as mural thrombus formation or mitral regurgitation.

Risk Stratification After Myocardial Infarction

Prognosis after MI is predominantly dependent on three factors: 1) left ventricular ejection fraction; 2) the presence of residual ischemia; and 3) the presence of ventricular arrhythmias. The left ventricular ejection fraction is inversely proportional to long-term survival and may be assessed by radionuclide ventriculography, contrast ventriculography, or echocardiography. An ejection fraction of less than 40% is associated with increased risk; however, this value is not an absolute cutoff, but a continuum. Recurrent symptoms or objective evidence of myocardial ischemia as demonstrated on a stress test (exercise or pharmacologic, with or without imaging), patients with significant ventricular ectopy, complex ectopy, or recurrent ventricular tachycardia on Holter monitoring also have a poor prognosis. Ironically, suppression of ventricular ectopy by antiarrythmic medications may increase the risk of death. A signal-average ECG that detects late potentials in the terminal portion of the QRS is useful for predicting the risk of sudden death after MI. Programmed electrical stimulation (EP study) has been used for risk stratification, but the value of a negative study is unclear.

Diagnosis of Pericardial Diseases

The electrocardiogram remains the most important test for the diagnosis of pericarditis, which is confirmed by the presence of diffuse concave ST segment elevation in multiple leads, and PR segment depression. There are no reciprocal changes in other leads, as would be expected in acute MI. Pericarditis should not be mistaken for an acute MI, because the risk of a hemopericardium is high if the patient were to receive thrombolytic therapy or heparin. Pericardial thickening also may be evaluated by CT or MRI.

Echocardiography is extremely sensitive for diagnosing pericardial effusions. Certain echocardiographic criteria suggest the diagnosis of tamponade, including right atrial or ventricular diastolic collapse, and augmented respiratory variation of diastolic flow through the mitral valve.

Assessment of Valvular Heart Disease

Echocardiography is ideally suited for assessment of valvular regurgitation and stenosis, demonstrating the morphology and anatomic relationships of the valves and related structures. Additionally, Doppler echocardiography provides a physiologic assessment of the severity of turbulent blood flow. In valvular stenosis, transvalvular gradients may be determined and valve areas calculated, with a high correlation with data obtained during cardiac catheterization. The degree of valvular incompetence also may be assessed, since Dopper flows demonstrate the extent of regurgitant flow. Radionuclide angiography allows serial assessment of ventricular function and has been used in conjunction with exercise testing for aortic insufficiency to assist in decisions regarding the timing of valve replacement surgery. Radionuclide angiography also is useful for quantitation of the regurgitant fraction and ventricular volume. Intraoperative TEE can be used to determine the need for valve replacement while the patient is undergoing another procedure, such as coronary artery bypass graft surgery. After implantation of a prosthetic valve, echocardiography may be used to assess function, although the acoustic window may mandate a transesophageal approach. Transthoracic and transesophageal echocardiography are often used to search for sources of emboli or the presence of vegetations in suspected endocarditis.

Preoperative Risk Stratification

The assessment of cardiac risk factors in patients undergoing noncardiac surgery is an important duty for most primary care physicians. The majority of indices for risk assessment have been devised for the general surgical population. However, these clinical parameters may be insufficient in many other patient cohorts, and additional information may be necessary [29]. Exercise stress testing remains useful for preoperative assessment, but many patients cannot undergo rigorous exercise. Pharmacologic testing, with dipyridamole, adenosine, or dobutamine, in conjunction with perfusion imaging has excellent prognostic value. Similarly, dobutamine stress echocardiography may effectively stratify patients based on operative risk [30].

References and Recommended Reading

Recently published papers of particular interest have been highlighted as:
• Of interest
•• Of outstanding interest

1. Cohen M, Hawkins L, Greenberg S, Fuster V: Usefulness of ST-segment changes in ≥ leads on the emergency room electrocardiogram in either unstable angina pectoris or non Q wave myocardial infarction in predicting outcome. *Am J Cardiol* 1991, 67:1368–1373.

2. Krone R, Greenberg H, Dwyer E, *et al.*: Long-term prognostic significance of ST segment depression during acute myocardial infarction. *J Am Coll Cardiol* 1993, 22:361–367.

3. Zehender M, Kasper W, Kauder E, *et al.*: Right ventricular infarction as an independent predictor of prognosis after acute inferior myocardial infarction. *N Engl J Med* 1993, 328:981–988.

4. Brugada P, Brugada J, Mont L, *et al.*: A new approach to the differential diagnosis of a regular tachycardia with a wide QRS complex. *Circulation* 1991, 83:1649–1659.

5. Casale P, Devereux R, Kligfeld P: Electrocardiographic detection of left ventricular hypertrophy: development and prospective validation of improved criteria. *J Am Coll Cardiol* 1985, 6:572–580.

6. Ghali J, Liao Y, Simmons B, *et al.*: The prognostic role of left ventricular hypertrophy in patients with and without coronary artery disease. *Ann Int Med* 1992, 117:831–836.

7.• Gibbons RJ, Balady GJ, Beasley JW, *et al.*: ACC/AHA guidelines for exercise testing: a report of the American College of Cardiology/American Heart Association task force on practice guidelines (committee on exercise testing). *J Am Coll Cardiol* 1996, 30:260–315.

8. Berman D, Kiat H, Friedman J, *et al.*: Separate rest thallium-201/stress technetium-99m sestamibi dual isotope myocardial perfusion single photon emission computed tomography: a clinical validation study. *J Am Coll Cardiol* 1993, 22:1455–1464.

9. Iskandrian A, Chae S, Heo J, *et al.*: Independent and incremental prognostic value of exercise single-photon emission computed tomographic (SPECT) thallium imaging in patients with coronary artery disease. *J Am Coll Cardiol* 1993, 22:665–670.

10. Machecourt J, Longere P, Fagret D, *et al.*: Prognostic value of thallium-201 single photon emission computed tomographic myocardial perfusion imaging according to extent of myocardial defect. *J Am Coll Cardiol* 1994, 23:1096–1106.

11. Chua T, Kiat H, German OG, *et al.*: Gated technetium-99m sestamibi for simultaneous assessment of stress myocardial perfusion, postexercise regional ventricular function and myocardial viability. *J Am Coll Cardiol* 1994, 23:1107–1114.

12.• Hachamovich R, Berman DS, Kiat H, *et al.*: Exercise myocardial perfusion SPECT in patients without known coronary artery disease. *Circulation* 1996, 93:905–914.

13. Dilsizian V, Bonow R: Current diagnostic techniques of assessing myocardial viability in patients with hibernating or stunned myocardium. *Circulation* 1993, 87:1–20.

14. Delbeke D, Videlefsky S, Patton JA, et al.: Rest myocardial perfusion metabolism imaging using simultaneous dual-isotope acquisition SPECT with technetium-99m-MIBI/fluorine-18FDG. *J Nucl Med* 1995, 36:2110–2119.

15. Lee K, Pryor D, Peiper K *et al.*: Prognostic value of radionuclide angiography in medically treated patients with coronary artery disease: a comparison with clinical and catheterization variables. *Circulation* 1990, 82:1705–1717.

16. Bonow R: Radionuclide angiography for risk stratification of patients with coronary artery disease. *Am J Cardiol* 1993, 72:735–739.

17. Anasari A: Transesophageal two-dimensional echocardiography: current perspectives. *Prog Cardiovasc Dis* 1993, 35:349–397.

18. Ryan T, Armstrong W, O'Donnell J, Feigenbaum H: Risk stratification after acute myocardial infarction by means of exercise two-dimensional echocardiography. *Am Heart J* 1987, 114:1305–1316.

19. Quinones M, Verani M, Haichin R, *et al.*: Exercise echocardiography versus thallium 201 single photon emission computed tomography in evaluation of coronary artery disease: analysis of 292 patients. *Circulation* 1992, 85:1026–1031.

20.• Marcovitz P, Shayna V, Horn R, *et al.*: Value of dobutamine stress echcardiography in determining the prognosis of patients with known or suspected coronary artery disease. *Am J Cardiol* 1996, 78:404.

21.• Vanoverschelde JJ, D'Hondt AM, Marwick T, et al.: Head-to-head comparison of exercise-redistribution-reinjection thallium single photon emission computed tomography and low dose dobutamine echocardiography for prediction of reversibility of chronic left ventricular ischemic dysfunction. *J Am Coll Cardiol* 1996, 28:432–442.

22.• Bikkina M, Larson M, Levy D: Prognostic implications of asymptomatic ventricular arrhythmias: the Framingham Heart Study. *Ann Int Med* 1992, 117:990–996.

23. Podrid PJ, Bumio F, Fogel R, *et al.*: Evaluating patients with ventricular arrhythmia: role of the signal averaged electrocardiogram, exercise test, ambulatory electrocardiogram, and electrophysiologic studies. *Cardiol Clin* 1992, 10:371–395.

24. Committee on Advanced Cardiac Imaging and Technology, Council on Clinical Cardiology, and Committee on Newer Imaging Modalities, Council on Cardiovascular Radiology, American Heart Association: potential value of ultrafast computed tomography to screen for coronary artery disease. *Circulation* 1993, 87:2071.

25.• Budoff MJ, Georgiou D, Broody A, *et al.*: Ultrafast computed tomography as a diagnostic modality in the detection of coronary artery disease: a multicenter study. *Circulation* 1996, 93:893.

26. Puleo P, Meyer D, Wathen C, *et al.*: Use of a rapid assay of subforms of creatine kinase MB to diagnose or rule out acute myocardial infarction. *N Engl J Med* 1994, 331:561–566.

27. Hamm C, Ravkilde J, Gerhardt W, *et al.*: The prognostic value of serum troponin T in unstable angina. *N Engl J Med* 1992, 327:146–150.

28.• Tatum J, Jesse R, Kontos M, *et al.*: Comprehensive strategy for the evaluation and triage of the chest pain patient. *Ann Emerg Med* 1997, 29:116–125.

29. Eagle K, Coley C, Newell J, *et al.*: Combining clinical and thallium data optimizes preoperative assessment of cardiac risk before major vascular surgery. *Ann Intern Med* 1989, 110:859–866.

30. Poldermans D, Fioretti PM, Foster E, *et al.*: Dobutamine stress echocardiography for assessment of perioperative cardiac risk in patients undergoing major vascular surgery. *Circulation* 1993, 87:1506–1512.

SELECT BIBLIOGRAPHY

American Heart Association/American College of Cardiology Task Force: Guidelines for clinical use of cardiac radionuclide imaging. *Circulation* 1995, 91:1278–1302.

American College of Cardiology/American Heart Association: Guidelines for the clinical application of echocardiography. *Circulation* 1997, 95:1686–1744.

American College of Cardiology/American Heart Association: Guidleines for exercise testing. *J Am Coll Cardiol* 1997, 30:260–315.

Pellikka PA, Roger VL, Oh JK, *et al.*: Stress echocardiography. Part II. Dobutamine stress echocardiography: techniques, implementation, clinical applications, and correlations. *Mayo Clin Proc* 1995, 70(1):16–27.

Pitt B: Evaluation of the postinfarct patient. *Circulation* 1995, 91:1855–1860.

Roger VL, Pellikka PA, Oh JK, *et al.*: Stress echocardiography. Part I. Exercise echocardiography: techniques, implementation, clinical applications, and correlations. *Mayo Clin Proc* 1995, 70(1):5–15.

Zaret BL, Wackers FJ: Nuclear cardiology. *N Engl J Med* 1993, 329:775–783, 855–863.

Evaluation of the Patient with Chest Pain 5

John A. Paraskos

Key Points

- Many of the economic and medical resources used in evaluating patients with chest pain are unnecessary.

- A carefully obtained history is crucial to assessing the likelihood of coronary disease before any testing is obtained (*ie*, the pretest likelihood for coronary disease).

- The pretest likelihood is assessed from the patient's age, gender, character of the pain or discomfort, and associated risk factors.

- Both the choice and interpretation of noninvasive tests to establish the diagnosis depend on the pretest likelihood and the perceived urgency or instability of the clinical scenario.

- The choice and timing of coronary arteriography depend on the urgency of the clinical scenario and the inability of noninvasive tests to establish the diagnosis reliably.

Evaluation of chest pain consumes a tremendous amount of economic and medical resources. Identification of patients whose chest pain results from myocardial ischemia is a challenging and important problem in clinical medicine, considering the potentially lethal consequences of error. Many of the resources expended in cardiac evaluation, however, are unnecessary.

The most important evaluative tool in most cases is a careful history augmented by physical examination and simple laboratory procedures. Angina pectoris is a diagnosis of history; an effective physician can often allay the patient's anxiety and prevent unnecessary diagnostic procedures by a careful history and a thorough knowledge of the likelihood of coronary artery disease (CAD) in a given population. Whenever a patient presents with chest pain, it is important to assess rapidly the likelihood of coronary disease in that individual, the likelihood that the character of the pain is cardiac in origin, and the multiplicity of other conditions that can produce similar symptoms. This differentiation is complicated by the overlap of signs and symptoms of myocardial ischemia with several noncardiac causes of chest pain (Table 1). Any of the thoracic structures can be a source of chest pain, as can structures outside the thorax, particularly the gastrointestinal tract. Because the heart and esophagus share the same spinal cord sensory innervation, myocardial ischemia and esophageal pain are sometimes indistinguishable [1,2]. A burning substernal discomfort typical of esophageal pyrosis is not uncommon in myocardial ischemia; conversely, substernal tightness or pressure or even crushing pain typical of angina pectoris, may be caused by esophageal disease. After a careful initial evaluation, many patients must be treated as if they have myocardial ischemia until the diagnostic dilemma is resolved by further observation, diagnostic studies, or response to therapy. If coronary disease is likely and the character of the pain is clearly or possibly ischemic, consultation with an internist or cardiologist is appropriate.

This chapter provides a useful method of determining the likelihood of coronary disease in any individual based on risk factors and pain characteristics. Physical findings associated with various causes of chest pain and procedures needed to confirm the diagnosis are also discussed.

CHEST PAIN AS A MANIFESTATION OF MYOCARDIAL ISCHEMIA

Angina pectoris is usually substernal and transient. It is often brought on by exercise and relieved by rest or nitrates. Angina may be provoked by a large meal and be mistaken for indigestion. If the coronary disease is stable, the pain episodes are usually short-lived (ie, 5 to 15 minutes) and provoked by exertion or meals.

Unstable angina is characterized by a less predictable prognosis, with a higher likelihood of acute myocardial infarction (MI) or sudden death. This instability is usually caused by a complication in the coronary artery (eg, plaque rupture, thrombosis, or spasm). Features that mark instability are new-

onset angina, accelerating angina (occurring more frequently or at lower workloads), rest angina, angina that wakes the patient from sleep, prolonged anginal episodes, anginal episodes not responsive to nitrates, and angina associated with severe nausea, weakness, dyspnea, sweating, palpitations, syncope, or pulmonary edema.

The pain of MI usually includes a number of these features of instability. It is usually not triggered by exertion and is not relieved by rest, antacids, or nitrates. The pain of MI is more often accompanied by nausea and sweating, and patients are often immobilized by a sense of impending doom.

Patients suspected of having acute MI must be admitted for intensive care monitoring, because short-term survival is enhanced by early intervention, especially for life-threatening ventricular arrhythmias. Patients with unstable angina also have a serious short-term prognosis and usually require hospitalization and consultation with a cardiologist so that therapeutic decisions can be made promptly.

When evaluating ischemic pain, the clinician should consider several questions. Is the chest pain typical for myocar-

---

TABLE 1 CAUSES OF CHEST PAIN

Cardiovascular
Coronary artery disease
  Obstructive, spastic, nonathero-
    sclerotic, and congenital
  Cocaine abuse
Severe aortic stenosis or aortic
  insufficiency
Hypertrophic cardiomyopathy
Aortic dissection
Pericarditis
Myocarditis
Dressler's syndrome
Pulmonary embolism
Pulmonary hypertension
Thoracic aneurysm
Hepatic engorgement
Mitral valve prolapse

Pulmonary
Pneumonitis
Pleurisy
Pulmonary infarction or hemorrhage
Pulmonary embolism or *in situ*
  thrombosis
Tracheitis and tracheobronchitis
Spontaneous pneumothorax
Intrathoracic tumor

Gastrointestinal
Hiatal hernia with reflux esophagitis
Esophageal spasm
Esophageal perforation
Esophagitis
Irritable esophagus
Mallory-Weiss syndrome
Peptic ulcer disease
Gastritis
Cholecystitis and biliary colic
Pancreatitis
Gas entrapment syndromes
  Gastric distention
  Hepatic or splenic flexure distention

Musculoskeletal
Costochondritis (Tietze's syndrome)
Costochondral or xiphisternal arthralgia
Sternoclavicular arthralgia
Manubriosternal arthralgia
Costovertebral arthritis
Epidemic myalgia
Fibromyalgia
Myositis
Thoracic outlet syndromes
Sternal or rib fractures
Slipping rib syndrome
Precordial catch syndrome (muscle spasm)
Muscle strain
Ostealgia from neoplasm, inflammation,
  or infarction
Sternal marrow pain (acute leukemia)
Trauma

Neurologic
Radicular syndrome
Thoracic disc disease
Brachial plexus syndrome
Intercostal neuritis
Reflex autonomic dysfunction
  (shoulder-hand syndrome)
Neurofibromatosis
Herpes zoster involving thoracic
  dermatome with postherpetic pain

Functional or psychiatric
Anxiety with periapical hyperesthesia
Hyperventilation with increased
  muscle tension
Panic attacks
Cardiac neurosis
Psychogenic regional pain syndrome
Malingering
Depression

Miscellaneous
Diaphragmatic spasm or flutter
Superficial thrombophlebitis
  (Mondor's syndrome)
Mediastinitis
Mediastinal emphysema
Mediastinal tumors

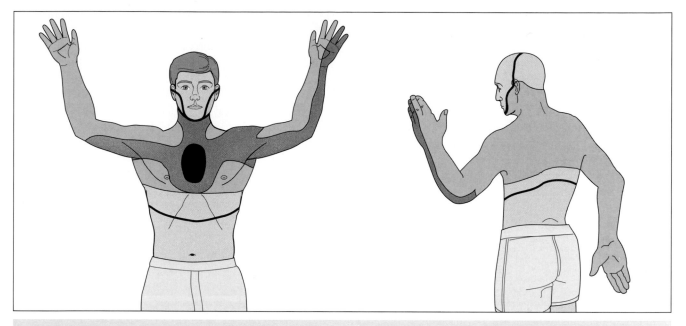

FIGURE 1 Location and radiation of ischemic pain. The *black area* represents the most frequent location of ischemic pain. *Dark shading* represents the most common sites of radiation, and *light* shading includes all but the rarest areas of sites of radiation (C3–T6). The *heavy lines* encompass the rarest sites of radiation (C2–T8). (*From* Richter [17]; with permission.)

dial ischemic pain, atypical for but possibly caused by ischemic pain, or clearly unlikely to be ischemic in origin? Also, is the pain likely to be of a serious nature? Even typical angina pectoris does not always indicate serious coronary disease; rather, it may be associated with less threatening causes (*eg*, mitral valve prolapse, nonthreatening stable coronary disease). Alternatively, chest pain may be caused by other life-threatening conditions that require immediate attention (*eg*, aortic dissection, critical aortic stenosis, accelerating hypertension, pulmonary thromboembolism, pulmonary hypertension). After addressing these questions, the clinician can judge whether intensive care unit monitoring is warranted and what emergency procedures are required. In answering these questions, a careful history is the most important tool [3,4].

Many episodes of myocardial ischemia and even MI are asymptomatic [5]. Others may be painless but provoke other symptoms such as profound weakness, severe diaphoresis, nausea, or malaise. These symptoms may be considered anginal equivalents and may alert the clinician to the correct diagnosis.

CHARACTERISTICS OF MYOCARDIAL ISCHEMIC PAIN

The location of myocardial ischemic pain is typically in the lower substernal area with radiation to either or both arms (more often the left than the right). Another typical site of radiation is to the anterior aspect of the neck or lower jaw. Ischemic pain rarely extends beyond the area from the pharynx and lower jaw to the epigastrium (C3–T6); the extreme possible limits are from the occiput to the epigastrium (C2–T8) (Fig. 1). In atypical presentations, myocardial ischemic pain may be localized in the jaw, teeth, mid or upper back, shoulder, elbow, or wrist, mimicking a dental or orthopedic problem. Ischemic pain is not so sharply localized,

however, that its area can be covered by a fingertip. Sharply localized inframammary pain is particularly unlikely to be ischemic in origin. Chest pain that radiates from the sternum to the back or vice versa may indicate aortic dissection.

Ischemic pain is usually described as heavy or constricting (ranging from crushing to mild pressure). It may also be described as expansible or burning, but rarely as sharp or stabbing. The pain is "deep" and "visceral" and is commonly associated with sweating, dyspnea, nausea, and hiccupping.

Duration of ischemic pain is useful to distinguish it from pain of other causes. A single episode of transient myocardial ischemia (angina pectoris) usually lasts 2 to 20 minutes, with extremes of 30 seconds to over 1 hour. Lightening-like stabs are clearly nonischemic. Episodes of discomfort lasting over 20 to 30 minutes should raise suspicion of MI or unstable angina. Therefore, if a patient has suffered for months from multiple episodes of pain lasting hours at a time and fails to demonstrate electrocardiographic (ECG) evidence for recent or remote MI, the pain is unlikely to be ischemic in origin.

The time-intensity curve of the pain may give helpful information. Typically, angina pectoris builds in intensity for several to 30 minutes, then wanes and disappears over several additional minutes. The pain of acute MI also waxes over the course of minutes. Chest pain that abruptly reaches a maximum intensity is unusual in ischemic pain and should raise suspicion of aortic dissection.

Inciting factors of the pain are often important clues to the correct diagnosis. Physical effort is the usual inciting factor for a transient episode of myocardial ischemia caused by fixed coronary obstructive disease. Exertion is more likely to cause angina early in the morning and with use of the arms or isometric activity. For many patients, working with the arms above shoulder level is more likely to provoke angina than other activities. Emotional stress, exposure to cold, walking up a grade or against the wind, and exertion after a large meal are other common initiating or contributing factors. Ischemic pain that develops at rest or wakes the patient from sleep is more suggestive of MI, unstable angina, or occasionally, coronary spasm (*ie,* variant angina).

Chest pain worsened by respiration is not ischemic. Such pain, brought on by a deep breath or cough, is usually sharp and either caused by pleural or pericardial inflammation or a chest-wall condition such as a fractured rib, costochondritis, or intercostal neuritis. Ischemic pain is not aggravated by a single motion of an arm, neck, or torso, and such a pattern strongly suggests a musculoskeletal cause. Pain that can be reproduced or worsened by local palpation is also not ischemic, although following MI, some patients may have local precordial tenderness of obscure cause.

Patterns of relief are also valuable in assessing the cause of chest pain. Prompt relief within 2 to 10 minutes of rest is most characteristic of effort-induced angina pectoris. Occasionally, effort-induced ischemic pain disappears while the activity continues; this is known as *walk-through* or *second-wind angina.* Relief within several minutes of the administration of sublingual nitrates is characteristic of MI; however, the pain of spastic gastrointestinal disorders also has been noted occasionally to respond dramatically to nitrates. Relief with food or antacids suggests esophagitis or peptic disease. Partial relief by sitting forward is more typical of pericarditis or pancreatitis. Occasionally, pericarditis develops as a complication of MI, and these patients can have pericardial chest pain with both pleuritic and positional components.

ATYPICAL ANGINA PECTORIS AND NONISCHEMIC CHEST PAIN

Nonischemic chest pain syndromes include sharply localized pain, especially costochondral or inframammary; pain radiating outside the limits of C2 to T8; momentary "catches" or stabs of pain; pain incited by motion, respiratory effort, or local pressure; and recurrent, long-lasting, unabating pain (many hours to days) in the absence of ECG evidence of ischemia or infarction.

Atypical angina pectoris is a phrase often used to refer to pain caused by myocardial ischemia with clinical features not typical of ischemic chest pain. Characteristics of a chest pain syndrome sometimes cannot be clearly classified as either nonischemic or typical for ischemia. Whether these patients are treated as coronary patients depends on the clinician's judgment.

The likelihood of significant coronary disease has been estimated at a pooled mean prevalence of 89% for all patients with chest pain typical for angina, 50% for those with chest pain atypical for angina, and 16% for all other subjects [6]. The prevalence was heavily influenced by age and gender (Fig. 2). The estimate of the prevalence of significant coronary disease has important implications for the interpretation of noninvasive tests for myocardial ischemia [7] (Figs. 3 and 4).

PHYSICAL EXAMINATION

The physical examination may be unremarkable during an episode of life-threatening myocardial ischemia or an evolving MI. More often, however, a careful physical examination provides useful clues to the diagnosis. For nonischemic causes of chest pain, it may help lead to the correct diagnosis. Cases of chest-wall tenderness, musculoskeletal disease, breast disease, thoracic outlet syndromes, or neurologic syndromes may be disclosed by abnormal physical findings. Disorders of the gastrointestinal tract often fail to provide characteristic findings; however, upper quadrant or epigastric tenderness or marked tympany suggests bowel distention or inflammation.

Cardiovascular examination may first call attention to a noncoronary cause for myocardial ischemia. The diagnosis of aortic dissection may be suggested by absent pulses or the inequality of blood pressure of the arms or legs. Suspicion of aortic dissection is heightened if aortic regurgitation or an enlarging pleural effusion exist. A late-peaking aortic systolic murmur associated with a diminished intensity of the second

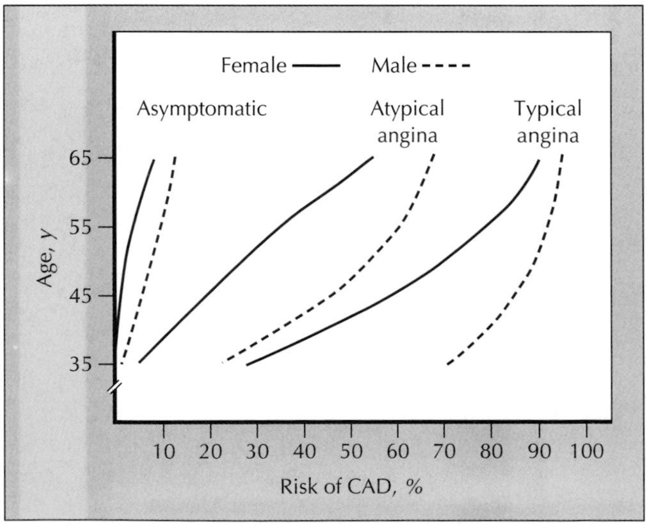

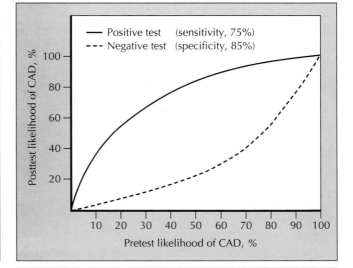

FIGURE 2 Influence of age, gender, and symptoms on risk of coronary artery disease (CAD). (*From* Epstein [7]; with permission.)

FIGURE 3 Influence of pretest likelihood of coronary artery disease (CAD) on the posttest likelihood of CAD for a test with 75% sensitivity and 85% specificity. (*From* Epstein [7]; with permission.)

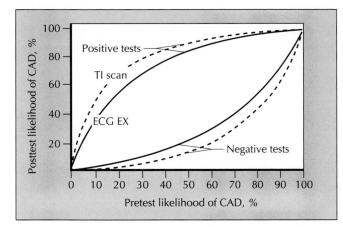

FIGURE 4 Influence of pretest likelihood of coronary artery disease (CAD) on the posttest likelihood of CAD for electrocardiographic exercise testing (ECG EX) and thallium perfusion scintigraphy (Tl scan). (*From* Epstein [7]; with permission.)

heart sound and a delayed carotid upstroke may provide the first clue to critical aortic stenosis. Hypertrophic cardiomyopathy also may be associated with angina pectoris in the absence of coronary occlusive disease and is likely to be manifested by a brisk carotid upstroke and a harsh systolic murmur at the left sternal edge, which typically increases with Valsalva's maneuver. The patient with mitral valve prolapse may be recognized by the characteristic nonejection click or mid to late systolic plateau or crescendo murmur at the apex or lower left sternal edge. Pericardial or pleural friction rubs may unmask underlying serosal inflammation. Friction rubs may occur with transmural MI or aortic dissection. Also, the presence of organic heart disease (*eg*, valvular lesion, hypertrophic cardiomyopathy) does not exclude concomitant CAD as a cause of the chest pain.

Although it is common for CAD to present without abnormal physical findings, it often gives evidence of ventricular dysfunction. The findings may present transiently during an episode of ischemia, or they may represent more prolonged changes caused by "stunned" myocardium or MI. Fourth heart sounds are ubiquitous in patients with significant symptomatic coronary disease, and they may become more prominent during ischemic episodes. Third heart sounds, paradoxically split second heart sounds, holosystolic murmurs, pulsus alternans, a fall in blood pressure, pulmonary congestion, pallor, as well as cold and clammy skin occasionally may be encountered during severe myocardial ischemia. Transient rises in blood pressure also may occur. Evidence for hypercholesterolemia (*eg*, xanthelasma, tuberous xanthoma) raises the suspicion of associated CAD, but does not confirm that the pain is ischemic. Femoral or carotid bruits or diminished peripheral pulses indicate the presence of atherosclerosis and, therefore, a higher likelihood of CAD.

Although tachycardia and tachypnea are nonspecific findings, they may be signs of left ventricular failure. Tachycardias may contribute to myocardial ischemia. Bradycardias often develop during the early stages of an inferior or posterior wall infarction.

During an acute ischemic episode, pulmonary congestion suggests a previously compromised left ventricle or severe ischemia involving a significant portion of the left ventricle. Severe ischemia may present dramatically as "flash" pulmonary edema in which the patient rapidly develops severe pulmonary congestion.

Dramatic presentations of ischemia with pulmonary edema, often with evidence of incipient shock, should alert the clinician to the possibility of a large MI or near-global ischemia. Left main coronary or very proximal left anterior descending obstruction, severe three-vessel disease, or severe aortic stenosis should be considered.

ELECTROCARDIOGRAPHIC, RADIOLOGIC, AND ECHOCARDIOGRAPHIC STUDIES

Electrocardiography

Electrocardiography performed at rest and in the absence of stress or ongoing chest pain, is an insensitive test for the presence of CAD. Most patients with CAD have normal resting ECGs. The presence of Q waves may indicate previous MI but is not found in most patients with CAD. ST-T wave abnormalities, arrhythmias, and conduction abnormalities are nondiagnostic findings.

Aside from the history and physical examination, ECG is the most valuable tool for initial patient assessment during chest pain. Evidence for ischemia may be in the form of horizontal or downsloping ST-segment depression of at least 1 mm (Fig. 5), with or without abnormally inverted or peaked hyperkalemic-appearing T waves (Fig. 6). More subtle findings include nonspecific T-wave flattening or inversion, straightened ST segments, or inverted U waves (Fig. 7). These latter findings are nonspecific and only mildly support the diagnosis of possible myocardial ischemia.

Myocardial injury or MI usually causes ST-segment elevation with eventual development of abnormal Q waves. Reciprocal changes (ST-segment depression) in V_1 to V_4 may represent true posterior-wall infarction. Posterior leads (V_7 and V_8) will demonstrate ST-segment elevation in these cases. In patients with inferior wall MI, ST-segment elevation in right precordial leads (V_4R) occurs with right ventricular involvement and is associated with higher rates of mortality and morbidity [8]. In all the multivariate analytic systems for the evaluation of chest pain, ECG plays a pivotal role. Nevertheless, while a normal ECG taken during an episode of chest pain is important testimony against ischemic disease, it does not exclude ischemia or infarction. If the history and patient setting are suggestive, the diagnosis must be seriously considered despite a normal ECG.

Electrocardiography may be helpful in supporting a diagnosis of acute pericarditis with diffuse ST elevations and possible PR-segment depression. Occasionally, the ECG suggests acute right ventricular strain, which in turn suggests a massive pulmonary embolism. In acute right ventricular strain, the QRS vector is often altered so that an S wave appears in lead I while a significant Q wave with T-wave inversion develops in lead III (S_1, Q_3, T_3 pattern of McGinn and White). T-wave inversion in leads II and aVF may also be present so that an inferior-wall MI is simulated. Inverted

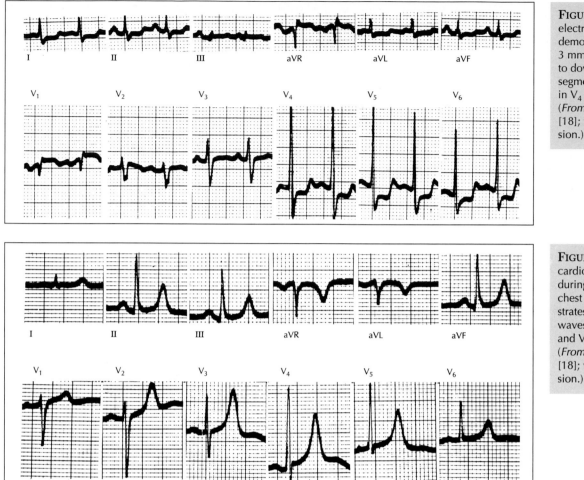

FIGURE 5 Exercise electrocardiogram demonstrating 2 to 3 mm of horizontal to downsloping ST segment depression in V₄ through V₆. (*From* Schamroth [18]; with permission.)

FIGURE 6 Electrocardiogram taken during ischemic chest pain demonstrates peaked T waves in II, III, aVF, and V₂ through V₆. (*From* Schamroth [18]; with permission.)

T waves in the right precordial leads (V_3 and V_4) may occur, but ST-segment deviations are absent or of small amplitude. Electrocardiography also may be valuable in the patient with chest pain by uncovering arrhythmias, conduction abnormalities, or hypertrophy patterns.

Chest Radiography

Chest radiographs are likely to be unremarkable during an acute ischemic episode or in an uncomplicated MI. Pulmonary vascular congestion, however, may occur in either. The heart shadow is usually normal. A large heart shadow during an ischemic episode or in the early stages of an infarct suggest antecedent myocardial damage, valvular disease, or pericardial effusion. Pulmonary infiltrates, pneumothorax, rib fractures, and metastatic lesions are other sources of chest pain that may be discovered by the chest film. A widened mediastinum on the posteroanterior view is nonspecific, but a normal mediastinal width makes aortic dissection much less likely.

Echocardiography

Echocardiography may be helpful in delineating the cause of cardiac chest pain. A transthoracic echocardiogram may reveal wall-motion abnormalities during an episode of ischemic heart pain and in the early stages of MI, even when the ECG is still normal. Unsuspected valvular disease, pericardial effusion, widened aortic root, and occasionally, dissection of the ascending aorta may be demonstrated. A transesophageal echocardiogram is useful and accurate in the early diagnosis of aortic dissection [9].

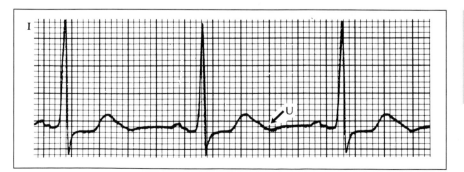

FIGURE 7 Electrocardiogram taken during ischemic chest pain demonstrates less than 1 mm horizontal ST depression associated with inverted U waves. (*From* Schamroth [18]; with permission.)

LABORATORY STUDIES

Laboratory studies are used as adjuncts in determining the presence of myocardial damage and in assessing the presence of associated and complicating factors.

Cardiac Biochemical Markers

Leakage of enzymes specific for injured myocardial tissue (creatine kinase-MB fraction, troponin I, and tropinin T) is usually relied upon to make the diagnosis of myocardial infarction. However, these enzymes take a number of hours to become abnormal after the onset of myocardial necrosis. Moreover, normal levels of these enzymes do not suggest that the patient is not suffering from myocardial ischemia. Levels of creatine kinase-MB are not expected to rise for 3 to 4 hours after the onset of myocardial necrosis. A ratio of isoenzyme $CK-MB_2$ to $CK-MB_1$ greater than 1.5 is a more sensitive early marker of myocardial necrosis and will occur before there is a measurable increase in total CK-MB [10]. Troponin I and T levels are very specific, very sensitive to myocardial damage, and may be elevated for as long as 14 days. They may also have prognostic value in unstable angina. Myoglobin levels are nonspecific but very sensitive and may rise within 1 hour [11]. Absence of myoglobin in the blood of a patient with chest pain suggests that an infarct is either not in progress or is very early in its course. Muscoloskeletal causes of chest pain (*eg*, skeletal muscle injury, myositis, thoracic outlet syndrome) can be expected to raise total creatine kinase levels as well as myoglobin levels. At this time, it appears that the newer assay of $CK-MB_{mass}$ is the best single marker, with a peak sensitivity of 99% at 12 hrs and early detection (93% at 7 hrs) [12].

Other Laboratory Studies

Arterial blood gases or pulse oximetry are at normal levels in acute ischemic heart disease, unless significant left ventricular dysfunction with pulmonary congestion develops or there is coexisting antecedent lung disease. Hypoxia with associated hypocapnia is a nonspecific finding common to pulmonary congestion, pulmonary embolism, and other acute respiratory problems.

A complete blood count may be valuable in the differential diagnosis of chest pain. Severe anemia is occasionally first manifested by angina. Both an acute MI and pulmonary embolism may be associated with a modest granulocytosis; however, a markedly elevated leukocyte count (> 15,000/mL) with a shift to the left should raise the suspicion of an infectious process.

EMERGENCY EVALUATION

In the initial diagnostic approach to the patient with recent or ongoing chest pain, emphasis is on rapid triage with simple but potent diagnostic tools. Central to the evaluation is the almost concurrent taking of a focused but careful history with a rapid determination of pertinent physical findings.

A rapid determination is made of the possibility of a life-threatening process. If there is a reasonable likelihood that the patient's pain is from myocardial ischemia, aortic dissection, or pulmonary embolism, the case must be considered a true medical emergency until proven otherwise. The administration of supplemental oxygen, the placement of the intravenous line, ECG monitoring, and arrangements for a full ECG are carried out expeditiously. Blood samples for initial laboratory tests are obtained wit th e positioning of the IV line. The possible need for chest radiography, echocardiography, or other noninvasive tests such as a perfusion lung scan or CT scan must also be considered at this time. Rapid diagnosis of MI and the exclusion of aortic dissection are imperative considering the importance of early thrombolytic therapy, rapid revascularization, or prompt surgical intervention.

If the patient has stable vital signs and the ECG does not give evidence of an acute MI, observation by monitoring in the emergency department is usually carried out until the diagnosis of an MI can be made or excluded. Nitrates, analgesics, and heparin anticoagulation are also administered in the absence of contraindication as clinically warranted. Features of the patient's presentation that suggest a potentially serious condition such as (but not limited to) coronary instability, aortic dissection, pulmonary embolism, or pericarditis, should initiate a prompt response. Hospitalization and early definitive evaluation and intervention are expedited [13–15].

NONINVASIVE EVALUATION

If the patient's history of chest pain more likely represents stable angina pectoris or is less likely caused by serious coronary disease, the work-up can proceed on an outpatient basis with noninvasive and provocative stress testing. If the patient is being evaluated in an emergency department for recent chest pain and an acute myocardial infarction has been excluded by serial enzyme analysis, additional noninvasive evaluation, including stress testing, is usually obtained before the patient is discharged home [15, 16]. Selection of the most appropriate test depends on the patient's exercise capacity, ability to tolerate pharmacologic intervention, and especially the pretest likelihood of significant coronary disease.

The choice of a suitable noninvasive test for ischemic disease is decided by the predictive accuracy of the test for the patient's age, gender, and clinical history [7]. Symptomatic coronary artery disease is rare before age 35, especially in women; however, its likelihood increases with each decade. Between ages 35 and 65, men have a higher likelihood of CAD; after 65, it is distributed equally between the sexes. The presence and number of associated risk factors also increases the likelihood of disease. Considering the age, gender, risk factors, and the character of the chest pain, a clinician can arrive at a level of suspicion (low, intermediate, or high) for CAD. Adding imaging techniques to provocative stress tests provides a greater degree of positive or negative confirmation of that pretest assessment.

RESTING ECHOCARDIOGRAPHY

Transthoracic echocardiography may demonstrate the regional wall motion abnormalities of ischemia, infarction, or even old scars, intracavitary thrombi, or aneurysms. Widening of the proximal aorta and aortic insufficiency may suggest ascending aortic dissection; occasionally an intimal flap may be demonstrated in these patients. Flattening of the interventricular septum suggests increased impedance to right ventricular outflow and is a sign of massive pulmonary embolism. Nevertheless, transthoracic echocardiography has not been shown to be useful as a screening tool in the rapid diagnostic evaluation for acute chest pain [16]. Transesophageal echocardiography has been shown to be particularly useful in the rapid diagnosis of patients suspected of having a possible aortic dissection.

Exercise Treadmill Test

The exercise treadmill test (ETT) or simple exercise ECG with treadmill (or bicycle ergometry) has the lowest predictive accuracy [7] and the least ability to quantitate the severity of ischemia. ETT is more likely to be valuable in those with a normal resting ECG, because resting ST-T abnormalities or left bundle-branch block interferes with interpretation of the test. ETT is best reserved for those with a somewhat moderate or intermediate pretest likelihood of disease, in whom the probability of a false-negative result is also low. A positive test carries a chance of being falsely positive and may require further testing with myocardial imaging.

If a patient develops anginalike chest pain associated with horizontal or downsloping ST-segment depression of more than 1 mm, the likelihood of CAD is markedly increased. If the test is positive with marked ST depression at a low level of exercise, widespread ischemia is suggested. Other features of widespread ischemia are ischemic changes associated with a drop in blood pressure while exercise continues and prolonged postexercise ischemic changes. For such patients, cardiac catheterization is usually the next step.

A person with high pretest likelihood of CAD still has a moderate possibility of disease, even in the absence of ischemic changes on the ETT. If it is necessary to establish the diagnosis of CAD, this person will require more sensitive tests with myocardial imaging or even coronary arteriography.

Exercise Perfusion Scintigraphy

Exercise perfusion scintigraphy with thallium or sestamibi carries a better predictive accuracy than simple ETT. These imaging methods improve the image quality and allows improved quantitative analysis of perfusion defects. A negative test, even in a patient with a high pretest likelihood of disease, decreases the possibility of myocardial ischemia considerably; other causes of chest pain should be strongly considered. Rarely is the pretest likelihood so compelling that coronary arteriography is needed to exclude a false-negative nuclear test.

Dipyridamole Perfusion Scintigraphy

Dipyridamole perfusion scintigraphy is often useful in those patients who are unable to exercise adequately on a treadmill. Dipyridamole causes maximum dilation of the coronary arteries. In the presence of significant CAD, coronary flow reserve is limited and disparities occur in the distribution of the thallium. Predictive accuracy is equivalent to an exercise scintigram. Patients with severe obstructive lung disease or asthma often cannot tolerate dipyridamole; in such patients, stress may be accomplished with dobutamine or adenosine.

Stress Echocardiography

Stress echocardiography can be accomplished with dipyridamole, dobutamine, or adenosine with excellent predictive accuracy. Treadmill or bicycle echocardiography also can be performed, but the exertion and hyperventilation involved may interfere with adequate imaging.

Other Noninvasive Techniques

Other noninvasive techniques including positron-emission tomography and 24-hour ambulatory ECG (Holter monitoring) are occasionally useful in the evaluation of ischemic chest pain. Holter monitoring is too insensitive to be used routinely as a diagnostic test for ischemia, but it may be particularly valuable in patients who experience pain only at rest or are strongly suspected of having episodes of silent ischemia.

When the likelihood of a cardiac cause is excluded or considered unlikely, further work-up of recurrent chest pain of obscure origin depends on the special characteristics of the patient and the pain. Esophageal manometry with or without provocation, ambulatory 24-hour esophageal monitoring of pH, and psychologic testing may be in order for the few patients who continue to be uncomfortable and in whom simple measures to treat esophageal disease fail [17].

CORONARY ARTERIOGRAPHY

The most reliable test for the diagnosis and quantitation of CAD is cardiac catheterization with selective coronary arteriography. Indications for coronary arteriography include chest pain suspicious for CAD undiagnosed by thorough noninvasive evaluation, chest pain thought to result from coronary disease but unresponsive to medical therapy, unstable angina, and postinfarction angina. The more unstable the angina, the more reasonable it is to use coronary arteriography early, even as one of the first diagnostic tests.

Coronary arteriography in at least two orthogonal views allows an excellent assessment of the extent of CAD as well as the potential for instability in the form of high-grade proximal stenoses, intraluminal thrombus, and ruptured or complicated plaques. Along with the patient's clinical course, this information is used to select medical therapy, angioplasty, or coronary artery bypass surgery in the management of the patient.

CONCLUSIONS

When a patient's chest pain has characteristics suspicious for myocardial ischemia and the patient's age, gender, and other risk factors make coronary disease possible, the clinician should exclude myocardial ischemia as a cause. If the characteristics suggest an unstable pattern of myocardial ischemia, the clinician should exclude acute or recent MI and assess the advisability of urgent antithrombotic therapy or the need for invasive diagnostic procedures. The patient's history, supported by simple physical examination and laboratory evaluation, is central to the process. The need for further consultation and more elaborate diagnostic procedures is determined by this initial evaluation. The more carefully the history is taken, the less likely it is that expensive procedures are ordered unnecessarily.

After the history, physical examination, and ECG, the choice of tests for diagnostic evaluation include ETT, ETT with imaging, and coronary arteriography. Imaging techniques with radionuclide or echocardiography greatly improve diagnostic accuracy. Although expensive, their use could limit the number of coronary arteriograms otherwise required.

REFERENCES

1. Richter JE, Bradley LA, Castell DO: Esophageal chest pain: current controversies in pathogenesis, diagnosis, and therapy. *Ann Intern Med* 1989, 110:66–78.

2. Davies HA: Anginal pain of esophageal origin: clinical presentation, prevalence, and prognosis. *Am J Med* 1992, 92(suppl 5A):5S–10S.

3. Goldman L, Weinberg M, Weisberg M, *et al.*: A computer-derived protocol to aid in the diagnosis of emergency room patients with acute chest pain. *N Engl J Med* 1982, 307:588–596.

4. Lee TH, Juarez G, Cook EF, *et al.*: Ruling out acute myocardial infarction: a prospective multicenter validation of a 12-hour strategy for patients at low risk. *N Engl J Med* 1991, 324:1239–1246.

5. Cohn PF: Silent myocardial ischemia. *Ann Intern Med* 1988, 109:312–317.

6. Diamond GA, Forrester JS: Analysis of probability as an aid in the clinical diagnosis of coronary artery disease. *N Engl J Med* 1979, 300:1350–1358.

7. Epstein SE: Implications of probability analysis on the strategy used for noninvasive detection of coronary artery disease: role of single or combined use of exercise electrocardiographic testing, radionuclide cineangiography and myocardial perfusion imaging. *Am J Cardiol* 1980, 46:491–499.

8. Zehender M, Kasper W, Kauder E, *et al.*: Right ventricular infarction as an independent predictor of prognosis after acute inferior myocardial infarction. *N Engl J Med* 1993, 328:981–988.

9. Hashimoto S, Kumada T, Osakada G, *et al.*: Assessment of transesophageal Doppler echography in dissecting aortic aneurysm. *J Am Coll Cardiol* 1989, 14:1253–1262.

10. Puleo PR, Meyer D, Wathen C, *et al.*: Use of a rapid assay of subforms of creatine kinase-MB to diagnose or rule out acute myocardial infarction. *N Engl J Med* 1994, 331:561–566.

11. Adams J, Abendschein D, Jaffe A: Biochemical markers of myocardial injury: is MB creatine kinase the choice for the 1990s? *Circulation* 1993, 88:750–763.

12. de Winter RJ, Koser RW, Sturk A, *et al.*: Value of myoglobin, troponin T, and CK-MB$_{mass}$ in ruling out an acute myocardial infarction in the emergency room. *Circulation* 1995, 92:3401–3407.

13. Pryor DB, Shaw L, Harrell FE Jr, *et al.*: Estimating the likelihood of severe coronary artery disease. *Am J Med* 1991, 90:553–562.

14. Lee TH, Ting HH, Shammash JB, *et al.*: Long-term survival of emergency department patients with acute chest pain. *Am J Cardiol* 1992, 69:145–151.

15. American College of Emergency Physicians: Clinical policy for the initial approach to adults presenting with a chief complaint of chest pain, with no history of trauma. *Ann Emerg Med* 1995, 25:274–299.

16. Gibler WB, Runyon JP, Levy RC, *et al.*: A rapid diagnostic and treatment center for patients with chest pain in the emergency department. *Ann Emerg Med* 1995, 25:1–8.

17. Richter J: Overview of diagnostic testing for chest pain of unknown origin. *Am J Med* 1992, 92(suppl 5A):41S–45S.

18. Schamroth L, ed.: *The Electrocardiology of Coronary Diseases*, edn 1. Philadelphia: JB Lippincott; 1975.

SELECT BIBLIOGRAPHY

Constant J: The clinical diagnosis of non-anginal chest pain: the differentiation of angina from non-anginal chest pain by history. *Clin Cardiol* 1983, 6:11–16.

Rude RE, Pool WK, Muller JE, *et al.*: Electrocardiographic and clinical criteria for recognition of acute myocardial infarction based on analysis of 3697 patients. *Am J Cardiol* 1983, 52:936–942.

Sampson JJ, Cheitlin MD: Pathophysiology and differential diagnosis of cardiac pain. *Prog Cardiovasc Dis* 1971, 23:507–531.

Evaluation of the Patient with Heart Failure

Carl V. Leier

6

Key Points

- Heart failure is a clinical presentation of an underlying cardiovascular disorder or disease.

- An effort should be made to diagnose the cause of heart failure, specifically to determine whether the heart failure is caused by a remedially reversible disorder or disease.

- The medical history, a good cardiovascular examination, electrocardiogram, chest roentgenogram, and two-dimensional Doppler echocardiogram are the essential components of the initial evaluation of the heart failure patient.

- Either cardiomegaly or a depressed ejection fraction alone is not indicative of inoperable underlying heart disease.

- Unclear etiology, possible underlying reparable heart disease, symptomatic dysrhythmias and conduction disturbances, New York Heart Association (NYHA) functional class III and IV classification, unstable course, and the need for specialized cardiovascular testing should prompt cardiology consultation or referral to a heart failure–transplantation center.

Heart failure is one of the cardiovascular conditions that is not decreasing in frequency. This chapter provides recommendations for the evaluation and follow-up of the heart failure patient; these recommendations are in general agreement with recently published guidelines [1•]. In this setting, optimal patient care and cost-effective management are inseparable because proper evaluation and therapy for heart failure keep patients alive, employed, out of hospitals, and off transplant lists.

INITIAL EVALUATION

The patient with ventricular dysfunction can present in several ways. Evaluation and therapy for each patient must be modified according to clinical presentation, acuity, and severity of heart failure; reversibility of the underlying disease process; and concomitant disease states. Nevertheless, general recommendations can be made to guide the optimal evaluation of the heart failure patient.

Medical History and Physical Findings

Important aspects of medical history

As in most conditions, the acuity and severity of symptoms determine the level of urgency in the evaluation and therapy for the patient with heart failure. A patient presenting with a 3-day history of orthopnea and 12 hours of resting dyspnea deserves more vigorous work-up and treatment than the patient with a 6-month history of steadily increasing pedal edema and easy fatigability, although both patients may ultimately undergo similar testing and often are placed on comparable long-term treatment.

Heart failure alone should never be considered a primary diagnosis. Heart failure is a symptom complex or syndrome; thus, it is always caused by some underlying cardiovascular disorder (*ie*, the primary diagnosis). On establishing the presence of heart failure by medical history and physical examination, the physician focuses on potential underlying causes, particularly reversible causes or those treatable with specific interventions (*eg*, coronary angioplasty and valvular repair or replacement). In general, intermittent symptoms of recent onset are more likely to be caused by reversible lesions (*eg*, occlusive coronary artery disease, ischemic papillary muscle dysfunction with episodic mitral regurgitation) than are long-standing symptoms. Although surgically treatable, chronic valvular stenosis or insufficiency often presents with long-standing symptoms. A history of major coronary risk factors (*eg*, smoking, diabetes mellitus, family history), concomitant angina pectoris, and intermittent or nocturnal symptoms should suggest occlusive atherosclerotic coronary artery disease and resultant disorders (*eg*, intermittent myocardial ischemia, diastolic or systolic dysfunction and papillary muscle dysfunction with mitral regurgitation). "Flash" pulmonary edema is usually caused by occlusive coronary artery disease, uncontrolled severe hypertension (often secondary to renal artery stenosis), periodic noncompliance to diet and drug therapy, or a combination of these factors.

Although a recent viral illness should raise the consideration of viral myocarditis in a patient with new onset heart failure, the symptoms of the viral event are often indistinguishable from those experienced during an episode of congestive heart failure. Serologic testing for virus and endomyocardial biopsy for signs of inflammation are usually unrevealing in this setting. Our ability to diagnose postviral cardiomyopathy should improve as better diagnostic techniques are developed for viral infections and retroviral DNA/RNA alterations.

As many as 30% to 40% of patients with idiopathic dilated cardiomyopathy have a family history of cardiomegaly, heart failure, or sudden death [2], suggesting that some patients with dilated cardiomyopathy develop their illness by genetic transmission. However, until these defects are more precisely defined and biotechnologically correctable, the clinical approach to these patients is still the same as that to other patients with dilated cardiomyopathy.

Increasing age, diabetes mellitus, and a history of systemic hypertension should suggest that diastolic dysfunction may play a pathophysiologic role, often the primary role, in the patient's heart failure.

Advancing age, clinical severity of heart failure, refractory response to optimal medical management, and a history of syncope or cardiac arrest are some of the major historical points that portend a less favorable prognosis [1•2–5].

Key physical findings

The initial physical examination is generally directed at evaluating the extent and severity of heart failure and looking for clues for an underlying cause.

Indicators of extent and severity of heart failure

The severity and general character of a patient's heart failure are cumulatively assessed on physical examination by the presence and degree of a general appearance of well-being, anxiety or distress, pallor, cyanosis, tachypnea, Cheyne-Stokes respiratory pattern, tachycardia, pulsus alternans, pulsus paradoxus, narrow pulse pressure, systemic hypotension, hypokinetic and laterally displaced apical impulse, ventricular gallop sounds, murmurs, pulmonary rales, pleural effusion, elevated jugular venous pressure (if absent, hepatojugular reflux), hepatomegaly with or without tenderness and ascites, and pedal edema. It is important to record the initial (*ie*, baseline) positive and pertinent negative findings because they, along with body weight and symptoms, are the principal means of guiding therapy.

Clues for underlying cause of heart failure

Most patients with chronic congestive cardiac failure have evidence of both right and left heart failure. Patients with decompensated nonischemic dilated cardiomyopathy and patients with predominant right heart dysfunction (*eg*, cor pulmonale, right ventricular dysplasia) usually present with prominent signs of right heart failure, including jugular venous distention, hepatomegaly with or without ascites, or peripheral edema. If the patient presents with predominant signs and symptoms of left heart failure, the primary considerations for differential diagnosis are systemic hypertension, occlusive coronary artery disease, and an aortic or mitral valvular disorder.

Evidence of systemic atherosclerotic vascular disease suggests occlusive coronary artery disease as the cause of the patient's heart failure.

Systemic hypotension unrelated to drug therapy in the patient with adequate or high ventricular filling pressures suggests considerable cardiac dysfunction and an unfavorable prognosis; vasodilator and converting enzyme inhibitor therapy are often difficult to administer in such a patient. Elevated blood pressure may be a consequence of the neurohormonal reaction to cardiac failure (particularly acute cardiac failure); however, long-standing or severe uncontrolled systemic hypertension is often a major contributor or the predominant cause of cardiac decompensation. The patient with hypertensive heart failure usually responds favorably to proper antihypertensive, afterload-reducing therapy.

Several systemic illnesses are associated with cardiac disease and failure; a few include various neuromuscular disorders (*eg*, muscular dystrophy, myotonia dystrophia, Friedreich's ataxia), thyroid disease, and amyloidosis. The presence of a hyperdynamic precordium and circulation (tachycardia and bounding, full pulses) raises the possibility of high-output heart failure and the various causes, including anemia, hyperthyroidism, and arteriovenous malformations; most of these conditions are treatable.

Blood/Serum Studies

Most patients with heart failure should have a baseline complete blood count, thyroid function studies, and measurement of serum electrolytes, urea nitrogen, creatinine, and magnesium. Hyponatremia, azotemia, and anemia of chronic disease are often indicative of a severe, advanced stage of heart failure. Other laboratory tests that may be indicated include sedimentation rate, C-reactive protein, and, occasionally, viral serology tests when myocarditis is suspected; coagulation studies (*ie*, prothrombin time, activated partial thromboplastin time, and platelet count) if anticoagulation therapy is anticipated; hepatic enzymes assessing the patient with severe heart failure and liver congestion; and arterial blood gas and pH in severe heart failure complicated by respiratory distress or problematic low cardiac output.

Chest Roentgenography

In addition to excluding unrelated but complicating conditions (*eg*, lung neoplasia) in a generally middle-aged to older population, the chest roentgenogram gives the physician a reasonable assessment of heart size, cardiac chamber enlargement, pulmonary congestion, and pleural effusion, and it can render clues regarding cause (Fig. 1). Along with the physical examination, the chest roentgenogram is the optimal (and least expensive) method of following heart size and pulmonary congestion during long-term management.

Electrocardiogram, Specialized Electrocardiographic Studies, and Electrophysiologic Testing

The electrocardiogram (ECG) establishes the cardiac rhythm for the period of the test and provides clues regarding chamber enlargement and conduction disturbances (Fig. 2). Infarct patterns suggest occlusive coronary artery disease as the cause or contributing condition, although nonischemic cardiomyopathies are the most common disorders causing "pseudoinfarct" patterns. Some studies have found atrial fibrillation and

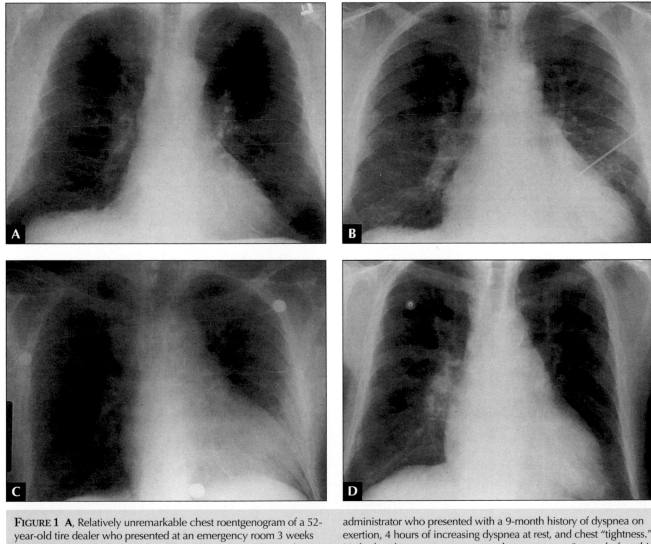

FIGURE 1 A, Relatively unremarkable chest roentgenogram of a 52-year-old tire dealer who presented at an emergency room 3 weeks earlier with acute "flash" pulmonary edema. At cardiac catheterization-angiography, high-grade obstructive lesions were noted along the proximal segments of the right coronary artery and left anterior descending coronary artery. **B**, Chest roentgenogram shows marked cardiomegaly, pulmonary venous engorgement, and pleural effusion of the base and minor fissure of the right chest; this 66-year-old salesman presented with decompensation of chronic heart failure secondary to nonischemic dilated cardiomyopathy. **C**, Moderate pulmonary edema on chest roentgenogram of a 49-year-old factory administrator who presented with a 9-month history of dyspnea on exertion, 4 hours of increasing dyspnea at rest, and chest "tightness." He had undergone coronary artery bypass surgery 8 years before this hospital admission. Electrocardiogram and cardiac enzyme analyses indicated an acute anterior myocardial infarction in the presence of a prior inferior wall infarction. **D**, Chest roentgenogram of a 78-year-old retired restaurant owner afflicted with 9 to 10 months of increasing dyspnea on exertion, orthopnea, and pedal edema. Mild to moderate left ventricular systolic dysfunction, marked biventricular diastolic dysfunction, and normal epicardial coronary arteries were noted at cardiac catheterization.

left ventricular conduction defects to be some of the predictors of a poor outcome in heart failure [3].

In the case of acute heart failure, an early ECG is invaluable in determining whether a patient might benefit from immediate thrombolytic therapy or urgent cardiac catheterization and an interventional procedure.

Although controversial, signal-averaged electrocardiography (SAE) appears to have little predictive power in nonischemic cardiomyopathy [3,6,7]. The prognostic value in ischemic cardiomyopathy is probably better, but the information is of limited practical value because therapeutic interventions have not yet been shown to significantly alter the clinical course of the heart failure patient with an abnormal SAE. The analysis of heart rate variability can provide a laboratory correlate of severity of heart failure and perhaps prognosis [8]. This methodology is currently limited in its clinical application by general non-availability, non-reimbursement, and multiple variables. The approach to an abnormal finding is still optimal congestive heart failure (CHF) therapy.

Holter ECG recordings are not recommended as a routine component of the initial evaluation of the heart failure patient, but are quite informative in directing antiarrhythmic therapy or defibrillator placement in patients experiencing dysrhythmia-induced symptoms [3,7,9,10]. ECG

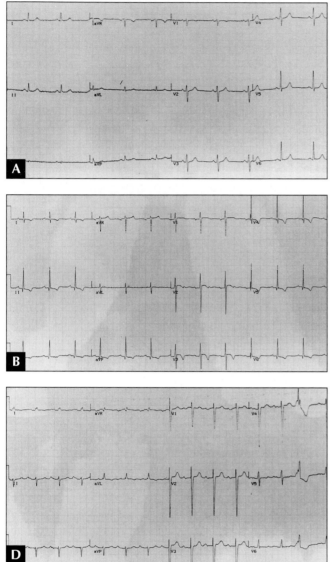

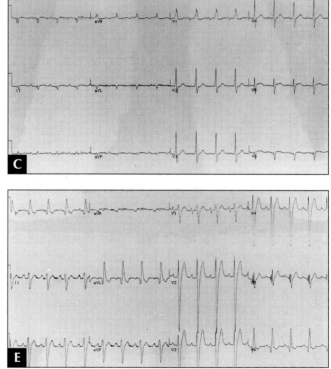

FIGURE 2 **A**, Normal electrocardiogram of a 68-year-old retired university professor who first presented with the sole complaint of 3 months of increasing dyspnea on exertion. Proximal high-grade obstructive coronary artery disease was noted at cardiac catheterization (*see* Fig. 4A). **B**, The electrocardiogram of a 52-year-old farmer with a 5-year history of increasing dyspnea on exertion, easy fatigability, and two episodes of severe decompensation (pulmonary edema). The left ventricular hypertrophy pattern noted on the electrocardiogram is a consequence of a 25- to 30-year history of inadequately controlled essential hypertension. **C**, Electrocardiogram of a 58-year-old laborer with a 3-week history of increasing weakness and pedal edema. Four weeks before admission, he experienced episodic severe chest pain and intermittent nausea and vomiting. The electrocardiogram shows an extensive posterolateral myocardial infarction, marked right axis deviation, and left posterior fascicular block. Physical examination, echocardiography, and cardiac catheterization further demonstrated moderate mitral regurgitation, elevated left and right ventricular end-diastolic and pulmonary artery pressures, depressed cardiac output, moderately increased left

ventricular diastolic volume, and reduced ejection fraction (24%) secondary to a large akinetic zone involving the inferior, posterior, and lateral regions of the left ventricle. Complete occlusions of the proximal right coronary artery and left circumflex coronary artery were seen on coronary angiography. **D**, This electrocardiogram, showing biventricular enlargement, left axis deviation, a premature ventricular beat, abnormal P waves, and prolonged PR interval, was taken of a 42-year-old housewife with a 3-year history of progressively symptomatic dilated cardiomyopathy. She was referred for further treatment and transplantation evaluation. **E**, Myocardial dystrophy is the likely explanation for the electrocardiographic changes observed in this 20-year-old patient with Duchenne muscular dystrophy. Sinus tachycardia, abnormal P waves, left axis deviation, intraventricular conduction delay, lateral wall "pseudoinfarct" pattern, and biventricular enlargement are represented on the recording. In addition to musculoskeletal limitations, he had been afflicted with advancing symptoms and signs of heart failure for 3 to 4 years before this admission. He was dyspneic at rest and had orthopnea, hepatomegaly, and pedal edema on admission.

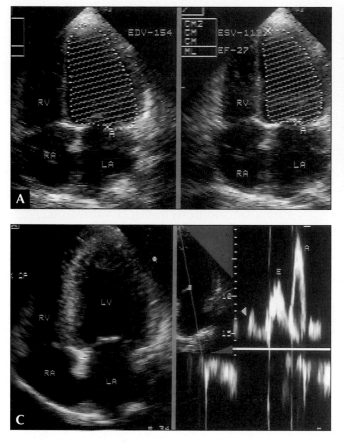

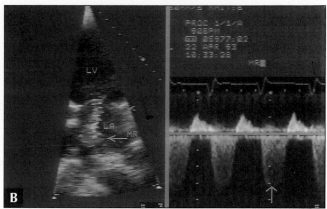

FIGURE 3 A, Two-dimensional echocardiographic apical four-chamber views in a 36-year-old patient who presented with congestive heart failure secondary to nonischemic dilated cardiomyopathy, demonstrating marked left ventricular (LV) enlargement and depressed systolic function with modest volume change from diastole (left) to systole (right). End-diastolic volume equals 154 cc; end-systolic volume, 111 cc; and ejection fraction (EF), 27%. **B,** Color Doppler (*left*) and continuous wave Doppler (*right*) images from a patient with dilated cardiomyopathy and considerable mitral regurgitation (*arrows*), which was barely audible on auscultation. (*See* Color Plate). **C,** Two-dimensional apical four-chamber view of a 53-year-old patient with long-standing hypertension and heart failure demonstrating (*left*) marked concentric left ventricular hypertrophy (wall thickness, 1.5 cm; LV mass index, 154 g/m²). Systolic function was normal (EF, 65%), but pulsed Doppler of mitral inflow (*right*) demonstrates markedly diminished early filling velocities (E) and enhanced atrial contribution to filling (A) consistent with impaired diastolic relaxation. (*See* Color Plate.)

event recorders with memory are useful in assessing patients with infrequent, dysrhythmia-induced symptoms.

The role of invasive electrophysiologic testing is currently somewhat limited in the setting of CHF. It is occasionally combined with upright tilt testing for the patient with unexplained near-syncope or syncope and non-diagnostic Holter or event ECG recordings, although the approach to suspected dysrhythmia-induced syncope in heart failure is steadily moving toward direct cardioverter-defibrillator insertion [11••].

Echocardiography

Echocardiography is a pivotal diagnostic study in the initial evaluation of the heart failure patient. In addition to providing information on the size and function of the four heart chambers, echocardiography is the test of choice to determine whether mitral or tricuspid regurgitation (both can be inaudible on examination) and ventricular diastolic dysfunction play a role in the patient's presentation (Fig. 3). Spontaneous echo contrast may identify patients particularly susceptible to intracavitary thrombus formation and embolization [12].

Exercise Testing

For patients who can adequately relate their symptoms to the physician, exercise testing is not an essential component of the initial evaluation. However, exercise testing can be helpful in corroborating a patient's symptoms, following the patient's therapy, assessing a patient's candidacy for employment or cardiac transplantation, and prescribing an exercise conditioning program [5,13–15]. Expiratory gas analysis is also not essential, but this technique provides a more precise evaluation of exercise capacity and effort [14]. A maximal exercise oxygen consumption of more than 20 mL/kg/min suggests that the patient and therapy are doing reasonably well. Oxygen consumption of less than 14 mL/kg/min indicates severe impairment of exercise capacity and the need to consider a patient's candidacy for cardiac transplantation, particularly if the patient has been receiving optimal heart failure therapy [15].

Cardiac Catheterization-Angiography

Most patients with heart failure deserve strong consideration for a diagnostic cardiac catheterization-angiography before their condition is declared irreparable. It is often impossible to distinguish nonischemic from ischemic forms of cardiac failure, and unless a reversible cause for heart failure is found, congestive heart failure has a grim long-term prognosis. An ejection fraction of 0.25 or less is no longer considered a contraindication to a revascularization procedure because revascularization can be effective in improving such a patient's ventricular dysfunction and heart failure if reversible myocardial ischemia, rather than infarction, is causing the ventricular dysfunction (Fig. 4) [16,17].

Patients with another end-stage illness limiting their overall clinical course and survival (*eg*, metastatic malignant neoplasia) and elderly patients who are not likely to survive a major surgical procedure may not benefit greatly from cardiac catheterization-angiography.

Patients who present with acute heart failure are more likely to have a remedially reparable cardiac lesion compared with patients with more chronic forms of heart failure. For patients presenting with acute pulmonary edema or cardiogenic shock, precise diagnostic definition of the cardiac lesions and urgent, specific intervention (eg, angioplasty or valvular repair or replacement) offer the optimal and, often, the only means of improving an otherwise dismal clinical course and reduced survival [18,19••].

Myocardial Biopsy

Without specific, proven-effective therapy as an end point for obtaining a specific diagnosis, there are no absolute indications for performing an endomyocardial biopsy in heart failure. On the other hand, transvenous endomyocardial biopsy is the best way of diagnosing or confirming several pathogenic cardiac conditions, including myocarditis, Löffler's eosinophilic endocarditis, amyloidosis, and other inflammatory and infiltrative disorders. Corticosteroid or any immunosuppressive therapy is not empirically indicated (ie, without an endomyocardial biopsy) for a patient who presents with dilated cardiomyopathy and suspected myocarditis. Most of these patients do not have myocarditis, and the risk–benefit ratio of empiric corticosteroid or any other immunosuppressive therapy in cardiomyopathic heart failure likely exceeds that of an endomyocardial biopsy and directed therapy. Endomyocardial biopsy is a principal means of following cardiac rejection after transplantation.

Pharmacohemodynamic Evaluation

Patients with apparently refractory heart failure should generally undergo intense pharmacohemodynamic study before being placed on a cardiac transplant list or being declared to have terminal, refractory congestive heart failure [20,21]. Such

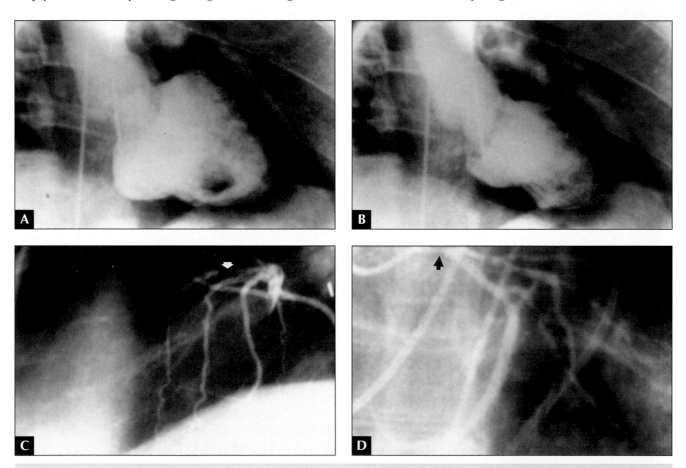

FIGURE 4 A through C, Angiographic frames of the patient presented in Figure 2A. Coronary artery bypass surgery was successful in bringing this patient from relative physical inactivity before surgery to a daily 2-mile run or 2000-yard swim within 9 months of his surgery. A, Contrast injection of left ventricle in diastole. Some chamber enlargement is present. B, Considerable anterior and apical hypokinesis are demonstrated in this end-systolic frame. The hypokinetic regions demonstrated thallium redistribution, indicating viable myocardium. The preoperative ejection fraction of 0.28 rose to 0.48 six months after surgery. C, Left lateral view of a left coronary artery injection demonstrating an occlusive lesion of the proximal left anterior descending coronary artery (arrow). Scattered plaques were noted along the proximal right coronary artery. The patient did not recall ever experiencing angina pectoris. D, Left coronary injection of a 76-year-old man who went to his local emergency room on two occasions with severe dyspnea, weakness, roentgenographic pulmonary edema, and transient electrocardiographic anterior ischemic changes. A high-grade obstructive lesion is present in the left main coronary artery (arrow) with additional obstructive disease in the proximal left anterior descending artery. A nondominant right coronary artery was completely occluded. He remains symptom-free (receiving only daily aspirin) with increased physical activity 18 months after coronary bypass surgery.

patients should be referred to a comprehensive heart failure center to take advantage of expertise in the use of standard heart failure medication, pharmacohemodynamic evaluation of standard and experimental agents, therapeutic application of experimental compounds, and assessment and treatment of transplant candidates.

Other Testing Modalities
Radionuclide studies
Resting or exercise radionuclide perfusion studies (*eg*, thallium studies) and positron emission tomography (PET) can help in determining myocardial viability in patients who present with occlusive coronary artery disease complicated by congestive heart failure [17,22]. A patient with operable occlusive coronary artery disease and a substantial amount of viable myocardium should be considered for a revascularization procedure.

Pulmonary function studies
Dyspnea and related symptoms of many patients are secondary to combined cardiac and pulmonic disease. After a patient's heart failure is optimally treated, pulmonary function studies are indicated in patients with any clinical evidence (*eg*, history of smoking, findings on physical examination) of lung disease. For patients with reduced expiratory flow rates, bronchodilators should be tested to determine the reversibility of impaired flow rates and whether certain patients need bronchodilators as part of their overall therapeutic plan.

FOLLOW-UP EVALUATION
The outpatient care of the patient with heart failure is facilitated by patient (and spouse) participation in the day-to-day management of the condition by adhering to dietary instructions, recording daily weights at home, promptly reporting new or worsening symptoms to the physician's office, continually learning about the condition and treatment, and, if feasible, joining a support group of heart failure patients.

General Clinical Evaluation
An immense amount of information can be quickly attained by observing the patient and spouse (or close family member or friend) during the initial greeting. A favorable or steady course and an unfavorable course (*eg*, worsening or new symptoms) can be sensed by the physician, then verified by further questioning and cardiovascular examination. The clinical impression extracted from this initial brief contact generally guides the direction, activities, and intensity of the outpatient visit.

The standard clinical question, "How are you doing?" is a reasonable way to start a focused recent medical history. Further questioning is then directed at the patient's (or spouse's) response, the course of prior symptoms, activity and sleep patterns, outpatient body weight recordings, dietary issues, and medications.

The focused follow-up cardiovascular examination in heart failure includes assessment of body weight, supine and upright heart rate and blood pressure, estimation of jugular venous pressure, palpation of carotid pulses and precordium, auscultation for the presence and intensity of gallop sounds and murmurs (particularly mitral and tricuspid regurgitation), palpation and measurement of the liver (vertical span along the right clavicular line), and palpation of the legs and ankles for edema and tenderness. General appearance and the respiratory rate pattern are gleaned from the patient during the examination. A careful lung examination for rales and pleural effusion follows a history of dyspnea at rest, increasing dyspnea, tachypnea, weight gain, and the finding of rales or effusion during a prior examination.

At this point, the clinician has most of the information needed to adjust the patient's activities, diet, and medication, order additional laboratory studies, and determine the timing of the subsequent visit. If the patient has recently experienced an unfavorable course, the decision is made to alter outpatient management or to admit the patient to the hospital.

Follow-up Laboratory Testing
A standard schedule of outpatient laboratory testing cannot satisfy the clinical needs of all patients with ventricular dysfunction and heart failure. Follow-up laboratory testing is best individualized to avoid inappropriate risk, expense, and use of laboratory time and resources for a low yield of useful information and clinical benefit. Common sense is the guiding principle. However, routine tests are necessary for patients receiving certain medications (*eg*, anticoagulation therapy) or are occasionally useful for patients with more symptomatic or advanced stages of heart failure.

Chronic stable mild heart failure (NYHA functional class I or II)
Patients in the NYHA class I or II category require fewer outpatient visits and less laboratory testing. After a stable course is achieved, an occasional (*eg*, every 6 to 12 months) serum potassium and urea nitrogen (or creatinine) determination is usually the maximal laboratory requirement. A chest roentgenogram to follow heart size or an echocardiogram to determine chamber size and function is reasonable at greater than 12-month intervals.

Chronic moderate to severe heart failure (NYHA functional class III or IV)
Patients with NYHA functional class III or IV heart failure require more frequent follow-up visits than patients with milder heart failure. As the severity of heart failure increases, symptoms and complications escalate in frequency and intensity, the overall clinical condition becomes more unstable, and the medication requirements and side effects increase. Functional class III or IV patients are generally seen in the outpatient setting at 2-week to 3-month intervals, with serum potassium and urea nitrogen (or creatinine) determinations made every 1 to 4 months. To avert hospitalization during a relatively unstable period, more frequent visits (as many as 1 to 2 per week) and laboratory testing may be required. Determining serum sodium and magnesium concentrations is informative in patients with advanced heart failure who are receiving vigorous diuretic therapy but is rarely required more than once every 2 to 3 months.

Unless the patient enters an unstable decompensated phase, optimal outpatient management includes an annual echocardiogram to assess cardiac chamber size and function and the degree of mitral and tricuspid regurgitation or an annual chest roentgenogram to simply assess heart size.

With effective history taking, intermittent exercise testing is not essential for the optimal treatment of most patients with chronic heart failure. An exercise study can be useful in assessing a patient with symptoms disparate from clinical or other laboratory findings, determining a prescription for a physical conditioning program, following a major change in therapy, and evaluating whether a patient should continue or seek employment, apply for employment disability, or undergo evaluation for cardiac transplantation.

Certain patients require other testing modalities to address specific complaints and problems. For example, Holter or event ECG recordings should be considered in the heart failure patient with palpitations and near-syncopal episodes, and ECG should be considered in a patient with a recent change in cardiac rhythm or a recent episode of prolonged angina. Repeat cardiac catheterization and coronary angiography should be considered in a heart failure patient whose remote catheterization showed nonocclusive coronary lesions but now presents with angina, angina-equivalent symptoms, or unexpected decompensation.

Decompensation

The patient whose symptoms are escaping a previously effective therapeutic plan deserves special, more intense consideration and, often, referral to a cardiologist or heart failure center.

After review of the patient's symptoms, inquiries should be made into changes in personal and home situations. Family or marital difficulties, financial problems, dietary alterations or indiscretions, and intentional or inadvertent changes in medications or dosing schedule often provide clues for the mechanisms of the clinical deterioration. A focused cardiovascular examination is then performed to establish physical evidence of clinical deterioration (eg, body weight, level of jugular venous distention, liver size, rales, pedal edema) and to reveal complications of heart failure (eg, new onset atrial fibrillation, recent development of mitral regurgitation) that may explain or significantly contribute to the deteriorating course. Decompensation is not uncommonly precipitated by noncardiovascular conditions (eg, respiratory infection or recent addition of a nonsteroidal antiinflammatory drug).

If the explanation for the unfavorable course is not apparent from history and physical examination and to further assess the extent of decompression, laboratory testing is indicated and generally includes assessment of serum electrolytes, urea nitrogen, creatinine, complete blood count and, occasionally, hepatic enzymes; chest roentgenogram to evaluate heart size and degree of pulmonary congestion; and two-dimensional Doppler echocardiography to assess changes in chamber size and function and the presence and degree of mitral and tricuspid regurgitation.

If the patient's deteriorating clinical condition is threatening or does not respond in a reasonable time (1 to 3 days) to a rational change in therapy, the patient should be hospitalized for monitored observation, intravenous therapy directed at improving symptoms and the patient's cardiovascular status (eg, intravenously administered diuretics, vasodilators, or dobutamine), additional diagnostic studies, and consideration for pharmacohemodynamic evaluation [20].

EVALUATING THE CARDIAC TRANSPLANTATION CANDIDATE

The complete evaluation of the heart failure patient for cardiac transplantation is best done via referral to a heart failure or transplantation specialist. Nevertheless, the referring internist or cardiologist can greatly assist in the preliminary assessment of the transplantation candidate. Basically, the typical candidate approved as a transplant recipient is a person younger than 60 years of age (65 years or younger at some centers) with symptomatic advanced heart failure refractory to optimal therapy. The patient is in otherwise good health without a chronic infection, infectious source, major chronic disease, or terminal illness. Compliance to physician and nurse instructions, stable psychological make-up, and an intact familial and social support structure are other important favorable features of an acceptable transplant-recipient candidate.

KEY REFERENCES

Recently published papers of outstanding interest, as identified in *References and Recommended Reading*, have been annotated.

•• Stevenson WG, Stevenson LW, Middlekauff HR, *et al.*: Improving survival for patients with advanced heart failure: a study of 737 consecutive patients. *J Am Coll Cardiol* 1996, 26:1417–1423.
This paper discusses the etiologic spectrum of death from heart failure and the means to counter the high mortality of this condition.

•• Holmes DR Jr, Bates EF, Kleiman NS, *et al.* for the GUSTO-I Investigators: Contemporary reperfusion therapy for cardiogenic shock: the GUSTO-I trial experience. *J Am Coll Cardiol* 1995, 26:668–674.
The results of this large multicenter trial were analyzed to determine which reperfusion interventions reduce mortality after myocardial infarction. While thrombolytic reperfusion reduced the incidence of shock, only PTCA lowered the mortality in patients whose infarction was complicated by cardiogenic shock.

REFERENCES AND RECOMENDED READING

Recently published papers of particular interest have been highlighted as:

• Of interest
•• Of outstanding interest

1.• Guidelines for the evaluation and management of heart failure: report of the American College of Cardiology/American Heart Association task force on practice guidelines (committee on evaluation and management of heart failure). *J Am Coll Cardiol* 1995, 26:1376–1398.

2. Unverferth DV, Wooley CF: Familial dilated cardiomyopathy. In *Dilated Cardiomyopathy*. Edited by Unverferth DV. Mt. Kisco, NY: Futura Publishing Co.; 1985:159–165.

3. Leier CV: The cardiomyopathies: mortality, sudden death, and ventricular arrhythmias. In *Cardiovascular Clinics: Contemporary Management of Ventricular Arrhythmias.* Edited by Greenspon AJ, Waxman HL. Philadelphia: FA Davis Co.; 1992:275–306.

4. Unverferth DV, Magorien RD, Moeschberger ML, *et al.*: Factors influencing the one-year mortality of dilated cardiomyopathy. *Am J Cardiol* 1984, 54:147–152.

5. Willens HJ, Blevins RD, Wrisley D, *et al.*: The prognostic value of functional capacity in patients with mild to moderate heart failure. *Am Heart J* 1987, 114:377–382.

6. Gonska B, Bethge K, Figulla H, *et al.*: Occurrence and clinical significance of endocardial late potentials and fractionations in idiopathic dilated cardiomyopathy. *Br Heart J* 1988, 59:39–46.

7. Turitto G, Ahuja RK, Caref EB, El-Sherif N: Risk stratification for arrhythmic events in patients with nonischemic dilated cardiomyopathy and nonsustained ventricular tachycardia: role of programmed ventricular stimulation and the signal-averaged electrocardiogram. *J Am Coll Cardiol* 1994, 24:1523–1528.

8. Brouwer J, Van Veldhuisen DJ, Man in't Veld AJ, *et al.* for the Dutch Ibopamine multicenter trial group: Prognostic value of heart rate variability during long-term follow-up in patients with mild to moderate heart failure. *J Am Coll Cardiol* 1996, 28:1183–1189.

9. Holmes J, Kubo SH, Cody RJ, *et al.*: Arrhythmias in ischemic and nonischemic dilated cardiomyopathy: prediction of mortality by ambulatory electrocardiography. *Am J Cardiol* 1985, 55:146–151.

10. Hofmann T, Meinertz T, Kasper W, *et al.*: Mode of death in idiopathic dilated cardiomyopathy: a multivariate analysis of prognostic determinants. *Am Heart J* 1988, 116:1455–1463.

11.•• Stevenson WG, Stevenson LW, Middlekauff HR, *et al.*: Improving survival for patients with advanced heart failure: a study of 737 consecutive patients. *J Am Coll Cardiol* 1996, 26:1417–1423.

12. Shen WF, Tribouilly C, Rida Z, *et al.*: Clinical significance of intracavitary spontaneous echo contrast in patients with dilated cardiomyopathy. *Cardiology* 1996, 87:141–146.

13. Leier CV, Huss P, Magorien RD, *et al.*: Improved exercise capacity and differing arterial and venous tolerance during chronic isosorbide dinitrate therapy for congestive heart failure. *Circulation* 1983, 67:817–822.

14. Weber KT, Kinasewitz GT, Janicki JS, *et al.*: Oxygen utilization and ventilation during exercise in patients with chronic cardiac failure. *Circulation* 1982, 65:1218–1223.

15. Mancini DM, Eisen H, Kussmaul W, *et al.*: Value of peak exercise oxygen consumption for optimal timing of cardiac transplantation in ambulatory patients with heart failure. *Circulation* 1991, 83:778–786.

16. Holmes DR Jr, Detre KM, Williams DO, *et al.*: Long-term outcome of patients with depressed left ventricular function undergoing PTCA. *Circulation* 1993, 87:21–29.

17. Di Carli MF, Asgarzadie F, Schelbert HR, *et al.*: Quantitative relation between myocardial viability and improvement in heart failure symptoms after revascularization in patients with ischemic cardiomyopathy. *Circulation* 1995, 92:3436–3444.

18. Lee L, Bates ER, Pitt B, *et al.*: Percutaneous transluminal coronary angioplasty improves survival in acute myocardial infarction complicated by cardiogenic shock. *Circulation* 1988, 78:1345–1351.

19.•• Holmes DR Jr, Bates EF, Kleiman NS, *et al.* for the GUSTO-I Investigators: Contemporary reperfusion therapy for cardiogenic shock: the GUSTO-I trial experience. *J Am Coll Cardiol* 1995, 26:668–674.

20. Stevenson LW, Dracup KA, Tillisch JH: Efficacy of medical therapy tailored for severe congestive heart failure in patients transferred for urgent cardiac transplantation. *Am J Cardiol* 1989, 63:461–464.

21. Haas GJ, Leier CV: Invasive cardiovascular testing in chronic congestive heart failure. *Crit Care Med* 1990, 18:51–54.

22. Mody FV, Brunken RC, Stevenson LW, *et al.*: Differentiating cardiomyopathy of coronary artery disease from nonischemic dilated cardiomyopathy utilizing positron emission tomography. *J Am Coll Cardiol* 1991, 17:373–383.

SELECT BIBLIOGRAPHY

ACC/AHA Guidelines Committee: American College of Cardiology/American Heart Association Guidelines for the Management of Heart Failure. Dallas, TX: American Heart Association; 1994.

Braunwald E, Grossman W: Clinical aspects of heart failure. In *Heart Disease.* Edited by Braunwald E. Philadelphia: WB Saunders; 1992:444–463.

Cohn JN: Approach to the patient with heart failure. In *Textbook of Internal Medicine*, edn 2. Edited by Kelley WN. Philadelphia: JB Lippincott; 1992:340–347.

Leier CV: The cardiomyopathies: mortality, sudden death and ventricular arrhythmias. In *Contemporary Management of Ventricular Arrhythmias, Cardiovascular Clinics 22/1.* Edited by Greenspon AJ, Waxman HL. Series Editor-in-Chief, Brest AN. Philadelphia: FA Davis; 1992:275–306.

Evaluation of the Patient with Hypotension and Shock

Richard C. Becker

7

> ### *Key Points*
> - Shock is a syndrome characterized by systemic hypotension and cellular hypoperfusion.
> - Profound vasodilation, arteriovenous shunting, and increased capillary permeability are features that typify septic, neurogenic, and anaphylactic shock.
> - Cardiogenic shock is caused by a marked reduction in overall cardiac performance (relative to existing metabolic demands).
> - In shock states, prompt stabilization, diagnosis, and definitive treatment are prerequisites for patient survival.

Hypotension is defined as a reduction in systemic blood pressure to lower than a mean arterial pressure of 70 mm Hg. It is important to recognize, however, that individuals with preexisting hypertension can, in fact, be relatively hypotensive at a higher mean arterial pressure.

Shock is a syndrome (*ie*, a recognizable collection of symptoms, signs, and laboratory abnormalities) that is characterized by hypotension and hypoperfusion. The latter feature is pathognomonic of shock states and is associated with widespread cellular and major organ dysfunction. Although this process is initially *reversible*, persistant hypoperfusion leads to *irreversible* cellular injury and ultimately death.

DETERMINANTS OF A NORMAL SYSTEMIC BLOOD PRESSURE

Systemic blood pressure is determined by the volume of blood ejected into the systemic circulation (cardiac output) and by the peripheral vascular resistance. Therefore, disturbances in blood pressure are caused by either a reduced cardiac output (the hallmark of cardiogenic shock) or a reduced peripheral vascular resistance (the hallmark of septic, neurogenic, and anaphylactic shock).

Peripheral Vascular Resistance

Peripheral vascular resistance varies inversely with the fourth power of the arteriolar (resistance vessels) radius. Therefore, vascular resistance is determined by vascular tone, which is directly influenced by:

1. Metabolic and mechanical autoregulatory mechanisms (adenosine is the primary metabolic regulator),
2. Neurogenic constrictor influences operating through norepinephrine,
3. Neurogenic vasodilator influences operating through acetylcholine and histamine, and
4. Circulating and locally released vasoactive substances, including catecholamines, angiotensin II, bradykinin, and prostaglandins.

The autonomic nervous system plays a particularly prominent role in the maintenance of systemic blood pressure, because it directly influences both cardiac output and peripheral vascular resistance.

Blood Volume

An adequate intravascular volume is required to maintain systemic blood pressure. This is accomplished primarily through the renin-angiotensin-aldosterone system; other contributors include arginine vasopressin and atrial natriuretic polypeptide.

Cardiac Performance

The three primary determinants of cardiac performance are preload, afterload, and contractility. As cardiac output is the product of heart rate and stroke volume, the former is considered to be a fourth determinant of cardiac performance (Table 1).

SHOCK STATE

When systemic hypotension is prolonged and severe, a series of compensating mechanisms are initiated in an attempt to restore blood volume, increase peripheral vascular resistance, and improve cardiac performance. Marked stimulation of the autonomic and renin-angiotensin-aldosterone systems occurs in patients with cardiogenic shock. If adequate end-organ perfusion is not restored, endogenous mediators (contraregulatory mechanisms) are released from monocytes, macrophages, and neutrophils. As in septic shock, these mediators may contribute directly to the perpetuation of the shock state and be responsible for end-organ damage (Fig. 1).

CLINICAL PRESENTATION

Hypotension and hypoperfusion are the two cardinal manifestations of shock states in general and of cardiogenic shock in particular. Hypotension is defined as a systolic blood pressure less than 90 mm Hg or a mean arterial blood pressure less than 70 mm Hg. As some patients experience end-organ (tissue) hypoperfusion at a higher blood pressure, a working definition of mean arterial pressure of 30 mm Hg or more below the baseline blood pressure may be preferred.

TABLE 1 DETERMINANTS OF CARDIAC PERFORMANCE

Preload (ventricular filling)
  Venous return
  Total blood volume
  Intrathoracic pressure
  Intrapericardial pressure
  Atrial contribution
  Atrioventricular synchony
Afterload (ventricular wall stress; impedance)
Contractility (intrinsic activity of myocardium)
  Sympathetic nervous system
  Circulating catecholamines
  Local environment (anoxia, ischemia, acidemia)
  Contractile mass
  Inotropic stimulation
Heart rate

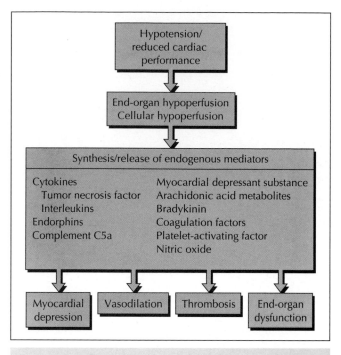

FIGURE 1 The shock state is initiated when tissue hypoperfusion stimulates the release of endogenous mediators, which in turn are responsible for myocardial depression, vasodilation, thrombosis, and end-organ dysfunction.

The presence of hypoperfusion can be determined indirectly from several key clinical observations: 1) altered mental status (agitation, restlessness, obtundation); 2) pale or mottled, cool, clammy skin; and 3) reduced urine output (< 30 mL/h). Most patients with cardiogenic shock are tachycardic (> 100 bpm). The peripheral pulses are typically weak and thready and tachypnea (> 20 respirations/min) is also common.

The common laboratory abnormalities are:
- Hypoxia, hypocarbia, metabolic acidosis
- Elevated blood lactate
- Leukocytosis (mild to moderate), thrombocytopenia (disseminated intravascular coagulation)
- Sinus tachycardia
- Pulmonary edema, adult respiratory distress syndrome
- Arterial hypotension, decreased cardiac output

INITIAL STABILIZATION

Care of critically ill patients is unique in many ways. Unlike other clinical situations that permit a series of diagnostic tests to be performed before instituting treatment, cardiogenic shock is imminently life-threatening; therefore, prompt stabilization is required before a thorough diagnostic evaluation can be performed (Table 2).

DIFFERENTIAL DIAGNOSIS

A number of common diseases of the heart can cause hypotension and cardiogenic shock (Table 3). The most common is abnormal myocardial function caused by severe

TABLE 2 RECOMMENDATIONS FOR STABILIZING CRITICALLY ILL PATIENTS

Assure adequate oxygenation (low threshold for tracheal intubation)
Obtain intravenous access (central access preferred)
Restore arterial pressure (mean, > 70 mm Hg)
  Volume replacement
  Vasopressor agents (dopamine, norepinephrine)
Correct acid–base abnormalities
Correct rhythm disturbances and conduction abnormalities

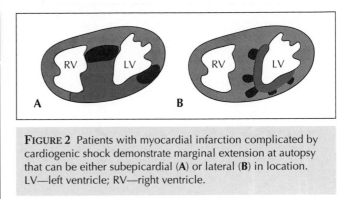

FIGURE 2 Patients with myocardial infarction complicated by cardiogenic shock demonstrate marginal extension at autopsy that can be either subepicardial (**A**) or lateral (**B**) in location. LV—left ventricle; RV—right ventricle.

coronary artery disease, multiple myocardial infarctions (MIs), or acute massive MI.

The incidence of cardiogenic shock complicating MI ranges from 5% to 15%. The degree of left ventricular compromise correlates closely with the overall extent of ventricular damage. The Starling mechanism of functional compensation fails when the surface area of necrosis exceeds 30% [1,2]. Smaller infarctions may cause complications associated with shock, including ventricular septal rupture, free-wall rupture, and papillary muscle rupture.

A consistent pathologic observation among patients with fatal cardiogenic shock is progressive myocardial necrosis (Fig. 2). Persistent occlusion of the infarct-related coronary artery is also common. Severe multivessel coronary artery disease, prior infarction, or compromised collateral circulation may cause shock in the absence of a large infarction.

TABLE 3 COMMON CAUSES OF CARDIOGENIC SHOCK

Acute myocardial infarction
Ventricular septal rupture
Acute mitral insufficiency
Right ventricular infarction
Myocarditis
Dilated cardiomyopathy
Advanced valvular heart disease
  Aortic stenosis
  Aortic insufficiency
  Mitral stenosis
  Mitral insufficiency
Tachy- and bradyarrhythmias
Cardiac tamponade
Pulmonary embolism
Hypertrophic cardiomyopathy
End-stage hypertensive heart disease

DIAGNOSTIC EVALUATION

Following initial stabilization of the patient, the clinician must promptly begin a thorough diagnostic evaluation. In many instances, a diagnosis can be secured through a careful physical examination, chest radiography, electrocardiography, and routine blood tests. At times, vital historical information can be provided by friends, family members, and medical records. Specialized testing, including echocardiography (transthoracic/transesophogeal), coronary angiography, computed tomography, magnetic resonance imaging, and pulmonary artery catheterization, may be required to confirm a diagnosis. The checklist in Table 4 should be helpful in making a diagnosis.

MANAGEMENT

Whenever possible, patients with cardiogenic shock should be managed in an intensive care unit. Close observation is an absolute prerequisite, and both intra-arterial and hemodynamic monitoring should be considered strongly.

Intra-arterial Monitoring

Direct blood pressure measurement is more accurate than noninvasive, indirect measurement in patients with hemodynamic instability and shock. Intra-arterial monitoring allows careful titration of vasoactive drugs and provides immediate access for frequent blood sampling, including blood gas analysis. The preferred cannulation site is the radial artery; however, other sites (femoral artery, dorsalis pedis artery, brachial artery) also may be used. Potential complications of intraarterial monitoring include bleeding, thrombosis, embolism, limb ischemia, pseudoaneurysm formation, infection, and peripheral neuropathy.

Hemodynamic Monitoring

Pulmonary artery catheterization for hemodynamic monitoring has four primary objectives (Table 5):

1. To assess left ventricular and right ventricular function,
2. To assess changes in hemodynamic status,
3. To guide treatment with pharmacologic and nonpharmacologic agents, and
4. To gather prognostic information.

TABLE 4 DIAGNOSTIC BENCHMARKS IN CARDIOGENIC SHOCK

	General physical appearance	Signs or history	Jugular venous pressure	Heart sounds	Lung examination	Chest radiograph	Electrocardiography	Other diagnostic tests
Myocardial infarction	Apprehensive Cool, moist skin Agitation	Symptom onset at rest Chest pain Dyspnea Hypotension Tachycardia	↑, ↔	S_3, S_4 gallops ± Holosystolic murmur (papillary muscle dysfunction)	Rales in > 50% of both lung fields	Pulmonary edema	ST-segment elevation ± Q waves Widespread ST-segment depression	Elevated creatine kinase Abnormal MB fraction (may not be elevated early) Focal wall motion abnormality on echocardiogram
Ventricular septal rupture	Anxious Diaphoretic	Recent MI (3–5 d)* Sudden change in clinical status Chest pain Dyspnea Tachycardia	↑	S_3, S_4 gallops Localized holosystolic murmur (new) Palpable systolic thrill (lower left sternal border)	Rales in > 50% of lung fields	Pulmonary edema	Persistent ST-segment elevation Pseudonormalization of T waves	L→R shunt on echocardiogram O_2 saturation "step-up"
Mitral insufficiency (acute)	Anxious Diaphoretic	Sudden dyspnea Recent inferior/ inferoposterior MI or History of mitral valve prolapse or History of blunt/ penetrating trauma	↑, ↔	S_1 decreased S_3 gallop Holosystolic murmur obscuring S_2 (A_2 component)	Rales in > 50% of lung fields	Pulmonary edema	Recent MI Nonspecific ST-T wave abnormality	Mitral insufficiency ± flail mitral leaflet on echocardiogram
Right ventricular infarction	Apprehensive Diaphoretic	Chest pain Nausea	↑↑	S_3, S_4 gallops (right sided)	Clear or basilar rales	Clear	Inferior injury pattern with posterior extension ≥0.5 mm ST elevation in V_3R, V_4R Bradyarrhythmias Conduction abnormalities (2°, 3° heart block)	Inferoposterior hypokinesis and right ventricular hypokinesis on echocardiogram
Myocarditis	Apprehensive Cool, moist skin	Viral prodrome Progressive shortness of breath Low-grade temperature Narrow pulse pressure	↑	S_3, S_4 gallops	Rales in > 50% of lung fields	Pulmonary edema Heart size normal or enlarged	Sinus tachycardia Nonspecific ST/T changes Pseudoinfarction pattern Bundle-branch block	Chamber dilation on echocardiogram Hypokinesis on echocardiogram
Dilated cardiomyopathy	Diaphoretic Cool Peripheral mottling	History of chronic heart failure Narrow pulse pressure Chronic venous stasis pigmentation-ulceration	↑↑	S_3, S_4 gallops Holosystolic murmur (mitral, tricuspid regurgitation)	Rales in > 50% of lung fields	Pulmonary edema Cardiomegaly	Sinus tachycardia/ tachyarrhythmias (atrial/ventricular) Low voltage Bundle-branch block Diffuse ST/T-wave changes	Four-chamber dilation on echocardiogram

*May occur earlier (24–48 hours) following thrombolytic therapy.

(Continued on next page)

TABLE 4 DIAGNOSTIC BENCHMARKS IN CARDIOGENIC SHOCK (CONTINUED)

	General physical appearance	Signs or history	Jugular venous pressure	Heart sounds	Lung examination	Chest radiograph	Electrocardiography	Other diagnostic tests
Hypertrophic cardiomyopathy	Anxious Diaphoretic	History of chest pain, dyspnea, syncope; Family history of sudden death; Apical "triple" beat; Rapid carotid upstroke	$\uparrow$, $\leftrightarrow$ (prominent A wave)	Prominent S_4 gallop; Holosystolic blowing murmur at apex; Holosystolic harsh murmur left sternal border ($\uparrow$ Valsalva)	Rales in > 50% of lung fields	Pulmonary edema	Left ventricular hypertrophy; Q waves inferolateral leads	Septal hypertrophy on echocardiogram; Outflow tract obstruction on Doppler studies
Aortic stenosis	Pale Diaphoretic	Carotid shudder, delayed upstroke	$\uparrow$	S_1 soft; single S_2 (P_2); S_3, S_4 gallops; Harsh, late-peaking systolic murmur (radiation to carotid arteries)	Rales in > 50% of lung fields	Pulmonary edema	Left ventricular hypertrophy	Aortic valve thickening; Reduced leaflet motion; Pressure gradient across aortic valve
Aortic insufficiency	Diaphoretic	History of hypertension, endocarditis, or trauma; Chest ± back pain; Dyspnea; Asymmetric blood pressure/pulses; Paralysis/sensory deficits	$\uparrow$, $\leftrightarrow$	S_1 soft or absent; S_2 (P_2) prominent; S_3, S_4 gallops; Early, low-pitch diastolic murmur	Rales in > 50% of lung fields	Pulmonary edema; "Calcium" sign with aortic dissection	Nonspecific ST/T-wave changes	Aortic dissection; Aortic insufficiency; Transesophogeal echocardiogram
Mitral stenosis	Diaphoretic Cyanotic	Progressive dyspnea; Frothy blood-tinged sputum; Prior thromboembolism	$\uparrow$ (prominent A wave)	S_1 prominent or reduced (immobile valve leaflets); P_2 prominent; Opening snap; Diastolic rumbling murmur	Rales in > 50% of lung fields	Pulmonary edema; Right ventricular prominence; Left atrial enlargement	Tachyarrhythmia (particularly atrial fibrillation); Right-axis deviation; Right ventricular hypertrophy; Atrial enlargement	Calcified, stenotic mitral valve
Pulmonary embolism	Anxious Cyanotic	Sudden pleuritic chest pain, dyspnea, cough, hemoptysis, or syncope; Risk factors for pulmonary embolism; Tachypnea (> 20 breaths/min)	$\uparrow$ (prominent A wave)	S_2 (P_2) increased; S_3, S_4 gallops (right sided); Holosystolic murmur (tricuspid regurgitation)	Clear	Oligemia; Elevated hemidiaphragm; Pleural effusion; "Wedge-shaped" infiltrate; Prominent hilar vessel	S_1, Q_3, T_3 pattern; Nonspecific ST/T-wave changes; Right bundle-branch block; Sinus tachycardia	V/Q mismatch; Abnormal pulmonary angiography; Right ventricular prominence on echocardiogram
Cardiac tamponade	Pale Anxious Apprehensive	Hypotension; Narrow pulse pressure; Distended neck veins; Pulsus paradoxus	$\uparrow\uparrow$ (absent Y descent)	Distant (if rapid pericardial fluid accumulation); ± Friction rub	Clear	Normal or enlarged cardiac silhouette	Low voltage; T-wave flattening	Pericardial effusion; Right atrial, right ventricular collapse on echocardiogram; Abnormal Doppler flow patterns

L→R—left to right; MI—myocardial infarction; P_2—pulmonic second heart sound; S_1—first heart sound; S_2—second heart sound; S_3—third heart sound; S_4—fourth heart sound; $\leftrightarrow$—normal; $\uparrow$—increased; $\uparrow\uparrow$—markedly increased.

The hemodynamic information obtained from pulmonary arterial catheterization can be used directly in both patient management and diagnosis (Tables 6 and 7).

Potential complications of catheterization include balloon rupture, knotting, pulmonary infarction, arterial perforation, thromboembolism, heart block, arrhythmias, myocardial perforation with tamponade, and infection.

Pharmacologic Therapy

Dopamine is an immediate precursor of norepinephrine. It has both α- and β-adrenergic agonist properties as well as dopaminergic-receptor agonism within the mesenteric and renal vascular beds. At doses required to increase mean arterial pressure and cardiac output (5 to 8 µg/kg body weight/min), heart rate and myocardial oxygen demand may be increased [3]. In the presence of acidemia, higher doses (up to 15 µg/kg/min) may be required to produce a hemodynamic improvement; at this dose, atrial and ventricular tachyarrhythmias may occur.

Dobutamine is a synthetic derivative of isoproterenol. It increases cardiac output at doses between 2.5 and 5.0 µg/kg/min without significantly increasing either heart rate or myocardial oxygen demand [4]. Therefore, in the setting of MI complicated by cardiogenic shock, dobutamine is considered the inotropic agent of choice.

Norepinephrine is a potent α-receptor agonist (increases peripheral vascular resistance). It exhibits some myocardial β_1-receptor agonism as well. Norepinephrine should be used in patients with hypotension refractory to other inotropic agents.

The efficacy of dopamine and dobutamine may decline with long-term administration. Tachyphylaxis may represent a downregulation of myocardial adrenergic receptors. Phosphodiesterase inhibitors increase cyclic AMP concentrations without relying directly on adrenergic receptors. Amrinone and milrinone have been used successfully in the treatment of cardiogenic shock [5].

Patients with increased left ventricular mass and diastolic dysfunction, hypertensive heart disease, or hypertrophic cardiomyopathy have unique requirements. In fact, inotropic agents may worsen their clinical condition. Calcium channel blockers (verapamil, diltiazem) or β-blockers given as a continuous intravenous infusion may improve ventricular distensibility and diastolic filling. In refractory congestive

TABLE 6 HEMODYNAMIC PARAMETERS IN PATIENTS WITH HYPOTENSION AND SHOCK (GUIDELINES FOR DIAGNOSIS)

	RA, *mm Hg*	RV, *mm Hg**	PA, *mm Hg**	PWP, *mm Hg*	AO, *mm Hg*	CI *L/min/m²*	SVR, *dyne/sec/cm⁻⁵*
Normal	0–6	25/0–6	25/6–12	6–12	120/80	≥2.5	1200–1500
Hypovolemia	0–2	15/0–2	15/2–6	2–6	≥ 90/60	< 2.0	> 1500
Cardiogenic shock	8	50/8	50/35	35	< 90/60	< 2.0	> 1500
Septic shock							
Early	0–2	25/0–2	25/0–6	0–6	< 90/60	< 2.5	< 1000
Late	0–4	25/4–10	25/4–10	4–10	< 90/60	< 2.0	> 1000
Massive PE	8–12	50/12	50/12	<12	< 90/60	< 2.0	> 1200
Tamponade	12–18	30/12–18	30/12–18	12–18	< 90/60	< 2.0	> 1200
Right ventricular infarction	12–20	30/12–20	30/12	<12	< 90/60	< 2.0	> 1200
Ventricular septal rupture	6	60/6–8	60/35	30	< 90/60	< 2.0	> 1500

*The first value represents the mean value; the second is the range.

AO—aortic pressure; CI—cardiac index; PA pulmonary artery; PE—pulmonary embolism; PWP—pulmonary wedge pressure; RA—right atrium; RV—right ventricle; SVR—systemic vascular resistance.

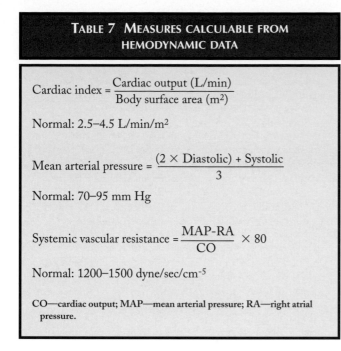

TABLE 7 MEASURES CALCULABLE FROM HEMODYNAMIC DATA

$$\text{Cardiac index} = \frac{\text{Cardiac output (L/min)}}{\text{Body surface area (m}^2)}$$

Normal: 2.5–4.5 L/min/m^2

$$\text{Mean arterial pressure} = \frac{(2 \times \text{Diastolic}) + \text{Systolic}}{3}$$

Normal: 70–95 mm Hg

$$\text{Systemic vascular resistance} = \frac{\text{MAP-RA}}{\text{CO}} \times 80$$

Normal: 1200–1500 dyne/sec/cm^{-5}

CO—cardiac output; MAP—mean arterial pressure; RA—right atrial pressure.

heart failure accompanied by hypotension, a pure α-agonist such as phenylephrine hydrochloride (Neo-Synephrine, Winthrop Pharmaceuticals, New York, NY), used in combination with supportive care, may be beneficial.

Thrombolytic therapy is useful in the treatment of massive pulmonary embolism. Intravenous tissue-plasminogen activator appears to be the agent of choice; however, urokinase has shown promise as well [6]. Unfortunately, while reducing the incidence of congestive heart failure and cardiogenic shock among patients with MI, thrombolytic therapy has not been shown to improve survival when administered in the presence of cardiogenic shock [7].

Antiarrhythmics (procainamide, lidocaine) or electrical cardioversion should be used as needed for patients with hemodynamically compromising supraventricular and ventricular tachyarrhythmias. Occasionally, intravenous amiodarone is required in the care of patients with cardiogenic shock and incessant ventricular tachycardia.

Mechanical Intervention

Intra-aortic balloon counterpulsation (IABP) can rapidly stabilize many patients with cardiogenic shock, particularly those with global myocardial ischemia or MI complicated by papillary muscle rupture or ventricular septal rupture. It is contraindicated in patients with severe aortic insufficiency. The observed hemodynamic changes following IABP insertion include:

1. A 10% to 20% increase in cardiac output,
2. A reduction in systolic and an increase in diastolic blood pressure (increased mean arterial pressure),

3. A diminution in heart rate, and
4. An increase in urine output.

In some patients, combined IABP and inotropic therapy is required to achieve and maintain an acceptable blood pressure (systolic, > 90 mm Hg systolic; mean, > 70 mm Hg) and cardiac index (> 2.2 L/min/m^2).

Recently, more powerful circulatory assist devices, such as the Hemopump (Johnson and Johnson Interventional Systems, Rancho Cordova, CA) and the percutaneous cardiopulmonary support system, have been used in the care of patients with cardiogenic shock caused by left heart failure [8,9]. As with IABP, these devices are designed for rapid clinical stabilization while preparations are made for definitive, corrective intervention.

Coronary angiography and urgent coronary angioplasty may improve survival for patients with MI complicated by cardiogenic shock [10,11,12•]. Although randomized trials have not been conducted, restoration of coronary arterial patency in retrospective studies and pooled series has been associated with a nearly 50% reduction in the mortality rate.

Alternative mechanical interventions include:

1. Pericardiocentesis for patients with cardiac tamponade,
2. Balloon valvuloplasty for those with critical aortic or mitral stenosis when surgical correction is not feasible, and
3. Pacemaker placement for patients with severe bradyarrhythmias, conduction disturbances, or right ventricular infarction refractory to fluid administration and inotropic support (atrioventricular pacing may be required with some patients).

The International Shock Registry results support early revascularization as an important tretment modality for patients with MI complicated by cardiogenic shock; however, a randomized clinical trail will be required to answer the question definitively [13•].

Surgical Intervention

Corrective surgery is most beneficial in patients with mechanical defects (papillary muscle rupture, ventricular septal rupture), critical valvular heart disease (aortic stenosis, aortic insufficiency, mitral stenosis), and severe coronary artery disease (three-vessel disease, left main disease). In a majority of cases, initial stabilization is achieved by inotropic support with or without a circulatory assist device. Overall, the best results are achieved when surgical intervention is undertaken promptly [14,15].

Cardiac transplantation is a therapeutic alternative for a small and highly selective group of individuals with cardiogenic shock. Mechanical circulatory support as a "bridge" to cardiac transplantation includes a total artificial heart and ventricular assist devices [16,17] (Table 8).

TABLE 8 TREATMENT OPTIONS IN CARDIOGENIC SHOCK

Pharmacologic	Mechanisms of action
Dobutamine	Inotropic support
Dopamine	Inotropic support
Norepinephrine	Inotropic support, vasopressor
Phenylephrine	Vasopressor
Tissue-plasminogen activator	Thrombolysis (pulmonary embolism ± MI)
Urokinase	Thrombolysis (pulmonary embolism ± MI)
Lidocaine, procainamide, amiodarone	Antiarrhythmic
Mechanical	
Intraaortic balloon pump	Improve cardiac output / Increase coronary artery perfusion
Hemopump	Improve cardiac output
Percutaneous cardio-pulmonary support	Improve cardiac output / Improve tissue perfusion
Pacemaker	Restore heart rate / Restore atrioventricular synchrony
Coronary angioplasty	Improve myocardial perfusion
Pericardiocentesis	Improve preload, ventricular filling
Surgery	Correct mechanical defects

REFERENCES AND RECOMMENDED READING

Recently published papers of particular interest have been highlighted as:
• Of interest
•• Of outstanding interest

1. Klein MD, Herman MV, Gorlin R: A hemodynamic study of left ventricular aneurysm. *Circulation* 1967, 35:614–630.
2. Page DL, Caulfield JB, Kastor JA, *et al.*: Myocardial changes associated with cardiogenic shock. *N Engl J Med* 1971, 285:133–137.
3. Mueller HS, Evans R, Ayres SM: Effect of dopamine on hemodynamics and myocardial metabolism in shock following acute myocardial infarction in man. *Circulation* 1978, 57:361–365.
4. Francis GS, Sharma B, Hodges M: Comparative hemodynamic effects of dopamine and dobutamine in patients with acute cardiogenic circulatory collapse. *Am Heart J* 1982, 103:995–1000.
5. Klocke RK, Mager G, Kux A, *et al.*: Effects of a 24-hour milrinone infusion in patients with severe heart failure and cardiogenic shock as a function of the hemodynamic initial condition. *Am Heart J* 1991, 121:1965–1973.
6. Goldhaber SZ, Kessler CM, Heit JA, *et al.*: Recombinant tissue-type plasminogen activator versus a novel dosing regimen of urokinase in acute pulmonary embolism: a randomized controlled multicenter trial. *J Am Coll Cardiol* 1992, 20:24–31.
7. Becker RC: Hemodynamic, mechanical and metabolic determinants of thrombolytic efficacy: a theoretic framework for assessing the limitations of thrombolysis in patients with cardiogenic shock. *Am Heart J* 1993, 125:919–929.
8. Smalling RW, Sweeney M, Lachterman B, *et al.*: Transvalvular left ventricular assistance in cardiogenic shock secondary to acute myocardial infarction. *J Am Coll Cardiol* 1994, 23:637–644.
9. Phillips SJ, Zeff RH, Kongtahworn C, *et al.*: Percutaneous cardiopulmonary bypass: application and indication for use. *Ann Thorac Surg* 1989, 47:121–123.
10. Abbottsmith CW, Topol EJ, George BS, *et al.*: Fate of patients with acute myocardial infarction with patency of the infarct-related vessel achieved with successful thrombolysis versus rescue angiography. *J Am Coll Cardiol* 1990, 16:770–778.
11. Lee L, Erbel R, Brown TM, *et al.*: Multicenter registry of angioplasty therapy of cardiogenic shock: initial and long-term survival. *J Am Coll Cardiol* 1991, 17:599–603.
12.• Eltchaninoff H, Simpfendorfer C, Franco I, *et al.*: Early and 1-year survival rates in acute myocardial infarction complicated by cardiogenic shock: a retrospective study comparing coronary angioplasty with medical treatment. *Am Heart J* 1995, 130:459–464.
13.• Hochman JS, Boland J, Sleeper LA, *et al.*: Current spectrum of cardiogenic shock and effect of early revascularization on mortality. Results of an international registry. *Circulation* 1995, 91:873–881.
14. Phillips SJ, Kongtahworn C, Slanner JR, Zeff MT: Emergency coronary artery reperfusion: a choice therapy for evolving myocardial infarction: results in 339 patients. *J Thorac Cardiovasc Surg* 1983, 86:679–688.
15. DeWood MA, Notske RN, Hensley GR, *et al.*: Intra-aortic balloon counterpulsation with or without reperfusion for myocardial shock. *Circulation* 1980, 61:1105–1112.
16. Joyce LD, Johnson KE, Pierce WS: Summary of the work experience with clinical use of total artificial hearts as heart support devices. *J Heart Transplant* 1986, 5:229–235.
17. Joyce LD, Kiser JC, Eales F, *et al.*: Experience with generally accepted centrifugal pumps. *Ann Thorac Surg* 1996, 61:287–290.

SELECT BIBLIOGRAPHY

Hibbard MD, Holmes DR, Bailey KR, *et al.*: Percutaneous transluminal coronary angioplasty in patients with cardiogenic shock. *J Am Coll Cardiol* 1992, 19:639–646.

Holmes DR Jr, Bates ER, Kleinman NS, *et al.* for the GUSTO-I Investigators: Contemporary reperfusion therapy for cardiogenic shock: the GUSTO-I Trial experience. *J Am Coll Cardiol* 1996, 26:668–674.

Kleiman NS, Terrin M, Meuller HS, *et al.* for the TIMI Investigators: Mechanisms of early death despite thrombolytic therapy: experience from the TIMI II study. *J Am Coll Cardiol* 1992, 19:1129–1135.

McCallister BD, Christian TF, Gersh BJ, Gibbons RJ: Prognosis of myocardial infarctions involving more than 40% of the left ventricle after reperfusion therapy. *Circulation* 1993, 88(part 1):1470–1475.

Evaluation of the Patient with Palpitations and Non–Life-Threatening Cardiac Arrhythmias

Kelly Anne Spratt
Mark N. Fiengo
Eric L. Michelson

8

> ## Key Points
> - Palpitations are a frequent but relatively nonspecific cardiac symptom.
> - Palpitations are not a reliable indicator of any particular cardiovascular finding or arrhythmia.
> - Palpitations are clinically important when there is associated functional incapacity or concern of the patient, when they cause severe hemodynamic sequelae, or serve as harbingers of life-threatening cardiac arrhythmias in selected patients.
> - A thorough history, physical examination, and judicious use of laboratory testing usually guides management.
> - Management must encompass the nature and severity of the palpitations, the patient's general medical and cardiac conditions, the mechanism of the arrhythmia, and an algorithm for risk stratification.

Palpitations are a common symptom and frequent cause of outpatient visits to generalists and cardiovascular subspecialists. This chapter emphasizes a holistic yet focused, practical, and cost-effective approach to evaluating patients with palpitations. It is a reference for initiating management strategies in most patients with palpitations and non–life-threatening cardiac arrhythmias.

PALPITATIONS

Definitions

In this discussion, *palpitation* is defined broadly as an uncomfortable or abnormal awareness of the heart beating. Symptoms vary and may be described as heavy beating of the heart, fluttering in the chest, skipped beats, rapid heart beating, irregular heart beating, pounding in the neck, or some other unpleasant sensation depending on the underlying cardiac rhythm and the patient. Palpitations are a relatively nonspecific symptom and are not a reliable indicator of any particular cardiovascular finding or arrhythmia.

Symptomatic Manifestations of Arrhythmias

Cardiac symptoms as a manifestation of arrhythmias can be very nonspecific. Patients may present with a variety of complaints. Among individuals with documented cardiac arrhythmias, some are completely asymptomatic, some have palpitations, and some have symptoms that may present as angina, dyspnea, fatigue, effort intolerance, near-syncope or syncope, or even noncardiac symptoms such as gastrointestinal upset [1,2].

Mechanisms

Arrhythmias can produce palpitations through multiple mechanisms. Arrhythmias can cause symptoms related to disorders of rhythm, disorders of rate, alterations in patterns of cardiac contractility, or alterations in cardiovascular hemodynamics. Intermittent disorders of rhythm such as paroxysmal supraventricular tachycardias, paroxysmal atrial fibrillation, atrial premature beats, and ventricular premature beats are frequent causes of palpitations. Disorders of rate also can be perceived as palpitations, and even sinus tachy- or bradycardia can cause symptoms (Fig. 1). In many cases, only normal sinus rhythm is found when using ambulatory electrocardiographic (ECG) recording techniques. This finding may suggest either a noncardiac origin or an awareness of increased contractility secondary to a surge in catecholamines (*eg*, before an interview, examination, or appearance on stage).

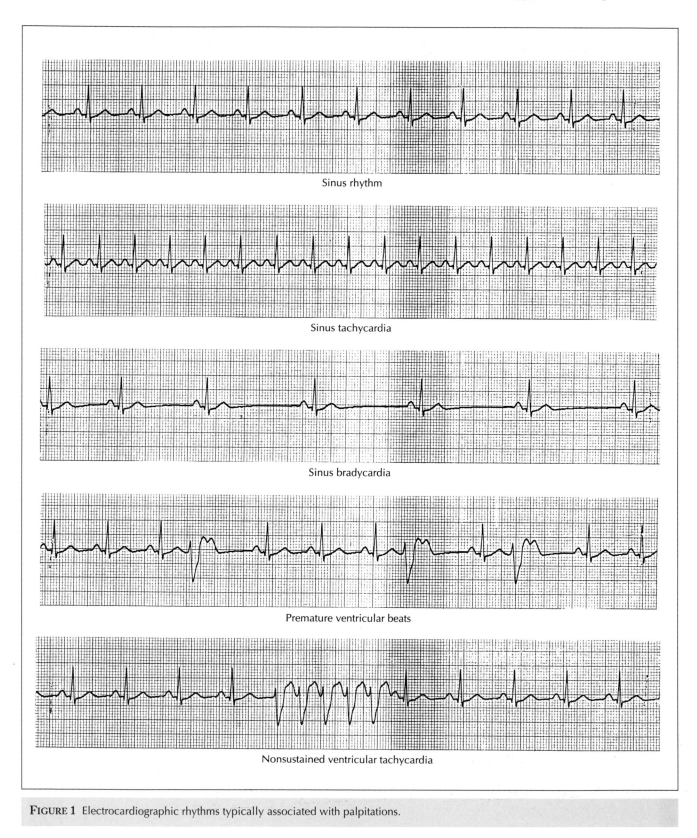

Sinus rhythm

Sinus tachycardia

Sinus bradycardia

Premature ventricular beats

Nonsustained ventricular tachycardia

FIGURE 1 Electrocardiographic rhythms typically associated with palpitations.

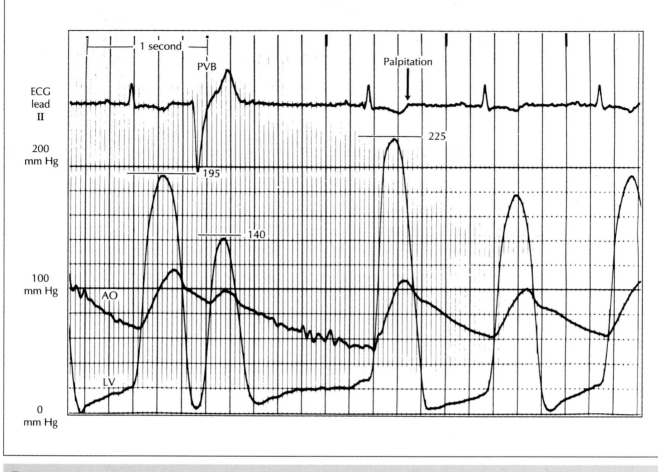

FIGURE 2 Increased left ventricular pressure (LV) after premature ventricular beat (PVB) in a patient with severe aortic stenosis and palpitations (*arrow*). AO—aortic pressure; ECG—electrocardiogram.

The alterations in cardiac contractility and increased stroke volume that occur after premature ventricular beats also may be interpreted as palpitations (Fig. 2). Any arrhythmia associated with atrioventricular (AV) dissociation or varying patterns of AV conduction may cause symptoms related to a variety of mechanisms including altered atrial contribution to ventricular filling, which affects cardiac output, or atrial contraction against closed AV valves, which causes engorgement and regurgitation of blood into the pulmonary veins and venae cavae (Fig. 3) and venous pulsations in the neck. Characteristically, AV nodal reentrant tachycardia causes a regular, rapid "pounding in the neck" related to (right) atrial contraction against the closed (tricuspid) AV valve with each heartbeat [3].

PATIENT EVALUATION

Initial Evaluation and Medical History

The ideal initial evaluation of the patient with palpitations is a thorough history and physical examination [4,5]. Most important to the general medical history is to determine the presence of common conditions (*eg*, hypertension or thyroid disease) that affect the cardiovascular system and possibly potentiate arrhythmias as well as to identify less common systemic disorders (*eg*, sarcoidosis) (Table 1). In adult noninsulin-dependent diabetic patients palpitations may be an indicator of poor glycemic control [6•]. Electrolyte abnormalities such as hypomagnezemia or hypokalemia may exacerbate the propensity for arrhythmias in both normal as well as structurally abnormal hearts. A thorough social history must be reviewed, and patients should be asked if they use tobacco, alcohol, caffeine or illicit drugs, as they will rarely volunteer this information. Family history should be reviewed regarding parents, siblings, and other family members with a history of cardiovascular disease, sudden cardiac death, or arrhythmias. As part of the initial history, it is also essential to determine the use of concomitant medications, whether prescription or over-the-counter drugs, that may affect the cardiovascular system (Table 2). Drugs associated with prolongation of the QT interval on the electrocardiogram in susceptible individuals may be associated with palpitations related to paroxysms of nonsustained ventricular tachyarrhythmias and may need to be discontinued.

It is also important to assess the patient's overall sense of well-being and probe thoroughly for clues to psychological

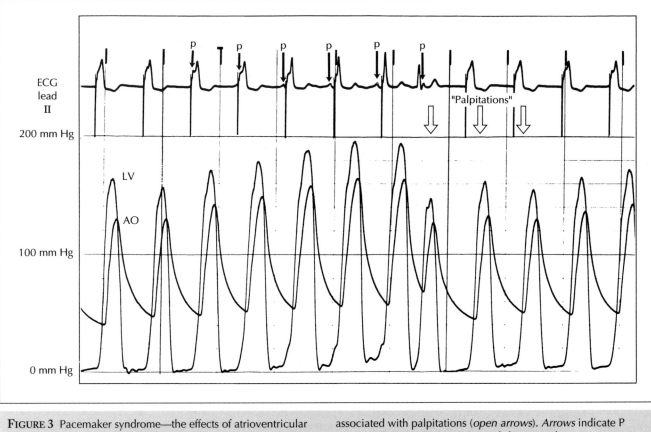

Figure 3 Pacemaker syndrome—the effects of atrioventricular dissociation on cardiac hemodynamics. There is a drop of 40 mm Hg in systemic blood pressure with atrioventricular asynchrony associated with palpitations (*open arrows*). *Arrows* indicate P waves. AO—aortic pressure; LV—left ventricular pressure.

illnesses such as depression and panic disorder as either may be the primary underlying affliction in many patients with palpitations. For example, patients with panic attacks are often exquisitely sensitive to heartbeat perception and an awareness of a change in heart rate may trigger further anxiety, which culminates in a vicious cycle of panic [7•]. The early identification of these patients is important as this can lead to avoidance of unnecessary testing and earlier initiation of treatment directed at the underlying problem. In such patients, recurrence of palpitations is frequent and may be associated with impaired work performance as well as a greater number of emergency medical visits [8•–10•].

Characteristics of Palpitations

Once a detailed, general medical history is obtained, the physician should characterize the patient's symptoms of palpitations qualitatively and quantitatively [11,12]. This includes establishing the frequency and duration of symptoms, the temporal pattern of symptoms, and the situations or circumstances that provoke or relieve symptoms (Table 3). The onset and termination of palpitations may help to identify the responsible arrhythmia. Symptoms that begin and terminate abruptly favor a reentrant or reciprocating tachycardia, such as AV reciprocating tachycardia or AV nodal reentrant tachycardia, whereas symptoms that begin abruptly but persist for days favor a diagnosis of paroxysmal atrial fibrillation [8•,13]. The rate and regularity, or irregularity,

are also important characteristics. For example, even in patients with otherwise normal cardiac function, supraventricular tachycardias are frequently disabling [14•]. Exacerbating or ameliorating factors, associated symptoms (*eg*, dyspnea, lightheadedness, syncope, and angina), and response to prophylaxis, avoidance of potentiating factors, or interventions all may provide clues to an effective arrhythmia evaluation and management strategy.

Physical Examination

The physical examination should focus on the stigmata of structural heart disease. It should also focus on recognition of noncardiac disorders and the systemic manifestations of diseases (*eg*, thyroid disorder and alcohol or drug abuse) known to affect the heart and predispose patients to arrhythmias.

Laboratory Testing

Initial routine laboratory testing should be limited to those tests likely to lead to a diagnosis or guide a management strategy. These may include a serum potassium or hemoglobin determination or an evaluation of thyroid function.

Electrocardiography is the cornerstone in the evaluation of patients with palpitations and is often useful in determining the mechanism of the responsible arrhythmia as well as the presence of underlying cardiac disease. The ECG can make the diagnosis of preexcitation syndrome,

TABLE 1 PATIENT HISTORY

General medical history
Hypertension
Thyroid disease
Electrolyte disorder
Neuropsychiatric disorder
   Depression
   Anxiety
   Panic disorder
Diabetes mellitus
Sarcoidosis
Amyloidosis
Hemochromatosis

Cardiovascular history
Ischemic heart disease
Hypertrophic heart disease
Mitral valve prolapse
Valvular heart disease
Preexcitation/Wolff-Parkinson-White Syndrome
Long-QT syndrome
Rheumatic heart disease
Heart failure/cardiomyopathy

Social history
Ethanol use
Caffeine use
Tobacco use
Illicit drug use
Stress

Family history
Cardiovascular disease
Sudden cardiac death
Arrhythmias

TABLE 2 NONCARDIAC DRUGS ASSOCIATED WITH PALPITATIONS*

α-Adrenergic agonist
Phenylpropanolamine
Phenylephrine

β-Adrenergic agonist
Terbutaline
Isoproterenol
Albuterol

Methylxanthine
Theophylline

Psychoactive
Phenothiazines†
Tricyclics†

Endocrine
Thyroxine

Gastrointestinal
Cisapride†

Anticholinesterase
Physostigmine
Neostigmine

Antimuscarinic
Atropine
Scopolamine

Illicit
Amphetamine
Cocaine

*Partial listing of more commonly associated drugs.
†Associated with QT interval prolongation.

TABLE 3 CHARACTERISTICS OF PALPITATIONS

Frequency	Rhythm regularity/irregularity
Temporal pattern	Exacerbating factors
Situations/circumstances	Ameliorating factors
Onset/termination	Associated symptoms
Duration	Response to prophylaxis or
Heart rate	interventions

long-QT syndrome, Mobitz type I or type II heart block, or other conduction system disease. Supraventricular or ventricular premature beats also may be identified, but the modern, computerized, multilead ECG often records only 12 to 15 seconds of rhythm, which is usually insufficient to diagnose rhythms that are not clearly present clinically when the recording begins. If a diagnosis is not made, ambulatory ECG monitoring is usually the next step. If symptoms are frequent (*ie*, daily), testing is by ambulatory ECG recording. However, if symptoms are intermittent, the diagnostic test of choice is often an event recorder. Event recorders are especially effective in patients in whom symptoms are brief and may not be present by the time they reach the emergency department [15•,16•]. In either case, correlation of symptoms with ECG findings is essential [1]. It is generally not sufficient merely to identify an arrythmia on ambulatory monitoring, but rather it is the close temporal relationship of a patient's typical symptom of palpitations with specific electrocardiographic findings that reveals the diagnosis. For example, the correlation of episodes of palpitations with normal sinus rhythm on the ambulatory or event record-

ing despite the presence of premature ventricular contractions at other times would be helpful in suggesting the diagnosis of anxiety rather than an arrythmia as the cause of the patient's symptoms. Figure 1 shows single-lead ECG strips of various rhythms typically documented by ambulatory ECG recording or event monitoring. Often, at least two leads are recorded simultaneously to facilitate interpretation.

The initial thorough history, physical examination, and routine laboratory testing are usually within the purview of the generalist in the evaluation of patients with palpitations. Exceptions may include patients known to have more advanced or specific cardiovascular disorders or those having palpitations associated with more severe or potentially life-threatening sequelae.

Risk Stratification

Although palpitations are a relatively frequent cause of outpatient visits to physicians, they are associated with serious cardiac arrhythmias in only a minority of cases [17••]. Risk stratification is critical to the evaluation of patients who present with palpitations. The physician must stratify patients as to those with symptomatic but benign arrhythmias, those with prognostically important arrhythmias, and those with potentially life-threatening or hemodynamically important tachy- or bradyarrhythmia.

In patients with unremarkable history, physical examination, ECG, and routine laboratory results and who experience minor symptoms without significant arrhythmia on ambulatory monitoring, no further cardiovascular evaluation is usually necessary. Reassurance for the patient is appropriate. Conversely, in patients whose findings are more remarkable and symptoms more incapacitating, or for whom an increased risk of sudden death is clearly suspected, more aggressive diagnostic evaluation is warranted, in some cases including cardiac catheterization or electrophysiologic studies (Table 4). These cases are usually referred to a cardiovascular specialist, and some highly specialized invasive tests (*eg*, electrophysiologic studies) are done by subspecialists. The challenge to the clinician is to identify those

TABLE 4 DIAGNOSTIC MODALITIES

Test	Clinical indication
Electrocardiography*	Initial test for patients with palpitations or suspected arrhythmia
24-hour electrocardiographic monitoring*	Frequent symptoms of palpitations or near-syncope
Ambulatory event recording*	Less frequent symptoms of palpitations or near-syncope
Echocardiography	Assessment of known or suspected structural heart disease and for evaluation of cardiac function or ischemic heart disease
Radionuclide studies	Assessment of known or suspected ischemic heart disease and less commonly for evaluation of cardiac function
Exercise stress testing*	Evaluation of exercise-induced arrhythmia or screening for ischemic heart disease
Head-up tilt testing	Evaluation of vasodepressor/vasovagal syncope
Signal-averaged electrocardiography	Risk stratification of patients with previous myocardial infarction
Invasive†	
Cardiac catheterization	Evaluation of cardiac/coronary anatomy and cardiac function in high-risk patients with known or suspected ischemic/ structural or valvular heart disease
Electrophysiologic testing	Evaluation of patients with life-threatening or hemodynamically important arrhythmias

*Initial testing modalities usually available to generalists
†Invasive diagnostic modalities done by cardiovascular specialists and subspecialists

TABLE 5 RISK STRATIFICATION OF PATIENTS WITH PALPITATIONS FOR LETHAL OR HEMODYNAMICALLY IMPORTANT ARRHYTHMIAS

Low risk
Patients without structural heart disease
Patients without a history of near-syncope or syncope
Patients without evidence of myocardial ischemia
Patients with preserved left ventricular function

High risk
Patients with structural heart disease
Patients with history of syncope
Patients with left ventricular ejection fraction < 40% or symptomatic heart failure
Patients with known coronary artery disease or myocardial infarction
Patients with conduction system disease
Patients with long-QT syndrome
Patients with Wolff-Parkinson-White syndrome

TABLE 6 EVALUATION OF ARRHYTHMIAS IN PATIENTS WITH PALPITATIONS

Benign arrhythmias that generally do not require extensive evaluation
Sinus bradycardia
Sinus arrhythmia
Isolated atrial premature beats
Isolated ventricular premature beats

Arrhythmias that may require more extensive evaluation
Tachy-brady syndrome
Atrioventricular nodal reentrant tachycardias
Atrioventricular reciprocating tachycardias
Nonsustained ventricular tachycardia
Prognostically important ventricular premature beats (couplets, triplets, multiform, R-on-T beats, very frequent beats)

Arrhythmias that generally require further evaluation
Persistent atrial or sinus tachycardia
Preexcitation/Wolff-Parkinson-White syndrome
Atrial fibrillation/atrial flutter
Sustained ventricular tachycardia

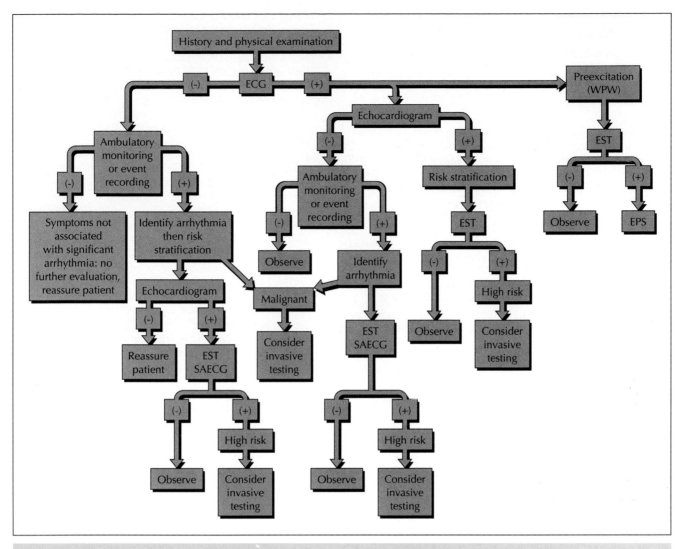

FIGURE 4 Diagnostic evaluation of palpitations. ECG—electrocardiography; EPS—electrophysiologic study; EST—exercise stress test; SAECG—signal-averaged ECG; WPW—Wolff-Parkinson-White syndrome.

individuals at increased risk for lethal or hemodynamically important arrhythmias from among those patients with intermediate findings and to choose the most appropriate diagnostic modality. In Table 5, low-risk patients are stratified as those who often require minimal evaluation, and high-risk patients are those who may require a more extensive work-up. Table 6 elaborates on several common rhythm abnormalities within these patient profiles, and based on this patient risk profile, Figure 4 presents an algorithm for the evaluation of patients with palpitations.

In managing patients with palpitations, cost-effectiveness of the evaluation must encompass several factors in addition to the direct cost of diagnostic testing. These include the adverse effect of palpitations on the patient's quality of life and productivity at work as well as the consequences of not recognizing a potentially lethal underlying cardiovascular problem.

CONCLUSION

Palpitations are a common symptom that can be frustrating for both the patient and physician. An optimal approach to evaluating the patient with palpitations is holistic; systematic with respect to the history, physical examination, and laboratory testing; and must include risk stratification. The evaluation strategy must be practical, cost-effective, and relevant to a well-defined algorithm for patient management.

KEY REFERENCES

Recently published papers of outstanding interest, as identified in *References and Recommended Reading*, have been annotated.

•• Weitz HH, Weinstock PJ: Approach to the patient with palpitations. *Med Clin North Am* 1995, 79:449–456.
This article provides a brief overview of the evaluation of the ambulatory patient with palpitations.

REFERENCES AND RECOMMENDED READING

Recently published papers of particular interest have been highlighted as:
• Of interest
•• Of outstanding interest

1. Zeldis SM, Levine BJ, Michelson EL, Morganroth J: Cardiovascular complaints: correlation with cardiac arrhythmias on 24-hour electrocardiographic monitoring. *Chest* 1980, 78:456–462.

2. Page RL, Wilkinson WE, Clair WK, *et al.*: Asymptomatic arrhythmia in patients with symptomatic paroxysmal atrial fibrillation and paroxysmal supraventricular tachycardia. *Circulation* 1994, 89:224–227.

3. Gursoy S, Steurer G, Brugada J, *et al.*: The hemodynamic mechanism of pounding in the neck in atrioventricular nodal reentrant tachycardia. *N Engl J Med* 1992, 327:772–774.

4. Goldman L, Braunwald E: Chest discomfort and palpitation. In *Harrison's Principles of Internal Medicine*, edn 13. New York: McGraw-Hill; 1994:60–61.

5. Braunwald E: The history. In *Heart Disease: A Textbook of Cardiovascular Medicine*. Philadelphia: WB Saunders; 1992:1–12.

6.• Karen JC, Curtis LG, Summerson JH: Symptoms and complications of adult diabetic patients in a family practice. *Arch Fam Med* 1996, 5:135–145.

7.• Ehlers A, Breuer P: How good are patients with panic disorder at perceiving their heartbeats? *Biol Psychol* 1996, 42:165•182.

8.• Barsky AJ, Cleary PD, Coeytaux RR, Ruskin JN: The clinical course of palpitations in medical outpatients. *Arch Intern Med* 1995, 55:1702–1708.

9.• Weber BE, Kapoor WN: Evaluation and outcomes of patients with palpitations. *Am J Med* 1996, 100:138–148.

10.• Barsky AJ, Ahern DK, Bailery ED, Delamates BA: Predictors of persistent palpitations and continued medical utilization. *J Fam Prac* 1996, 42:465–472.

11. Pritchett ELC, MaCarthy EA, Lee KL, Wildinson WE: The clinical presentation of paroxysmal supraventricular tachycardia in untreated patients. In *Cardiac Electrophysiology*. Edited by Zipes DP, Jalife J. Philadelphia: WB Saunders; 1990:703–707.

12. Kastor JA: Atrial fibrillation. In *Arrhythmias*. Philadelphia: WB Saunders; 1994:25–34.

13. Kannel WB, Wolf PA: Epidemiology of atrial fibrillation. In *Atrial Fibrillation: Mechanisms and Management*. Edited by Falk FH, Podrid PJ. New York: Raven Press; 1992:81–93.

14.• Wood KA, Drew BJ, Scheinmann MM: Frequency of disabling symptoms in supraventricular tachycardia. *Am J Cardiol* 1997, 79:145–149.

15.• Fogel RI, Evans JJ, Prystowsky EN: Utility and cost of event recorders in the diagnosis of palpitations, presyncope, and syncope. *Am J Cardiol* 1997, 79:207–208.

16.• Kinlay S, Leitch JW, Neil A, *et al.*: Cardiac event recorders yield more diagnoses and are more cost-effective than 48-hour Holter monitoring in patients with palpitations. *Ann Intern Med* 1996, 124:16–20.

17.•• Weitz HH, Weinstock PJ: Approach to the patient with palpitations. *Med Clin North Am* 1995, 79:449–456.

9

Evaluation of the Patient with Syncope

Charles M. Blatt
Thomas B. Graboys

Key Points

- Five percent to 10% of emergency visits and hospitalizations involve investigation and management of patients with syncope.
- Patient history is key in defining the cause of the syncopal event; a witness is often a critical historian.
- Patient history must focus on a detailed setting for the syncopal event and should define any situational relationships.
- The physical examination must assess orthostatic potential and focus on potential cardiac and carotid obstructive lesions.
- Multiple unwitnessed syncopal events under curious circumstances should be suspected as factitious.
- Over-the-counter medications may interact with prescribed medications, especially in the elderly, and must be considered as a cause of syncope.
- Referral to a specialist is warranted when either neurologic or cardiac brady- or tachyarrhythmic causes are suggested by preliminary testing.

Syncope accounts for 5% to 10% of emergency room visits and hospitalizations. Traditionally, syncope is viewed as either cardiac or neurologic in origin. These processes overlap, however, because of the dominant role of the vagus nerve and myocardial mechanoreceptors in the generation of neurocardiogenic syncope. Intense peripheral vasodilation followed by bradycardia is mediated by inhibition of sympathetic efferents and enhancement of parasympathetic efferent activity. Psychogenic syncope bridges the gap between cardiac and neurogenic syncope by many inadequately defined mechanisms. Causes of syncope are listed in Table 1; a diagnostic approach is shown in Figure 1.

HISTORY

Patient history is the key to determining the origin of the syncopal event. Physical examination and laboratory tests are important in a minority of events. The clinician should establish a clinical description of the syncopal event with questions such as the following:

Was the syncope witnessed or unwitnessed?
Does the patient have a memory of the event?
Was the event prodromal?
Was it a singular or recurrent episode?
Were injuries associated with the syncopal event?
Can a situational relationship be established?
    Did the patient rise abruptly [1]?
    Did the patient urinate (postmicturition) [2]?
    Did the patient defecate [3]?
    Did the patient eat a meal (postprandial) [4]?

Did the patient cough?

Did the patient swallow?

Was the patient exposed to intense pain?

Was the patient exposed to the sight of blood?

Has the patient recently started a new drug regimen?

The physician must first exclude potential polypharmaceutic drug–drug interactions that might induce either a brady- or tachycardiac event. For the elderly patient, β-adrenergic and calcium-blocking agents may induce sinoatrial block, and benign drugs (*eg*, the popular antihistamines astemizole and terfenadine) may induce ventricular tachyarrhythmia. Aggravation of ventricular arrhythmia or "proarrhythmia" by antiarrhythmic drugs, a concept introduced by our group a decade ago [5], should also be excluded among patients with syncope who are receiving these agents.

Witnesses

The witness to the syncopal event fills in the history that the patient cannot provide. If episodes of syncope are multiple and all unwitnessed with curious circumstances in which a witness could not be present, factitious syncope must be considered. Witnesses should be located and interviewed to focus the inquiry and lead to a more cost-effective diagnostic approach. Panic attacks, anxiety episodes, and conversion reactions may be diagnosed with the aid of a witness, thus eliminating the need for further testing that would delay introduction of therapy [6].

Patient Memory

How the patient remembers the syncopal event may be helpful, and the patient should be asked to recreate in detail the circumstances leading to the event. A postictal confusion, with or without evidence of urinary or fecal incontinence, clearly points to a neurologic cause, whereas clearheadedness immediately after the event points away from seizure as a cause. A completely prodromal event, independent of body position or activity, may focus diagnostic events to uncovering complete heart block, especially for the older patient in whom a sclero-

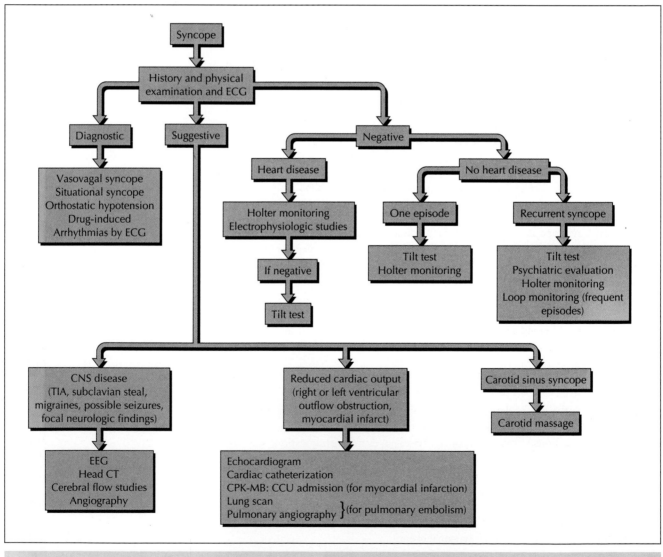

FIGURE 1 Diagnostic approach to syncope. CCU—coronary care unit; CNS—central nervous system; CPK-MB—creatine phosphokinase-muscle brain units; CT—computed tomography; ECG—electrocardiography; EEG—electroencephalography; TIA—transient ischemic attack. (*From* Kapoor [8]; with permission.)

TABLE 1 CAUSES OF SYNCOPE	
Arrhythmia	Situational
Bradyarrhythmia	Coughing
Tachyarrhythmia	Defecation
Supraventricular	Eating
Ventricular	Micturition
Carotid sinus sensitivity	Swallowing
Cerebrovascular disease	Valvular
Drug induced	Aortic stenosis
Vasodilation	Pulmonic stenosis
Arrhythmogenic	Miscellaneous
Neurocardiogenic	Idiopathic hypertrophic
Orthostatic	subaortic stenosis
Pulmonary embolism	Atrial myxoma (right
Psychogenic	or left)
Anxiety	
Conversion	
Panic	

TABLE 2 PHYSICAL EXAMINATION FINDINGS
Orthostatic vital signs
Blood pressure
Supine, sitting, standing after 30 and 60 seconds
Heart rate
Appropriate rise
Persistent decline with standing
Cardiac bruits
Cardiac obstructive murmurs
Aortic stenosis
Mitral stenosis
Hypertrophic cardiomyopathy
Ectopy
Neurologic examination

calcific process may affect the cardiac conduction system. The nature of the prodrome, if witnessed or recalled, is likely to help define a vagally mediated event, including pallor, diaphoresis, nausea, and suggestive historical details.

Multiple Events

Multiple syncopal episodes may define a patient with a benign process or point to a psychogenic cause [7]. In general, the clinical history tends to be more valuable in distinguishing vasodepressor syncope from syncope caused by either atrioventricular block or ventricular tachycardia [8].

Setting the Stage

The history obtained from the patient and any witnesses should set the stage of the syncopal event in detail, with precise definition of the time of day; altitude; relation to meals; events of the preceding 24 hours; change in routine patterns of sleep, bowel movement, and food intake; coincident medication, including novel combinations of prescription and over-the-counter medication; and preceding breathlessness, palpitations, and chest discomfort. The witness must be questioned for evidence of seizure activity; was the patient postictal or incontinent? In addition to the obvious tonic-clonic grand mal activity, evidence of petit mal must be sought. Pulmonary embolism is often overlooked as a cause of syncope, and a conducive historical setting for this problem must be considered. This history includes recent inactivity, travel, or surgery.

PHYSICAL FINDINGS

Although a meticulous history is the cornerstone of defining the cause of syncope, physical findings also may contribute to the correct diagnosis (Table 2). Foremost is the demonstration of any abnormalities in orthostasis. Blood pressure readings

should be taken in both arms while the patient is supine, sitting, and standing. A normal response is a slight decrease in pressure when assuming the upright posture, but blood pressure is maintained within 30 to 60 seconds and a slight increase in heart rate occurs. Among older patients complaining of postural dizziness or near loss of consciousness, orthostatic hypotension induced by antihypertensive drugs is a frequent cause of postural dizziness of frank syncope. Potent antihypertensive drugs may induce a decrease of 20 to 30 mm Hg in blood pressure when assuming an upright posture.

Autonomic Dysfunction

While standing, patients with idiopathic orthostatic hypotension experience a gradual decrease in blood pressure without a commensurate increase in heart rate. This type of autonomic dysfunction also may be a sign of Shy-Drager's disease. Individuals with high vagal tone not only may demonstrate changes in heart rate while obtaining postural blood pressures but also profound sinus bradycardia. Slow heart rates as a manifestation of vagotonia may indicate the patient's predisposition to vasodepressor or vasovagal syncope.

Auscultation of the Carotid Vessels and Heart

Careful examination of the carotid vessels for bruits and auscultation of the heart determine the presence of aortic stenosis or obstructive cardiomyopathy. The presence of a high density of ectopic beats also may help to define arrhythmia as a potential cause of syncope. Central nervous system examination can exclude evidence for focal neurologic deficit. In most patients, however, physical findings are not helpful and not nearly as critical to the diagnosis as a proper history.

LABORATORY EVALUATION

Ambulatory and Transtelephonic Electrocardiographic Monitoring

Laboratory evaluation of a patient with syncope (Table 3) should focus on where the diagnosis will most likely be found.

Any historical suggestion of cardiac arrhythmia, either tachycardia or bradycardia, demands 48 to 72 hours of ambulatory monitoring. A transtelephonic device with loop memory capacity may be the only practical means of documenting cardiac rhythm when events are infrequent [9]. Also, the exercise tolerance test may provide invaluable information regarding the ability to provoke ventricular tachycardia of hemodynamic significance as well as bradycardia or advanced atrioventricular block [10].

Carotid Sinus Massage

The coincidence of coronary artery disease may be demonstrated by an exercise test, and the application of carotid sinus massage during the routine 12-lead electrocardiogram may provide information regarding carotid bulb sensitivity. A sensitive carotid may be stimulated by a tight collar when the neck is rotated, thus generating a syncopal event [11].

Signal-Averaged Electrocardiogram

The signal-averaged electrocardiogram [12] is used to demonstrate the presence of high-frequency, low-amplitude electrical activity at the terminal portion of the QRS complex and may indicate susceptibility to ventricular arrhythmia. Electrophysiologic provocation studies [13] may provide further clues regarding the ease of stimulating a brady- or tachyarrhythmia and help to define the sinoatrial recovery time, which may be helpful under well-defined circumstances [14]. The tachy-brady syndrome, wherein the abrupt termination of rapid supraventricular tachycardia (including atrial fibrillation) produces a prolonged sinus pause, may give rise to prolonged asystole and near or complete syncope. Whether to pursue invasive studies depends on exclusion of the more obvious causes of syncope. Our practice is to defer electrophysiologic study until a full noninvasive evaluation is completed [15].

Autonomic Testing

Autonomic testing using head-up tilt and an isoproterenol infusion has been studied in detail [16,17,18]. The appearance

---

TABLE 3 LABORATORY EVALUATION

By the generalist
Carotid sinus massage
Electrocardiography
Ambulatory electrocardiographic monitor
Transtelephonic "loop memory"
Exercise tolerance test
Electroencephalography
If indicated by physical examination:
    Echocardiography
    Carotid arterial noninvasive tests

By the specialist
Signal-averaged electrocardiography
Cardiac electrophysiologic study
Tilt-table autonomic testing

---

of intense bradycardia and hypotension during head-up tilt, with or without the infusion of isoproterenol, and the induction of near syncope or syncope suggestive of the clinical scenario are diagnostic of neurocardiogenic syncope. An increase in myocardial contractility and a coincidental decline in left ventricular end diastolic dimension precede the onset of syncope [19]. A vagus-mediated slowing of the heart rate appears to play a secondary role to vasodepression in inducing a hypotensive syncopal episode. This appears to explain the inefficacy of cardiac pacing in the management of patients with neurocardiogenic syncope [20].

Echocardiography

Echocardiography occasionally supplements and clarifies issues raised on physical examination. Systolic murmurs may require further clarification regarding the potential for hemodynamically critical aortic stenosis, pulmonary stenosis, idiopathic hypertrophic subaortic stenosis (IHSS), or atrial myxoma to be the source of syncope. The patient with unsuspected IHSS receiving a diuretic may experience a syncopal episode; with rehydration the patient may have no further symptoms. Ventricular or atrial tachyarrhythmia in the setting of IHSS also may cause syncope.

MANAGEMENT

Single Event

Typically, the first episode of lost consciousness is based on a vasovagal event; however, this diagnosis is one of exclusion. Patient history is typical, with an absence of neurologic prodrome or sequelae and a spontaneous resumption of consciousness without the need for resuscitation. These features define the diagnosis and determine further management. In many cases, a solitary episode of lost consciousness suggests either cardiac or neurologic syncope and requires further evaluation.

Multiple Episodes

There is more concern if the patient experiences two or more syncopal episodes, particularly if they share historical characteristics. At times, several days of hospitalization are needed to define the syncope as neurologic, which may only be disclosed through a sleep-deprived electroencephalogram, for example, or a cardiac rhythm disorder that may either have been a brady- or tachycardiac event. Evaluation of the patient with syncope depends on the unique nature and frequency of the event and the clinical condition of the patient.

WHEN TO REFER

The generalist should maintain responsibility for the overall care of the patient and integration of the evaluation and therapy for syncope with the patient's preexisting medical and social problems. It is often the valued role of the generalist to maintain a critical perspective on results of the general and specialized testing. If one test does not fit a scenario that the bulk of the other diagnostic tests support, it may need to be discarded. One test result should not countermand the weight of clinical sensibility if the other objective tests lean away from the diagnosis supported by that single test.

Under most circumstances, the generalist proceeds with a thorough history and physical examination, including carotid sinus massage, an electrocardiogram and a 24-hour ambulatory monitor. If the physical examination suggests an obstructive lesion of the carotid arteries, referral for carotid noninvasive testing is indicated. If the vascular obstruction is reported as significant, referral to a neurologist or vascular surgeon is warranted. The neurologist also should be consulted when the history suggests a seizure disorder.

Cardiac murmurs suggestive of valvular obstructive disease or hypertrophic obstructive cardiomyopathy require prompt referral. Consultation with a cardiologist is indicated if pathology is defined or the murmur remains enigmatic and the history suggests a cardiac source of syncope.

Referral to the cardiologist also is advised when the 24-hour ambulatory monitor provides various types of data. An unambiguous, complete atrioventricular block requires pacemaker implantation. Tachyarrhythmia, particularly ventricular, requires referral to the cardiologist to determine the need for further assessment with electrocardiographic signal averaging or arrhythmia provocation (electrophysiologic studies).

REFERENCES

1. Lipsitz LA: Orthostatic hypotension in the elderly. *N Engl J Med* 1989, 321:952–956.

2. Kapoor WN, Peterson JR, Karpf M: Micturition syncope. *JAMA* 1985, 253:796–798.

3. Kapoor WN, Peterson J, Karpf M: Defecation syncopes: a symptom with multiple etiologies. *Ann Intern Med* 1986, 146:2377–2423.

4. Lipsitz LA, Pluchino FC, Wei JY, *et al.*: Cardiovascular and norepinephrine responses after meal consumption in elderly (older than 75 years) persons with postprandial hypotension and syncope. *Am J Cardiol* 1986, 58:810–815.

5. Velebit V, Podrid PJ, Lown B, *et al.*: Aggravation and provocation of ventricular arrhythmias by antiarrhythmic drugs. *Circulation* 1982, 65:886–894.

6. Linzer M, Pontinen M, Gold DT, *et al.*: Impairment of physical and psychosocial health in recurrent syncope. *J Clin Epidemiol* 1991, 44:1037–1044.

7. Linzer M, Felder A, Hackel A, *et al.*: Psychiatric syncope: a new look at an old disease. *Psychosomatics* 1990, 31:181–188.

8. Kapoor WN: Diagnostic evaluation of syncope. *Am J Med* 1991, 90:91–106.

9. Cumbee SR, Pryor RE, Linzer M: Cardiac loop ECG recording: a new noninvasive diagnostic test in recurrent syncope. *South Med J* 1990, 83:39–43.

10. Podrid PJ, Graboys TB, Lampert S, Blatt CM: Exercise stress testing for exposure of arrhythmia. *Circulation* 1987, 75:60–65.

11. Lewis T: A lecture on vasovagal syncope and the carotid sinus mechanism. *BMJ* 1932, 1:873–876.

12. Kuchar DL, Thorburn CW, Sammel NL: Signal-averaged electrocardiogram for evaluation of recurrent syncope. *Am J Cardiol* 1986, 58:949–953.

13. Krol RB, Morady F, Flaker CG, *et al.*: Electrophysiologic testing in patients with unexplained syncope: clinical and noninvasive predictors of outcome. *J Am Coll Cardiol* 1987, 10:358–363.

14. Linzer M, Prystowsky EN, Divine GW, *et al.*: Predicting the outcome of electrophysiologic studies in syncope: validation of a derived model. *J Gen Intern Med* 1991, 6:113–120.

15. Lown B: Management of patients at high risk of sudden death. *Am Heart J* 1982, 103:689–697.

16. Almquist A, Goldenberg IF, Milstein S, *et al.*: Provocation of bradycardia and hypotension by isoproterenol and upright posture in patients with unexplained syncope. *N Engl J Med* 1989, 320:346–351.

17. Grubb BP, Temesy-Armos P, Han H, Elliot L: Utility of upright tilt-table testing in the evaluation and management of syncope of unknown origin. *Am J Med* 1991, 90:6–10.

18. Kapoor WN, Brant N: Evaluation of syncope by upright tilt testing with isoproterenol: a nonspecific test. *Ann Intern Med* 1992, 116:358–363.

19. Shalev Y, Gal R, Tchou PJ, *et al.*: Echocardiographic demonstration of decreased left ventricular dimensions and vigorous myocardial contraction during syncope induced by head-up tilt. *J Am Coll Cardiol* 1991, 18:746–751.

20. Sra JS, Jazayeri MR, Avitall B, *et al.*: Comparison of cardiac pacing with drug therapy in the treatment of neurocardiogenic (vasovagal) syncope with bradycardia or asystole. *N Engl J Med* 1993, 328:1085–1090.

SELECT BIBLIOGRAPHY

Bendit DG, *et al.*: ACC expert consensus document: tilt table testing for assessing syncope. *J Am Coll Cardiol* 1996, 28:263.

Kinlay S, Leitch JW, Neil A, *et al.*: Cardiac event recorders yield more diagnosis and are more cost-effective than 48 hour Holter monitoring in patients with palpitations. A controlled clinical trial. *Ann Intern Med* 1996, 124:16–20.

Low PA, Gilden JL, Freeman R, *et al.*: Efficacy of midodrine vs placebo in neurogenic orthostatic hypotension: a randomized, double-blind multicenter study. *JAMA* 1997, 277:1046–1051.

Martin TP, Hanusa BH, Kapour WN: Risk stratification of patients with syncope [comment]. *Ann Emerg Med* 1997, 29:459–466.

Ooi WL, Barrett S, Hossain M, *et al.*: Patterns of orthostatic blood pressure change and their clinical correlates in a frail, elderly population. *JAMA* 1997, 277:1299–1304.

Evaluation of the Patient Resuscitated from Cardiac Arrest

10

Eric N. Prystowsky

Key Points

- Sudden cardiac death is the most common cause of mortality in adults less than age 65 years of age.
- Coronary artery disease is the most common cause of cardiac arrest.
- Survivors of cardiac arrest should undergo a complete history and physical examination as well as cardiac catheterization and electrophysiologic testing.
- An implantable cardioverter defibrillator (ICD) is often necessary to prevent sudden cardiac death.
- Antiarrhythmic drug therapy, alone or with the ICD, is often useful.
- Survivors of cardiac arrest are at a high risk for a recurrent episode if not treated properly, so referral to a clinical electrophysiologist is suggested.

Sudden cardiac death is the most common cause of mortality in adults less than 65 years of age [1]. It is estimated that sudden cardiac death claims a patient approximately every 1 to 2 minutes [2]. There are various cardiac causes for sudden death (Table 1). In a relatively small percentage of patients, bradycardia may be the first arrhythmia identified in the cardiac arrest victim, but ventricular fibrillation or rapid sustained ventricular tachycardia (VT-S) is more common (Fig. 1) [3–7].

Cobb and coworkers [8] were pioneers in establishing community-based intervention for cardiac arrest victims. They developed a rapid response system for emergency services in Seattle using the Seattle Fire Department. Approximately 60% of Seattle residents 12 years of age and older have had some training in cardiopulmonary resuscitation. Even in such an emergency care system, only approximately 30% of cardiac arrest victims are discharged from the hospital alive. Most communities, especially in more rural areas of the United States, have far fewer successful resuscitations. In Memphis, approximately 10% to 13% of patients with cardiac arrest and out-of-hospital ventricular tachycardia or ventricular fibrillation who are given emergency care are discharged from the hospital alive [9]. Because survival rates are so poor in patients with out-of-hospital cardiac arrest caused by ventricular fibrillation or VT-S, physicians should determine who is at greatest risk for these arrhythmias in order to prevent the first episode and decrease sudden death.

CAUSES OF SUDDEN CARDIAC DEATH

Heart Disease

Sudden cardiac death because of ventricular fibrillation occurs most commonly in patients with heart disease. By far, coronary artery disease is the most common condition associated with sudden cardiac death [10,11], and it is important to identify whether cardiac arrest occurred at the time of acute myocardial infarction (MI) (Fig. 2). Cobb and coworkers [12] reported a 1-year mortality rate of 2% in patients with an acute MI at the time of cardiac arrest compared with 22% in patients without acute MI. Coronary artery spasm can cause ventricular fibrillation, but it has been documented as the cause of cardiac arrest in only a small percentage of patients [13].

Some patients with hypertrophic or dilated cardiomyopathy as well as those with certain forms of congenital heart disease (*eg*, postoperative tetralogy of Fallot) also can be at risk for sudden cardiac death [14]. There is sometimes a familial pattern of sudden cardiac death, especially in certain idiopathic dilated cardiomyopathies or in hypertrophic cardiomyopathy.

Electrophysiologic Abnormalities

Patients with the Wolff-Parkinson-White syndrome rarely have cardiac arrest [15]. The most common form of tachycardia in this syndrome is paroxysmal supraventricular tachycardia, which is usually a regular, narrow QRS-complex tachycardia. In some patients, atrial fibrillation may cause a rapid ventricular rate because of conduction from the atrium to the ventricle over the accessory pathway; this can subsequently degenerate into ventricular fibrillation (Fig. 3) [15].

Patients with the idiopathic long-QT syndrome are at risk for syncope and cardiac arrest [16]. Typically, these patients have torsades de pointes, a polymorphic ventricular tachycardia, which can degenerate into ventricular fibrillation. Long-QT syndrome has a strong familial pattern, with autosomal dominant and recessive modes of inheritance. The hallmark is a prolonged QT interval, although this is not present in every electrocardiogram. Therapy can usually prevent cardiac arrest. It is important to make an accurate diagnosis and to evaluate other family members who may be at risk.

Infrequently, patients with no evidence of structural heart disease can have ventricular fibrillation. In a recent series of 19 patients with idiopathic ventricular fibrillation, six had a history of syncope and two had presyncope before cardiac arrest [17]. However, ventricular tachyarrhythmias are an uncommon cause for syncope in patients with no identifiable structural heart disease. Thus, it is not advisable to pursue aggressively this cause for syncope in most patients, unless a strong suspicion exists for the presence of ventricular tachycardia.

Iatrogenic Causes

Aggressive diuresis with subsequent marked hypokalemia can lead to cardiac arrest because of ventricular fibrillation. A more common iatrogenic cause of cardiac arrest is proarrhythmia resulting from drug use, especially antiarrhythmic drugs. Several types of ventricular proarrhythmias exist, including drug-associated ventricular fibrillation, new-onset VT-S, incessant ventricular tachycardia, and torsades de pointes. Patients with depressed left ventricular function and those with a history of VT-S are more likely to develop proarrhythmia during antiarrhythmic drug treatment.

An example of torsades de pointes ventricular proarrhythmia is shown in Figure 4. This patient had heart disease and atrial fibrillation. Intravenous procainamide failed to terminate atrial fibrillation, and electrical cardioversion restored sinus rhythm. The QT interval was markedly prolonged immediately after cardioversion. Approximately 10 minutes later, the patient developed torsades de pointes and required resuscitative efforts. Because ventricular proarrhythmia often occurs during the first few days of therapy, we recommend starting antiarrhythmic drugs in-hospital for patients with heart disease.

APPROACH TO SURVIVORS OF CARDIAC ARREST

Evaluation

Survivors of cardiac arrest should undergo a complete history and physical examination. The history may reveal data suggesting a long-term problem with cardiac dysfunction, such as exertional shortness of breath. Alternatively, the patient may relate a history of chest pain that has increased in severity over several weeks before cardiac arrest. In our experience, patients almost always have some degree of retrograde amnesia when they awaken after cardiac arrest. This usually precludes any useful information regarding events that immediately preceded the cardiac arrest, unless an observer can provide these data. It should be ascertained whether the patient took any new prescription or over-the-counter drugs. Some aggressive diets,

TABLE 1 COMMON CAUSES OF CARDIAC ARREST
Heart disease
Coronary artery disease
Cardiomyopathy
Congenital heart disease
Electrophysiologic abnormalities
Wolff-Parkinson-White syndrome
Long-QT syndrome
Idiopathic ventricular fibrillation
Iatrogenic
Proarrhythmia with drugs
Electrolyte derangements

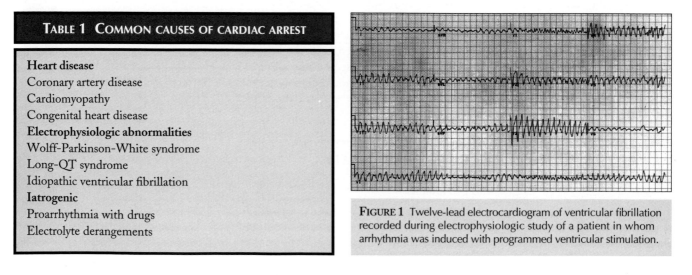

FIGURE 1 Twelve-lead electrocardiogram of ventricular fibrillation recorded during electrophysiologic study of a patient in whom arrhythmia was induced with programmed ventricular stimulation.

(*eg*, liquid protein diets) can lead to marked abnormalities in electrolytes and development of ventricular tachyarrhythmias. When appropriate, one should investigate and screen for use of illicit drugs, especially cocaine.

Physical examination may reveal the presence of atherosclerosis, detected by findings of peripheral vascular disease such as a decreased arterial pulse or the presence of xanthomas or xanthelasma. Cardiac examination may disclose a ventricular

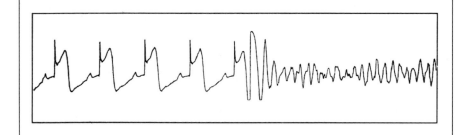

FIGURE 2 Emergence of ventricular fibrillation during the first hour of acute myocardial infarction. (*From* Prystowsky [23]; with permission.)

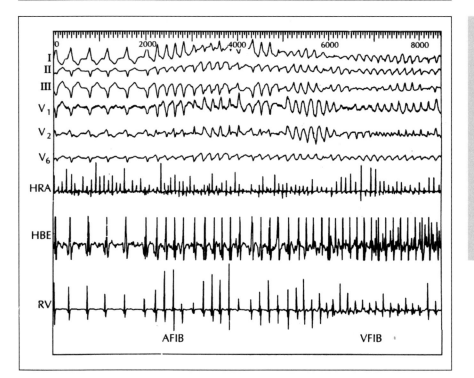

FIGURE 3 Atrial fibrillation (AFIB) initiated during electrophysiologic study of a patient with anterograde conduction over the accessory pathway. Simultaneous tracings are from electrocardiographic leads I, II, III, V_1, V_2, and V_6 as well as from intracardiac leads in the high right atrium (HRA), His bundle area (HBE), and right ventricle (RV). Atrial fibrillation is evidenced by the rapid, irregular rhythm recorded on the HRA lead. At the left, the wide, grossly irregular QRS complexes are caused by conduction over the accessory pathway. At the right, ventricular fibrillation (VFIB) has occurred. (*From* Prystowsky *et al.* [24]; with permission.)

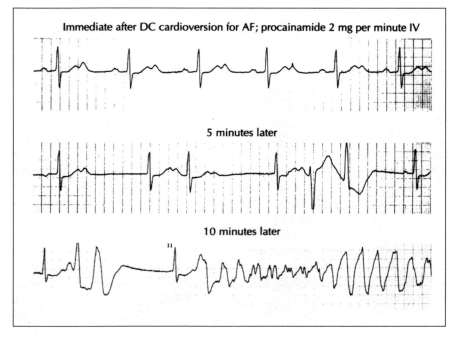

FIGURE 4 Development of torsades de pointes ventricular proarrhythmia in a patient treated with procainamide for atrial fibrillation (AF). IV—intravenous. (*From* Prystowsky and Klein [18]; with permission.)

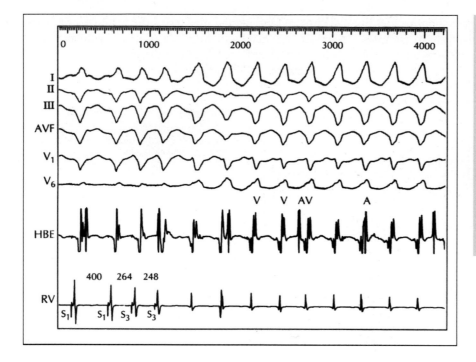

FIGURE 5 Initiation of sustained rapid ventricular tachycardia during programmed ventricular stimulation. Simultaneous tracings are electrocardiogram leads I, II, III, aVF, V_1, V_6, and intracardiac electrograms from the His bundle (HBE) and right ventricle (RV). The RV is paced at cycle length 400 msec (150/min) for eight beats, and two premature stimuli (S_2, S_3) are introduced with coupling of intervals of 264 and 248 msec, respectively. After the second premature stimulus, sustained ventricular tachycardia occurs and ventriculoatrial dissociation is noted on the HBE lead, with more ventricular (V) than atrial (A) electrograms.

(S_3) or atrial gallop (S_4), suggesting the possibility of systolic or diastolic dysfunction. Significant cardiac murmurs may be heard, and evidence for systemic diseases (*eg*, thyrotoxicosis) that affect the heart also may be present.

Extensive laboratory investigation is required. Serial cardiac enzymes and electrocardiograms are necessary to diagnose an acute myocardial infarction. The electrocardiogram also may uncover the long-QT syndrome, a previous MI, nonspecific findings that suggest cardiomyopathy, or the presence of ventricular preexcitation. Serum electrolyte testing may diagnose severe hypokalemia. Other blood tests are usually unrevealing but are occasionally helpful; for example, a substantially elevated erythrocyte sedimentation rate may suggest acute myocarditis or vasculitis.

Echocardiography is a requisite part of the work-up. Myocardial size and function as well as valvular abnormalities are easily evaluated with this technique. Cardiac catheterization should be performed in all patients unless the cause of cardiac arrest is obvious, for example, an acute MI [18•]. Treadmill exercise testing may be useful in patients with suspected coronary artery disease to evaluate functional status or in those who had cardiac arrest during exertion. In my experience, VT-S rarely emerges during the exercise test in patients who are referred for cardiac arrest [19].

A complete electrophysiologic evaluation should be done for patients in whom an unequivocal precipitating cause of cardiac arrest has not been identified. Atrial pacing tests sinus node function and atrioventricular (AV) conduction, as well as evaluates the inducibility of supraventricular tachycardia. Most importantly, pacing the ventricle with introduction of premature beats may initiate VT-S or ventricular fibrillation [20] (Fig. 5). Sustained monomorphic ventricular tachycardia is induced more commonly in patients with coronary artery disease compared with other forms of heart disease or idiopathic ventricular fibrillation [20]. In a review of 1233 survivors of cardiac arrest who underwent electro-

physiologic evaluation, 42% had sustained monomorphic ventricular tachycardia initiated, whereas 16% had sustained polymorphic ventricular tachycardia or ventricular fibrillation induced [20].

Treatment

An approach to therapy is summarized in Figure 6. Patients with a clearly reversible etiology for cardiac arrest are given specific therapy for that condition. An example is routine post-MI care for patients with ventricular fibrillation that occurred within the first 48 hours after MI. Most patients do not have an obvious cause for the cardiac arrest, and treatment depends on the type of heart disease present. The overwhelming majority of patients have either coronary artery disease or cardiomyopathy. Data are sparse on patients with idiopathic ventricular fibrillation, however, but early defibrillator implantation should be considered in these cases [17]. The accessory pathway should be ablated in cardiac arrest survivors with Wolff-Parkinson-White syndrome and rapid preexcited ventricular rates during atrial fibrillation induced at electrophysiologic study [18•]. This is usually accomplished with endocardial catheter ablation techniques. Patients with cardiomyopathy should undergo electrophysiologic evaluation; results may affect the choice of antiarrhythmic therapy. Little information is available regarding the accuracy of serial electrophysiologic–pharmacologic drug testing to determine the efficacy of treatment in patients with cardiomyopathy; thus, I recommend an implantable cardioverter defibrillator (ICD) as part of their therapy [18•].

Patients with coronary artery disease are dichotomized into those with and those without sustained ventricular tachyarrhythmias initiated at electrophysiologic study. These patients are further divided by the need for coronary artery bypass graft (CABG) surgery. The approach to the cardiac arrest survivor is multifactorial, and the need for coronary revascularization should be considered. However, it is uncommon for revascularization alone to prevent recurrent cardiac arrest.

For patients in whom VT-S or ventricular fibrillation is not induced, an ICD is recommended as initial therapy for all patients except those with no evidence of myocardial dysfunction [20]. This is a small subgroup who tend to have severe three-vessel coronary artery disease and well-preserved left ventricular function. The assumption is that these patients had an ischemic cardiac arrest without MI, although proof is almost always lacking in these instances. Few patients fall into this category, but I have had success with revascularization only in these individuals.

Patients who have VT-S or VF initiated and require CABG surgery are recommended for ICD therapy at the time of surgery. However, with the more recent use and high success of nonthoracotomy lead systems, one may want to delay ICD implantation in some patients until after CABG. If CABG or other cardiac surgery is not required, these patients are subgrouped according to the left ventricular ejection fraction. Wilbur and coworkers [21] demonstrated that recurrence of cardiac arrest was unacceptably high in patients with lower ejection fractions, who had suppression of their ventricular arrhythmias during serial electrophysiologic– phar-

macologic drug testing. For this reason, I recommend early consideration for an ICD in these individuals; however, I do routinely begin with antiarrhythmic drug therapy in patients with ejection fractions of 40% or more. Efficacy is evaluated with electrophysiologic testing. In these individuals, programmed ventricular stimulation is repeated in the presence of antiarrhythmic drugs. The patient is discharged and receives the drug if only a few repetitive ventricular beats can be initiated with an aggressive pacing protocol. Overall, most cardiac arrest survivors are treated with an ICD.

PREVENTION OF CARDIAC ARREST

Patients often have symptoms that are possibly related to an arrhythmia. These include palpitations, presyncope, dizziness, and syncope. The aggressiveness of the work-up depends not only on the symptom but also on the underlying cardiac condition; an approach to these patients is demonstrated in Figure 7. Patients without any structural heart disease and no electrocardiographic abnormalities should undergo ambulatory electrocardiographic monitoring, usually with a handheld or loop event recorder, to evaluate palpitations. Syncope or presyncope in patients without heart disease is often caused by neurally mediated syncope, which is

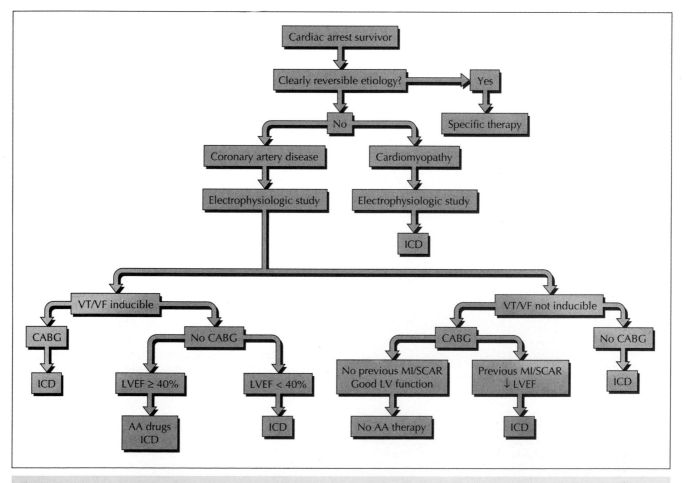

FIGURE 6 Approach to therapy for cardiac arrest survivors. AA—antiarrhythmic; CABG—coronary artery bypass graft surgery; ICD—implantable cardioverter defibrillator; LVEF—left ventricular ejection fraction; MI—myocardial infarction; SCAR— myocardial scar; VF—ventricular fibrillation; VT—sustained ventricular tachycardia.

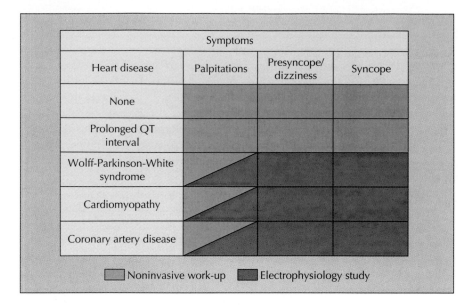

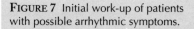

Symptoms			
Heart disease	Palpitations	Presyncope/ dizziness	Syncope
None			
Prolonged QT interval			
Wolff-Parkinson-White syndrome			
Cardiomyopathy			
Coronary artery disease			

☐ Noninvasive work-up   ■ Electrophysiology study

best uncovered during tilt-table evaluation. Patients with a prolonged QT interval and potential arrhythmic symptoms should undergo electrocardiographic monitoring to correlate symptoms with an electrocardiographic tracing. Electrophysiologic study is usually not helpful in these individuals; causes other than arrhythmias for dizziness or syncope should be sought. Therapy should be initiated if any suspicion exists that the symptoms relate to a ventricular arrhythmia. β-blockers are the initial treatment of choice.

Patients with WPW syndrome, cardiomyopathy, or coronary artery disease likely have an arrhythmic cause for their symptoms. Presyncope, dizziness, or syncope in these individuals requires electrophysiologic evaluation. If palpitations are present, either a noninvasive or invasive work-up may be done, depending on the characteristics of the palpitations. For example, if the patient relates a rapid, long-lasting episode of palpitations, electrophysiologic study is recommended. Alternatively, a patient may report skipped beats, in

Arrhythmia	PVCs, VT-NS	PVCs / VT-NS		VT-S, VF
Heart disease	Absent	Present		Present
LV dysfunction	Absent	Absent	Present	Present
Potential risks for SCD	Minimal	Intermediate		High

FIGURE 8 Risk stratification to identify patients most likely to have cardiac arrest. The first column (*light*) includes patients with premature ventricular complexes (PVCs) and nonsustained ventricular tachycardia (VT-NS) who have no heart disease. Patients in the far righthand column (*dark*) have a history of sustained ventricular tachycardia (VT-S) or ventricular fibrillation (VF). Risk stratification involves the patients in the middle column (*shaded*). LV—left ventricular; SCD—sudden cardiac death. (*From* Prystowsky [22]; with permission.)

which case ambulatory electrocardiographic recordings are the initial recommendation. Therapy is directed by the findings of the work-up.

Few patients with out-of-hospital cardiac arrest are resuscitated early enough to allow survival and discharge from the hospital with minimal brain damage. Thus, risk stratification is a reasonable attempt to prevent the first cardiac arrest event in asymptomatic individuals; an approach to risk stratification is shown in Figure 8. The concept of risk stratification is to determine which individuals most closely resemble patients who have already had a cardiac arrest because of VT-S or VF [22]. Factors considered are the arrhythmia, heart disease, and left ventricular dysfunction. Asymptomatic patients without heart disease are at minimal risk for sudden cardiac death. Survivors of cardiac arrest and patients with a history of VT-S are at high risk for sudden cardiac death. Heart disease, often with marked left ventricular dysfunction, is usually present. Individuals having either premature ventricular complexes or nonsustained ventricular tachycardia with variable degrees of heart disease and left ventricular dysfunction are at intermediate risk for sudden cardiac death. This is the group for which risk stratification is suggested. In this intermediate group, the risk for sudden cardiac death increases as left ventricular dysfunction worsens, a shift from the left to the right in Figure 8. On the righthand side of the column, the patients have similar characteristics to individuals who have already suffered a VT-S or VF.

Although reasonable, risk stratification still requires further investigation. No data have been published demonstrating that any type of prophylactic therapy prolongs life in these individuals.

WHEN TO REFER

If not treated properly, survivors of cardiac arrest are usually at high risk for a recurrent episode. These individuals should be referred to a clinical electrophysiologist. Patients with long-QT syndrome may be evaluated initially by a cardiologist, but they also may require input from a clinical electrophysiologist, especially if defibrillator therapy is contemplated. Patients with syncope or presyncope who have heart disease or WPW syndrome should be referred to an electrophysiologist. Palpitations thought to be primarily extrasystoles can be evaluated by the primary-care physician or cardiologist. If the clinician is concerned about a more serious arrhythmia, the patient should be referred to an electrophysiologist.

REFERENCES AND RECOMMENDED READING

Recently published papers of particular interest have been highlighted as:
• Of interest
•• Of outstanding interest

1. Cupples LA, Gagnon DR, Kannel WB: Long- and short-term risk of sudden coronary death. *Circulation* 1992, 85:11–18.

2. Gillum FR: Sudden coronary death in the United States, 1980–1985. *Circulation* 1989, 79:756–765.

3. Prystowsky EN, Heger JJ, Zipes DP: The recognition and treatment of patients at risk for sudden death. In *Cardiac Emergencies.* Edited by Eliot RS, Saenz A, Forker AD. Kisco, NY: Futura Publishing; 1982:353–384.

4. Cobb LA, Werner JA, Trobaugh GB: Sudden cardiac death. I. A decade's experience with out-of-hospital resuscitation. *Mod Concepts Cardiovasc Dis* 1980, 49:31–36.

5. Liberthson RR, Nagel EL, Hirschman JC, Nussenfeld SR: Pre-hospital ventricular defibrillation. Prognosis and follow-up course. *N Engl J Med* 1974, 291:317–321.

6. Myerburg RJ, Conde CA, Sung RJ, *et al.*: Clinical, electrophysiologic and hemodynamic profile of patients resuscitated from pre-hospital cardiac arrest. *Am J Med* 1980, 68:568–576.

7. Luu M, Stevenson WG, Stevenson LW, *et al.*: Diverse mechanisms of unexpected cardiac arrest in advanced heart failure. *Circulation* 1989, 80:1675–1680.

8. Cobb LA, Weaver WD, Fahrenbruch CE, *et al.*: Community-based interventions for sudden cardiac death. Impact, limitations, and changes. *Circulation* 1992, 85(I):98–102.

9. Kellermann AL, Hackman BB, Somes G, Kreth TK: Impact of first-responder defibrillation in an urban emergency medical services system. *JAMA* 1993, 270:1708–1713.

10. Liberthson RR, Nagel EL, Hirschman JC, *et al.*: Pathophysiologic observations in pre-hospital ventricular fibrillation and sudden cardiac death. *Circulation* 1974, 49:790–798.

11. Reichenbach DD, Moss NS, Meyer E: Pathology of the heart in sudden cardiac death. *Am J Cardiol* 1977, 39:865–872.

12. Cobb LA, Werner JA, Trobaugh GB: Sudden cardiac death. II. Outcome of resuscitation; management, and future directions. *Mod Concepts Cardiovasc Dis* 1980, 49:37–42.

13. Myerburg RJ, Kessler KM, Mallon SM, *et al.*: Life-threatening ventricular arrhythmias in patients with silent myocardial ischemia due to coronary artery spasm. *N Engl J Med* 1992, 326:1451–1455.

14. Maron BJ, Roberts WC, Epstein SE: Sudden death in hypertrophic cardiomyopathy: a profile of 78 patients. *Circulation* 1982, 65:1388–1394.

15. Klein GJ, Prystowsky EN, Yee R, *et al.*: Asymptomatic Wolff-Parkinson-White. Should we intervene? *Circulation* 1989, 80:1902–1905.

16. Moss AJ, Robinson J: Clinical features of the idiopathic long QT syndrome. *Circulation* 1992, 85(I):140–144.

17. Wever EFD, Hauer RNW, Oomen A, *et al.*: Unfavorable outcome in patients with primary electrical disease who survived an episode of ventricular fibrillation. *Circulation* 1993, 88:1021–1029.

18.• Prystowsky EN, Klein GJ: *Cardiac arrhythmias: an integrated approach for the clinician.* New York: McGraw-Hill; 1994.

19. Evans JJ, Skale BT, Windle JR, *et al.*: Comparison of ventricular tachycardia induction between exercise and electrophysiologic testing in patients with ventricular tachycardia [abstract]. *Circulation* 1984, 70:423.

20. Knilans TK, Prystowsky EN: Antiarrhythmic drug therapy in the management of cardiac arrest survivors. *Circulation* 1992, 85:118–124.

21. Wilbur DJ, Garan H, Finkelstein D, *et al.*: Out-of-hospital cardiac arrest: use of electro-physiologic testing in the prediction of long-term outcome. *N Engl J Med* 1988, 318:19–24.

22. Prystowsky EN: Antiarrhythmic therapy for asymptomatic ventricular arrhythmias. *Am J Cardiol* 1988, 61:102A–107A.

23. Prystowsky EN: Tachyarrhythmias: the role of antiarrhythmic drugs in the therapeutic hierarchy. In *Tachycardias: Mechanisms and Management.* Edited by Josephson ME, Wellens HJJ. 1993, 375–389.

24. Prystowsky EN, Knilans TK, Evans JJ: Diagnostic evaluation and treatment strategies for patients at risk for serious cardiac arrhythmias. Part 2: Ventricular tachyarrhythmias and Wolff-Parkinson-White syndrome. *Mod Concepts Cardiovasc Dis* 1991, 60:55–59.

SELECT BIBLIOGRAPHY

Cummins RO, Ornato JP, Thies WH, Pepe PA: Improving survival from sudden cardiac arrest: the "chain of survival" concept. *Circulation* 1991; 83:1832–1847.

Mirowski M, Reid PR, Mower MM, *et al.*: Termination of malignant ventricular arrhythmias with an implanted automatic defibrillator in human beings *N Engl J Med* 1980; 303:322–324.

Maron BJ, Shirani J. Poliac LC, *et al.*: Sudden death in young competitive athletes: clinical, demographic and pathological profiles. *JAMA* 1996; 276:199–204.

Gilman JK, Naccarelli GV: Evaluation and management of sudden death survivors. *J Intensive Care Med* 1997; 12:1–11.

Evaluation of the Patient with Edema **11**

Michael H. Humphreys

Key Points

- Edema formation occurs from localized causes such as inflammation or lymphatic or venous obstruction, or in a generalized manner, usually in the setting of cardiac, liver, or renal disease.

- In cardiac and liver disease, edema is the result of sodium retention because of sensed arterial underfilling.

- Nephrotic edema usually results from primary renal sodium retention usually without any evidence of arterial underfilling.

- The management of generalized edema is directed at the underlying disease as well as at the edema itself.

- General measures useful in the management of generalized edema include restriction of dietary salt intake and administration of diuretics.

- Specific measures such as abdominal paracentesis in patients with cirrhotic ascites may also be useful.

- The therapeutic approach to the treatment of generalized edema should be based on the severity of the edema and the symptoms it causes.

Edema comes from the Greek word for swelling. Rather than being a disease process itself, edema is a reflection of some underlying condition; its management must therefore be placed in the larger context of the management of this condition [1•].

EDEMA FORMATION

Edema is the accumulation of excess extravascular, extracellular fluid. The filtration of plasma, water, and electrolytes occurs across virtually all capillaries in the body. The rate of filtration is determined by the magnitude of the Starling forces, the differences in hydrostatic and oncotic pressures between the capillary lumen and the interstitium, and by the permeability and surface area of the capillary wall. This filtered fluid is returned to the circulation by the lymphatics, so that the overall constancy of plasma volume is maintained. Edema results when the rate of capillary filtration exceeds the rate of lymphatic return. This can occur with a large increase in capillary hydrostatic pressure, with a large reduction in oncotic pressure, or with increased capillary permeability or surface area. Different types of edema can thus be characterized by one or more of these abnormalities; to a limited extent, recognition of the primary abnormality may offer a rationale for specific therapeutic interventions, such as the infusion of hyperoncotic albumin solutions to patients with hypoalbuminemia.

TYPES OF EDEMA

Edema may be classified as localized edema, which is confined to a specific region or extremity of the body, or as generalized edema, which reflects a widespread increase

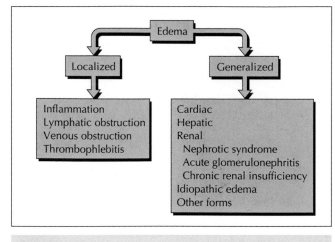

FIGURE 1 Causes of localized and generalized edema.

in extracellular fluid. Generalized edema usually has a dependent component; ankle and leg edema may be only mild after overnight recumbency, when the edema fluid has redistributed to the trunk, but it becomes much more noticeable after prolonged standing. Anasarca is generalized edema so severe that it can be detected in nearly all regions of the body by the indentation caused by the pressure of an applied finger (pitting edema).

EVALUATION AND TREATMENT OF THE PATIENT WITH LOCALIZED EDEMA

Localized edema results from a disturbance in the balance of fluid filtration and return that is confined to a localized region or vascular bed. Localized edema is readily recognized: it is restricted to a discrete area of the body, is asymmetric, and may be accompanied by other features such as pigmentary changes, redness, heat, and pain. Causes of localized edema are listed in Figure 1. Inflammatory edema results from localized tissue injury, usually from infection. Signs of inflammation, including erythema, heat, and pain, are present. The tissue edema results from a cytokine-mediated increase in capillary permeability and from hyperemia, which increases the capillary surface area by opening previously nonperfused capillaries. Angioneurotic edema is a special case of inflammatory edema.

Lymphatic obstruction leads to localized edema by blocking the route of return of normally filtered capillary fluid. The mechanism of the edema accumulation relates to an increase in tissue compliance as tissue hydrostatic pressure increases. Lymphatic obstruction typically occurs from tumor blockade or after surgery involving lymph node dissection. Venous obstruction increases capillary hydrostatic pressure, leading to a rate of capillary filtration that exceeds the rate of lymphatic return. Chronic venous insufficiency in the lower extremities leads to hyperpigmentation and venous stasis ulcers. When thrombophlebitis is the cause of the venous obstruction, the characteristic inflammatory signs of this condition are present.

The recognition of localized edema generally poses no problem for the clinician. For the most part, its management rests with the management of the underlying condition.

EVALUATION OF THE PATIENT WITH GENERALIZED EDEMA

Generalized edema may prove to be more vexing. The major conditions leading to generalized edema are also listed in Figure 1. Unlike localized edema, generalized edema reflects a widespread disturbance in sodium metabolism whereby the kidneys retain sodium, which leads to a positive sodium balance. This is true even in the absence of structural renal disease, as is generally the case in cirrhosis of the liver and congestive heart failure.

The initial evaluation of the patient with generalized edema, like that of the patient with localized edema, is straightforward. The goal at this stage is to define the disease process responsible for the edema formation—the standard database obtained from the history taking, the physical examination, and screening laboratory studies is usually sufficient for this purpose.

Cardiac Edema

Cardiac edema occurs in patients with a history of heart disease; these patients usually have orthopnea, shortness of breath, dyspnea on exertion, and other symptoms of left ventricular failure. Peripheral edema in such patients is accompanied by elevated venous pressure, passive hepatic congestion, hepatojugular reflux, and other signs of right ventricular failure, as well as by cardiac findings of ventricular gallop rhythm; occasional patients with severe chronic lung disease and cor pulmonale exhibit signs of right-sided heart failure alone.

Laboratory studies in patients with cardiac edema should determine whether renal insufficiency coexists with the heart failure. If renal insufficiency, manifested by elevated blood urea nitrogen and serum creatinine concentrations, is present, the clinician must determine if it reflects renal hypoperfusion resulting from severe left ventricular failure or structural renal disease resulting from some related condition (*eg*, hypertensive nephrosclerosis or diabetes) or an unrelated process. Urinalysis is the best way to make this determination. Patients with prerenal azotemia usually have only modest proteinuria (trace to 1+) and a bland urinary sediment, whereas patients with structural renal disease are likely to have higher-grade proteinuria and formed elements (cells, casts, and oval fat bodies) in the sediment. The distinction is important because the management of heart failure in the setting of chronic renal disease becomes more complicated, and consultation with a nephrologist may be necessary.

The renal and hormonal responses to heart failure are similar to the responses in true hypovolemic situations. The sympathetic nervous system is activated, as is the renin-angiotensin-aldosterone axis [1•,2]. Plasma levels of the natriuretic hormone, atrial natriuretic peptide, are elevated in heart failure, but this hormone only blunts the vasoconstrictor and antinatriuretic actions of the heightened sympathetic and renin-angiotensin-aldosterone systems; it does not overcome them. The management of cardiac edema in part focuses on the interruption of these antinatriuretic systems.

TABLE 1 DIAGNOSIS OF HEPATIC EDEMA

Evidence of chronic liver disease
Spider angiomata
Palmar erythema
Jaundice

Presence of portal hypertension and ascites
Prominent venous pattern on abdominal wall
Esophageal varies

Peripheral edema (usually, but not always, present)

TABLE 2 MAJOR FINDINGS IN THREE FORMS OF EDEMA

	Cardiac	Hepatic	Renal
Dependent edema	++++	+++	++
Facial edema	–	–	Present
Ascites	+	++++	+
Hypoalbuminemia	–	++	++++
Proteinuria	0–Trace	0–Trace	++++

Hepatic Edema

Generalized edema resulting from chronic liver disease likewise poses few diagnostic difficulties. This edema typically occurs in patients who exhibit signs of chronic liver disease, such as spider angiomata and palmar erythema, and jaundice is often present as well (Table 1).

Most patients with cirrhosis of the liver and moderate to severe ascites have reduced creatinine clearance even if the serum creatinine level is normal. This is because the muscle wasting that accompanies chronic liver disease reduces daily creatinine production so that diminished renal clearance may not be reflected in a rise in the serum concentration [3]. It follows that cirrhotic patients should have their creatinine clearance determined directly if nephrotoxic or renally excreted drugs are prescribed. Functional renal insufficiency in patients with hepatic cirrhosis exists along a continuum of progressive renal hypoperfusion that culminates ultimately in the pattern of functional renal failure called the hepatorenal syndrome; although these patients are universally edematous, management is directed at preserving renal function rather than at treating the edema. Urinalysis findings in uncomplicated cirrhosis with ascites are indicative of a lack of structural renal disease: proteinuria is minimal, and the sediment is usually bland. However, in jaundiced patients who have bile in the urine, renal epithelial cells can be observed in the urinary sediment. This finding does not indicate tubular toxicity, as it does in other settings.

The pathogenesis of cirrhotic ascites involves arterial vasodilation leading to renal hypoperfusion and activation of the same antinatriuretic systems that occurs in congestive heart failure [1•,2]. Recent studies suggest that increased production of the potent vasodilator nitric oxide may be responsible for the arterial underfilling that results in sodium retention [4•]. Although the treatment of hepatic edema would logically involve interruption of these antinatriuretic systems, this approach has not been very successful in management (*see* later discussion).

Renal Edema

Generalized edema resulting from intrinsic renal disease occurs in three different settings (Fig. 1). In patients with nephrotic syndrome, edema is one of the hallmarks, as it is in acute glomerulonephritis, in which proteinuria is usually present but may not be of nephrotic magnitude (> 3.5 g/24h). Finally,

edema is often present in patients with chronic renal insufficiency, which usually but not always results from chronic glomerular disease. The mechanisms underlying sodium retention in these conditions may differ, but growing evidence suggests that "nephrotic" sodium retention resulting from hypovolemia and renal hypoperfusion due to reduced serum albumin concentration and plasma volume is actually quite rare. Additionally, evidence suggests that "nephritic" edema arising from primary sodium retention may be a common mechanism in proteinuric renal disease [5•]. Sodium retention in chronic renal insufficiency is a special case of nephritic edema resulting from impaired sodium excretion caused by the renal disease.

The evaluation of the patient with renal edema involves the development of the clinical database from the history taking and physical examination. Clues from the physical examination include the distribution of the edema: whereas cardiac and hepatic edema are dependent, renal edema has a special predilection for facial and periorbital areas, as well as a dependent component. Narrow, pale transverse bands appear in the nail beds of hypoalbuminemic patients (Muehrcke's lines); although these bands are not specific for nephrotic syndrome, they are most prominent in nephrotic patients. Urinalysis invariably reveals the presence of proteinuria (3+ to 4+), and the urine sediment provides clues as to the nature of the underlying renal disease.

Findings of nephrotic syndrome include hyaline casts, oval fat bodies, and lipid; the last can appear in several forms, including free lipid droplets, lipid-laden casts, and cholesterol esters viewed as "Maltese crosses" with the aid of polarizing filters on the microscope stage and eyepiece and often seen in oval fat bodies. Evidence of glomerular inflammation is indicated by hematuria, particularly if the bulk of the erythrocytes have a characteristic dysmorphic appearance, and erythrocyte casts. Occasionally, glomerulonephritis with a marked exudative component may cause pyuria and leukocyte casts to be present. Chronic renal insufficiency is suggested by broader, waxy casts. The evaluation should also include a 24-hour urine collection for the measurement of creatinine clearance and the quantitation of proteinuria. These data should enable the renal edema to be characterized as belonging to one of these three broad categories. Renal imaging with diagnostic ultrasonography is usually carried out to identify renal size and echodensity: kidneys from patients with acute glomerulonephritis and many forms of nephrotic syndrome are swollen and enlarged and have normal echodensity, whereas kidneys from patients with chronic renal insufficiency are characteristically reduced in size and have increased echodensity.

Table 2 summarizes some of the major characteristics of edema in cardiac, hepatic, and renal disease.

Idiopathic Edema

A fourth form of generalized edema has been termed *idiopathic edema* [6]. This puzzling and controversial entity is observed solely in women, nearly all of whom are of childbearing age. Many of these women view themselves as overweight even when this view is not shared by others, and the condition has been associated with eating disorders. Clinical identification of this entity rests with complaints of edema (usually dependent but also involving the face), abdominal bloating, and in many women, a dependency on diuretics. The patient's description of the severity of the edema often appears exaggerated, and the abdominal bloating is more likely to be related to bowel distention than to ascites. The standard clinical database is adequate to rule out other forms of generalized edema. The pathophysiology of this condition has remained enigmatic, and no agreement exists about the separate roles of the renin-angiotensin system, altered capillary permeability, estrogen and progesterone production, and several other factors that have sometimes been thought to participate in idiopathic edema formation. Many women who complain of this disorder take diuretics, and it has been suggested that edema can be reproduced in susceptible individuals by the combination of diuretic withdrawal and "binge" eating of carbohydrate and sodium after a period of near-fasting [7].

Other Forms of Edema

Other forms of generalized edema occur. These forms, which are usually mild in severity and often warrant no specific treatment, are listed in Table 3.

TREATMENT OF THE PATIENT WITH GENERALIZED EDEMA

In patients with generalized edema, a goal of therapy is often the management of the edema itself, even though edema is only a sign of an underlying condition. This section focuses on some of the measures that have been used in managing generalized edema.

Indications

In the management of edema, as in the management of any other condition, the physician must determine that the benefits of therapy outweigh its risks and complications. In many patients, generalized edema is mild and poses no major difficulty for the patient; in such cases, its management need not be a major therapeutic focus. In other patients, edema is so severe and disabling that it must be addressed as a major target of therapy, particularly if complications directly attributable to the edema itself are present. Table 4 lists some of these complications.

General Measures

Because generalized edema indicates a disturbance in sodium metabolism reflecting an underlying primary disease (usually cardiac, liver, or renal disease), the management of edema must be regarded as only symptomatic therapy, and the physician must direct attention toward the management of the underlying disease itself in an effort to get at the root cause of the edema formation. Often, this requires consultation with the appropriate specialist; a full discussion of this management is beyond the scope of this chapter.

In cardiac failure, inotropic agents and preload- and afterload-reducing drugs are the main pharmacologic tools for improving left ventricular function. Angiotensin-converting enzyme (ACE) inhibitors may have particular benefit in this setting because of the activation of the renin-angiotensin-aldosterone system in heart failure: in addition to exerting favorable effects on preload and afterload, ACE inhibitors improve renal hemodynamics and may thereby potentiate the effect of diuretics in heart failure [8]. They also appear to be effective in improving survival. The management of chronic liver disease offers fewer options, and the major goal of therapy is to stabilize this condition, chiefly by behavioral modifi-

TABLE 3 OTHER FORMS OF GENERALIZED EDEMA	
Type	**Comments**
Cyclic edema	Can develop in women of childbearing age just before the monthly menstrual period; is self-limited and does not require treatment other than counseling; can be confused with idiopathic edema
Myxedema	Is the characteristic brawny edema that resists pitting; develops in patients with hypothyroidism
Edema due to the use of vasodilators	Results from sodium retention (with agents such as minoxidil and hydralazine) and may also result from altered capillary permeability (with nifedipine and possibly other calcium channel blockers of the dihydropyridine class); usually requires the addition of a diuretic to the therapeutic regimen
Edema of pregnancy	Is rarely a problem for the general internist, but its treatment often benefits from a nephrology consultation
Capillary leak syndrome	Develops in critically ill patients who are usually septic
Inferior vena cava obstruction	Rarely causes generalized edema
Protein-losing enteropathy	Rarely causes generalized edema

cation to eliminate alcohol intake in patients with alcoholic cirrhosis. Promising therapies for chronic hepatitis are being developed. The management of nephrotic edema offers a wider array of approaches, including disease-specific interventions such as the administration of glucocorticoids, immunosuppressive agents, and antiplatelet drugs, and nonspecific measures such as a modest restriction of dietary protein intake (0.8 g/kg/24h) and the use of ACE inhibitors. These latter measures reduce the severity of the proteinuria and may thereby facilitate the management of the edema; they may also arrest or retard the progressive renal insufficiency that accompanies many forms of nephrotic syndrome [9].

In addition to the management of the underlying disease, several other measures have general applicability in the management of edema. Bed rest has long been recognized as an adjunc-

tive treatment of edema, presumably because of the reduction in antinatriuretic stimuli associated with upright posture and, in patients with heart failure, the lowered demand on cardiac output. However, in most cases, it is too impractical to be very useful. Restriction of dietary sodium intake is another measure of general utility in the management of edema. Theoretically, if sodium intake could be reduced to a level below the prevailing rate of sodium excretion, a negative sodium balance would ensue and the edema would clear. In practice, this is usually impossible to achieve. Most patients in the phase of avid sodium retention associated with edema formation excrete less than 10 mEq/d of sodium. Reducing sodium intake to this level can be accomplished only on a metabolic ward with strict supervision of dietary intake. More modest degrees of sodium restriction (30–50 mEq/d, which is equivalent to roughly 1.5–2 g of sodium) can be achieved in the outpatient setting by motivated, compliant patients, and this intake may be adequate to balance excretion in edematous patients with less avid sodium retention. However, in most patients, dietary restriction to this level retards but does not prevent further edema formation, and other measures are necessary to reduce its severity.

Diuretic administration is the mainstay of edema management and is used in virtually all forms of generalized edema. The three groups of diuretics most commonly used in the management of edema are presented in Table 5. In clinical practice, the milder-acting thiazide diuretics are usually the agents of first choice in approaching the management of edema with diuretics. It is rational to initiate therapy in cirrhosis with spironolactone because of the hyperaldosteronism that is usually associated with cirrhotic edema. The effective dose can be determined by monitoring urine sodium and potassium concentrations: when the sodium-to-potassium ratio rises above 1, inhibition of aldosterone's tubular action has been achieved [10]. Doses of up to 400 mg/d may be required. Spironolactone has also been shown to be effective in some nephrotic patients [11].

The potassium-sparing diuretics should not be used in patients with moderate to advanced renal insufficiency, nor

TABLE 5 SELECTED DIURETICS IN THE TREATMENT OF EDEMA

Class	Initial dose, *mg*	Maximum daily dose, *mg*	Duration of action, *h*
Thiazides			
Chlorothiazide	250	1000	6–12
Hydrochlorothiazide	25	100	6–12
Chlorthalidone	25	100	48
Metolazone	2.5	20	12–24
Loop diuretics			
Bumetanide	0.5	10	4–6
Ethacrynic acid	25	200	6–8
Furosemide	20	400	6–8
Potassium-sparing agents			
Amiloride	5	20	24
Spironolactone	25	400	48
Triamterene	50	300	6–12

should potassium supplements be administered with them, in order to reduce the risk of producing potentially serious hyperkalemia. However, the response to diuretic therapy varies from patient to patient depending on the stage of the disease and the pattern of tubular sodium reabsorption. Many patients with moderate to severe edema are unresponsive to thiazides or potassium-sparing agents and require more potent high-ceiling diuretics or combinations of agents acting at different nephron sites [8].

Because the renal sodium retention leading to edema formation may reflect the normal renal compensation to sensed circulatory inadequacy, diuretic therapy can be viewed as a pharmacologic interruption of a normal compensatory response. This contributes to the complications of diuretic administration on the one hand and to "escape" from the action of the diuretics on the other. Resistance to the diuretic's effects can occur for various reasons, including inadequate or ineffective treatment of the primary disease, delayed drug absorption (which may result from edematous gastrointestinal mucosa), and inadequate dosage [12]. However, escape most commonly reflects intravascular volume depletion with a decreased glomerular filtration rate and increased reabsorption of sodium at nephron sites proximal to the site of action of the diuretic.

Excess circulating antidiuretic hormone, aldosterone, or both may also contribute to enhanced tubular reabsorption of sodium and water. If renal plasma flow is sufficiently impaired, an inadequate amount of diuretic may be transported to the tubular cell. An older study indicated that reabsorption of up to 900 mL of ascites per day is possible in patients with liver disease undergoing diuretic treatment without causing an impairment in renal function [13]. Consequently, diuresis of the cirrhotic patient with no peripheral edema should not exceed this rate in order to avoid plasma volume depletion and worsened renal hypoperfusion. In nephrosis, the binding of furosemide by protein in the tubular fluid may interfere with its action; consequently, higher doses may be required [12].

A continuous intravenous infusion of bumetanide has been shown to have greater diuretic efficacy in patients with chronic renal failure than does the same total dose of drug given in intermittent intravenous injections [14]. Combination therapy consisting of a loop diuretic such as furosemide and a more distally acting drug such as metolazone may help to restore natriuresis in patients who have developed resistance to the loop agent alone [8].

Specific Measures

The plethora of treatments in addition to those outlined previously is testimony to the fact that general measures are not always effective in treating edema. Some of these additional treatments are listed in Table 6. Pleurocentesis and paracentesis can be used for the direct removal of edema fluid accumulated in thoracic and abdominal cavities. If no other treatment is provided at the same time, the fluid usually reaccumulates. The indications for these procedures are related to symptoms caused by them, although small volumes may be removed for diagnostic purposes.

Pleurocentesis should be undertaken when the pleural effusion is large and compromises respiration, either through the sense of dyspnea or through impairment of gas exchange by the compression of lung parenchyma. Paracentesis may be carried out for relief of tense ascites, which can also interfere with respiratory function by limiting diaphragmatic excursion. In the cirrhotic patient, paracentesis may have the added benefit of improving systemic hemodynamics. The elevated intra-abdominal pressure from tense ascites compresses the inferior vena cava and limits venous return to the heart. Removal of as little as 500 mL of ascites is sufficient to obviate this problem and improve cardiac filling pressures and output [15]. In recent years, large-volume paracentesis has gained favor in the management of intractable cirrhotic ascites [15,16]. With careful monitoring and aseptic technique, this approach does not lead to deteriorating renal function, particularly if it is accompanied by the concurrent infusion of albumin. However, because the fluid usually reaccumulates, paracentesis must be repeated periodically.

A number of plasma volume expansion maneuvers have been tried for the management of cirrhotic and nephrotic edema in an effort to correct the renal hypoperfusion state that may characterize these conditions. Plasma and hyperoncotic albumin infusions preferentially expand the plasma compartment while maintaining or increasing plasma oncotic pressure, and they may transiently improve renal function, even to the point of increasing sodium excretion. In the case of liver

---

TABLE 6 TREATMENT OF EDEMA

General measures
Treatment of the primary disease
Bed rest
Sodium restriction
Diuretic administration

Specific measures
Fluid removal
   Pleurocentesis (heart failure, cirrhosis, nephrosis)
   Paracentesis (heart failure, cirrhosis, nephrosis)
Plasma volume expansion
   Infusion of plasma or hyperoncotic albumin solutions (cirrhosis, nephrosis)
   Ascitic fluid reinfusion (cirrhosis)
   Insertion of a peritoneovenous shunt (cirrhosis)
   Head-out water immersion (cirrhosis, nephrosis)
Pharmacologic therapy
   Vasodilators (heart failure)
   Angiotensin-converting enzyme inhibitors (heart failure, nephrosis)
   Vasoconstrictors (cirrhosis)
Continuous arteriovenous hemofiltration (heart failure, nephrosis)

Adapted from Gines *et al.* [1•]; with permission.

disease, fresh frozen plasma infusions may also provide depleted clotting factors. However, this approach has limited utility in the management of edema. The infusions are expensive, and their effects on renal function are at best transient; moreover, they have no effect on the underlying disease process. In addition, the portal pressure in cirrhotic patients is higher after volume expansion [17], increasing the risk for gastrointestinal bleeding, and the infused protein is rapidly excreted into the urine in nephrotic patients. For these reasons, alternative approaches to volume expansion therapy have been advocated.

In cirrhotic patients, ascitic fluid reinfusion reduces the volume of ascites and restores it to the plasma compartment. This technique has improved renal function and promoted natriuresis in the short term, particularly if it is accompanied by the administration of high-ceiling diuretics. However, this cumbersome procedure, which has a high risk of infection and sepsis, air embolism, and activation of the clotting system, is no longer carried out, particularly because large-volume paracentesis is an acceptable alternative in the management of intractable ascites. A method of chronic ascitic fluid infusion is achieved with the surgical insertion of a peritoneovenous (LeVeen) shunt. Tubing containing a one-way valve is placed with one end in the peritoneal cavity. It is tunneled subcutaneously, and the other end is inserted into the right atrium through the internal jugular vein. Whenever intra-abdominal pressure exceeds right atrial pressure, ascitic fluid is delivered by this route into the bloodstream.

Although the initial, uncontrolled experience with this technique was favorable in the management of intractable ascites, data from controlled studies have not indicated a clear-cut utility of the technique, particularly in view of the high percentage of shunt failure, sepsis, and activation of the clotting cascade. A controlled trial comparing shunting with repeated paracentesis found no differences in the morbidity and survival rates between these two approaches to the management of ascites [18].

Head-out water immersion, in which the patient is immersed to the neck in a tub of thermoindifferent water for 4 or 5 hours, is another form of central blood volume expansion that has been used in treating cirrhotic and nephrotic edema. The water pressure redistributes blood volume from the periphery to the great veins of the thorax, thereby correcting sensed underfilling and reflexly acting on the kidneys to lead to natriuresis. Although the increase in sodium excretion during immersion is impressive, patients revert to their avid sodium-retaining state after they come out of the immersion tub. The benefit is thus only transitory, and no report to date has commented on the use of this technique in the long-term management of edema. Rather, its utility lies in the ability to explore some of the pathophysiologic mechanisms that lead to sodium retention and edema formation in these conditions.

Pharmacologic therapy (in addition to diuretic use) has been used in the management of edema. The agents used include both vasocontrictor and vasodilator compounds, as well as agents to inhibit renin secretion or angiotensin II production. With the notable exception of the use of afterload- and preload-reducing agents in the treatment of congestive heart failure, this approach has resulted in only limited benefit in the management of edema [8].

The technique of continuous arteriovenous hemofiltration affords a means of fluid removal over the short term in patients with congestive heart failure. Extracorporeal circulation is used, and arterial blood pressure provides the force for the ultrafiltration of plasma water through a semipermeable membrane contained in a small cartridge. Ultrafiltration rates can be extremely high with this system. Its major drawback is the requirement for an extracorporeal circuit, but it can be used to assist volume control until other measures improve cardiac function sufficiently to allow the native kidneys to resume their homeostatic function. It has also been advocated in the management of severe nephrotic edema. It is obviously reserved for desperate situations and is carried out, usually in the critical care setting, by an experienced nephrologist.

REFERENCES AND RECOMMENDED READING

Recently published papers of particular interest have been highlighted as:
• Of interest
•• Of outstanding interest

1.• Gines P, Humphreys MH, Schrier RW: Edema. In *Textbook of Nephrology*, edn 3. Edited by Massry SG, Glassock RJ. Baltimore: Williams & Wilkins; 1995: 582–589.

2. Schrier RW: Pathogenesis of sodium and water retention in high-output and low-output cardiac failure, nephrotic syndrome, cirrhosis, and pregnancy. *N Engl J Med* 1988, 319:1065–1072, 1127–1134.

3. Papadakis MA, Arieff AI: Unpredictability of clinical evaluation of renal function in cirrhosis. *Am J Med* 1987, 82:945–952.

4 Martin P-Y, Schuer RW: Pathogenesis of water and sodium retention in cirhosis. *Kidney Int* 1997, 51:(suppl 59):S-43-S-49.

5.• Humphreys MH: Mechanisms and management of nephrotic edema. *Kidney Int* 1994, 45:266–281.

6. MacGregor GA, de Wardener HE: Idiopathic edema. In *Diseases of the Kidney*, edn 6. Edited by Schrier RW, Gottschalk CW. Boston: Little, Brown; 1997:2343–2351.

7. Macgregor GA, Roulston JE, Markandu ND, *et al.*: Is "idiopathic" oedema idiopathic? *Lancet* 1979, i:397–400.

8. Abraham WT, Schrier RW: Edematous disorders: pathophysiology of renal sodium and water retention and treatment with diuretics. *Curr Opin Nephrol Hypertens* 1993, 2:798–805.

9. de Zeeuw D, Apperloo AJ, de Jong P: Management of chronic renal failure. *Curr Opin Nephrol Hypertens* 1992, 1:116–123.

10. Eggert RC: Spironolactone diuresis in patients with cirrhosis and ascites. *Br Med J* 1970, 4:401–403.

11. Shapiro M, Hasbargen J, Hensen J, Schrier RW: Role of aldosterone in the sodium retention of patients with nephrotic syndrome. *Am J Nephrol* 1990, 10:44–48.

12. Brater DC: Resistance to diuretics: mechanisms and clinical implications. *Adv Nephrol* 1993, 22:349–369.

13. Shear L, Ching S, Gabuzda GJ: Compartmentalization of ascites and edema in patients with hepatic cirrhosis. *N Engl J Med* 1970, 282:391–396.

14. Rudy DW, Voelker JR, Greene PK, *et al.*: Loop diuretics for chronic renal insufficiency: a continuous infusion is more effective than bolus therapy. *Ann Intern Med* 1991, 115:360–366.

15. Simon DM, McCain JR, Bonkovsky HL, *et al.*: Effects of therapeutic paracentesis of systemic and hepatic hemodynamics and on renal and hormonal function. *Hepatology* 1987, 7:423–429.

16. Kellerman PS, Linas SL: Large-volume paracentesis in treatment of ascites [editorial]. *Ann Intern Med* 1990, 112:889–891.

17. Boyer JL, Chatterjee C, Iber FL, Basu AK: Effect of plasma-volume expansion on portal hypertension. *N Engl J Med* 1966, 275:750–755.

18. Gines P, Arroyo V, Vargas V, *et al.*: Paracentesis with intravenous infusion of albumin as compared with peritoneovenous shunting in cirrhosis with refractory ascites. *N Engl J Med* 1991, 325:829–835.

SELECT BIBLIOGRAPHY

Seldin DW, Giebisch G: *Diuretic Agents: Clinical Physiology and Pharmacology.* Academic Press; 1997.

Seldin DW, Giebisch G, eds.: *The Regulation of Sodium and Chloride Balance.* New York: Raven Press; 1990.

Staub NC, Taylor AE, eds.: *Edema.* New York: Raven Press; 1984.

DeSanto NG, Capasso G, Papalia T, De Napoli N: Edema: pathophysiology and therapy. *Kidney Int* 1997, 51(59).

Risk Factors for and Prevention of Atherosclerotic Cardiovascular Disease 12

Pantel S. Vokonas
William B. Kannel

> ### Key Points
> - Atherosclerotic cardiovascular disease (CVD), in all its clinical manifestations, represents the leading cause of disability and mortality throughout much of the industrialized world.
> - Epidemiologic studies have identified several important risk factors for CVD including hypertension, hyperlipidemia, cigarette smoking, diabetes, obesity, and physical inactivity.
> - Cardiovascular risk is assessed in the outpatient setting using standard clinical procedures and simple laboratory tests followed by appropriate measures to modify relevant factors.
> - Information available from intervention studies has already validated the efficacy and safety of preventive management of several risk factors in reducing the toll of CVD in the population.

Atherosclerotic cardiovascular disease (CVD) encompasses a broad spectrum of disease conditions of the heart and circulation that include coronary heart disease (CHD), cerebrovascular disease, and peripheral vascular disease (PVD). Because congestive heart failure often shares antecedents of atherosclerotic and hypertensive heart disease, it is also included under the heading of CVD.

The incidence of almost all cardiovascular events increases dramatically with advancing age (Fig. 1), serving to emphasize the heavy toll of disability and death attributable to CVD throughout life as well as the need for preventive attention for persons of all ages.

Because these conditions represent leading causes of morbidity and mortality in the United States and throughout much of the industrialized world, a working knowledge of risk factors for CVD and potential benefits of their modification on the part of primary care physicians and other health care professionals would make an important contribution to the future clinical and preventive management of this constellation of diseases.

RISK FACTORS FOR CARDIOVASCULAR DISEASE

Evidence from epidemiologic investigations indicates that a number of identifiable factors are associated with enhancement or acceleration of the underlying atherosclerotic process [1] and thus, contribute to the development of clinical manifestations of CVD. This represents the central concept of the so-called risk-factor hypothesis, which constitutes the mainstay of modern cardiovascular prevention.

In this context, advanced age and male gender are two of the most important such risk factors; however, both factors are considered irremediable. Attention, therefore, focuses on attributes that can be potentially modified. These factors can be broadly classified in two categories: 1) atherogenic personal traits such as hypertension, hyperlipidemia, and glucose intolerance; or 2) lifestyle influences

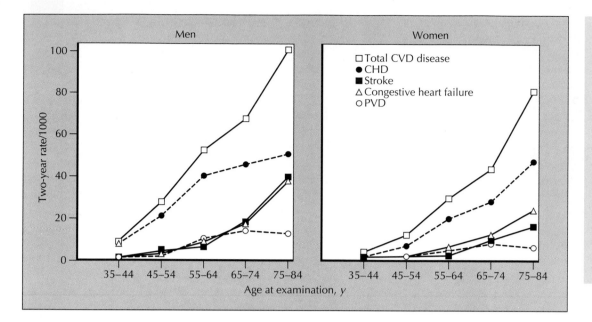

FIGURE 1 Age trends in incidence of total cardiovascular disease (CVD) and component CVD outcomes including coronary heart disease (CHD), stroke, congestive heart failure, and peripheral vascular disease (PVD) for men and women. Framingham Study, 26-year follow-up.

such as smoking, physical inactivity, and dietary patterns. Several well-established risk factors for CVD are considered in detail below.

Blood Pressure and Hypertension

Although conventional clinical wisdom emphasizes hypertensive risk related to elevations of diastolic blood pressure (diastolic hypertension), evidence from Framingham and other studies indicates an equal if not more potent risk for CVD associated with elevations of systolic blood pressure [2]. This is particularly relevant in older persons in whom progressive vascular stiffening results in significant elevations of systolic blood pressure and high prevalence of isolated systolic hypertension.

Relations between CVD occurrence and systolic and diastolic components of blood pressure are illustrated in Figures 2 and 3, respectively. Absolute risk, based on CVD incidence rates, is usually two to three times higher in older persons at corresponding levels of blood pressure, and tends to be higher in men than in women.

Risk gradients for CVD are generally similar in direction and magnitude when individuals are classified according to hypertensive status instead of absolute levels of blood pressure (Table 1). Overall risk of CVD tends to be two to three times higher in subjects with definite hypertension than in normotensive subjects, whereas risk is intermediate for those patients with mild hypertension. Similar patterns of risk attributable to hypertension have been documented specifically for CHD, stroke, congestive heart failure, and PVD (Table 2). When considered alone, isolated systolic hypertension also confers substantial risk of CVD events.

Previous data from randomized clinical trials have established a strong case for the efficacy of treating combined elevations of systolic and diastolic blood pressure in hypertensive patients at all ages, although considerable uncertainty remained regarding the treatment of isolated systolic hypertension. The findings of the Systolic Hypertension in the Elderly Program (SHEP) [3] and other studies [4••], however, have served to dispel much of this uncertainty.

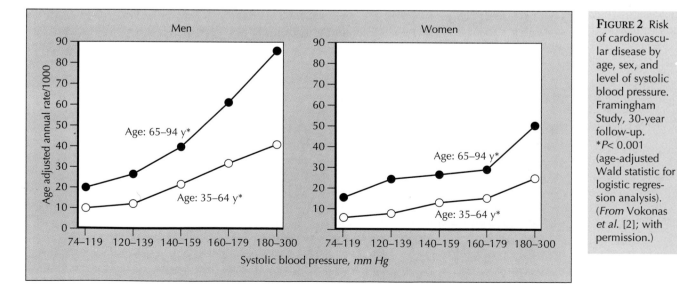

FIGURE 2 Risk of cardiovascular disease by age, sex, and level of systolic blood pressure. Framingham Study, 30-year follow-up. *$P< 0.001$ (age-adjusted Wald statistic for logistic regression analysis). (*From* Vokonas et al. [2]; with permission.)

In addition to substantial reductions in cerebrovascular events and congestive heart failure, the majority of such studies performed in older persons to date have consistently demonstrated beneficial trends or significant reductions in CHD events and mortality. Such results appear to be considerably less apparent in clinical therapeutic trials in predominantly middle-aged hypertensive patients [4••].

Blood Lipids

Abnormalities of blood lipids represent well-established risk factors for at least two components of CVD, namely CHD and PVD. Regarding CHD, evidence from population studies indicate that overall incidence rates for CHD correlate well with serum total cholesterol levels [5,6,7,8••]. The character of this relation further suggests that a change in serum choles-

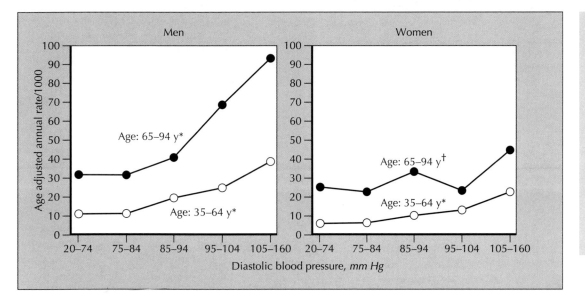

FIGURE 3 Risk of cardiovascular disease by age, sex, and level of diastolic blood pressure. Framingham Study, 30-year follow-up. *$P < 0.001$, †$P < 0.05$ (age-adjusted Wald statistic for logistic regression and analysis. *From* Vokonas *et al.* [2]; with permission.)

TABLE 1 RISK OF CARDIOVASCULAR DISEASE BY HYPERTENSIVE STATUS ACCORDING TO AGE AND SEX: FRAMINGHAM STUDY, 30-YEAR FOLLOW-UP

	Average annual age-adjusted rate per 1000, CVD			
	35–64 y*		65–94 y*	
Hypertensive status	Men	Women	Men	Women
Normal (<140/90 mm Hg)	11	5	22	19
Mild (140–160/90–95 mm Hg)	20	10	40	26
Definite (>160/95 mm Hg)	31	17	73	35

*All trends significant at $P<0.001$.
From Vokonas *et al.* [2]; with permission.

TABLE 2 RISK OF CARDIOVASCULAR EVENTS BY HYPERTENSIVE STATUS: FRAMINGHAM STUDY, 30-YEAR FOLLOW-UP

	Age-adjusted risk ratio*			
	35–64 y		65–94 y	
Cardiovascular event	Men	Women	Men	Women
Coronary heart disease	2.6§	3.3§	2.9§	2.0§
Stroke	6.0§	3.0§	3.1§	3.0§
Peripheral vascular disease	2.5§	3.0§	1.5	1.7‡
Congestive heart failure	3.0§	3.0§	3.8§	2.0§
CVD†	2.8§	3.4§	3.3§	1.8§

*Ratio of definite hypertension: normotension; hypertension defined as blood pressure greater than 160/95 mm Hg.
†In persons free of any CVD at the initial visit: ‡$P<0.05$, §$P<0.001$, hypertensives versus normotensives.
From Kannel *et al.* [14]; with permission.

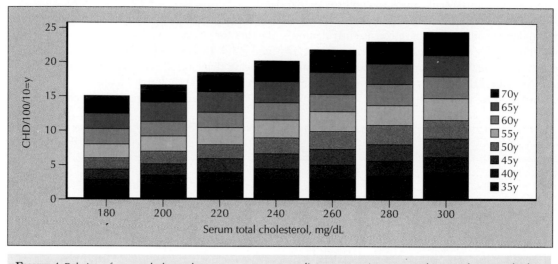

FIGURE 4 Relation of serum cholesterol to coronary heart disease (CHD) in men who have systolic blood pressures of 120 mm Hg or less, no diabetes, no left ventricular hypertrophy as determined by electro-cardiogram, no cigarette smoking, and average high-density lipoprotein cholesterol levels at 45 mg/dL. (*Adapted from* Castelli *et al.* [7]; with permission.) *Data from* Anderson *et al.* [28].)

terol of 1% corresponds to a directionally similar change in CHD incidence of approximately 2%. Data from the Framingham Study that illustrate this relation for men and women at varying ages are shown in Figures 4 and 5.

Although useful in screening large populations for dyslipidemias, serum cholesterol cannot be considered the sole measure of risk for CHD attributable to serum lipids. This is based on our current understanding of lipoprotein cholesterol subfractions and the availability of standardized laboratory methods to measure them in clinical practice [8••]. Serum total cholesterol tends to index low-density-lipoprotein (LDL) cholesterol, which varies directly with CHD risk (Fig. 6) and is considered atherogenic. High-density-lipoprotein (HDL) cholesterol varies inversely with CHD incidence (Fig. 7) and is considered anti-atherogenic

or protective. This lipid moiety adds substantial precision in assessing coronary risk at limited additional cost. Construction of a serum cholesterol–to-HDL ratio provides a highly accurate characterization of CHD risk in subjects of the Framingham Study, as illustrated in Figure 8. Indeed, additional data from Framingham and other studies confirm the overall reliability of the cholesterol/HDL ratio in assessing CHD risk in younger and older persons, and also in men and women. The rationale for this approach is that the ratio reliably captures the effect of a dynamic equilibrium of lipid transport into and out of body tissues, possibly including the intima of blood vessels.

Data from several studies, including the Framingham Study, suggest that serum triglycerides may be important predictors for CHD in men or women, but not consistently in

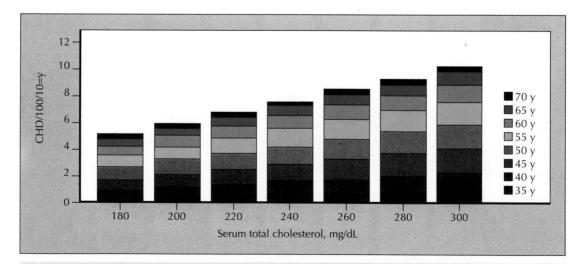

FIGURE 5 Relation of serum cholesterol to coronary heart disease (CHD) in women with systolic blood pressures of 120 mm Hg or less, no diabetes, no left ventricular hypertrophy as determined by electrocar-diogram, no cigarette smoking, and average high-density lipoprotein cholesterol levels at 55 mg/dL. (*Adapted from* Castelli *et al.* [7]; with permission. *Data from* Anderson *et al.* [28].)

both sexes. Despite these observations, the current consensus holds that elevated levels of serum triglycerides represent a risk marker for obesity, glucose intolerance, and low HDL levels, all of which confer risk for CHD and, to the extent possible, deserve preventive attention [9].

Data from intervention studies using dietary or drug therapy demonstrate the benefit of lipid alteration in reducing risk of CHD events [8••,10••]. Because nearly all such investigations have been conducted in middle-aged men, considerable uncertainty remains regarding the efficacy and safety of such

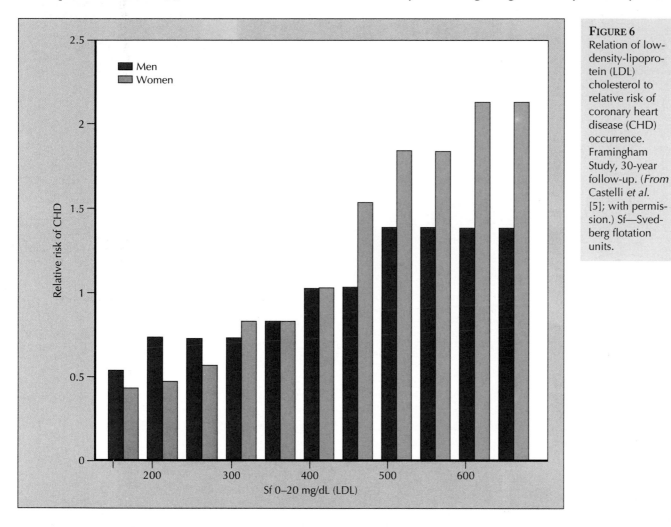

FIGURE 6
Relation of low-density-lipoprotein (LDL) cholesterol to relative risk of coronary heart disease (CHD) occurrence. Framingham Study, 30-year follow-up. (*From* Castelli *et al.* [5]; with permission.) Sf—Svedberg flotation units.

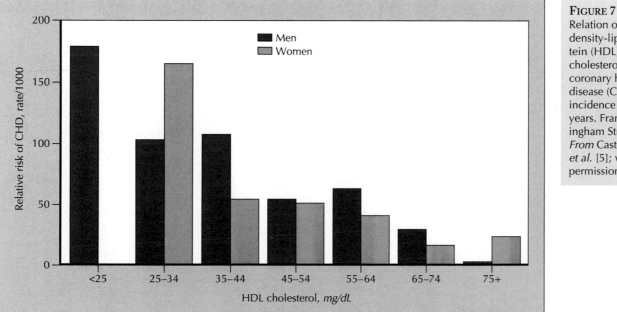

FIGURE 7
Relation of high-density-lipoprotein (HDL) cholesterol to coronary heart disease (CHD) incidence in 4 years. Framingham Study. *From* Castelli *et al.* [5]; with permission.)

Risk Factors for and Prevention of Atherosclerotic Cardiovascular Disease

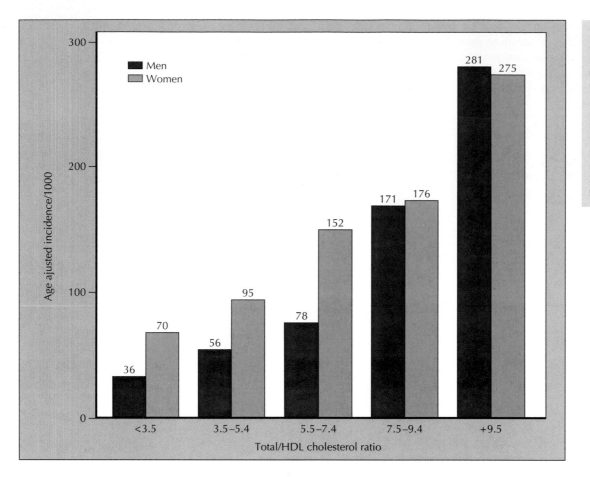

FIGURE 8 Risk of coronary heart disease (CHD) by total to high-density lipoprotein (HDL) cholesterol ratios among men and women 50 to 90 years of age. Framingham Study, 26-year follow-up.

measures in women and in older persons of both sexes. Information from two recent large clinical trials, however, makes a compelling case for reducing elevated or even average levels of LDL cholesterol with drugs in patients with established angina pectoris or following myocardial infarction (MI) [11••,12••]. These effects of drug therapy in the secondary prevention of CHD events, *ie*, in persons with pre-existing CHD, appear to be beneficial irrespective of age in both sexes. Current management of hyperlipidemia in a person considered to be at risk therefore, should consist of a highly individualized approach beginning with appropriate dietary measures and weight control before initiating a trial of specific drug therapy to achieve a carefully monitored lipid-lowering effect. Details regarding the treatment of dyslipidemias appear elsewhere in this volume.

Cigarette Smoking

Carbon monoxide derived from cigarette smoke reduces the oxygen-carrying capacity of hemoglobin. In addition, nicotine and other substances are known to exert potent effects on vascular smooth muscle and blood platelets, possibly initiating thrombotic events in persons whose circulation has already been compromised by underlying atherosclerosis [13•]. Smoking is also suspected of triggering ventricular arrhythmias, resulting in sudden death in vulnerable persons presumably by enhancing sympathetic tone and reducing the threshold to ventricular fibrillation.

Data from Framingham and other studies are quite consistent with the effects of such mechanisms and actually docu-

ment strong risk associations between cigarette smoking and an array of CVD outcomes including CHD (Fig. 9), stroke, PVD, and death [14,15].

Glucose Tolerance and Diabetes Mellitus

A number of clinical measures are employed in the Framingham Study to identify impaired glucose tolerance, nearly all of which demonstrate significant risk associations with CVD [15]. These measures include blood glucose levels, glycosuria, and the composite risk categories designated as glucose intolerance and diabetes mellitus. Although diabetes mellitus confers enhanced risk in men, overall risk increases dramatically for younger and older women. Similar patterns of risk are noted specifically for CHD, stroke, and PVD as well as coronary and cardiovascular mortality. Diabetes also emerges as an important risk factor in the development of congestive heart failure, particularly in older women with insulin-dependent diabetes mellitus. Presumably, the microvascular disease unique to diabetes, as well as other mechanisms, serves to produce progressive damage to heart muscle, ultimately resulting in compromised ventricular function and heart failure.

There is limited evidence that control of hyperglycemia by oral hypoglycemic agents or insulin effectively forestalls the development or complications of CVD, although encouraging trends in this regard were identified in the recently completed Diabetes Control and Complications Trial [16]. Available information would, therefore, continue to support the concept that there is more to be gained in reducing risk by correcting associated cardiovascular risk factors in persons with diabetes than by attention confined to early detection and control of hyperglycemia.

Left Ventricular Hypertrophy

Left ventricular hypertrophy as determined by the electro-cardiogram emerges as a strong risk factor for CHD in both sexes. Modest increases in CHD incidence are noted for voltage criteria for LVH alone with marked additional risk conferred by definite LVH which, in addition to voltage criteria, includes repolarization (ST and T wave) abnormalities consistent with LVH. These ECG findings presumably reflect derangements of myocardial structure and function related to early compromise of the underlying coronary circulation that appear before the development of clinical manifestations of CHD [17•].

In this context, LVH (LV mass) as determined by cardiac echocardiography has emerged as an extremely potent independent predictor of CHD as well as other CVD events, especially in older persons [18].

Body Weight

Progressive increases in body weight resulting in obesity represent important risk factors for CVD in men and women at all ages. Increases in body weight translate into directionally similar changes in several risk factors considered to be more directly related to the pathogenesis of atherosclerosis than obesity [19]. These include increases in blood pressure, serum cholesterol and triglycerides, and blood glucose. The exception is HDL cholesterol, which varies inversely with body weight. Recent data from Framingham and other studies, however, document the independent contribution of obesity in the development of CVD and its component outcomes [15,20]. Such observations serve to emphasize the need to incorporate measures ultimately designed to control or, if necessary, to gradually reduce body weight as part of comprehensive risk management. When coupled with appropriate dietary measures, weight control is particularly useful in the initial management of patients with hypertension, dyslipidemia, and diabetes or combinations of these conditions.

Recent studies also indicate that character of fat distribution is as important as total adiposity in conferring risk for developing CVD. Thus, the pattern of increased abdominal or truncal obesity, which appears to be closely related to the phenomenon of insulin resistance, is also associated with hypertension, hyperlipidemia, and glucose intolerance, all factors that enhance CVD risk [21••].

Physical Activity

Accumulating evidence now suggests that lifetime vigorous physical activity may forestall CHD in men, although similar evidence is not yet available for women [22,23]. Previously reported data from the Framingham Study indicating that overall mortality (including coronary mortality) was inversely related to level of physical activity in middle-aged men support these findings. Although a program of regular physical activity coupled with appropriate dietary and weight-control measures should be strongly encouraged for

persons of all ages, it would be unwise to place undue emphasis on this approach alone in attempting to reduce the risk for CVD.

Other Risk Factors

Several hematologic or hemostatic factors are described as risk variables in the Framingham Study. Hematocrit appeared to contribute to CVD in middle-aged men and women, but not in older persons [15]. White blood cell count—which is strongly correlated with the number of cigarettes smoked per day, hematocrit, and vital capacity—is also associated with enhanced risk for CVD in men (both smokers and nonsmokers), but only in women smokers [24]. These data are consistent with reports from other studies. Plasma fibrinogen showed strong risk associations for CVD in men similar to findings from other studies [25]. Significant risk associations, however, are not apparent in women.

An extensive array of psychosocial, occupational, dietary, and other factors are described as putative risk parameters for CVD in the Framingham Study; however, limited information is available regarding specific associations of these factors with CVD in young or older persons. A recent report characterized the independent contribution of parental history as a risk factor for CHD in the Framingham Study [26].

CARDIOVASCULAR RISK PROFILES

Although associations between a specific risk factor and CVD can be considered in isolation as a single relation, in

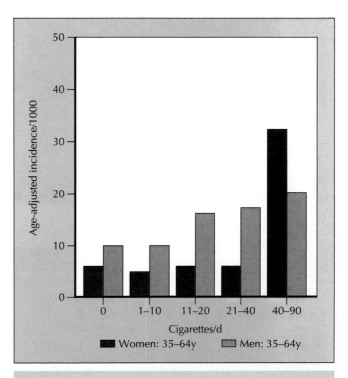
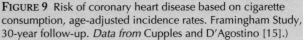

FIGURE 9 Risk of coronary heart disease based on cigarette consumption, age-adjusted incidence rates. Framingham Study, 30-year follow-up. *Data from* Cupples and D'Agostino [15].)

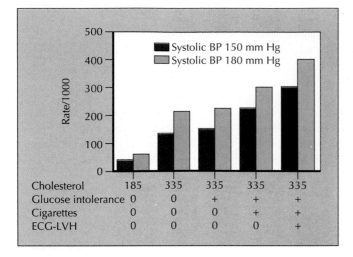

FIGURE 10 Risk of coronary heart disease in 8 years at systolic blood pressures (BPs) of 150 and 180 mm Hg according to the intensity of other factors, men 45 years of age. Framingham Study, 26-year follow-up. ECG-LVH—left ventricular hypertrophy as determined by electrocardiogram.

many instances combinations of several risk factors may constitute the observed risk profile. In such instances, risk of CVD can be reliably estimated by synthesizing a number of risk factors into a composite score, based on a multiple logistic function [27]. Risk factors are assessed by standard clinical procedures (smoking history, blood pressure, and ECG) and by routine laboratory studies (serum total cholesterol, HDL cholesterol, and blood glucose). This type of composite index permits detection of individuals at relatively high risk on the basis of marked elevation of a single factor or because of marginal abnormalities of several risk factors.

This multivariate risk scenario is illustrated in Figure 10, which characterizes the risk of CHD at two predefined levels of systolic blood pressure and then considers changes in the levels or values of other risk factors toward worsening risk. Note that CHD incidence increases progressively with the additional impact of other risk factors for both categories of blood pressure.

Specially prepared charts incorporating this multivariate approach can be used to assess risk in the clinical setting; Table 3 is used to predict the probability of CHD [28].

PERSPECTIVES FOR PRIMARY PREVENTION OF CARDIOVASCULAR DISEASE

Effective prevention of a specific disease or cluster of diseases such as CVD often requires two basic approaches, and primary care physicians can play important roles in implementing both. The first approach focuses on individuals identified to be at risk for CVD. These persons usually require additional assessment of risk factors, extensive counselling, and the initiation of appropriate measures to reduce the probability of CVD outcomes. Continued medical surveillance is necessary to maintain long-term control of operative risk factors. The objective is to delay or prevent the development of disease in that individual.

The second approach addresses a defined population. In this approach, community-based screening programs focus-ing on risk factors such as hypertension or hyperlipidemia are used to identify susceptible persons for individualized medical attention. Public education efforts and other techniques are employed to curb cigarette smoking and to encourage less atherogenic diets, regular exercise, and other beneficial measures. The objective with this approach is to shift the overall distribution of risk factors to one favoring a lower rate of occurrence of CVD in the population.

Such considerations are more relevant today than ever before. Recently, a marked and progressive decline in mortality due to CHD and CVD has occurred in the United States and several other industrialized nations. Age-specific trends indicate decreasing mortality due to CVD, including CHD and stroke, across the entire age span. Similar trends in cardiovascular mortality have been identified in the Framingham population [29]. At the same time, the prevalence of several CVD risk factors such as untreated hypertension, elevated serum cholesterol levels, and cigarette smoking has diminished in the general population, while impressive improvements have occurred in the diagnosis and treatment of CVD. Although the available information supports the contention that both of these potentially beneficial effects have contributed to the observed decline in mortality from CVD, the current consensus gives greater weight to the success of widespread primary preventive strategies, resulting in lowered levels of major risk factors that contribute to disease, rather than to improved diagnosis and treatment of established disease [30].

ACKNOWLEDGMENT

The authors thank Ms. Claire Chisholm for her invaluable assistance in preparing this manuscript. This work was supported by the Health Services Research and Development Service of the Department of Veterans Affairs, the Visiting Scientist Program of the Framingham Heart Study and grant nos. N01-HV-92922, N01-HV52971, and 5T32-HL-07374-13 of the National Institutes of Health.

TABLE 3 CORONARY HEART DISEASE RISK FACTOR PREDICTION TABLE

1. Find points for each risk factor

Age (if female)		Age (if male)		HDL-cholesterol		Total-cholesterol		Pressure			
Age (y)	n	Age (y)	n	HDL-C	n	Total-C	n	SBP	n	Other	n
30	-12	30	-2	25–26	7	139–151	-3	98–104	-2	Cigarettes	4
31	-11	31	-1	27–29	6	152–166	-2	105–112	-1	Diabetic–male	3
32	-9	32–33	0	30–32	5	167–182	-1	113–120	0	Diabetic–female	6
33	-8	34	1	33–35	4	183–199	0	121–129	1	ECG-LVH	9
34	-6	35–36	2	36–38	3	200–219	1	130–139	2		
35	-5	37–38	3	39–42	2	220–239	2	140–149	3	0 points for each NO	
36	-4	39	4	43–46	1	240–262	3	150–160	4		
37	-3	40–41	5	47–50	0	263–288	4	161–172	5		
38	-2	42–43	6	51–55	-1	289–315	5	173–185	6		
39	-1	44–45	7	56–60	-2	316–330	6				
40	0	46–47	8	61–66	-3						
41	1	48–49	9	67–73	-4						
42–43	2	50–51	10	74–80	-5						
44	3	52–54	11	81–87	-6						
45–46	4	55–56	12	88–96	-7						
47–48	5	57–59	13								
49–50	6	60–61	14								
51–52	7	62–64	15								
53–55	8	65–67	16								
56–60	9	68–70	17								
61–67	10	71–73	18								
68–74	11	74	19								

2. Sum points for all risk factors

$$\overline{\text{Age}} + \overline{\text{HDL-C}} + \overline{\text{Total-C}} + \overline{\text{SBP}} + \overline{\text{Smoker}} + \overline{\text{Diabetes}} + \overline{\text{ECG-LVH}} = \overline{\text{Point Total*}}$$

3. Look up risk corresponding to point total

	Probability			Probability	
n	5-y (%)	10-y (%)	n	5-y (%)	10-y (%)
≤1	<1	<2	17	6	13
2	1	2	18	7	14
3	1	2	19	8	16
4	1	2	20	8	18
5	1	3	21	9	19
6	1	3	22	11	21
7	1	4	23	12	23
8	2	4	24	13	25
9	2	5	25	14	27
10	2	6	26	16	29
11	3	6	27	17	31
12	3	7	28	19	33
13	3	8	29	20	36
14	4	9	30	22	38
15	5	10	31	24	40
16	5	12	32	25	42

4. Compare to average 10-y risk

	Probability	
Age (y)	Women (%)	Men (%)
30-34	<1	3
35-39	<1	5
40-44	2	6
45-49	5	10
50-54	8	14
55-59	12	16
60-64	13	21
65-69	9	30
70-74	12	24

These tables were prepared with the help of William B. Kannel, MD, Ralph D'Agostino, PhD, Keaven Anderson, PhD, Daniel McGee, PhD. Framingham Heart Study.

*Minus points subtract from total.

ECG-LVH—left ventricular hypertrophy as determined by electrocardiogram; HDL—high-density lipoprotein; SBP—systolic blood pressure.

From Anderson *et al.* [28]; with permission.

KEY REFERENCES

Recently published papers of outstanding interest, as identified in *References and Recommended Reading*, have been annotated.

•• Mulrow CD, Cornell JA, Herrera CR, *et al.*: Hypertension in the elderly: implications and generalizability of randomized trials. *JAMA* 1994, 272:1932–1938.

Outstanding review of nearly all significant randomized clinical trials of drug therapy for hypertension in elderly persons using meta-analytic methods to effect comparisons with similar studies in younger subjects. Results indicate that five-year morbidity and mortality benefits of drug therapy for hypertension are actually greater for older than younger subjects.

•• Levine GN, Keaney JF Jr, Vita JA: Cholesterol reduction in cardiovascular disease: clinical benefits and possible mechanisms. *N Engl J Med* 1995, 332:512–519.

Excellent review of complex interrelationships between hypercholesterolemia, atherosclerosis and endothelial dysfunction as well as the effects of cholesterol reduction by drug therapy in ameliorating these interactions and, in turn, reducing the rate of cardiovascular events.

•• Shepherd J, Cobbe SM, Ford I, *et al.*: for the West of Scotland Coronary Prevention Study Group. Prevention of coronary heart disease with pravastatin in men with hypercholesterolemia. *N Engl J Med* 1995, 333:1301–1307.

Important study in the primary prevention of CHD events. This clinical trial conducted in the West of Scotland randomized 6595 middle-aged men with hypercholesterolemia and no history of MI to receive either pravastatin or placebo. After an average follow-up period of nearly 5 years, there was a 31% reduction in definite coronary events (nonfatal MI or death attributed to CHD) in the active treatment compared to the placebo group. Of interest, there was no excess of deaths from noncardiovascular causes in the active treatment group. Such findings in prior studies, particularly those aimed at primary prevention of CHD, have raised concerns regarding the long-term safety of dietary and drug measures in reducing cholesterol in persons free of CHD.

•• Scandinavian Simvastatin Survival Study Group. Randomized trial of cholesterol lowering in 4444 patients with coronary heart disease: The Scandinavian Simvastatin Survival Study (4S). *Lancet* 1994, 344:1383–1389.

Important study in the secondary prevention of CHD events. This clinical trial randomized 4444 men and women with hypercholesterolemia and either angina pectoris or prior MI to simvastatin or placebo. After a median follow-up of 5.4 years, there were impressive reductions in all-cause mortality and multiple cardiovascular and CHD outcomes, including myocardial revascularization procedures, in the active treatment as compared to the placebo group. There was no excess of deaths due to noncardiovascular causes observed in this study. Of interest, subgroup analysis showed that older men and women benefited from simvastatin therapy to a similar degree as their younger counterparts.

•• Sacks FM, Pfeffer MA, Moye LA, *et al.*: for the Cholesterol and Recurrent Events Trial Investigators. The effects of pravastatin on coronary events after myocardial infarction in patients with average cholesterol levels. *N Engl J Med* 1996, 335:1001–1009.

This clinical trial has redefined the target level of cholesterol meriting therapeutic intervention particularly in patients following MI. A total of 4159 men and women with total cholesterol levels below 240 mg/dl were randomized to either pravastatin or placebo between 3 and 20 months following MI. After 5 years of follow-up, there was a 24% reduction in the primary end point (fatal coronary event or nonfatal MI) in the pravastatin as compared to the placebo group. The rate of myocardial revascularization procedures was also reduced in the active treatment group. There were no significant differences in either overall mortality or mortality from noncardiovascular causes between the two groups.

•• Reaven GM, Lithell H, Landsberg L: Hypertension and associated metabolic abnormalities: the role of insulin resistance and the sympathoadrenal system. *N Engl J Med* 1996, 334:374–381.

Comprehensive review of the role of insulin resistance in hypertension including the complex relationships between hypertension, hyperinsulinemia, glucose intolerance, and dyslipidemia that enhance risk for CHD.

REFERENCES AND RECOMMENDED READING

Recently published papers of particular interest have been highlighted as:
• Of interest
•• Of outstanding interest

1. Ross R: The pathogenesis of atherosclerosis: a perspective for the 1990s. *Nature* 1993, 362:801–809.
2. Vokonas PS, Kannel WB, Cupples LA: Epidemiology and risk of hypertension in the elderly: the Framingham Study. *J Hypertens* 1988, 8(suppl I):53–59.
3. SHEP Cooperative Research Group: Prevention of stroke by antihypertensive drug treatment in older persons with isolated systolic hypertension: final results of the Systolic Hypertension in the Elderly Program (SHEP). *JAMA* 1991, 265:3255–3264.
4.•• Mulrow CD, Cornell JA, Herrera CR, *et al.*: Hypertension in the elderly: implications and generalizability of randomized trials. *JAMA* 1994, 272:1932–1938.
5. Castelli WP, Wilson PW, Levy D, Anderson K: Cardiovascular risk factors in the elderly. *Am J Cardiol* 1989, 63:12H–19H.
6. Pikkanen J, Linn S, Heiss G, *et al.*: Ten-year mortality from cardiovascular disease in relation to cholesterol level among men with and without preexisting cardiovascular disease. *N Engl J Med* 1990, 322:1700–1707.
7. Castelli WP, Anderson K, Wilson PWF, *et al.*: Lipids and risk of coronary heart disease. The Framingham Study. *Ann Epidemiol* 1992, 2:23–28.
8. •• Levine GN, Keaney JF Jr, Vita JA: Cholesterol reduction in cardiovascular disease: clinical benefits and possible mechanisms. *N Engl J Med* 1995, 332:512–519.
9. Gotto AM Jr: Hypertriglyceridemia: risks and perspectives. *Am J Cardiol* 1992, 70:19H–25H.
10. •• Shepherd J, Cobbe SM, Ford I, *et al.*: for the West of Scotland Coronary Prevention Study Group: Prevention of coronary heart disease with pravastatin in men with hypercholesterolemia. *N Engl J Med* 1995, 333:1301–1307.
11.•• Scandinavian Simvastatin Survival Study Group: Randomized trial of cholesterol lowering in 4444 patients with coronary heart disease: The Scandinavian Simvastatin Survival Study (4S). *Lancet* 1994, 344:1383–1389.
12. •• Sacks FM, Pfeffer MA, Moye LA, *et al.*: for the Cholesterol and Recurrent Events Trial Investigators. The effects of pravastatin on coronary events after myocardial infarction in patients with average cholesterol levels. *N Engl J Med* 1996, 335:1001–1009.
13.• Muller JE, Abela GS, Nesto RW, *et al.*: Triggers, acute risk factors and vulnerable plaques: the lexicon of a new frontier. *J Am Coll Cardiol* 1994, 23:809–813.
14. Kannel WB, Higgins M: Smoking and hypertension as predictors of cardiovascular risk in population studies. *J Hypertens* 1990, 8(suppl 5):S3–S8.
15. Cupples LA, D'Agostino RB: Some risk factors related to the annual incidence of cardiovascular disease and death using pooled repeated biennial measurements: Framingham Heart Study, a 30-year follow-up. In *The Framingham Study: An Epidemiological Investigation of Cardiovascular Disease.* Edited by Kannel WB, Wolf PA, Garrison RJ: National Heart, Lung and Blood Institute; 1987: NIH Publication No. 87–2703.

16. Diabetes Control and Complications Trial Research Group: The effect of intensive treatment of diabetes in the development and progression of long-term complications in insulin-dependent diabetes mellitus. *N Engl J Med* 1993, 329:997–986.

17.• Levy D, Salomon M, D'Agostino RB, *et al.*:Prognostic implications of baseline electrocardiographic features and their serial changes in subjects with left ventricular hypertrophy. *Circulation* 1994, 90:1786–1793.

18. Levy D, Garrison RJ, Savage DD, *et al.*: Prognostic implications of echocardiographically determined left ventricular mass in the Framingham Heart Study. *N Engl J Med* 1990, 322:1561–1566.

19. Borkan GA, Sparrow D, Wisnieski C, *et al.*: Body weight and coronary risk: patterns of risk factor change associated with long-term weight change. The Normative Aging Study. *Am J Epidemiol* 1986, 124:410–419.

20. Manson JE, Colditz GA, Stampfer MJ, *et al.*: A prospective study of obesity and risk of coronary heart disease in women. *N Engl J Med* 1990, 322:882–889.

21.•• Reaven GM, Lithell H, Landsberg L: Hypertension and associated metabolic abnormalities: the role of insulin resistance and the sympathoadrenal system. *N Engl J Med* 1996, 334:374–381.

22. Berlin JA, Colditz GA: A meta-analysis of physical activity in the prevention of coronary heart disease. *Am J Epidemiol* 1990, 132:612–628.

23. Paffenbarger RS Jr, Hyde RT, Wing AL, *et al.*: The association of changes in physical activity level and other lifestyle characteristics with mortality among men. *N Engl J Med* 1993, 328:533–537.

24. Kannel WB, Anderson K, Wilson PWF: White blood cell count and cardiovascular disease. *JAMA* 1992, 267:1253–1256.

25. Ernst E: Fibrinogen: its emerging role as a cardiovascular risk factor. *Angiology* 1994, 45:87–93.

26. Myers RH, Kiely DK, Cupples LA, *et al.*: Parental history is an independent risk factor for coronary artery disease: The Framingham Study. *Am Heart J* 1990, 120:963–969.

27. Chambless LE, Dobson AJ, Patterson CC, *et al.*: On the use of a logistic risk score in predicting risk of coronary heart disease. *Stat Med* 1990, 9:385–396.

28. Anderson KM, Wilson PWF, Odell PM, *et al.*: An updated coronary risk profile. A statement for health professionals. *Circulation* 1991, 83:357–363.

29. Sytkowski PA, Kannel WB, D'Agostino RB: Changes in risk factors and the decline in mortality from cardiovascular disease. The Framingham Heart Study. *N Engl J Med* 1990, 322:1635–1641.

30. Goldman L: Cost-effectiveness perspectives in coronary heart disease. *Am Heart J* 1990, 119:733–739.

SELECT BIBLIOGRAPHY

Hunninghake DB: Diagnosis and treatment of lipid disorders. *Med Clin North Am* 1994, 78:247–257.

Pinkney JH, Yudkin JS: Antihypertensive drugs: issues beyond blood pressure control. *Prog Cardiovasc Dis* 1994, 36:397–415.

Schaefer EJ: New recommendations for the diagnosis and treatment of plasma lipid abnormalities. *Nutr Rev* 1993, 51:246–253.

Summary of the Second Report of the National Cholesterol Education Program (NCEP) Expert Panel on Detection, Evaluation, and Treatment of High Blood Cholesterol in Adults (Adult Treatment Panel II). *JAMA* 1993, 269:3015–3023.

The Fifth Report of the Joint National Committee on Detection, Evaluation, and Treatment of High Blood Pressure. National High Blood Pressure Education Program, National Heart, Lung, and Blood Institute; 1993: NIH Publication No. 93–1088.

The Effect of Exercise on the Heart and the Athlete's Heart

13

Barry A. Franklin
Gerald F. Fletcher

Key Points

- The maximal oxygen consumption or aerobic capacity is considered the best single index of cardiorespiratory fitness.
- Exercise training reduces the rate-pressure product at any given submaximal workrate; however, the effects of regular exercise on myocardial perfusion, regional wall motion abnormalities, and ejection fraction are less clear.
- Exercise may benefit the heart by favorably modifying many of the risk factors that are associated with the development of coronary artery disease.
- A low level of aerobic fitness has been shown to be a powerful and independent risk factor for cardiovascular and all-cause mortality.
- Pathophysiologic evidence suggests that the increased myocardial demands of vigorous exercise may precipitate cardiac arrest or acute myocardial infarction in persons with known or occult cardiovascular disease, especially if they are habitually sedentary.
- Endurance-trained athletes often demonstrate enhanced left ventricular dimension and performance, a significantly higher aerobic capacity compared with similarly aged control subjects, and electrocardiographic anomalies that are generally considered normal variants.

Exercise training appears to play an important role in the primary and secondary prevention of coronary artery disease (CAD). The salutary effects of chronic exercise training are well documented. Recent studies also suggest that exercise, when incorporated as part of an intensive multifactorial intervention, can stabilize or even reverse the otherwise inexorable progression of atherosclerotic CAD [1••,2].

There are, however, limitations to the benefits that exercise offers relative to the prevention and rehabilitation of patients with CAD. Contrary to the speculation of some observers [3], regular exercise training, regardless of the intensity, duration, or both, does not confer "immunity" to CAD [4]. Moreover, recent reports [5–7] suggest that vigorous physical activity may actually trigger cardiovascular events in persons with a diseased or susceptible heart.

This chapter reviews the physiologic effects of endurance exercise on the heart, with specific reference to cardiorespiratory fitness, cardiac function and pathophysiology, coronary risk factors, all-cause mortality, cardiovascular events, and the athlete's cardiovascular system.

CARDIORESPIRATORY FITNESS

Aerobic capacity, which is physiologically defined as the highest rate of oxygen transport and utilization achieved at peak effort, may be expressed in terms of a modification of the Fick equation: $\dot{V}O_2 = HR \times SV \times (CaO_2 - C\bar{v}O_2)$, where $\dot{V}O_2$ is somatic oxygen consumption in mL per minute, HR is heart rate in beats per minute, SV is stroke volume in mL per beat, and $(CaO_2 - C\bar{v}O_2)$ is the arteriovenous oxygen difference in mL of oxygen per dL of blood.

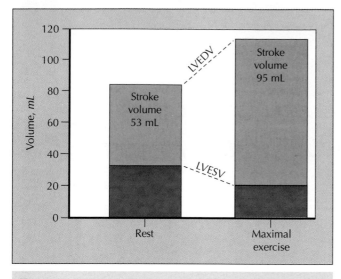

FIGURE 1 Changes in stroke volume from rest to maximal upright exercise are shown in young, healthy men. LVEDV—left ventricular end-diastolic volume; LVESV—left ventricular end-systolic volume. (*From* Poliner *et al.* [8].)

respectively. Interindividual variations in aerobic capacity are primarily due to marked differences in maximal cardiac output rather than the peripheral extraction of oxygen. Because there is little variation in maximal systemic arteriovenous oxygen difference with training, $\dot{V}O_2$max virtually defines the pumping capacity of the heart. Therefore, it is of major importance in the evaluation of cardiovascular disease.

Most exercise studies on persons with and without heart disease have demonstrated 10% to 30% increases in preconditioning values of $\dot{V}O_2$max, with the greatest improvements among the most unfit [9•]. The enhancement in $\dot{V}O_2$max is achieved by central or peripheral adaptations; the latter also provides a distinct hemodynamic advantage at submaximal and maximal exercise (Table 2). Because a given submaximal task or workrate requires a relatively constant aerobic requirement (mL/kg/min), the cardiac patient who has undergone an exercise training program works at a lower percentage of $\dot{V}O_2$max, with greater reserve.

For most deconditioned adults and patients with CAD, the threshold intensity for exercise training probably lies between 40% and 60% $\dot{V}O_2$max; however, considerable evidence suggests that it increases in direct proportion to the pretraining $\dot{V}O_2$max or level of habitual physical activity [10]. The interrelationship among the training intensity, frequency, and duration may permit a low to moderate training intensity to be quite effective through increases in the exercise frequency, duration, or both. Although it is widely believed that aerobic benefits from exercise accrue only from *continuous* workouts of 30 minutes or more, recent studies have shown similar improvements in cardiorespiratory fitness in subjects who completed three 10-minute bouts of moderate exercise on a workout day [11]. Thus, it appears that the improvement in $\dot{V}O_2$ max may depend more on the total amount of exercise accomplished or kilocalories expended than on the specific exercise frequency, intensity, or duration.

Within physiologic limits, enhanced venous return increases the heart's end-diastolic volume, stretching cardiac muscle fibers and increasing their force of contraction. During exercise there is an increase in ejection fraction resulting from both the Frank-Starling mechanism and a decreased end-systolic volume (Fig. 1) [8]. The latter is due to increased ventricular contractility, secondary to catecholamine-mediated sympathetic stimulation.

Typical circulatory data at rest and during maximal exercise in a healthy sedentary man, a patient with CAD, and a world-class endurance athlete are shown in Table 1. The 10-fold increase in oxygen consumption at maximal exercise ($\dot{V}O_2$max) in the sedentary man is contrasted by six- and 23-fold increases in the cardiac patient and endurance athlete,

TABLE 1 HYPOTHETICAL CIRCULATORY DATA AT REST AND DURING MAXIMAL EXERCISE FOR A SEDENTARY MAN, A PATIENT WITH HEART DISEASE, AND A WORLD-CLASS ENDURANCE ATHLETE

Condition	Oxygen consumption, L/min	mL/kg/min	Cardiac output, L/min	Heart rate, bpm	Stroke volume, mL/beat	Arteriovenous oxygen difference, mL/dL blood
Sedentary man (70 kg)						
Rest	0.25	3.5*	6.1	70	87	4.0
Maximal exercise	2.50	35.0	17.7	190	93	14.0
Cardiac Patient (70 kg)						
Rest	0.25	3.5*	6.1	82	74	4.0
Maximal exercise	1.50	21.5	10.4	165	66	13.6
World-class endurance athlete (70 kg)						
Rest	0.25	3.5*	6.1	45	136	4.0
Maximal exercise	5.60	80.0	35.0	190	184	16.0

*3.5 mL/kg/min = 1 metabolic equivalent; average resting metabolic rate expressed per unit body weight.

TABLE 2 MECHANISMS RESPONSIBLE FOR THE INCREASE OF $\dot{V}O_2MAX$ WITH PHYSICAL CONDITIONING

Central

Increased cardiac output and stroke volume at maximal exercise (predominantly normal patients)

Increased central blood volume and total hemoglobin

Peripheral

Increased size and number of skeletal muscle mitochondria

Increased myoglobin (increased O_2 storage)

Increased oxidative enzymes (*eg*, succinic dehydrogenase, cytochrome oxidase)

Increased skeletal muscle capillary density

The above peripheral mechanisms lead to:

Decreased cardiac output (decreased muscle blood flow) at a given submaximal workload

Increased CaO_2 - $C\bar{v}O_2$ at submaximal and maximal workrates

CaO_2 - $C\bar{v}O_2$—arteriovenous oxygen difference in mL O_2/dL blood;
 $\dot{V}O_2max$—maximal oxygen consumption.

CARDIAC FUNCTION: PATHOPHYSIOLOGY

The effects of chronic aerobic exercise training on the autonomic nervous system reduce myocardial demands at rest and during exercise, even when low-to-moderate training intensities are used [12]. Vagal tone appears to be increased at rest, whereas sympathoadrenergic drive (circulating catecholamines, particularly norepinephrine) is decreased during exercise [13]. The result is a reduction in the rate-pressure product at any given oxygen uptake or submaximal workrate, especially when the muscle groups used during training are employed (Fig. 2). [14]. Reduced myocardial demands presumably allow the cardiac patient to perform at a higher "symptom-limited" workload before reaching the reproducible rate-pressure product that evokes ischemic ST-segment depression, anginal symptoms (Fig. 3), or both.

The effects of physical conditioning on myocardial perfusion, regional wall motion abnormalities, and ejection fraction are less clear. However, limited data support the benefit of high-intensity exercise training in improving left ventricular ejection fraction in men with CAD [15•]. Studies describing changes in ventricular arrhythmias following exercise rehabilitation have also produced inconsistent results [1••]. Some investigators have used thallium exercise testing and multiple-gated image acquisition scans on subjects before and after exercise training programs to assess changes in cardiac function.

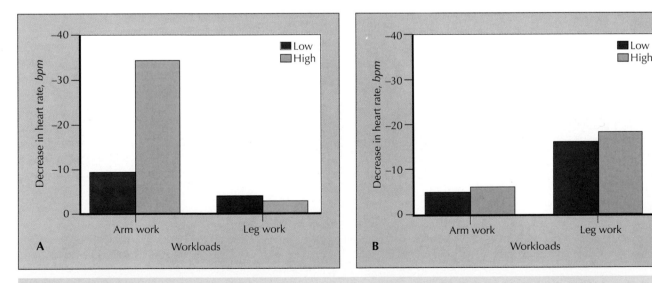

FIGURE 2 A, Arm training using a cycle ergometer markedly decreased the heart rate response during arm exercise at low and high workloads, whereas the heart rate reduction during leg work was small. **B**, Similarly, leg training markedly decreased the heart rate during leg work, whereas the heart rate reduction during arm work was minimal. (From Clausen *et al.* [14]; with permission.)

Although the findings have been generally unimpressive, modest improvements have been reported with and without vigorous exercise training regimens [10]. In contrast, angiographic studies in group trials have failed to confirm the appearance of new coronary collateral vessels following exercise training [16]. Today it is widely believed that the proliferation of collaterals often stems, at least in part, from a compromised

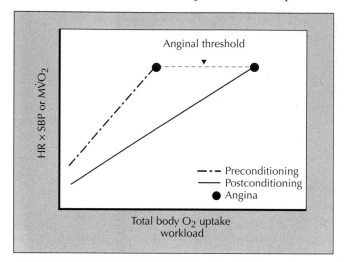

Anginal threshold

HR × SBP or MV̇O₂

— · — Preconditioning
——— Postconditioning
● Angina

Total body O₂ uptake
workload

FIGURE 3 Effect of physical conditioning on the heart rate times systolic blood pressure product (HR x SBP) and myocardial oxygen consumption (MV̇O₂) at submaximal and peak exercise. Peak body oxygen uptake and workload are augmented by exercise training. Myocardial oxygen requirements are reduced at a given workload or oxygen uptake, but angina occurs at the same HR x SBP product, indicating that the major mechanism of beneficial action of exercise therapy is reduction of MV̇O₂ rather than an increased myocardial oxygen supply.

coronary circulation secondary to the progression of CAD [17].

Improvements, if any, in coronary blood flow may perhaps be related to the conditioning bradycardia or reduced norepinephrine release at submaximal exercise. Because coronary blood flow predominates during diastole, coronary perfusion time is increased (Fig. 4). Thus, decreased heart rate with exercise training appears to play a critical role in patients with ischemic heart disease in view of the potential for increased coronary blood flow and reduced oxygen demands on the myocardium.

Exercise training as a sole intervention does not necessarily halt the progression of CAD or, for that matter, prevent restenosis or reinfarction. However, intensive multifactorial intervention (including exercise) can result in regression or limitation of progression of angiographically documented coronary atherosclerosis [1••]. One study [2], which included a low-fat, low-cholesterol diet (fat < 20% of energy; cholesterol < 200 mg/day) showed that a minimum of 1600 kcal per week of physical activity may halt the progression of CAD, whereas regression may be achieved with an energy expenditure of 2200 kcal per week (Fig. 5). For many patients, these goals would require walking 15 and 20 miles per week, respectively.

CORONARY RISK FACTORS

Regular exercise may indirectly benefit the heart by favorably modifying many of the risk factors that are associated with the development of CAD [9•,10,18••,19•]. Aerobic exercise training can promote modest decreases in body weight, fat stores, blood pressure (particularly in hypertensive patients) [20], total blood cholesterol, serum triglycerides, and low-density lipoprotein (LDL) cholesterol, and increases in the "antiatherogenic" high-density lipoprotein (HDL) cholesterol

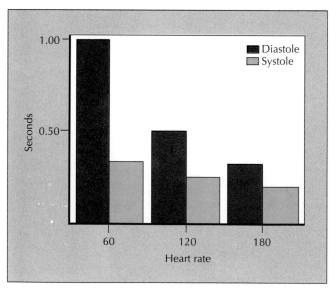

■ Diastole
□ Systole

Seconds

1.00
0.50

60   120   180
Heart rate

FIGURE 4 Relationship of systolic and diastolic time to heart rate. Since coronary blood flow predominates during diastole, with increased heart rate, as during exercise, diastolic (perfusion) time is disproportionately shortened. Reduction of heart rate at rest and during exercise becomes critical to the prevention of ischemia in patients with coronary artery disease.

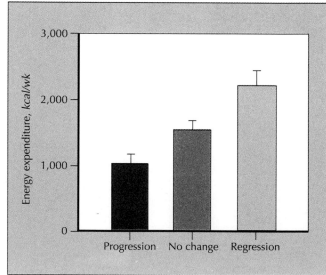

3,000

2,000

1,000

0

Energy expenditure, kcal/wk

Progression   No change   Regression

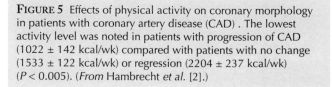

FIGURE 5 Effects of physical activity on coronary morphology in patients with coronary artery disease (CAD). The lowest activity level was noted in patients with progression of CAD (1022 ± 142 kcal/wk) compared with patients with no change (1533 ± 122 kcal/wk) or regression (2204 ± 237 kcal/wk) (*P* < 0.005). (*From* Hambrecht *et al.* [2].)

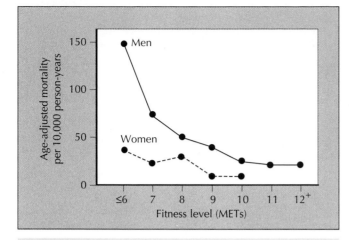

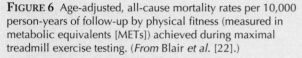

FIGURE 6 Age-adjusted, all-cause mortality rates per 10,000 person-years of follow-up by physical fitness (measured in metabolic equivalents [METs]) achieved during maximal treadmill exercise testing. (*From* Blair *et al.* [22].)

subfraction. Exercise-mediated reductions in total cholesterol and LDL cholesterol are greatest when concomitant body weight losses occur [21]. Diabetes mellitus may also be favorably affected by regular physical activity [9•,19•].

FITNESS AND MORTALITY

Recent studies [22,23•,24••,25•,26–28,29•] have shown that a low level of aerobic fitness is an independent risk factor for all-cause mortality. In one investigation [22] researchers prospectively studied 10,224 men and 3120 women who were given a preventive medical examination and a maximal treadmill exercise test to assess their aerobic fitness. Over an average follow-up period of slightly more than 8 years, 240 men and 43 women died. In general, the higher the initial level of fitness, the lower was the subsequent death rate from cancer and heart disease (Fig. 6). This was so even after statistical adjustments were made for age, coronary risk factors, and family history of heart disease. Moreover, there appeared to be no additional benefit (*ie*, lower mortality) associated with fitness levels higher than 9 to 10 metabolic equivalents (METs). For men,

the greatest reduction in risk occurred as one progressed from the lowest level of fitness (≤ 6 METs) to the next lowest level (7 METs), suggesting that even a modest improvement in fitness among the most unfit confers a substantial health benefit. The investigators concluded that the fitness levels associated with a plateau in death rates, 9 to 10 METs, can be attained by most men and women who walk briskly on a regular basis.

Subsequently, these investigators examined the relationship between changes in aerobic fitness and the risk of death in men [23•]. Participants were 9777 men (20 to 82 years of age) who were given two preventive medical examinations, which included an assessment of aerobic fitness by maximal exercise testing, about 5 years apart. Approximately 5 years after the second examination, deaths from all causes and from cardiovascular disease were determined. The highest death rate occurred in men who were unfit at both examinations (122.0/10,000 man-years); the lowest death rate was in men who were physically fit at both examinations (39.6/10,000 man-years). Men who improved from the *untrained* to the *trained* category between the first and second examinations had an intermediate death rate (67.7/10,000 man-years), even after adjustments were made for age, health status, and other risk factors. For each minute increase in treadmill test time between examinations, there was a corresponding 7.9% decrease in risk of mortality.

Recently Blair and coworkers [24••] reported the relative risk for all-cause mortality for several mortality predictors (Table 3), including low fitness (20% least trained). Untrained men and women were approximately twice as likely to die during an 8-year follow-up period compared with their exercised-trained counterparts. Moreover, the protective effect of training held for smokers and nonsmokers as well as for those with and without elevated cholesterol levels or hypertension. In a related analyses [25•], moderate-to-high trained men with a body mass index (BMI) greater than 30 kg/m² had approximately one third the age-adjusted death rate of lean (< 27 BMI) untrained men. Collectively, these findings and other recent reports [26–28,29•] support the hypothesis that regular physical activity improves health and delays death

Mortality predictor	Relative risk*	
	Men	Women
Low fitness (20% less fit)	2.03	2.23
Current or recent cigarette smoker	1.89	2.12
Systolic blood pressure ≥ 140 mmHg	1.67	0.89
Cholesterol ≥ 240 mg/dL	1.45	1.16
Body mass index ≥ 27 kg/m²	1.33	1.18

TABLE 3 RELATIVE RISK FOR ALL-CAUSE MORTALITY FOR SELECTED MORTALITY PREDICTORS, MEN AND WOMEN, AEROBICS CENTER LONGITUDINAL STUDY, 1970—1989

*Adjusted for age and examination year.
From Blair *et al.* [24••].

in persons with and without documented CAD. This effect seems to be especially important in those who exercise more vigorously and achieve higher levels of training capacity as evidenced by greater levels of $\dot{V}O_2$max [28].

CARDIOVASCULAR EVENTS

Pathophysiologic evidence suggests that the increased myocardial demands of vigorous exercise may precipitate cardiovascular events in persons with known or occult CAD. By increasing myocardial oxygen consumption and simultaneously shortening diastole and coronary perfusion time, exercise may evoke a transient oxygen deficiency in the subendocardial tissue, which may be exacerbated by a decrease in venous return secondary to an abrupt cessation of exercise. In addition to symptomatic or silent myocardial ischemia [30], sodium-potassium imbalance, increased catecholamine excretion, and circulating free fatty acids may all be arrhythmogenic. The additional risk of cardiac arrest during vigorous exercise, compared with that at other times, may be more than 100-fold during or soon after heavy physical exertion [5].

These data, however, contradict the widely held belief that regular exercise reduces the risk of cardiovascular disease [19•]. The critical question, however, is whether or not the cardiovascular benefits of regular exercise outweigh the transient, additional risk. The relative risk of cardiac arrest during exercise compared with that at other times is 56 times greater among sedentary men but only 5 times greater among men with high levels of habitual physical activity [31]. However, the total risk of cardiac arrest among habitually active men was only 40% of that for sedentary men. Thus, these findings agree with the hypothesis that vigorous physical activity both protects against but may provoke sudden cardiac death under certain conditions [32].

The notion that strenuous physical exertion can precipitate acute myocardial infarction, particularly in persons who are habitually sedentary (Table 4), has been supported by two recent studies [6,7]. This may occur with abrupt increases in heart rate and blood pressure that disrupt vulnerable atherosclerotic plaque and lead to thrombotic occlusion of a coronary vessel [33]. An increase in platelet activation and hyperreactiv-ity, which could contribute to (or even initiate) coronary thrombosis, has also been reported in inactive subjects but not in physically trained ones who engaged in sporadic high-intensity exercise [34].

THE ATHLETE'S HEART

Certain electrocardiographic findings are common and usually "normal" in athletes or those who are "endurance trained." These include sinus bradycardia (heart rate < 60 bpm), sinus arrhythmia, sinus pauses, first-degree atrioventricular (AV) block, second-degree AV block (Mobitz type I), wandering atrial pacemaker, AV junctional rhythms, incomplete right bundle branch block, rightward QRS axis, ventricular hypertrophy, minor ST segment depression or elevation (early repolarization), and altered T waves [35–37]. The amplitude of the QRS complex may also be at or above the upper limit of normal. Such anomalies in highly trained athletes likely result from changes in sympathetic or parasympathetic tone, increases in left ventricular (LV) mass, dimensions, or both, rather than from pathologic alterations in the cardiovascular system. Most atrial and ventricular premature complexes and atrial tachycardias are also considered normal variants and are nonspecific for heart disease [38]. However, complex ventricular ectopy, including runs of ventricular tachycardia, may require extensive cardiologic evaluation before medical clearance for athletic participation.

The cardiac profile of individuals who participate regularly in vigorous, isotonic exercise is characterized by LV volume overload with increased LV internal dimension, end-diastolic volume, stroke volume, and myocardial mass [39]. These changes are associated with enhanced LV performance and a significantly higher aerobic capacity compared with similarly aged control subjects. $\dot{V}O_2$max values in national class and championship athletes vary from a high of 94 mL/kg/min, now reported in a cross-country skier, to values between 40 and 45 mL/kg/min for athletes participating in anaerobic-type sports. Although intense physical training may increase the $\dot{V}O_2$max by 25% or more, it has become increasingly apparent that natural endowment (ie, genetics or family history) rather than training per se, plays a major role in producing a gold medal winner in an Olympic endurance event [40].

Fortunately, sudden death events in athletes are extremely rare occurrences. The prevalence of athletic-related deaths appears to be about one in 200,000 high school-age athletes and is higher in older athletes [41••,42]. CAD is the most frequent autopsy finding in athletes over the age of 35 years who die during competition or training [43]. In contrast, inherited structural cardiovascular abnormalities, including hypertrophic cardiomyopathy, idiopathic left ventricular hypertrophy, myocardial bridging, and anomalous origin of the left coronary artery, are the major causes of sudden death during exercise in younger athletes [44•].

The primary goal of cardiac preparticipation screening should be to determine whether the athlete has a history of syncope or chest pain. This information can be economically assessed with a questionnaire [45] designed to specifically identify a family history of sudden cardiac death, hypertrophic

TABLE 4 RELATIVE RISK OF EXERTION-RELATED MYOCARDIAL INFARCTION ACCORDING TO THE USUAL FREQUENCY OF STRENUOUS PHYSICAL EXERTION*

Study	Frequency of exertion, *times/wk*	Relative risk
German [7]	< 4	6.9
	≥ 4	1.3
United States [6]	< 1	107
	1–2	19.4
	3–4	8.6
	≥ 5	2.4

*≥ 6 metabolic equivalents (METs) (1 MET = 3.5 mL O$_2$/kg/min).

cardiomyopathy, Marfan's syndrome, or premature CAD. In such cases, additional studies are clinically warranted. Recently, an expert panel appointed by the American Heart Association issued the US's first set of standardized recommendations for the screening of young athletes for potentially fatal cardiovascular disease [41••]. When cardiac abnormalities are diagnosed, physicians should use established guidelines to formulate recommendations for continued participation or disqualification from competitive sports [46•].

ACKNOWLEDGMENT

The authors thank Brenda White for her assistance in preparing this manuscript.

KEY REFERENCES

Recently published papers of outstanding interest, as identified in *References and Recommended Reading*, have been annotated.

•• Wenger NK, Froelicher ES, Smith LK, *et al.*: Clinical Practice: Guideline: Cardiac Rehabilitation. Rockville, MD: U.S. Department of Health Service, Agency for Health Care Policy and Research and National Heart, Lung, and Blood Institute; 1995.
The definitive reference on the physiologic and psychosocial outomes that are associated with an exercise-based cardiac rehabilitation program.

•• Fletcher GF, Balady G, Froelicher VF, *et al.*: Exercise standards. *Circulation* 1995, 91:580–615.
This document represents a major update on the role of exercise testing and prescription in the primary and secondary prevention of cardiovascular disease.

•• Blair SN, Kampert JB, Kohl HW III, *et al.*: Influences of cardiorespiratory fitness and other precursors on cardiovascular disease and all-cause mortality in men and women. *JAMA* 1996, 276:205–210.
A classic study highlighting the important role of physical inactivity (low aerobic fitness) as a major, independent risk factor for heart disease.

•• Maron BJ, Thompson PD, Puffer JC, *et al.*: Cardiovascular preparticipation screening of competitive athletes. *Circulation* 1996, 94:850–856.
The first definitive US guidelines and recommendations for the appropriate preparticipation screening of competitive athletes.

REFERENCES AND RECOMMENDED READING

Recently published papers of particular interest have been highlighted as:
• Of interest
•• Of outstanding interest

1.•• Wenger NK, Froelicher ES, Smith LK, *et al.*: Clinical Practice Guideline: Cardiac Rehabilitation. Rockville, MD: U.S. Department of Health Service, Agency for Health Care Policy and Research and National Heart, Lung, and Blood Institute; 1995.

2. Hambrecht R, Niebauer J, Marburger C, *et al.*: Various intensities of leisure time physical activity in patients with coronary artery disease: effects on cardiorespiratory fitness and progression of coronary atherosclerotic lesions. *J Am Coll Cardiol* 1993, 22:468–477.

3. Bassler TJ: Marathon running and immunity to heart disease. *Physician Sportsmed* 1975, 3:77–80.

4. Noakes TD, Opie LH, Rose AG, *et al.*: Autopsy-proved coronary atherosclerosis in marathon runners. *N Engl J Med* 1979, 301:86–89.

5. Cobb LA, Weaver WD: Exercise: a risk for sudden death in patients with coronary heart disease. *J Am Coll Cardiol* 1986, 7:215–219.

6. Mittleman MA, Maclure M, Tofler GH, *et al.*: Triggering of acute myocardial infarction by heavy physical exertion: protection against triggering by regular exertion. *N Engl J Med* 1993, 329:1677–1683.

7. Willich SN, Lewis M, Löwel H, *et al.*: Physical exertion as a trigger of acute myocardial infarction. *N Engl J Med* 1993, 329:1684–1690.

8. Poliner LR, Dehmer GJ, Lewis SE: Left ventricular performance in normal subjects: a comparison of the responses to exercise in the upright and supine position. *Circulation* 1980, 62:528–534.

9.• Balady GJ, Fletcher BJ, Froelicher ES, *et al.*: Cardiac rehabilitation programs. A statement for healthcare professionals from the American Heart Association. *Circulation* 1994, 90:1602–1610.

10. Franklin BA, Gordon S, Timmis GC: Amount of exercise necessary for the patient with coronary artery disease. *Am J Cardiol* 1992, 69:1426–1431.

11. DeBusk RF, Stenestrand U, Sheehan M, *et al.*: Training effects of long versus short bouts of exercise in healthy subjects. *Am J Cardiol* 1990, 65:1010–1013.

12. Franklin BA, Besseghini I, Golden LH: Low intensity physical conditioning: effects on patients with coronary heart disease. *Arch Phys Med Rehabil* 1978, 59:276–280.

13. Ferguson RJ, Taylor AW, Côté P, *et al.*: Skeletal muscle and cardiac changes with training in patients with angina pectoris. *Am J Physiol* 1982, 24:H830–H836.

14. Clausen JP, Trap-Jensen J, Lassen NA: The effects of training on the heart rate during arm and leg exercise. *Scand J Clin Lab Invest* 1970, 26:295–301.

15.• Oberman A, Fletcher GF, Lee J, *et al.*: Efficacy of high-intensity exercise training on left ventricular ejection fraction in men with coronary artery disease (the training level comparison study). *Am J Cardiol*, 1995, 76:643–647.

16. Franklin BA: Exercise training and coronary collateral circulation. *Med Sci Sports Exerc* 1991; 23:648–653.

17. Price SA, Wilson LM: *Pathophysiology: Clinical Concepts of Disease Processes*, edn 3. St. Louis: C.V. Mosby; 1986.

18.•• Fletcher GF, Balady G, Froelicher VF, *et al.*: Exercise standards. *Circulation* 1995, 91:580–615.

19.• Fletcher GF, Balady G, Blair SN, *et al.*: Statement on exercise: benefits and recommendations for physical activity programs for all Americans. *Circulation* 1996, 94:857–862.

20. Franklin BA, Gordon S, Timmis GC: Exercise prescription for hypertensive patients. *Ann Med* 1991, 23:279–287.

21. Vu Tran Z, Weltman A: Differential effects of exercise on serum lipid and lipoprotein levels seen with changes in body weight: a meta-analysis. *JAMA* 1985, 254:919–924.

22. Blair SN, Kohl HW III, Paffenbarger RS, *et al.*: Physical fitness and all-cause mortality: a prospective study of healthy men and women. *JAMA* 1989, 262:2395–2401.

23.• Blair SN, Kohl HW III, Barlow CE, *et al.*: Changes in physical fitness and all-cause mortality: a prospective study of healthy and unhealthy men. *JAMA* 1995, 273:1093–1098.

24.•• Blair SN, Kampert JB, Kohl HW III, *et al.*: Influences of cardiorespiratory fitness and other precursors on cardiovascular disease and all-cause mortality in men and women. *JAMA* 1996, 276:205–210.

25.• Barlow CE, Kohl HW III, Gibbons LW, *et al.*: Physical fitness, mortality and obesity. *Intl J Obesity* 1995, 19:S41–S44.

26. Paffenbarger RS, Hyde RT, Wing AL, *et al.*: The association of changes in physical-activity level and other lifestyle characteristics with mortality among men. *N Engl J Med* 1993, 328:538–545.

27. Sandvik L, Erikssen J, Thaulow E, *et al.*: Physical fitness as a predictor of mortality among healthy, middle-aged Norwegian men. *N Engl J Med* 1993, 328:533–537.

28. Lee I-M, Hsieh C-C, Paffenbarger RS Jr: Exercise intensity and longevity in men: The Harvard Alumni Heath Study. *JAMA* 1995, 273:1179–1184.

29.• Vanhees L, Fagard R, Thijs L, *et al.*: Prognostic significance of peak exercise capacity in patients with coronary artery disease. *J Am Coll Cardiol* 1994, 23:358–363.

30. Hoberg E, Schuler G, Kunze B, *et al.*: Silent myocardial ischemia as a potential link between lack of premonitoring symptoms and increased risk of cardiac arrest during physical stress. *Am J Cardiol* 1990, 65:583–589.

31. Siscovick DS, Weiss NS, Fletcher RH, *et al.*: The incidence of primary cardiac arrest during vigorous exercise. *N Engl J Med* 1984, 311:874–877.

32. Thompson PD, Mitchell JH: Exercise and sudden cardiac death: protection or provocation [editorial]. *N Engl J Med* 1984, 311:914–915.

33. Richardson PD, Davies MJ, Born GV: Influence of plaque configuration and stress distribution on fissuring of coronary atherosclerotic plaques. *Lancet* 1989, 2:941–944.

34. Kestin AS, Ellis PA, Barnard MR, *et al.*: Effect of strenuous exercise on platelet activation state and reactivity. *Circulation* 1993, 88:1502–1511.

35. Knowlan DM: The electrocardiogram in the athlete. In *Cardiovascular Evaluation of Athletes*. Edited by Walter BF and Harvey WP. Newton: Laennec Publishing; 1993:43.

36. Huston TP, Puffer JC, Rodney WM, *et al.*: The athletic heart syndrome. *N Engl J Med* 1985, 313:24–32.

37. Lichtman J, O'Rourke RA, Klein A, *et al.*: Electrocardiogram of the athlete. *Arch Intern Med* 1973, 132:763–770.

38. Pantano JA, Oriel RJ: Prevalence of cardiac arrhythmias in apparently normal well trained runners. *Am Heart J* 1982, 104:762–768.

39. Kaimal KP, Franklin BA, Moir TW, *et al.*: Cardiac profiles of national-class race walkers. *Chest* 1993, 104:935–938.

40. Bouchard C, Lesage R, Lortie G, *et al.*: Aerobic performance in brothers, dizygotic and monozygotic twins. *Med Sci Sports Exerc* 1986, 18:639–646.

41.•• Maron BJ, Thompson PD, Puffer JC, *et al.*: Cardiovascular preparticipation screening of competitive athletes. *Circulation* 1996, 94:850–856.

42. Maron BJ, Poliac JC, Roberts WC: Risk for sudden cardiac death associated with marathon running. *J Am Coll Cardiol* 1996, 28:428–431.

43. Waller BF, Roberts WC: Sudden death while running in conditioned runners aged 40 years or over. *Am J Cardiol* 1980, 45:1292–1300.

44.• Maron BJ, Shirani J, Poliac LC, *et al.*: Sudden death in young competitive athletes: clinical, demographic, and pathological profiles. *JAMA* 1996, 276:199–204.

45. Ades PA: Preventing sudden death: cardiovascular screening of young athletes. *Physician Sportsmed* 1992, 20:75–89.

46.• Maron BJ, Isner JM, McKenna WJ: 26th Bethesda Conference: Recommendations for determining eligibility for competition in athletes with cardiovascular abnormalities. Task Force 3: Hypertrophic cardiomyopathy, myocarditis and other myopericardial diseases and mitral valve prolapse. *J Am Coll Cardiol* 1994, 24:880–885.

SELECT BIBLIOGRAPHY

Fletcher GF: Holter recording in athletes: purposes and indication. In *Cardiovascular Evaluation of Athletes*. Edited by Walter BF, Harvey WP. Newton: Laennec Publishing; 1993:87.

Franklin BA, Almany SL, Hauser AM: Cardiovascular evaluation of the athlete. In *Sports Injuries: Mechanisms, Prevention, and Treatment*. Edited by Fu FH, Stone DA. Baltimore: Williams & Wilkins Co.; 1994:111–121.

Approach to the Patient with Hyperlipidemia

14

Neil J. Stone

Key Points

- Damage to the endothelium initiates a cascade of events leading to cholesterol-rich, atherosclerotic plaque.

- Both total and high-density lipoprotein (HDL) cholesterol should be measured in all adults over 19 years of age at least once every 5 years; the intensity of the evaluation and treatment depends on coronary risk status and other health conditions.

- Intervention focuses on low-density lipoprotein (LDL) cholesterol calculated by measurement of fasting cholesterol, triglycerides, and HDL.

- Risk factors include age, menopausal status, hypertension, diabetes mellitus, cigarette smoking, and family history of premature cardiovascular disease (before 65 years of age in female and 55 in male relatives); sedentary lifestyle and obesity are targets for intervention that should improve one or more risk factors.

- Secondary causes of hyperlipidemia should always be ruled out before treatment begins; diet, drugs, and diseases affecting lipid levels should be reviewed.

- Diet is the initial treatment, emphasizing low fat (< 30% of calories), low saturated fat, and low dietary cholesterol; calories should be restricted and regular aerobic exercise encouraged for overweight patients.

- In patients with coronary disease, significantly lowering LDL cholesterol can slow progression or cause regression of existing atherosclerotic plaques as seen by angiography. This lowering is associated with a marked improvement in coronary event rates. In secondary prevention trials encompassing a wide range of LDL cholesterol values, aggressive lowering of LDL cholesterol reduces subsequent risk of myocardial infarction as well as all-cause mortality.

- Major drugs to lower elevated LDL cholesterol in high-risk patients include bile-acid sequestering resins, niacin, and hydroxymethylglutaryl–coenzyme A reductase inhibitors (or statins); in the other drug category is gemfibrozil, which is used to treat severe triglyceride excess.

The atherosclerotic process begins with a cholesterol-rich fatty streak that can be seen in coronary arteries as early as the second decade of life. In patients with risk factors for atherosclerosis, this streak can progress to a fibrous plaque whose main components are intra- and extracellular cholesterol, smooth muscle cells, and cellular elements from the vessel wall contained by a thin fibrous cap. This fibrous plaque can evolve into a complicated plaque with hemorrhage, necrosis, calcification, and overlying thrombosis.

The initiating event of atherosclerosis is endothelial injury caused by turbulence of blood flow (explaining the predilection for atherosclerotic worsening at the branch points) or merely hypercholesterolemia resulting in excess low-density lipoprotein (LDL). The damaged surface attracts platelets that release growth factors leading to the involvement of smooth muscle cells. The hallmark of accelerated atherosclerotic syndromes is damaged intimal and medial layers, as seen in venous coronary bypass grafts, angioplasty, and heart transplantation.

Low-density lipoprotein oxidation is critical in this process, which allows the LDL to be taken up easily by monocytes and macrophages that become foam cells.

Even in minimally modified form, the usual LDL-receptor mechanism does not function to limit excess cholesterol uptake by the cell. Steinberg and coworkers [1] showed the interrelationships between theories about lipids and response to injury.

The Multiple Risk Factor Intervention Trial studied 360,000 men and showed convincingly that risk of coronary death correlates with serum cholesterol over a wide range of values [2]. The lowest risk was seen in those with cholesterol values under 200 mg/dL, and there was increasing risk with values above 240 mg/dL. Other risk factors also may be implicated in the atherosclerotic process (Table 1). Every patient evaluated for hyperlipidemia should have a checklist of risk factors on his or her chart. Not only are risk factors associated with dyslipidemia (*eg*, lipid abnormalities are more likely in patients with diabetes, hypertension, and obesity), but the presence of associated risk factors increases cardiac risk.

Nonmodifiable risk factors include age and gender (*ie*, men and postmenopausal women are at increased risk).

Modifiable risk factors include excess LDL, low levels of high-density lipoprotein (HDL), hypertension (including systolic hypertension in elderly patients), diabetes mellitus, cigarette smoking, sedentary lifestyle, and abdominal or male-pattern obesity. Femoral-gluteal obesity is primarily a cosmetic problem, whereas abdominal obesity is associated with hyperinsulinemia and attendant hypertension, hyperglycemia, low HDL cholesterol (HDL-c), and hypertriglyceridemia [3]. Figure 1 shows the value of assessing cholesterol in light of associated risk factors [2]. For example, a nonsmoker with cholesterol in the 221 to 244 range has a lower risk than a smoker with hypertension and cholesterol in the 182 to 202 range. Hence, a high-risk individual would be one with two or more risk factors or the presence of coronary or vascular disease elsewhere.

Secondary causes of elevated blood lipids should always be determined. A useful mnemonic is to think of the three *D*'s: *diet*, *drugs*, and *diseases* (Table 2). If secondary causes are not seen, consider primary hyperlipidemia and screen the patient's family.

TABLE 1 HOW RISK FACTORS AFFECT ATHEROSCLEROSIS

Biology	Hyperlipidemia	Hypertension	Smoking	Genetics	Other
Endothelial injury	Excess LDL	+	+	Homocystinuria	Immune complexes
Lipoproteins, monocytes	++	–	–	++	
Platelets	+	–	++	–	
Smooth cell proliferation	+	+	–	++	
Plaque disruption	++	+	–	++	
Thrombosis	+	–	++	+	
Associated with oxidized LDL	Low HDL		Depletes vitamin C	Small, dense LDL	

HDL—high-density lipoprotein; LDL—low-density lipoprotein; -—mild reductions; ——moderate reductions; +—mild increments; ++—moderate increments.

Adapted from Badimon *et al.* [36]; with permission.

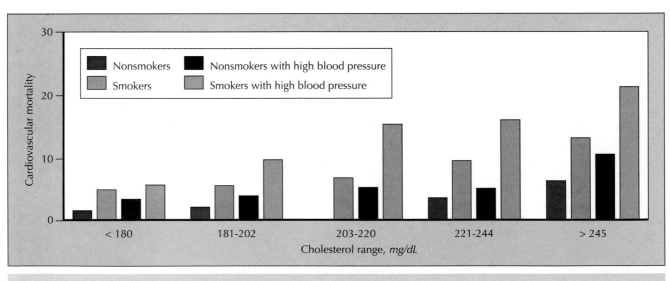

FIGURE 1 Effect of risk factors on modifying risk of cardiovascular mortality in the Multiple Risk Factor Intervention Trial (MRFIT) Study.

MEASUREMENT OF LIPIDS AND LIPOPROTEINS

Serum cholesterol can be obtained in the nonfasting state and has been recommended as a screening test. Many patients with desirable cholesterol values but low HDL-c will be missed using the original Adult Treatment Panel's criteria: 240 mg/dL or greater is high, 200 to 239 mg/dL is borderline, and under 200 mg/dL is desirable [4]. This is important, because low serum cholesterol levels (< 200 mg/dL) and low HDL-c (< 35 mg/dL) are frequently seen in those who either have or are suspected of having coronary artery disease (CAD). This combination is often noted in men with a family history of premature CAD [5]. Thus, screening may be best accomplished with nonfasting cholesterol and HDL-c. If abnormal values are found, repeat the tests. This should be done in the fasting state 12 to 14 hours after the meal. This allows measurement of triglycerides, which are so highly variable that the patient should be fasting and at a steady weight. A nonfasting value is only useful in the patient with abdominal pain and suspected pancreatitis; here, values over 1000 mg/dL suggest chylomicronemia as a cause of the pancreatitis. Measurement of total cholesterol and HDL-c is also performed. Laboratories can then calculate LDL cholesterol (LDL-c) by the following formula:

LDL-c = Total cholesterol − HDL-c − (Triglycerides/5)

This formula is valid if triglycerides are less than 400 mg/dL and the rare type III abnormality is not present. LDL-c values are used to determine risk and if further evaluation and therapy are needed (Table 3). As with lipids, these values need to be repeated at least once to establish a true baseline.

Secondary causes of hyperlipidemia also need to be considered. Dietary causes include a diet too rich in saturated fat, cholesterol, and excess calories. Drugs implicated in hyperlipidemia include steroids, androgens, diuretics, beta-blockers, and retinoic-acid derivatives. Diseases commonly found to cause hyperlipidemia include hypothyroidism (measure thyroid-stimulating hormone to find subclinical hypothyroidism that can elevate cholesterol levels), obstructive liver disease, chronic renal disease, nephrosis, and diabetes mellitus.

Family screening is mandatory if lipid levels are diet-resistant, because several familial syndromes such as familial hypercholesterolemia and familial combined hyperlipidemia may be present. The former often has cholesterol deposits in tendons, most notably the Achilles tendons, called *xanthomas*. The latter is associated more with abnormalities of triglyceride metabolism.

Low HDL-c (< 35 mg/dL) increases coronary risk and is also a target for therapy. Excess body weight, cigarette smoking, hypertriglyceridemia, and sedentary lifestyle (which are often interrelated) should be corrected so that elevated HDL-c may result. Exercise must be regular and sustained over many months before elevated HDL-c is seen. Alcohol raises HDL-c, but it cannot be recommended for this purpose because of the negative aspects associated with excess usage (especially in women and younger persons). High HDL-c (> 70 mg/dL) is linked to longevity syndromes, and in a low-risk person, it suggests a more conservative approach to drug therapy.

Hypertriglyceridemia drops out as an independent risk factor in multivariate analysis, yet triglycerides are a valuable indicator that associated metabolic abnormalities may be present. Dense, triglyceride-rich LDL particles characterize those patients with greater coronary artery disease by angiography [6]. Those with small, dense LDL usually have triglyceride levels over 150 mg/dL (Table 4). The clinician should have a clue that triglycerides will be elevated, because the serum is often turbid (*eg*, you cannot read newsprint clearly through it)

TABLE 2 SECONDARY CAUSES OF HYPERCHOLESTEROLEMIA AND HIGH TRIGLYCERIDES

Cause	Procedure or test
Hypercholesterolemia	
Diet	Dietary history (focus on saturated fats, dietary cholesterol)
Drugs	Diuretics, steroids, anabolic steroids
Hypothyroidism	TSH test
Nephrotic syndrome	Urine analysis, serum albumin
Obstructive liver disease	Abnormal alkaline phosphatase and enzymes
Diabetes mellitus	FBS, glycated hemoglobin
Transplantation	Multiple causes including drugs like steroids
High triglycerides	
Diet	Dietary history (focus on calorie excess, alcohol)
Drugs	Diuretics, steroids, estrogens, retinoic acid, beta-blockers
Hypothyroidism	TSH test
Nephrotic syndrome (severe)	Urine analysis, serum albumin
Chronic renal disease	BUN, creatinine
Diabetes mellitus	FBS, glycated hemoglobin

BUN—blood urea nitrogen; FBS—fasting blood sugar; TSH—thyroid-stimulating hormone.

TABLE 3 LOW-DENSITY LIPOPROTEIN CHOLESTEROL DECISION CUTOFFS

LDL-c, *mg/dL*	Impression	Comments
≥ 160	High-risk	Evaluate for therapy
130–159	Borderline	Evaluate if risk factors
< 130	Desirable	Goal if no evidence of CAD
100	Optimal	Goal for those with CAD

CAD—coronary artery disease.

TABLE 4 TRIGLYCERIDE DECISION CUTOFFS

Triglyceride, *mg/dL*	Significance
< 200	Desirable; some think coronary risk is less if under 150
200–399	Borderline; if associated with low HDL-c, high LDL-c, diabetes or personal/family history of CAD, it is significant
≥ 400	High; avoid estrogens, steroids, and excess alcohol as they can trigger marked triglyceride rise and pancreatitis

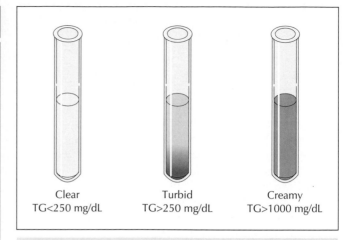

Clear	Turbid	Creamy
TG<250 mg/dL	TG>250 mg/dL	TG>1000 mg/dL

FIGURE 2 Visual inspection of triglyceride-rich lipoproteins. Turbidity shows if large, triglyceride-rich lipoproteins are present. TG—triglycerides.

(Fig. 2). If triglycerides exceed 1000 mg/dL, the serum is often creamy, representing chylomicronemia. The cream means that the patient is either nonfasting (triglycerides mildly elevated) or has a major disorder of triglyceride removal with increased risk of pancreatitis (triglycerides > 1000 mg/dL).

How accurate are these measurements? Most laboratories now show a precision and accuracy level of 95% or more for cholesterol. Table 5 shows factors that must be considered when the clinician evaluates lipid measurements. Screening values can be nonfasting because one is only trying to see if a potential lipid/lipoprotein problem exists. For detailed evaluation or determining response to therapy, it is useful to require the individual to fast for 12 to 14 hours and not consume alcohol within the preceding 24 hours. Also, the individual should be at a stable weight and without intercurrent illness or stress. Lipids should be determined in outpatients using the sitting position without an overly tight tourniquet. Nonetheless, there can be significant sources of error; Table 5 gives a brief listing [7]. A common source of confusion occurs when an individual starts total fat and saturated fat restriction but HDL-c decreases along with LDL-c. The LDL:HDL ratio, however, is improved, and it may improve more if regular aerobic exercise is added.

It has been known for two decades that cholesterol levels decrease and triglyceride levels increase over a several-week period after a myocardial infarction (MI). Cholesterol measured within the first 24 hours does reflect pre-event lipid values [8], yet cholesterol values decrease markedly in the week after MI [9]. How soon after MI should plasma lipid values be assessed? In one study, cholesterol fell 31% and LDL-c 48% in the week after MI [10]. Physicians and patients often are first aware of lipids in the post-MI state. Every patient with MI requires a fasting lipoprotein profile before discharge, but the patient should be cautioned that it may take 2 to 3 months before lipid values return to their pre-event stage. Because these patients generally undergo dietary and activity counseling before leaving the hospital (with the goal of achieving LDL-c values of approximately 100 mg/dL and HDL-c values of over 45 mg/dL), in many cases the patient and physician will never learn how bad the lipids were if no previous values are available.

Patients with CAD who are admitted electively have lipid and lipoprotein values that must be interpreted critically as well. HDL (and also apolipoprotein A-I) values are lower at cardiac catheterization [11]. This is significant, because HDL-c values are important predictors of the presence and extent of CAD [12].

TABLE 5 SOURCES OF LABORATORY VARIATION IN LIPID MEASUREMENTS

Behavioral		Sampling sources	
Diet	Fats raise TC, HDL; saturated fats raise LDL	Fasting	Essential for triglycerides
Obesity	Increases TG; lowers HDL	Nonfasting	After eating, see increased VLDL and lower LDL; total cholesterol changes to small degree
Smoking	Decreases HDL (*eg*, 11% in one study)		
Exercise	Lowers TG; increases HDL	Posture	Approximately 9% higher for TC and LDL and 10% for HDL-c when lying down compared with standing
Alcohol	Increases TG; increases HDL		
		Fingerstick	Can see unreliable values if technician not well trained or machine not calibrated regularly

HDL—high-density lipoprotein; LDL—low-density lipoprotein; TC—total cholesterol; TG—triglyceride; VLDL—very-low-density lipoprotein.

DIETARY THERAPY

Nonpharmacologic Modification Trials

The Oslo Dietary and Smoking Intervention Trial studied men without overt CAD and showed that those randomized to a modified fat diet and counseling to reduce smoking had a 47% lower incidence of sudden death and heart attack than those in the control group [13]. Further analysis showed that the net difference of 10% in serum cholesterol between the intervention and control groups was the main cause for the 47% reduction in first events of CAD. At 5 years, the difference between both groups in total mortality became significant, with a 33% lower mortality in the intervention group.

The Multiple Risk Factor Intervention Trial (MRFIT) studied 12,866 high-risk men from 35 to 57 years of age who were hypercholesterolemic, hypertensive, or smokers [14]. There was an insignificant difference of 7.1% in mortality between special-intervention and usual-care groups after 8 years. Although quit rates for cigarette smokers clearly improved in the trial and dietary change was evident, the mean net differences between special intervention and usual care for diastolic blood pressure was only 4%, and for serum cholesterol was only 2%. A possibly unfavorable response to high-dose, diuretic, antihypertensive medication in the treated group (especially those with electrocardiographic abnormalities at baseline) may explain some of the differences as well. At 10 years, the small differences achieved in risk factors finally resulted in significant differences between clinical end points.

The Los Angeles Veterans Administration Study randomized patients to a treatment group with an intake of 50% less cholesterol and significantly lower saturated fat than the control group [15]. At the end of the study, the treatment group had 12.7% lower cholesterol and significantly lower coronary and cerebrovascular events ($P < 0.01$) than the control group.

Ornish and coworkers [16] looked at a selected (randomization here was really a failed effort) group of individuals who on a strict, very low-fat diet demonstrated regression on quantitative coronary angiography performed at 1 year. LDL levels decreased from 152 to 95 mg/dL in the treatment group. Other interventions in this trial included exercise, meditation, stress management, and smoking cessation.

The St. Thomas Atherosclerosis Regression Trial showed the benefits of diet on coronary dimensions in patients with CAD [17]. After 39 months, the proportion showing an increased luminal diameter was 4% for the usual-care group, 38% for the diet group, and 33% for the diet-and-cholestyramine-resin group. The mean absolute width of the coronary segments correlated independently and significantly with LDL-c change during the trial.

Practical Aspects of Diet

A diet with a low percentage of calories derived from total fat and saturated fat and low in dietary cholesterol has been recommended for the American public. Current dietary figures are from the US Surgeon General's report in 1988 [18] (Table 6).

The diet recommended for the general population is the Step 1 Diet. The MRFIT trial showed that certain high-fat eating behaviors are easier for patients to alter than others. Those changes made with relative ease include increasing consumption of fish and poultry, having less red meat, using skim or low-fat milk products, using margarine instead of butter, and reducing egg yolks. Those that were much harder were decreasing the quantity of meat consumption to 6 or 7 ounces daily and avoiding high-fat cheese, snacks, crackers, chips, processed sausage, and luncheon meats [19]. Patients also should be advised that before they add psyllium, modified fat foods, or even garlic, they must subtract dietary fat from their diet. These items can help to lower cholesterol as adjuncts, not substitiutes, to a low-saturated-fat diet [20].

The lipid-lowering therapeutic diet is the Step 2 Diet, and it is particularly recommended for patients at high risk of CAD. Here, a dietitian is required to help the patient not only achieve a very low saturated fat intake but also to choose and prepare balanced, nutritious, and nonrepetitious meals.

Dietary assessment is required to determine progress and can be used to involve the patient in behavioral change. Ask if the patient has the specific skills needed to be on a good cholesterol-lowering diet, such as knowing how to read labels, order when dining out, prepare low-fat foods, and alter familiar recipes to comply with the diet. If the patient cannot do these things, referral to a dietitian is crucial. You may wish to have the patient bring a written, 24- to 72-hour dietary diary to the next visit; with this, it is easy to tell at a glance if the patient understands the diet. Another option is having the patient fill out a food-frequency questionnaire designed to review dietary adherence. A useful one is the MEDICS questionnaire; the letters of this mnemonic stand for the sources of dietary fat (Table 7).

Soluble fiber is a useful adjunct to a cholesterol-lowering therapy and can be obtained in oatmeal, oatbran, or in fruits and vegetables. In addition, fruits and vegetables are a good source of antioxidants. Finally, a good diet can make it easier for a given dosage of medication to facilitate the attainment of LDL-c goals [21]. Drugs should be added to the diet and never prescribed in place of it.

TABLE 6 CURRENT AND RECOMMENDED US DIETS			
	Current diet	Step 1	Step 2
Total fat, %		< 30	< 30
Men	36		
Women	37		
Saturated fat, %		< 10	< 7
Men	13		
Women	13		
Dietary cholesterol, *mg*		< 300	< 200
Men	435		
Women	304		

DRUG TREATMENT

Clinical Intervention Trials

Primary-prevention clinical trials have shown that lipid-lowering drugs can affect the incidence of CAD. The first was the Lipid Research Clinics Primary Prevention Trial, which showed that using cholestyramine resin for every 1% that the cholesterol was lowered resulted in a 2% lowering of coronary risk [22]. The Helsinki Heart Trial used a different medication, gemfibrozil, which raised HDL-c as much as it lowered LDL-c [23]; this trial also showed a significant reduction in fatal and nonfatal MI. Most of the benefit in this trial occurred in men with a lipid profile characterized by high cholesterol, high triglycerides, and low HDL-c. Although the above-mentioned trials showed that lipid-lowering could reduce the risk of a first MI, they were not sufficiently powered to show whether or not total mortality was affected by lipid lowering (Table 8). The West of Scotland trial had sufficient numbers to answer whether or not aggressive lipid lowering in high-risk men without a prior MI was indeed both beneficial and safe [24••]. In those men randomized to the diet and pravastatin arm, there was a significant reduction in fatal and nonfatal events of CAD. Moreover, overall mortality was improved by 22%, which almost reached statistical significance ($P = 0.051$). Because the average age for the high-risk men in this trial was 55, these results cannot be generalized to younger men or women. The Simvastatin Scandinavian Trial was a placebo-controlled, randomized trial of simvastatin in 4444 survivors of MI [25••]. This landmark study showed that LDL-c lowering from an average of 190 mg/dL to 130 mg/dL not only reduced rates if fatal and nonfatal CAD, but also lowered total mortality as well. The benefits of treatment with simvastatin extended to older as well as younger subjects. Women also had significant reductions in cardiovascular end points. Because hospital admissions were significantly reduced in the treatment group, calculation of the resultant reduction in hospital costs over the 5.4 years of the trial lowered the effective cost of simvastatin 88% to $0.28 per day [26••]. The CARE trial enrolled 4159 survivors of MI, but the average LDL-c was only 139 mg/dL [27••]. Encompassing a spectrum of patients with more "average" values for LDL-c, this CARE trial showed that treatment with pravastatin resulted in a highly significant reduction in the primary end point of death from CAD and nonfatal MI. Lipid reduction in women had a pronounced effect: they enjoyed a 45% reduction in the primary end point as compared with their male counterparts. Patients who entered the trial with LDL-c below 125 mg/dL did not show significant benefit from lipid lowering.

The Post Coronary Artery Bypass Graft Trial (Post CABG) examined the benefit of aggressive LDL-c lowering in 1249 men and 102 women with a history of coronary artery bypass surgery [28••]. The aggressive treatment group received lovastatin (and, if needed, cholestyramine resin) to keep the mean LDL-c under 100 mg/dL. The moderate treatment group received less lipid-lowering therapy to keep the LDL-c in the 132–136 mg/dL range. The aggressive treatment group had only a 27% rate of progression as contrasted with a rate of 39% for those who received moderate treatment ($P < 0.001$). The aggressively treated group also had a lower rate of revascularization at 4 years—6.5% as contrasted with a rate of 9.2% in those with the moderate lowering of LDL-c. This study validated the NCEP goal of achieving an LDL-c less than 100 mg/dL for those with documented CAD.

Drug studies using angiography as an end point have shown that aggressive, lipid-lowering therapy can reduce progression or even cause regression. The Cholesterol-Lowering Atherosclerosis Study (CLAS) evaluated 162 post–coronary bypass patients randomly assigned to placebo or treatment with colestipol and niacin [29]. Combined

TABLE 7 THE MEDICS QUESTIONNAIRE*	
Meats	How often and how much red meat, sausage, and organ meats? Fried foods? Know how to order when dining out?
	Advise more fish, skinless poultry. Have meats broiled with sauces on the side. Avoid high-fat meats, hot dogs, sausage, and organ meats. Try to keep total meat quantity to under 6 oz daily.
Eggs	How many egg yolks per week?
	Use egg yokes sparingly; egg whites are preferred.
Dairy	How many high-fat cheese, milk, and cream products per week? Do you add cheese to burgers or nachos?
	Low-fat cheese and milk products are advised.
Invisible fats	How many baked goods per week?
	Stick with whole-grain products and avoid high-fat doughnuts, coffee cakes, croissants, and muffins.
Cooking dairy fats	What cooking or table fat do you use and how much?
	Avoid butter; use soft margarine, avoiding hardened forms. Avoid fried foods. Use canola, safflower, corn oil, and olive oil. Avoid coconut, palm, and palm kernel oils, which are highly saturated. Know how to modify recipes.
Snacks	What snacks and how often?
	Advise fruits, vegetables, pretzels; avoid high-fat dips, candy bars.
	Physician may add questions about distilled spirits (hard liquor, wine, or beer) and salt, if applicable.

*Can be given to patients at each visit to fill out and circle those lipid-lowering habits (in italics) that they need to work on.

Clinical Trial	Patient sample	Years, n	Mean pretrial LDL-c, mg/dL	Intervention	%Δ LDL	% Δ HDL
Primary prevention						
LRC-PPT	3806 men	7.4	204	Cholestyramine, 24 g/d	-20.3	1.6
Helsinki	4081 men	5	206	Gemfibrozil, 600 mg bid	-10	10
WOSCOP	6595 men	4.9	192	Pravastatin, 40 mg/d	-26	5
Secondary prevention						
4S	4444 men and women	5.4	189	Simvastatin, 20 mg; 37% took 40 mg	-35	8
CARE	4159 men and women	5	139	Pravastatin, 40 mg/d	-28	2
Post CABG (Aggressive treatment arm)	676 men and women	4.3	155 After 1 year, those treated aggressively lowered to 93 *vs.* 136 in moderate arm	Lovastatin (mean, 76 mg/d); 30% took 8 g/d of cholestyramine resin to further lower LDL-c	-37 to -40	7.5

4S—Simvastatin Scandinavian Survival Study; CARE—Cholesterol and Recurrent Events Trial; Helsinki—Helsinki Primary Prevention Trial; LRC-PPT—Lipid Research Clinics Primary Prevention Trial; Post CABG—Post Coronary Artery Bypass Graft Trial; WOSCOP—West of Scotland Primary Prevention Trial.

coronary, femoral, and carotid angiograms were obtained initially and after 2 years. Drug treatment resulted in a 26% decrease in cholesterol, 43% decrease in LDL-c, and 37% increase in HDL-c. Of the treatment group, 61% showed favorable outcomes (either nonprogression of coronary lesions or reversal) versus 39% of the placebo group. Atherosclerosis regression was observed in 16.2% of the drug group versus 2.4% of the placebo group ($P < 0.002$). Results were even more impressive at 4-year follow-up.

The Familial Atherosclerosis Treatment Study (FATS) [30] used quantitative coronary angiography in 146 patients with hypercholesterolemia treated in a double-blind, randomized trial with lovastatin and colestipol, niacin and colestipol, or placebo and colestipol over a 2-year period. The two treatment groups had less progression and more regression, and clinical cardiac events were markedly reduced.

In the University of California–San Francisco Familial Hypercholesterolemia trial, Kane and coworkers [31] showed that aggressive LDL-lowering therapy involving two and even three drugs resulted in decreased progression and even regression on serial angiography in asymptomatic men and women with familial hypercholesterolemia. This study was the first to show a significant effect from lipid lowering on atherosclerosis in women. These patients were heterozygous for familial hypercholesterolemia. This is a diet-resistant genetic syndrome in which untreated cholesterol values average approximately 360 mg/dL.

The Program on the Surgical Control of the Hyperlipidemias (POSCH) investigated the effect of partial ileal bypass on blood cholesterol reduction, coronary morbidity, and mortality in 838 survivors of MI and followed for a mean of 9.7 years [32]. These patients were not chosen on the basis of their lipids. Cholesterol reduction was greater in the treatment group, and at repeat coronary arteriography, progression of coronary disease was significantly reduced in the surgery group ($P < 0.001$). This was almost a pure trial of LDL-c lowering, because HDL-c values were not greatly affected.

In summary, these coronary angiographic trials show that regression and stabilization are 1.5 to 2.0 times more common in patients with intervention than in control patients, and progression is likewise reduced by approximately 50% in those with intensive lipid lowering. Lesions with a narrowing of 50% luminal diameter or greater at baseline seem to be more responsive, but reduction in subsequent coronary events is related to the stabilization of lesions to less than 50% luminal narrowing [33].

Choice of Drugs

Before starting drug therapy, determine if the patient has made a concerted effort regarding diet and exercise. Referral to a dietitian may provide the information necessary to obtain a good dietary response. Consumption of food and especially alcohol may be underreported, and physical activity may be overestimated. Also, check if menopausal women have been prescribed estrogens, which can reverse the menopausal changes of raised LDL-c and lowered HDL-c. Estrogen treatment may lower LDL-c by 10% or more, but this may not occur if progestins are used as well. Available evidence suggests that protection of postmenopausal estrogens against CAD, however, is not dependent on the lipid effects.

Finally, review the benefits, disadvantages, and risks of drug therapy with the patient. Drug therapy will most likely benefit those at highest risk of coronary disease, such as patients with known vascular disease or a risk factor status putting them at risk in the short-term for coronary events. Men under 45 years of age and women under 55 years are thought to have a lower immediate risk of a coronary event. Therefore, gender is a risk factor when a man is 45 years or older and a woman is 55 years or older. (An exception is when the woman has an early menopause and then is at higher risk.) A young patient with elevated total cholesterol and LDL-c but a normal HDL-c and no other risk factors may be managed better with diet. Those at highest risk (eg, positive family history, two or more risk factors, familial hypercholesterolemia with LDL over 225 mg/dL despite diet, or known vascular disease) should be considered for drug therapy if the LDL-c is over 190 mg/dL and the HDL-c less than 35 mg/dL. An overview of drug therapy is given in Table 9.

Bile-acid sequestrants (eg, cholestyramine, colestipol) are used primarily for patients with hypercholesterolemia and normal triglyceride levels. Bile-acid sequestrants must be started slowly (one scoop daily), and the patient must have a clear understanding of the anticipated gastrointestinal side effects such as constipation. Those on a high-fiber diet seem to do best. Low-dose resin therapy is a useful choice, because it is well tolerated and results in LDL-c lowering in the 15% to 20% range.

Fibric-acid derivatives such as gemfibrozil (600 mg twice daily) can be employed in patients with hypertriglyceridemia and low HDL-c but elevated total cholesterol, or in the patient with marked triglyceride excess (> 500 mg/dL). Do not prescribe gemfibrozil if renal or hepatic function is impaired. While not as lithogenic as the first-generation fibric acid clofibrate, it does present a small, increased risk for gallstones.

Nicotinic acid preparations offer excellent lipid-lowering alternatives, because they raise HDL-c and lower LDL-c and triglycerides. These drugs must be given slowly and incrementally. Very low-dose initial therapy (100 mg) with increasing of the initial dose two or three times daily may be required every 2 to 4 weeks for up to 6 months, until the therapeutic dose has been achieved. At low doses, HDL-c is favorably affected, but higher doses are needed to lower LDL-c [34]. Concomitant aspirin ingestion helps to prevent flushing, which is a prostaglandin-mediated reaction. Patients should be warned about this flushing; they should take niacin with food, one aspirin approximately 30 minutes before, and slowly increase the dose. This may allow many to avoid the more expensive (and possibly with more gastrointestinal side effects) sustained-release preparations. A recent report noted that using sustained-release niacin to lower LDL-c resulted in a high incidence of hepatotoxicity. Immediate-release niacin was preferred and recommended for patients who agree to be monitored by health professionals [35]. Niacinamide is another form of the vitamin, but it is not a lipid-lowering drug and should not be substituted for niacin. Niacin may cause gout in patients with hyperuricemia. It also can aggravate mild

TABLE 9 OVERVIEW OF LIPID-LOWERING THERAPY

Drug	Lipid effects	Negative aspects	Comments
Bile-acid sequestrants Cholestyramine Colestipol	TC, LDL–; TG+; HDL+	At higher dosages, gastrointestinal side effects (eg, constipation, rectal bleeding)	Avoid if TG > 250 mg/dL; use psyllium if constipation a problem; low-dose resin (two scoops per day) most useful
Fibric-acid derivative Gemfibrozil	TC, LDL–; TG––; HDL++	May predispose to gallstones May raise LDL-c. Not recommended as first-line drug for secondary prevention.	Drug of choice for those with marked hypertriglyceridemia; shown to be of value in primary prevention trial for those with combined high TC and TG and low HDL-c.
Niacin Nicotinic acid or vitamin B₃ Niacinamide is *not* a substitute for niacin (minimal lipid lowering)	TC, LDL–; TG––; HDL++	Flushing in all initially; must monitor liver function tests; can exacerbate ulcer disease, elevates glucose, and cause gout; acanthosis nigricans can be seen—abates if niacin stopped	Unmodified form is inexpensive; an aspirin can be used to mitigate flushing; avoid in diabetics, if possible; if niacin well tolerated, don't change brands!
HMG-CoA reductase inhibitors Lovastatin, pravastatin Simvastatin, fluvastatin, atorvastatin	TC, LDL––; TG–; HDL+	Few side effects at low doses; liver function tests should be monitored; myositis risk in certain situation (eg, with cyclosporine or gemfibrozil)	Expensive, but may be most cost-effective; lovastatin should be taken with food (not so with the others)
Combination therapy Niacin and resin Statin and resin	TC, LDL––; TG–; HDL++	Must still watch individual drug's effects	May be better for those with combined hyperlipidemia or severe hyperlipidemia

HDL—high-density lipoprotein; HMG-COA—hydroxymethylglutaryl-coenzyme A; LDL—low-density lipoprotein; TC—total cholesterol; TG—triglycerides; +—mild increments; ++—moderate increments; +++—largest increments; - —mild reductions; – —moderate reductions; —— largest reductions.

type 2 diabetes, because it increases hepatic glucose output and thus should be avoided in most diabetics.

The most powerful drugs to lower LDL-c are HMG-CoA reductase inhibitors. For the patient with multiple risk factors or coronary disease, they may be the most cost-effective, because a low dose may allow the LDL-c goal to be met. With increasing dosage, there is less incremental lipid lowering. As a rough guide, 20 mg of lovastatin or pravastatin offers similar LDL-c lowering as 10 mg of simvastatin or 40 mg of fluvastatin. Also atorvastatin, recently released, is roughly twice as potent as simvastatin. When considering a further increase in dosage above the equivalent of 40 mg of lovastatin, the addition of low-dose resin therapy is often more useful and less expensive. Myositis can be seen when these agents are combined with gemfibrozil, cyclosporine, and less often, niacin. This can lead to rhabdomyolysis if not caught early, so this combination should not be used routinely. The dosage of reductase inhibitors must be kept low if used with cyclosporine (ie, under 20 mg of lovastatin).

Combination therapy is most valuable in several specific situations. First, when LDL-c is so high that very large dosages of a single drug would be needed, possibly increasing toxicity, a resin and niacin or a resin and hydroxymethylglutaryl–coenzyme A (HMG-CoA) reductase inhibitor are useful combinations for the marked excess LDL-c (eg, in familial hypercholesterolemia). Second, when lower doses of two drugs would minimize cost or side effects, or multiple lipid abnormalities prevent a single lipid-lowering drug from sufficing, combination therapy is indicated. This is often seen in familial combined hyperlipidemia. Combinations such as niacin and resin, niacin and an HMG-CoA reductase inhibitor, and niacin and gemfibrozil have been used. There is increased risk of liver toxicity with niacin and HMG-CoA reductase inhibitors (as well as increased myositis), so these patients must be watched carefully. If diet and exercise regimens to control triglycerides and HDL-c are strictly adhered to, combination therapy is sometimes not needed.

Treatment of isolated, low HDL-c is a controversial subject. Although these individuals may be at risk, not all with low HDL-c are at increased risk. Vegetarians are a good example; they have both low HDL-c and LDL-c. If low HDL-c is not accompanied by hypertriglyceridemia, the benefit from drug therapy is uncertain. A possible approach is to keep LDL-c low with a low-saturated-fat diet rich in fruits and vegetables (a good source of antioxidants) and to reserve niacin therapy (for those with coronary disease) or gemfibrozil or niacin (if triglycerides are also elevated).

KEY REFERENCES

Recently published papers of outstanding interest, as identified in *References and Recommended Reading*, have been annotated.

•• Shepherd J, Cobbe SM, Ford I, *et al.* for the West of Scotland Coronary Prevention Study Group: *N Engl J Med* 1995, 333:1301–1307.
A primary prevention trial with a large enough sample size to determine if lipid lowering was associated with overall benefit as well as improvement in cardiovascular end points. In the high-risk men studied, treatment with pravastatin-lowered LDL-c on average 26% and significantly reduced fatal and nonfatal myocardial infarction.

•• Scandinavian Simvastatin Survival Study Group: Randomised trial of cholesterol lowering in 4444 patients with coronary heart disease: the Scandinavian Simvastatin Survival Study (4S). *Lancet* 1994, 344:1383–1389.
This important secondary prevention trial established aggressive lipid lowering as important therapy in hypercholesterolemic men and women who had sustained an acute myocardial infarction. Total mortality as well as cardiovascular endpoints and the need for revascularization were favorably influenced by treatment with simvastatin, which lowered LDL-c approximately 35%.

•• Pedersen TR, Kjerkshus J, Berg K, *et al.* for the Scandinavian Survival Study Group: Cholesterol lowering and the use of health care resources: results of the Scandinavian Simvastatin Survival Study. *Circulation* 1996, 93:1796–1802.
This paper provides and interesting look at potential cost savings from effective secondary prevention in hypercholesterolemic men and women after myocardial infarction.

•• Sacks FM, Pfeffer MA, Moye LA, *et al.*: The effect of pravastatin on coronary events after myocardial infarction in patients with average cholesterol levels. *N Engl J Med* 1996, 335:1001–1009.
This study extended the conclusions of the 4S trial to those with lower cholesterol and LDL-c values at entry. Benefit extended down to those whose LDL-c was 125 mg/dL or higher after myocardial infarction.

•• The Post Coronary Artery Bypass Graft Trial Investigators: The effect of aggressive lowering of low-density lipoprotein cholesterol levels and low-dose anticoagulation on obstructive changes in saphenous-vein coronary artery bypass grafts. *N Engl J Med* 1997, 336:153–162.
Clinical trial examining value of aggressive LDL-c lowering in those with saphenous vein coronary artery bypass grafts. Aggressive treatment group had less progression and lower rates of revascularization than those treated less intensively. Low dose warfarin was not effective therapy.

REFERENCES AND RECOMMENDED READING

Recently published papers of particular interest have been highlighted as:

• Of interest
•• Of outstanding interest

1. Steinberg D, Parthasarathy S, Carew TE, *et al.*: Beyond cholesterol: modifications of low density lipoprotein that increase its atherogenicity. *N Engl J Med* 1989, 320:915–924.

2. Stamler J, Wentworth D, Neaton JD, *et al.*: Is the relationship between serum cholesterol and risk of premature death from coronary heart disease continuous and graded? *JAMA* 1986, 256:2823–2826.

3. Kaplan NM: The deadly quartet: upper-body obesity, glucose intolerance, hypertriglyceridemia, and hypertension. *Arch Intern Med* 1989, 149:1514–1520.

4. Expert Panel on Detection, Evaluation, and Treatment of High Blood Cholesterol in Adults: Summary of the Second Report of the National Cholesterol Education (NCEP) Expert Panel on Detection, Evaluation, and Treatment of High Blood Cholesterol in Adults (Adult Treatment Panel II). *JAMA* 1993, 269:3015–3023.

5. Ginsburg GS, Safran C, Pasternak RC: Frequency of low serum high density lipoprotein cholesterol levels in hospitalized patients with "desirable" total cholesterol levels. *Am J Cardiol* 1991, 68:187–192.

6. Tornvall P, Bavenholm P, Landou C, *et al.*: Relation of plasma levels and composition of apolipoprotein B–containing lipoproteins to angiographically defined coronary artery disease in young patients with myocardial infarction. *Circulation* 1993, 88(part 1):2180–2189.

7. Cooper GR, Myers GL, Smith J, Schlant RC: Blood lipid measurements: variations and practical utility. *JAMA* 1992, 267:1652–1660.

8. Gore JM, Goldberg RJ, Matsumoto AS, *et al.*: Validity of serum total cholesterol level obtained within 24 hours of acute myocardial infarction. *Am J Cardiol* 1984, 54:722–725.

9. Ryder REJ, Hayes TM, Mulligan IP, *et al.*: How soon after myocardial infarction should plasma lipid values be assessed? *BMJ* 1984, 289:165–173.

10. Avogaro P, Bon GB, Cazzolato G, *et al.*: Variations in apolipoproteins B and A1 during the course of myocardial infarction. *Eur J Clin Invest* 1978, 8:121–129.

11. Genest JJ, Corbett HM, McNamara JR, *et al.*: Effect of hospitalization on high-density lipoprotein cholesterol in patients undergoing elective coronary angiography. *Am J Cardiol* 1988, 61:998–1000.

12. Hearn JA, DeMaio SJ, Roubin GS, *et al.*: Predictive value of lipoprotein (a) and other serum lipoproteins in the angiographic diagnosis of coronary artery disease. *Am J Cardiol* 1990, 66:1176–1180.

13. Hjermann I, Holme I, Velve Byre K, Leren P: Effect of diet and smoking intervention on the incidence of coronary heart disease. *Laucet* 1981, ii:1303–1310.

14. The Multiple Risk Factor Intervention Trial Research Group: Mortality rates after 10.5 years for participants in the multiple risk factor intervention trial: findings related to a priori hypotheses of the trial. *JAMA* 1990, 263:1795–1801.

15. Dayton S, Pearce ML, Hashimoto S, *et al.*: A controlled clinical trial of a diet high in unsaturated fat in preventing complications of atherosclerosis. *Circulation* 1969, 40(suppl II):II-1–II-63.

16. Ornish D, Brown SE, Scherwitz LW, *et al.*: Can lifestyle changes reverse coronary heart disease? The Lifestyle Heart Trial. *Lancet* 1990, 336:129–133.

17. Watts GF, Lewis B, Brunt JNH, *et al.*: Effects on coronary artery disease of lipid-lowering diet, or diet plus cholestyramine, in the St. Thomas Atherosclerosis Regression (STARS) Study. *Lancet* 1992, 339:563–569.

18. *The Surgeon General's Report on Nutrition and Health* U.S. Department of Health and Human Services. Public Health Service. USDHHS (PHS) Publication No. 88-50210, 1988.

19. Gorder DD, Dolecek TA, Coleman GG, *et al.*: Dietary intake in the Multiple Risk Factor Intervention Trial (MRFIT): nutrient and food group changes over 6 years. *J Am Diet Assoc* 1986, 86:744–751.

20. Pearson TA: The quest for a cholesterol-decreasing diet: should we subract, substitute, or supplement? *Ann Intern Med* 1993, 119:627–628.

21. Cobb MM, Teitelbaum HS, Breslow JL: Lovastatin efficacy in reducing low-density lipoprotein cholesterol levels on high- vs. low-fat diets. *JAMA* 1991, 265:997–1001.

22. Lipid Research Clinics Program: The Lipid Research Clinics Coronary Primary Prevention Trial Result. I. Reduction in incidence of coronary heart disease. *JAMA* 1984, 251:351–364.

23. Frick MH, Eto O, Haapa K, *et al.*: Helsinki Heart Study: primary prevention trial with gemfibrozil in middle-aged men with dyslipidemia. *N Engl J Med* 1987, 317:1237–1245.

24.•• Shepherd J, Cobbe SM, Ford I, *et al.* for the West of Scotland Coronary Prevention Study Group: Prevention of coronary heart disease with pravastatin in men with hypercholesterolemia. *N Engl J Med* 1995, 333:1301–1307.

25.•• Scandinavian Simvastatin Survival Study Group: Randomised trial of cholesterol lowering in 4444 patients with coronary heart disease: the Scandinavian Simvastatin Survival Study (4S). *Lancet* 1994, 344:1383–1389.

26.•• Pedersen TR, Kjerkshus J, Berg K, *et al.* for the Scandinavian Survival Study Group: Cholesterol lowering and the use of health care resources: results of the Scandinavian Simvastatin Survival Study. *Circulation* 1996, 93:1796–1802.

27.•• Sacks FM, Pfeffer MA, Moye LA, *et al.*: The effect of pravastatin on coronary events after myocardial infarction in patients with average cholesterol levels. *N Engl J Med* 1996, 335:1001–1009.

28.•• The Post Coronary Artery Bypass Graft Trial Investigators: The effect of aggressive lowering of low-density lipoprotein cholesterol levels and low-dose anticoagulation on obstructive changes in saphenous-vein coronary artery bypass grafts. *N Engl J Med* 1997, 336:153–162.

29. Cashin-Hemphill L, Mack WJ, Pogoda JM, *et al.*: Beneficial effects of colestipol-niacin on coronary atherosclerosis. A 4-year follow-up. *JAMA* 1990, 264:3013–3017.

30. Brown G, Albers JJ, Fisher LD, *et al.*: Regression of coronary artery disease as a result of interim lipid-lowering therapy in men with high levels of apolipoprotein B. *N Engl J Med* 1990, 323:1289–1298.

31. Kane JP, Malloy MJ, Ports TA, *et al.*: Regression of coronary atherosclerosis during treatment of familial hypercholesterolemia with combined drug regimens. *JAMA* 1990, 264:3007–3012.

32. Buchwald H, Varco RL, Matts JP, *et al.*: Effect of partial ileal bypass surgery on mortality and morbidity from coronary heart disease in patients with hypercholesterolemia. *N Engl J Med* 1990, 323:946–955.

33. Blankenhorn DH, Hodis HN: Arterial imaging and atherosclerosis reversal. *Arterioscler Thromb* 1994, 14:177–192.

34. Squires RW, Allison TG, Gau GT, *et al.*: Low-dose, time-release nicotinic acid: effects in selected patients with low concentrations of high-density lipoprotein cholesterol. *Mayo Clin Proc* 1992, 67:855–860.

35. McKenney JM, Proctor JD, Harris S, Chinchili VM: A comparison of the efficacy and toxic effects of sustained vs. immediate-release niacin in hypercholesterolemic patients. *JAMA* 1994, 271:672–677.

36. Badimon JJ, Fuster V, Chesebro JH, Badimon L: Coronary atherosclerosis. A multifactorial disease. *Circulation* 1993, 87(suppl II):II-3–II-16.

Select Bibliography

Badimon JJ, Fuster V, Chesebro JH, Badimon L: Coronary atherosclerosis. A multifactorial disease. *Circulation* 1993, 87(suppl II):II-3–II-16.

Byington RP, Jukema JW, Salonen JT, *et al.*: Reduction in cardiovascular events during pravastatin therapy: pooled analysis of clinical events of the pravastatin atherosclerosis intervention program. *Circulation* 1995, 92:2419–2425.

Herd JA, Ballantyne CM, Farmer JA, *et al.*: Beneficial effects of fluvastatin on coronary atherosclerosis in patients with mild to moderate cholesterol elevations: the Lipoprotein and Coronary Atherosclerosis Study (LCAS). In press.

MAAS Investigators: Effect of simvastatin on coronary atheroma: the Multicentre Anti-Atheroma Sudy (MAAS). *Lancet* 1994, 344:633–638.

Rath M, Niendorf A, Reblin T, *et al.*: Detection and quantification of lipoprotein (a) in the arterial wall of 107 coronary bypass patients. *Arteriosclerosis* 1989, 9:579–592.

Waters D, Higginson L, Gladstone P, *et al.*: Effects of monotherapy with an HMGCoa reductase inhibitor on the progression of coronary atherosclerosis as assessed by serial quantitative arteriography: the Canadian Coronary Atherosclerosis Intervention Trial. *Circulation* 1994, 89:959–968.

Evaluation of the Patient with Hypertension

Robert G. Luke

15

> ### *Key Points*
> - The primary care physician plays the key role in the detection, assessment, and treatment of essential (primary) hypertension. Screening is cost-effective.
> - Ninety percent of all hypertension is primary; 5% to 10% is secondary.
> - Secondary hypertension mainly results from renal or renovascular disease. Clinical features identify a minority of patients for work-up for these and other causes.
> - High normal blood pressures and mild hypertension respond well to nonpharmacologic measures, such as dietary modifications and exercise.
> - Pharmacologic intervention is lifelong.
> - Most patients can now be treated with a single daily dose of a single drug with no or minimal side effects.

This chapter deals with the diagnosis, initial work-up, and approach to treatment of patients with hypertension. A more detailed discussion of antihypertensive drug therapy and of the diagnosis of secondary causes of hypertension is provided in Chapter 28. This chapter alone, however, should facilitate the initial management of hypertension in the ambulatory setting.

ROLE OF THE GENERALIST

About one in four adults in the United States has hypertension, which is defined as blood pressure of greater than or equal to 140/90 mm Hg. Hypertension is the major risk factor for stroke, cardiac failure, and nephrosclerosis and one of the most important risk factors for atherosclerosis. The generalist must screen for, diagnose, and treat hypertension in all patients. In addition, the generalist selects 5% to 10% of such patients to undergo detailed study for secondary causes of high blood pressure, some of which cause curable high blood pressure. Treatment of hypertension in the past three decades has reduced the prevalence of fatal stroke by 60% and that of fatal myocardial infarction by about 40%, and it has very much reduced the prevalence of hypertensive heart failure and malignant hypertension [1•]. Although this effect has not yet been documented, it is likely that the prevalence of hypertensive nephrosclerosis, which causes 30% of all end-stage renal disease, will also be reduced considerably. Surveys show that only two thirds of patients are being treated, and only half of those have a blood pressure of 140/90 mm Hg [2].

Thus, the role of the generalist in hypertension is important and clear in detection, prevention, and treatment. Treatment is cost-effective, and with patience and skill, the primary care physician can manage hypertension, when indicated, with antihypertensive drugs in the majority of patients. This is true preventive therapy mainly in asymptomatic patients. With the large array of efficacious medications now available, the physician's goal can be control of

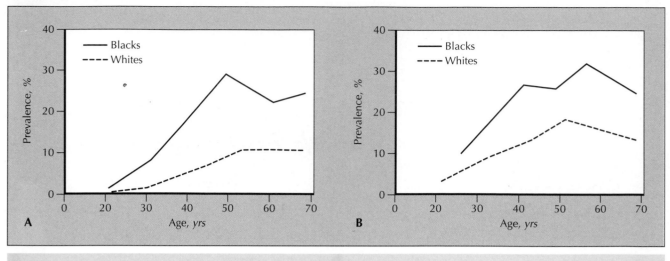

FIGURE 1 Percent prevalence of diastolic blood pressure greater than 95 mm Hg in black and white women (**A**) and men (**B**). *Adapted from* Troyler [29]; with permission.)

blood pressure within the indicated range, with virtually no side effects, and even improvement in quality of life [3].

EPIDEMIOLOGY OF ESSENTIAL HYPERTENSION

Hypertension is either primary (essential) or, in approximately 10% of patients, secondary. Secondary hypertension mainly results from renal disease or renovascular hypertension. The latter condition, and the small number of cases (about 1%) due to endocrine causes, are potentially curable. Essential hypertension usually develops between 35 and 55 years of age and is associated with a family history of the condition.

Screening for hypertension is cost-effective for all adults [4]. Blood pressure should be measured at all initial contacts with the physician, no matter how brief. Healthy adults with normal blood pressure should have their blood pressure rechecked in the absence of other reasons for medical visits perhaps every 2 to 3 years. Patients with high-normal blood pressures (130 to 139/85 to 89 mm Hg), however, should have at least yearly blood pressure measurements thereafter and should have a screen for other cardiovascular risk factors (*see* Table 9).

High blood pressure is more common in men. Both its prevalence and untreated hypertension in individual patients increases with age. In African-Americans, hypertension is more common, develops at an earlier age, is more severe, and more often causes target organ damage (especially stroke and renal failure) (Fig. 1).

Systolic blood pressure is as important a risk factor for cardiovascular events as is diastolic blood pressure. Isolated systolic hypertension (systolic pressure, > 160 mm Hg; diastolic pressure, ≤ 90 mm Hg) is common in the elderly and also benefits from treatment [5].

Hypertension in children less than 16 years of age (> 140/90 mm Hg) is usually secondary [6]. Drug treatment for essential hypertension in this age group is rarely indicated, except in children with associated type I diabetes mellitus or in

controlled prospective trials.

DIAGNOSTIC APPROACH

The physician's initial goal is to attempt to answer the questions raised in Table 1. Hypertension cannot be diagnosed based on a single blood pressure reading or in a single visit, unless severe hypertension (≥ 180/110 mm Hg) or target organ damage is present (Table 2).

Blood pressure should be taken carefully and according to protocol (Fig. 2) [7]. In patients with blood pressure of less than 160/100 mm Hg and without target organ damage, a diagnosis of hypertension should not be made until a mean blood pressure of more than (or equal to) 140/90 mm Hg is confirmed on at least two further visits (*see* Fig. 6).

This judicious approach to diagnosis is important. Labeling a patient "hypertensive" is not without some potentially negative effects [8]. The patient's concept of himself or herself may change from one of being well to one of being ill, leading, for example, to absenteeism from work. Similarly, many nonspecific symptoms (*eg*, headache and dizziness) are often

TABLE 1 DECISION POINTS IN EVALUATING THE HYPERTENSIVE PATIENT
Does the patient
Have sustained hypertension?
Take relevant drugs?*
Have hypertensive disease (effects on target organs)?
Have other risk factors for cardiovascular disease?
Need lifestyle modification?
Need antihypertensive drugs? Is therapy emergent or urgent? Which drug or drugs?
Need the minimum work-up or a more extensive search for a secondary cause or causes?
*See **Table 3**.

TABLE 2 TARGET ORGAN DAMAGE
Cardiac
Paroxysmal nocturnal dyspnea
Exertional dyspnea
Angina
History of myocardial infarction
Left ventricular hypertrophy
Central nervous system
Transient ischemic attack
Stroke
Retinal
Severe vasospasm
Exudates
Hemorrhages
Papilledema
Renal
Proteinuria
Microalbuminuria*
Hematuria
Serum creatinine level of > 1.4 mg/dL
Vascular
Peripheral vascular disease
*Especially in diabetes mellitus

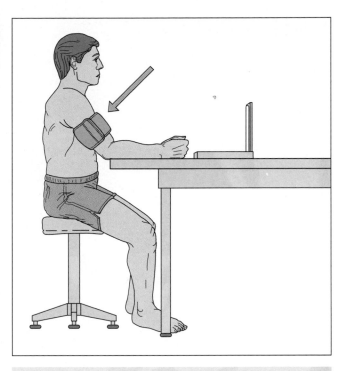

FIGURE 2 Patients seated, resting 5 minutes. Arm supported by table, unrestricted by tight clothing. Cuff bladder at least 80% of arm circumference. Take blood pressure twice in the same arm 2 minutes apart. Check blood pressure in other arm and also with the patient standing.

wrongly blamed on mild to moderate hypertension—by both patients and physicians [9]! Only severe essential hypertension is associated with symptoms, and essential hypertension usually evolves over many years before becoming severe.

With secondary hypertension, however, it is the *rate of rise* of the blood pressure rather than the actual blood pressure level itself that determines severity. For example, a patient with acute glomerulonephritis and a previously normal blood pressure may become ill with target organ damage at a blood pressure of approximately 160/100 mm Hg. The same is true in preeclampsia.

The history and physical examination findings will aid greatly in answering all of the issues in Table 1 (Fig. 3). Symptoms and signs of hypertensive disease should be sought (*see* Table 2). Discontinuance of therapy with certain drugs may ameliorate or correct high blood pressure (Table 3). At the first visit, even if the patient's blood pressure is only high-normal (130 to 140/80 to 89 mm Hg), a minimum work-up should be performed. This work-up consists of urinalysis; measurement of serum levels of creatinine, potassium, calcium, and lipids (low-density lipoprotein, high-density lipoprotein, and triglycerides); and electrocardiography. Even slight hypertension may be an initial presentation of underlying primary renal disease, such as adult dominant polycystic disease or chronic glomerulonephritis.

An electrocardiogram may reveal left atrial or ventricular hypertrophy or evidence of ischemic heart disease. Left ventricular hypertrophy is an independent cardiovascular risk factor. Clinical, radiologic, and electrocardiographic findings (Fig. 4) are less sensitive indicators of left ventricular hypertrophy than is echocardiography. The latter is still too expensive for routine assessment of hypertension but can be a useful test when determining the need for drug therapy is difficult [11].

CLASSIFICATION OF PATIENT'S HYPERTENSION

After one or several visits, as described previously, the physician should be able to answer the questions in Table 1 and to classify the patient's condition tentatively according to the guidelines in the fifth report of the Joint National Committee on Detection, Evaluation and Treatment of High Blood Pressure, and by evidence of target organ damage, the need for a more extensive search for secondary causes, and the important but unusual requirement for immediate drug treatment, admission to the hospital, or both (Tables 2, 4, 5, and 6 and Fig. 5) [13•].

INITIATION OF TREATMENT

Lifestyle Modifications

Lifestyle modifications (nonpharmacologic therapy) can be implemented in all patients with high-normal blood pressure and above (Table 7). All of these interventions, including weight loss, salt restriction, increased dietary potassium (fruits and vegetables) (Table 8), and exercise have been docu-

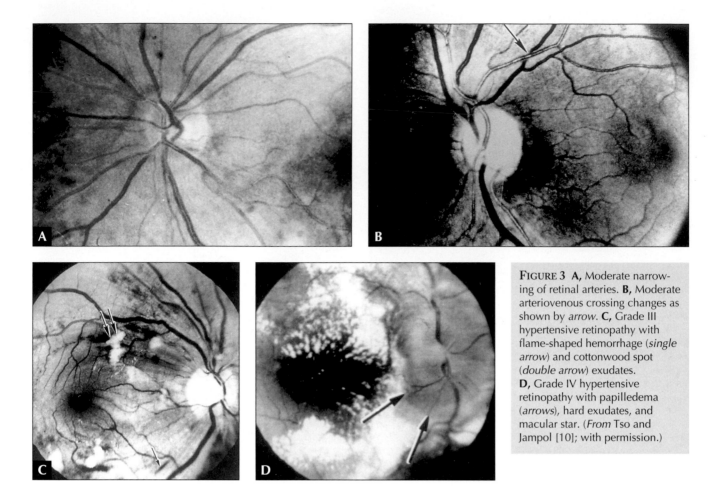

FIGURE 3 A, Moderate narrowing of retinal arteries. **B,** Moderate arteriovenous crossing changes as shown by *arrow*. **C,** Grade III hypertensive retinopathy with flame-shaped hemorrhage (*single arrow*) and cottonwood spot (*double arrow*) exudates. **D,** Grade IV hypertensive retinopathy with papilledema (*arrows*), hard exudates, and macular star. (*From* Tso and Jampol [10]; with permission.)

mented to have beneficial and independent effects on blood pressure [14–16,17••,18]. The physician should persist with them in the compliant patient for 3 to 6 months before concluding that they are ineffective.

The most difficult decision is when to initiate antihypertensive drug therapy in mild hypertension if nonpharmacologic treatment fails. Both patients and physicians *must* understand that such drug treatment is a lifelong commitment unless lifestyle modifications are subsequently more effective. Occasional drug samples taken intermittently when the patient believes his or her blood pressure is high will not work. The presence of any associated cardiovascular risk factor swings the balance toward treatment because the risks are additive (Table 9). Patients with type I diabetes mellitus or renal disease should be treated for even slight elevations in blood pressure, especially if microalbuminuria is present [19,20••]. If all risk factors listed in Table 5 are absent, it is reasonable to observe the patient for 6 to 12 months, especially if their readings are in the lower blood pressure range of mild hypertension (Fig. 6). Semiautomatic home and work blood pressure measuring devices cost in the $50 to $100 range and are quite useful with careful calibration and instruction in their use. Ambulatory blood pressure monitoring is not suitable for routine use in primary care.

Significant errors in blood pressure measurement and therefore in the classification of hypertension can be caused by very stiff vessels in elderly arteriosclerotic patients (pseudohypertension); by "white coat" hypertension, in which ambulatory at-home blood pressure measurements are much lower than blood pressure measurements obtained at the physician's office, although this finding is not necessarily always benign; and by cuff inflation hypertension [21–23]. Discrepancies between target organ damage and blood pressure levels or unexpected hypotensive reactions to monotherapy should bring these possible errors to mind.

Drug Selection and Goals of Treatment

A high proportion of patients with mild or moderate hypertension can be treated by single drugs from the six now-

TABLE 3 DRUGS THAT CAUSE OR INTERFERE WITH THERAPY FOR HYPERTENSION
Alcohol
Oral contraceptive agents
Nonsteroidal antiinflammatory drugs
Cyclosporine
Steroids
Nasal decongestants
Amphetamines
Erythropoietin
Monoamine oxidase inhibitors

recommended classes of drug; each individual drug can control blood pressure in approximately 50% of such hypertensive patients, and some patients who do not respond to one drug in a particular class will respond to a single drug from another class [13•,24]. A list of clinical indicators for selection among these six classes of medication is given in Table 10. Target blood pressure should be 140/90 mm Hg or less. In younger patients with diabetes mellitus or primary renal

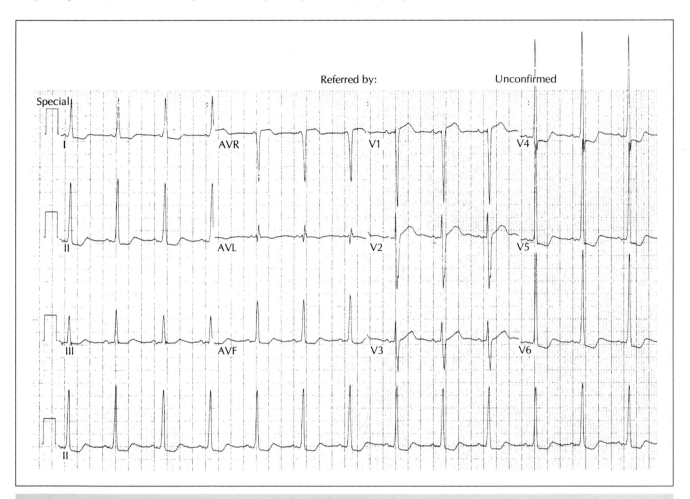

FIGURE 4 Electrocardiogram showing left ventricular hypertrophy by voltage criteria (SV_1 plus RV_5 or $RV_6 \geq 35$ mm) with secondary ST and T wave changes.

	Systolic pressure, *mm Hg*	Diastolic pressure, *mm Hg*
TABLE 4 CLASSIFICATION OF BLOOD PRESSURE FOR ADULTS AGED 18 YEARS AND OLDER		
Category		
Normal	< 130	< 85
High-normal	130–139	85–89
Hypertension		
Stage 1 (mild)	140–159	90–99
Stage 2 (moderate)	160–179	100–109
Stage 3 (severe)	180–209	110–119
Stage 4 (very severe)	≥ 210	≥ 120

From Joint National Committee on Detection, Evaluation and Treatment of High Blood Pressure [13•]; with permission.

TABLE 5 INDICATIONS OF THE NEED TO SEARCH FOR SECONDARY CAUSES OF HYPERTENSION

General

Age of onset at < 30 or > 55 years

Severe hypertension (systolic pressure, > 180 mm Hg; diastolic pressure, > 110 mm Hg)

Abrupt onset, rapid increase in severity, or development of resistance to previously effective therapy

Specific

Symptoms of pheochromocytoma

Unexplained hypokalemia (primary aldosteronism)

Signs of Cushing's syndrome

Palpable kidneys, renal bruit, or abnormal urinalysis results (renal or renovascular hypertension)

Delayed or absent femoral pulses (coarctation)

TABLE 6 INDICATIONS FOR IMMEDIATE OR EARLY TREATMENT IN PATIENTS WITH HYPERTENSION*

Hypertensive emergency (immediate treatment)
Hypertensive encephalopathy
Acute left ventricular failure
Severe preeclampsia
Renal failure
Cerebral hemorrhage
Hypertension with dissecting aortic aneurysm
Unstable angina
Myocardial infarction

Hypertensive urgency (early treatment)
Hypertensive grade III or IV retinal changes
Severe preoperative or perioperative hypertension

Immediate means within 1 hour; *early*, within 24 hours.

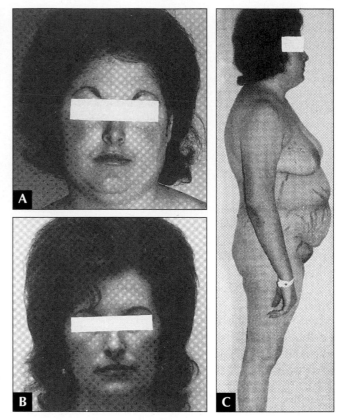

FIGURE 5 Patient with Cushing's disease (**A** and **C**) and 1 year after removal of an adrenal adenoma (**B**). (*From* Tyrrell [12]; with permission.)

disease, the goal should be to achieve blood pressure that is as near as possible to 120/80 mm Hg as is tolerated [25]; angiotensin-converting enzyme inhibitors are now the drug of choice for hypertension in diabetes mellitus and in many patients with primary renal disease. Diastolic blood pressure should not be lowered below 85 mm Hg in older patients with coronary artery or cerebrovascular disease or marked left ventricular hypertrophy. In patients with postural hypotension (*eg*, from diabetic autonomic neuropathy), the standing blood pressure must be targeted for symptomatic reasons.

A single daily dose is most convenient for the patient. Care must be taken, however, to ensure that blood pressure control is still adequate in the awakening period between 6:00 and 10:00 AM, because this is a period of increased sudden death from stroke and myocardial infarction [26].

Thiazide diuretics have been used for 40 years and remain cheap and effective drugs, either as initial therapy or as an addition to other medications, especially angiotensin-converting enzyme inhibitors or α-blockers. For hydrochlorothiazide, a dose of 12.5 to 25 mg is initially used; 50 mg is the maxi-

mum daily dose. Most of the long-term trials have used diuretics; recent trials have demonstrated their effectiveness in isolated systolic hypertension and in elderly persons with hypertension [5,27]. Before these agents are prescribed, fasting blood glucose, serum potassium, and uric acid levels should be checked as a baseline; the serum potassium levels should be checked again in about 1 month. Unless the patient is receiving digoxin or has another cause of potassium loss, the use of routine potassium supplements or a potassium-sparing diuretic is not necessary. Vasodilators such as hydralazine and

TABLE 7 LIFESTYLE MODIFICATIONS FOR PATIENTS WITH HIGH-NORMAL AND HIGHER BLOOD PRESSURE

Modification	Comments
Stop smoking*	Might allow avoidance of antihypertensive drug therapy in mild hypertension if smoking is the only associated cardiovascular risk factor
Restrict daily alcohol intake	< 2 oz of liquor, 8 oz of wine, or 24 oz of beer
Moderately restrict daily salt intake	6 g (100 mmol) of sodium chloride [18]
Eat a diet high in potassium	Beneficial in the absence of renal insufficiency or hyperkalemia [17••]; pleasant because high in vegetables and fresh fruit; salt substitutes containing potassium may be useful
Reduce weight by at least 10 lb (obese patients)	Often reduces blood pressure significantly [15,18]
Engage in moderate, regular isotonic exercise	For example, walking briskly at least 3 times per week for 30 to 45 min [16]

*Smoking does not cause chronic hypertension but is an important associated risk factor for cardiovascular disease.

TABLE 8 EQUIVALENT POTASSIUM RATIONS*

Legumes

Beans (dry): 40 g
Broad beans (dry): 50 g
Peas (fresh): 260 g
Canned beans: 230 g
Frozen peas: 260 g
Lentils (dry): 70 g
Chick peas (dry): 60 g
Broad beans (fresh): 160 g
Canned lentils: 250 g

Vegetables

Greenhouse asparagus: 200 g
String beans: 200 g
Mushrooms: 100 g
Peppers: 450 g
Turnip: 200 g
Squash: 300 g
Carrots: 250 g
Fennel: 200 g
Potatoes: 100 g
Radicchio: 300 g
Cabbage: 200 g
Artichoke globe: 150 g
Cauliflower: 150 g

Eggplant: 300 g
Green tomatoes: 250 g
Spinach: 100 g
Broccoli: 150 g
Chicory: 150 g
Lettuce: 200 g
Green peppers: 400 g
Prickly lettuce: 200 g

Fresh fruit

Apricots: 160 g
Cherries: 180 g
Peaches: 200 g
Oranges: 200 g
Pears: 400 g
Grapes: 200 g
Orange juice: 250 g
Apples: 450 g
Plums: 170 g
Bananas: 150 g
Grapefruit: 200 g

Dairy

Milk (skimmed): 350 g

*Each ration contains approximately 10–12 mmol of potassium; patients in the intervention group were advised to eat three to six rations per day. The amount of each ration is reported as "net weight."
From Siani *et al.* [14]; with permission.

TABLE 9 ASSOCIATED RISK FACTORS FAVORING ANTIHYPERTENSIVE DRUG THERAPY

Hyperlipidemia
Diabetes mellitus
Renal disease
Black race
Coronary artery disease
Left ventricular hypertrophy
Cerebrovascular disease
Family history of premature cardiovascular events
Smoking

stances can precipitate ischemic events, and the immediate goal of treatment should not be to restore normal levels but rather to reduce diastolic blood pressure initially by about 15 to 20 mm Hg or to the 160 to 170/100 to 110 mm Hg range. Very high blood pressure alone is not a reason to treat emergently in the absence of symptoms or target organ damage. Restarting therapy with previously effective medications in noncompliant patients may be all that is necessary: blood pressure may increase markedly after sudden cessation of central α_2 blockers (*eg*, clonidine), but this rise usually responds to the restarting of therapy. In patients with severe hypertension but no emergent or urgent indication to treat, reasonable regimens are a β-blocker plus hydralazine with or without (depending on severity) a thiazide diuretic, or an angiotensin-converting enzyme inhibitor plus a thiazide or a calcium channel blocker.

minoxidil may cause reflex tachycardia and edema and are not suitable for monotherapy.

In the case of a hypertensive medical emergency or urgency in the office, oral nifedipine, captopril, clonidine, and labetalol are rapidly acting and useful while the physician arranges admission to a hospital special care unit, which is usually necessary in such patients (*see* Table 6). Overly rapid correction of blood pressure in these circum-

SECONDARY HYPERTENSION

Routine screening of all hypertensive patients for secondary causes of hypertension is not cost-effective, except for performing urinalysis and measuring serum creatinine levels to screen for primary renal disease, by far the most common cause of secondary hypertension. Proteinuria before hypertension usually indicates primary renal disease. Hypertensive nephrosclerosis is associated with only modest proteinuria (< 2

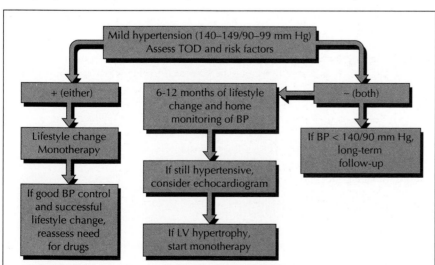

FIGURE 6 Algorithm for mild hypertension. BP—blood pressure; LV—left ventricular; TOD—target organ damage, as in Table 2.

Drug Class*	Indications	Contraindications/Problems
Thiazide diuretic (hydrochlorothiazide)	Very cheap, long-term efficacy established, potentiate other drug groups, isolated systolic hypertension, CHF, older and black patients	Gout. Hypokalemia, diminished glucose tolerance and hyperlipidemia—minimal clinical importance if HCTZ dose does not exceed 50 mg.
Loop diuretic (furosemide)	Serum creatinine level >2 mg/dL; resistant edema	Readily cause extracellular fluid volume depletion
ß-Blocker (atenolol)	CAD, younger whites	Asthma, RD, PVD, CHF, IDDM
Angiotensin-converting enzyme inhibitor (captopril, enalapril)	RD, LVH, CHF†, diabetes mellitus; whites	Renal artery stenosis, hyperkalemia
Angiotensin II-blocker (Losartan)	Same as ACE inhibitor (use if cough prevents use of ACE inhibitor)	Same as ACE inhibitor
Calcium channel blockers	CAD, RD, PVD; blacks	CHF†
Dihydropyridines (amlodipine)	Cyclosporine-induced (long-acting nifedipine) CAD, RD, PVD; blacks	Use long-acting only [28•]
Other (diltiazem)		Bradycardia, heart block
alpha-Blocker (prazosin)	Hyperlipidemia; prostatism	Postural hypotension

*The examples in parentheses are prototypes

†Angiotensin-converting enzyme inhibitors are used for CHF with systolic dysfunction; calcium channel blockers like diltiazem are being used for patients with CHF due to diastolic dysfunction (normal LV ejection fraction), as in some hypertensives.

CAD—coronary artery disease; CHF—congestive heart failure; IDDM—insulin-dependent diabetes mellitus; LVH—left ventricular hypertrophy; PVD—peripheral vascular disease; RD—renal disease.

g/24h), and only after many years of hypertension. It is more frequent in the fourth and fifth decades of life in blacks, and it usually only occurs in whites older than 60 years of age in the absence of malignant hypertension.

Renovascular hypertension is the most common cause of correctable hypertension. Urinalysis and serum creatinine levels are of no value in screening for renovascular hypertension; indeed, no single screening test is adequate, and if clinical suspicion warrants a search for it, the gold standard remains renal arteriography, which is, unfortunately, an expensive and invasive procedure. In the age group of 35 to 55 years for whites and 25 to 55 for blacks, a search is required only for patients with initially severe hypertension, those with a renal bruit, or those whose hypertension is resistant to therapy with two concurrently used antihypertensive agents. An imperfect but reasonable screening test for functional renal artery stenosis is the captopril isotope renogram. If structural renal disease (polycystic kidneys, obstruction, reflux nephropathy) is suspected, renal ultrasound (noninvasive) is indicated.

Table 11 provides information on referring patients with secondary causes of hypertension.

TABLE 11 GUIDELINES FOR REFERRAL OF PATIENTS WITH SECONDARY CAUSES OF HYPERTENSION

Condition	Specialist referred to	Comments
Suspected renal disease	Nephrologist	
Suspected renal artery stenosis	Renovascular group*	Clinical and angiographic study by this group offers the most cost-effective outcome
Renovascular renal failure (ischemic renal failure)†	Renovascular group*	This problem is seen with increasing frequency; it should be suspected in elderly patients who often smoke and who have diffuse evidence of atherosclerotic disease, hypertension, and an elevated serum creatinine level without evidence of another primary renal disease
Unexplained hypokalemia; symptoms suggestive of pheochromocytoma, elevated urinary catecholamine levels, or clinical findings suggestive of Cushing's syndrome	Specialist in hypertension (nephrologist, cardiologist, or endocrinologist)	Use a "hypertensologist" with experience in cost-effective work-up

*Ideally, a nephrologist, a radiologist-angioplaster, and a vascular surgeon.

†Bilateral severe renal artery stenosis with renal atrophy or an absent or atrophic kidney plus contralateral severe renal artery stenosis.

KEY REFERENCES

Recently published papers of outstanding interest, as identified in *References and Recommended Reading*, have been annotated.

•• Appel LJ, Moore TJ, Obarzanek E, *et al.*: A clinical trial of the effects of dietary patterns on blood pressure. *N Engl J Med* 1997, 336:1117–1124.

The results of the DASH (Dietary Approaches to Stop Hypertension) study are important. A high fruit and vegetable, low dairy fat diet at constant (3g) sodium intake and body weight reduced BP by 11.4 systolic and 5.5 mmHg diastolic in stage 1 hypertension—as effective as drug monotherapy!

•• Pontremoli R: Microalbuminuria in essential hypertension—its relation to cardiovascular risk factors. *Nephrol Dial Transplant* 1996, 11:2113–2134.

Screening for microalbuminuria is well established to detect early, often reversible diabetic renal disease. This finding in essential hypertension clearly indicates increased cardiovascular risk and can be useful in guiding the generalist to either introduce antihypertensive drug therapy or to intensify it to better control hypertension.

REFERNCES AND RECOMMENDED READING

Recently published papers of particular interest have been highlighted as:

• Of interest

•• Of outstanding interest

1.• Cutler JA, Psaty BM, MacMahon S, *et al.*: Public health issues in hypertension control: what has been learned from clinical trials. In *Hypertension: Pathophysiology, Diagnosis, and Management*, 3rd edn. Laragh JH, Brenner BM, eds. New York: Raven Press, Ltd.; 1995:253–270.

2. Burt VL, Cutler JA, Higgins M, *et al.*: Trends in the prevalence, awareness, treatment and control of hypertension in the adult US population. *Hypertension* 1995, 26:60–69.

3. Grimm RJ, Grandits GA, Cutler MA, *et al.*: Relationships of quality-of-life measures to long-term lifestyle and drug treatment in the treatment of mild hypertension study. *Arch Intern Med* 1997, 157:638–648.

4. Littenberg B, Garber AM, Sox HC: Screening for hypertension. *Ann Intern Med* 1990, 112:192–202.

5. SHEP Cooperative Research Group: Prevention of stroke by antihypertensive drug treatment in older persons with isolated systolic hypertension. *JAMA* 1991, 265:3255–3264.

6. Task Force on Blood Pressure Control in Children: Report of the second task force on blood pressure control in children—1987. *Pediatrics* 1987, 79:1–25.

7. American Society of Hypertension: Recommendations for routine blood pressure measurement by indirect cuff sphygmomanometry. *Am J Hypertens* 1992, 5:207–209.

8. Haynes RB, Sackett DL, Taylor DW, *et al.*: Increased absenteeism from work after detection and labeling of hypertensive patients. *N Engl J Med* 1978, 299:741–744.

9. Weiss NA: Relation of high blood pressure to headache, epistaxis, and selected other symptoms. *N Engl J Med* 1972, 287:631–633.

10. Tso O, Jampol L: Hypertensive retinopathy, choroidopathy, and optic neuropathy of hypertensive ocular disease. In *Hypertension: Pathophysiology, Diagnosis, and Management*, vol. 1. Laragh JH, Brenner BM, eds. New York: Raven Press; 1990:433–465.

11. Frolich ED, Chobanian AV, Devereau RB, *et al.*: The heart in hypertension [review article] . *N Engl J Med* 1992, 327:998–1008.

12. Tyrrell JB: Cushing's syndrome. In *Cecil Textbook of Medicine*, edn 19. Wyngaarden JB, Smith LH, Bennett JC, eds. Philadelphia: WB Saunders; 1992:1284–1288.

13.• Joint National Committee on Detection, Evaluation and Treatment of High Blood Pressure: The sixth report of the Joint National committee on detection, evaluation, and treatment of high blood pressure (JNC V). *Arch Intern Med* 1997, in press.

14. Siani A, Strazzullo P, Giacco A, *et al.*: Increasing the dietary potassium intake reduces the need for antihypertensive medication. *Ann Intern Med* 1991, 113:753–759.

15. Reisin E, Abel R, Modan M, *et al.*: Effect of weight loss without salt restriction on the reduction of blood pressure in overweight hypertensive patients. *N Engl J Med* 1978, 298:1–6.

16. Boyer JL, Kasch FW: Exercise therapy in hypertensive men. *JAMA* 1970, 211:1667– 671.

17.•• Appel LJ, Moore TJ, Obarzanek E, *et al.*: A clinical trial of the effects of dietary patterns on blood pressure. *N Engl J Med* 1997, 336:1117–1124.

18. The Trials of Hypertension Prevention Collaborative Research Group: Effects of weight loss and sodium reduction intervention on blood pressure and hypertension incidence in overweight people with high-normal blood pressure. The Trials of Hypertension Prevention, phase II. *Arch Intern Med* 1997, 157(6):657–667.

19. Bennett PH, Haffner S, Kasiske BL, *et al.*: Screening and management of microalbuminuria in patients with diabetes mellitus. *Am J Kidney Dis* 1995, 107–112.

20.•• Pontremoli R: Microalbuminuria in essential hypertension—its relation to cardiovascular risk factors. *Nephrol Dial Transplant* 1996, 11:2113–2134.

21. Mejiia AD, Egan BR, Schork NJ, *et al.*: Artefacts in measurement of blood pressure and lack of target organ involvement in the assessment of patients with treatment-resistant hypertension. *Ann Intern Med* 1990, 112:270–277.

22. Pickering TG, James GD, Boddie C, *et al.*: How common is white coat hypertension? *JAMA* 1988, 259:225–228.

23. Cardillo C, De Felice F, Campia U, *et al.*: Psychophysiological reactivity and cardiac end-organ changes in white coat hypertension. *Hypertension* 1993, 21:836–844.

24. Materson BJ, Reda DJ, Cushman WC, *et al.*: Single-drug therapy for hypertension in men. *N Engl J Med* 1993, 328:914–921.

25. Peterson JC, Adler S, Burkart JM, *et al.*: Arterial pressure control proteinuria and the progression of renal disease. The modification of diet in renal disease study. *Ann Intern Med* 1995, 1234:754–762.

26. Quyyumi AA: Circadian rhythms in cardiovascular disease. *Am Heart J* 1990, 130:726–733.

27. Mulrow CD, Cornell JA, Herrera CR, *et al.*: Hypertension in the elderly. *JAMA* 1994, 272:1932–1938.

28.• Alderman MH, Cohen J, Roque R, Madhavan S: Effect of long-acting and short-acting calcium antagonists on cardiovascular outcomes in hypertensive patients. *Lancet* 1997, 349:495–598.

29. Troyler H: Socioeconomic status, age, and sex in the prevalence and prognosis of hypertension in blacks and whites. In *Hypertension Pathophysiology, Diagnosis, and Management*, vol. 1. Laraugh JH, Brenner BM, eds. New York: Raven Press; 1990:159–174.

SELECT BIBLIOGRAPHY

Kaplan NM: *Clinical Hypertension*, edn 4. Collins N, ed. Baltimore: Williams & Wilkins; 1986.

Laraugh JH, Brenner BM: *Hypertension*, vol 2. New York: Raven Press; 1990.

Secondary Hypertension 16

Thomas G. Pickering

Key Points

- Secondary hypertension occurs in less than 5% of cases, but its diagnosis is important because of the possibility of a permanent cure.
- Routine screening of all hypertensive patients is not recommended and should be reserved for those in whom clinical clues are present.
- Renovascular hypertension is the commonest type and should be suspected in two populations: young women with severe or recent hypertension, and older patients with evidence of atherosclerotic disease.
- Captopril renography is one of the best noninvasive tests for diagnosing renovascular hypertension.
- Although both aldosterone-secreting tumors and pheochromocytomas may be diagnosed biochemically, an anatomic diagnosis may be difficult to make because aldosteronomas may be very small, and pheochromocytomas occur outside the adrenal glands.

In about 5% of cases, hypertension can be attributed to a secondary cause, such as a renal or endocrine disorder. The diagnosis of such cases is important not only because of the potential for a permanent cure but also because, if untreated, the underlying disorder may cause other problems, such as renal failure [1]. Hypertension may be the presenting manifestation of these conditions, or it may be one of a variety of signs and symptoms in patients with systemic disease (Table 1).

WHEN TO SCREEN FOR SECONDARY HYPERTENSION

Routine screening of all hypertensive patients for secondary causes is not recommended because the expense and unreliability of the available screening tests make it uneconomical. Two general indications for screening are the severity of the hypertension and the presence of clinical clues detected during routine examination. Renovascular hypertension has a prevalence of less than 5% in the general hypertensive population but is as high as 30% in patients with accelerated hypertension [2]. Essential hypertension occurs rarely before the age of 15 years, and young hypertensive children should be investigated thoroughly for a secondary cause.

Renovascular Hypertension

Renovascular hypertension is by far the most common secondary cause of hypertension and is often difficult to diagnose. It has two main causes—fibromuscular dysplasia and atheromatous stenosis. In younger patients (< 50 years of age), fibromuscular dysplasia of the renal arteries predominates, and in older patients renovascular hypertension usually results from atheroma [3,4•]. Fibromuscular dysplasia is usually confined to the renal arteries, where it is characterized by one or more fibrous bands that partly occlude the lumen (Fig. 1). Its etiology is unknown, although smoking may contribute. Most patients do not have a family history of

TABLE 1 CAUSES OF SECONDARY HYPERTENSION

Causes presenting as hypertension	Causes presenting as systemic disease
Renal artery stenosis (fibromuscular dysplasia or atheroma)	Cushing's disease
Renal parenchymal disease	Scleroderma
Aldosterone-secreting tumor	Collagen disease (systemic lupus erythematosus, polyarteritis)
Glucocorticoid-remediable aldosteronism	Hypothyroidism
Pheochromocytoma	
Coarctation of the aorta	
Drug-induced hypertension	

hypertension. Atheromatous stenoses commonly are bilateral and associated with stenosis in other arteries. Because essential hypertension accelerates the development of atheroma, lesions in the renal arteries could be both a cause and a consequence of the hypertension.

To cause hypertension, a renal artery stenosis must be of sufficient severity to impair blood flow to the kidney, which responds by increasing renin secretion. This response activates angiotensin and aldosterone and hence raises blood pressure (Fig. 2). When the stenosis is limited to one renal artery, there is no accompanying sodium retention because the increased arterial pressure in the unaffected kidney results in a pressure natriuresis (Fig. 3A). When only one kidney is present and its artery is stenosed, the renin is normal and the hypertension largely results from sodium retention (Fig. 3B). When both arteries are stenosed, there also may be sodium retention because both kidneys are protected from the high systemic pressure as a result of the stenosis, and no pressure natriuresis occurs (Fig. 3C) [5].

Clinical clues suggestive of renovascular hypertension are shown in Table 2. If these clues are present, further work-up of the patient may be appropriate. The only viable office screening tests are renin-sodium profiling and an oral captopril test. Renin-sodium profiling is performed by relating the plasma renin activity to the 24-hour urinary sodium excretion. A high or normal renin level is compatible with renovascular hypertension, whereas a low renin level excludes it. The captopril test is performed by taking blood for plasma renin activity before and 1 hour after the administration of captopril, 25 mg, by mouth [6]. In patients with normal renin levels, an increase of renin of more than 150% is very suggestive of renovascular disease (Fig. 4); however, false-positive results are common in high-renin patients [7•].

When there is a moderate level of suspicion that renovascular disease is present, the best screening test is probably a renal scan performed with mercaptoacetyl triglycine (MAG_3) (Fig. 5) after a single oral dose of captopril [8]. This test is more reliable than a conventional scan because the captopril reduces the glomerular filtration rate in the presence of a renal artery stenosis. If the index of suspicion is very high, or if the captopril scan results are positive, arteriography is indicated.

Revascularization is the preferred form of treatment. If possible, this should be done by angioplasty or, alternatively, by surgery (eg, by a hepatorenal artery bypass for the

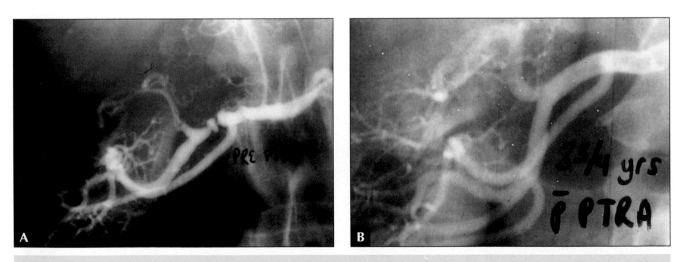

FIGURE 1 Renal angiogram showing fibromuscular dysplasia before (**A**) and after (**B**) renal angioplasty, which in this case cured the hypertension.

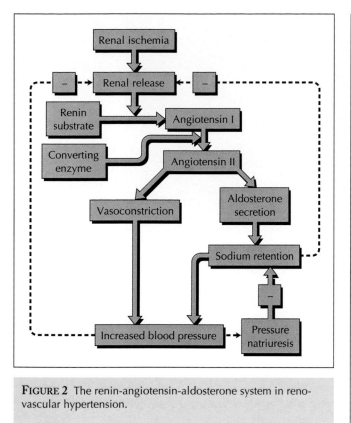

FIGURE 2 The renin-angiotensin-aldosterone system in reno-vascular hypertension.

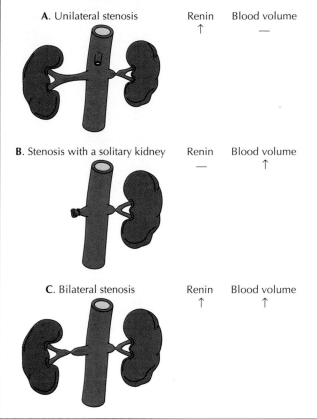

FIGURE 3 Three models of renovascular hypertension: **A**, Unilateral renal artery stenosis. **B**, Stenosis with a solitary kidney. **C**, Bilateral stenoses.

right kidney or a splenorenal artery bypass for the left). In younger patients with fibromuscular disease, angioplasty often cures the hypertension [5]; in older patients, the cure rates are lower no matter which form of revascularization is used [1]. If the ischemic kidney is small and functionless, nephrectomy may be indicated. Medical treatment is reserved generally for patients who are judged to be ineligible for one of these procedures.

Aldosteronoma

In patients whose serum potassium level is low in the absence of thiazide diuretics, an aldosterone-secreting tumor should be suspected [9]. A 24-hour urine collection for electrolytes and aldosterone should be obtained; high urine potassium, high aldosterone, and low plasma renin activity are characteristic. Differentiation from bilateral adrenal hyperplasia is obtained by computed tomography scan of the adrenal glands (Fig. 6).

TABLE 2 CLINICAL CLUES SUGGESTIVE OF RENOVASCULAR HYPERTENSION
Severe or refractory hypertension in any patient
Moderate or severe hypertension in a young white woman
Vascular bruits
Azotemia; high renin; hypokalemia; proteinuria
Sudden onset of hypertension

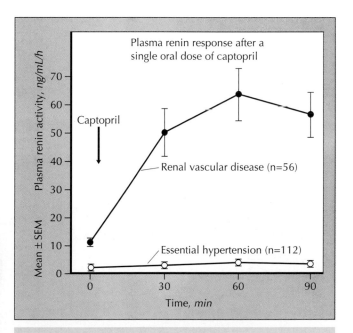

FIGURE 4 The increase of plasma renin activity after a single oral dose of captopril may distinguish patients with essential hypertension from patients with renovascular hypertension.

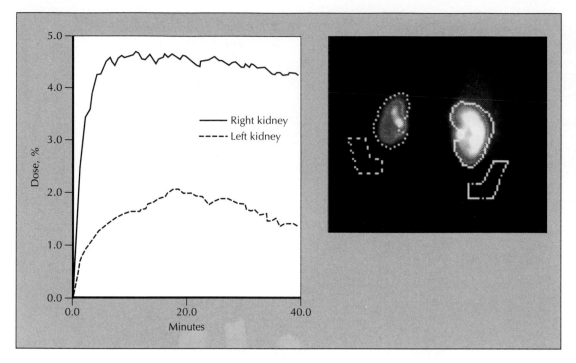

FIGURE 5 Renal scan in an azotemic patient suggests renal artery stenosis of the left kidney. Note the asymmetry of kidney size and delayed uptake of isotope by the left kidney. (*See* Color Plate.)

Aldosteronomas may be difficult to localize because of their small size (Fig. 7). Adrenalectomy usually is curative.

Glucocorticoid-Remediable Aldosteronism

Although exceedingly rare, this condition is of great interest because it represents the only form of hypertension for which a specific genetic mutation has been identified [10]. Its inheritance is autosomal dominant and the condition clinically presents in the same way as aldosterone-secreting tumor, with hypertension and hypokalemia. However, the increased aldos-

terone secretion is corticotropin-dependent and hence reversible by administration of glucocorticoids (dexamethasone, which suppresses corticotropin).

Pheochromocytoma

Although it accounts for less than 1% of hypertensive cases, pheochromocytoma is important to diagnose because, if undetected, it potentially is fatal; it is easily curable once detected [11]. Characteristic findings are shown in Table 3. A 24-hour urine collection for cate-

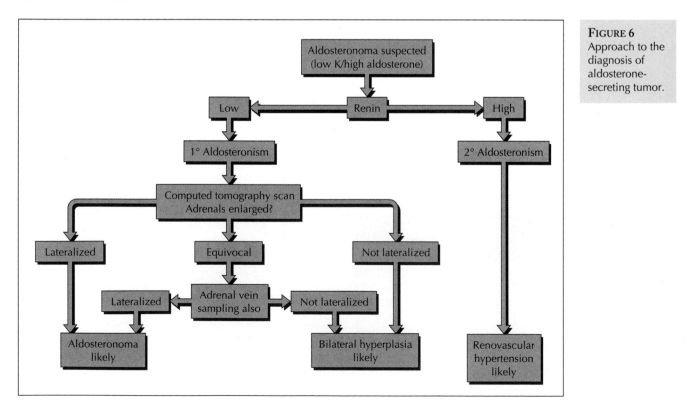

FIGURE 6 Approach to the diagnosis of aldosterone-secreting tumor.

Cardiology for the Primary Care Physician

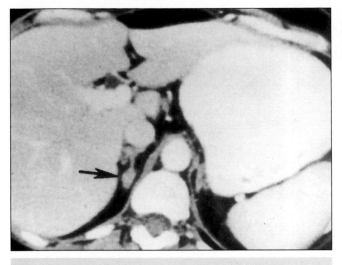

FIGURE 7 Computed tomography scan showing aldosterone-secreting tumor (*arrow*).

TABLE 3 CLINICAL ASPECTS OF PHEOCHROMOCYTOMA

Five H's*
Hypertension
Headache
Hyperhidrosis
Hypermetabolism
Hyperglycemia

Rule of 10
10% familial
10% bilateral (adrenal)
10% malignant
10% multiple (extra-adrenal)
10% occur in children

*95% will have headache, hyperhidrosis, or palpitations.

cholamines and metanephrines may provide biochemical confirmation; in doubtful cases, plasma catecholamines also may be measured (*see* Table 4). The tumors usually can be localized by an abdominal computed tomography scan; extra-adrenal tumors may be detected by metaiodobenzylguanidine (MIBG) scans (Fig. 8) [12]. Treatment is by adrenalectomy following α-adrenergic blockade with phenoxybenzamine.

COARCTATION OF THE AORTA

Coarctation usually is diagnosed in childhood but occasionally remains undetected until adulthood. The diagnosis can be made from the routine physical examination [13]. The most striking finding is a systolic murmur best heard over the back, between the left scapula and the spine; there also may be an aortic ejection murmur arising from a bicuspid aortic valve. The femoral pulses are weak and delayed, and the blood pressure is lower in the legs than in the arms. The coarctation itself usually is situated at the site of the ductus arteriosus, just below the origin of the left subclavian artery. The diagnosis can be confirmed by echocardiography. Treatment is by surgical correction

TABLE 4 URINE AND BLOOD TESTS FOR PHEOCHROMOCYTOMA

Test	Upper limit of normal
Urine metanephrines	1.8 mg/24 h
Urine catecholamines	1.0 mg/24 h
Urine vanillylmandelic acid	11 mg/24 h
Plasma catecholamines (norepinephrine and epinephrine)	950 pg/mL
Plasma catecholamines (after clonidine)	500 pg/mL

of the stenosis, which usually is performed after the child reaches 5 years of age.

Renal Parenchymal Disease

The discovery of a small kidney in a hypertensive patient does not necessarily signify renal artery stenosis but may occur with unilateral parenchymal disease, which is commonly attributed to pyelonephritis, although glomerulonephritis is just as likely [14]. The main renal artery is small but patent; removal of the shrunken kidney may cure the hypertension. Chronic pyelonephritis typically is bilateral, but whether it actually causes hypertension is uncertain. On the other hand, chronic glomerulonephritis, which causes more parenchymal disease than pyelonephritis, certainly can. Proteinuria is more pronounced with glomerulonephritis than with pyelonephritis.

Hypertension may be the presenting feature of adult polycystic disease. Clinically, patients with this condition also may

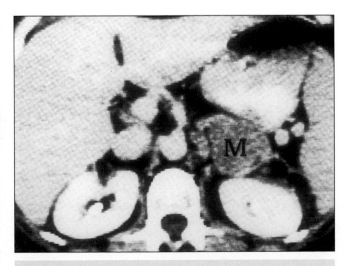

FIGURE 8 Computed tomography scan showing pheochromocytoma (*M*).

experience abdominal pain and hematuria, and the renal or associated hepatic cysts may be palpable on physical examination. The hypertension is associated with high plasma renin activity [15].

Cushing's Disease

Most patients with Cushing's disease are hypertensive, although it rarely is the presenting feature [16]. The diagnosis is established by elevated plasma or urinary levels of cortisol. Treatment of the underlying condition usually cures the hypertension.

Thyroid Disorders

About 20% of hypothyroid patients have associated diastolic hypertension, which can be improved by thyroid supplementation. Systolic hypertension is characteristic of hyperthyroidism [17].

Scleroderma

In the later stages of this condition the kidneys may be affected, causing very high renin levels and severe hypertension.

REFERENCES AND RECOMMENDED READING

Recently published papers of particular interest have been highlighted as:
- Of interest
- • Of outstanding interest

1. Rimmer JM, Gennari FJ: Artherosclerotic renovascular disease and progressive renal failure. *Ann Intern Med* 1993, 118:712–719.
2. Davis BA, Crook JE, Vestal RE, Oates JA: Prevalence of renovascular hypertension in patients with Grade II or IV hypertensive retinopathy. *N Engl J Med* 1979, 301:1273–1276.
3. Mann SJ, Pickering TG: Detection of renovascular hypertension: state of the art: 1992. *Ann Intern Med* 1992, 117:845–853.
4.• Derkx FHM, Schalekam P: Renal artery stenosis and hypertension. *Lancet* 1994, 334:237–239.
5. Pickering TG: Renovascular hypertension: medical evaluation and non-surgical treatment. In *Hypertension: Pathology, Diagnosis, and Management.* Edited by Laragh JH, Brenner BM. New York: Raven Press; 1990:1539–1560.
6. Müller FB, Sealey JE, Case CB, *et al.*: The Captopril test for identifying renovascular disease in hypertensive patients. *Am J Med* 1986, 80:633–644.
7.• Gerber LM, Mann SJ, Muller FB, *et al.*: Response to the captopril test is dependent on the baseline renin profile. *J Hypertens* 1994, 12:173–178.
8. Mann SJ, Pickering TG, Tos TA, *et al.*: Captopril renography in the diagnosis of renal artery stenosis: accuracy and limitations. *Am J Med* 1991, 90:30–40.
9. Bravo EL: Primary aldosteronism: new approaches to diagnosis and management. *Cleve Clin J Med* 1993, 60:379–386.
10. Lifton RP, Dluhy RG, Powers M, *et al.*: A chimaeric 11 beta-hydroxylase/aldosterone synthase gene causes glucocorticoid-remediable aldosteronism and human hypertension. *Nature* 1992, 355:262–265.
11. Sheps SG, Jiang N-S, Klee GG, van Heerden JA: Recent developments in the diagnosis and treatment of pheochromocytoma. *Mayo Clin Proc* 1990, 65:88–95.
12. Clesham CL, Kennedy A, Lavender JP, *et al.*: Meta-iodobenzylguanidine (MIBG) scanning in the diagnosis of phaeochromocytoma. *J Hum Hypertens* 1993, 7:353–356.
13. Rocchini A: Coarctation of the aorta. In *Hypertension Primer.* Edited by Izzo JL, Black HR. Dallas: American Heart Association; 1993:107–108.
14. Brown MA, Whitworth JA: Hypertension in human renal disease. *J Hypertens* 1992, 10:701–712.
15. Chapman AB, Johnson A, Gabow PA, Schrier RW: The renin-angiotensin-aldosterone system and autosomal dominant polycystic kidney disease. *N Engl J Med* 1990, 32:1091–1096.
16. Carpenter PC: Cushing's syndrome: update of diagnosis and management. *Mayo Clin Proc* 1986, 61:49–58.
17. Klein I, Ojamaa K: Thyroid diseases and hypertension. In *Hypertension Primer.* Edited by Izzo JL, Black HR. Dallas: American Heart Association; 1993:108–109.

Pheochromocytoma 17

Vincent DeQuattro
Deping Lee

Key Points
- Pheochromocytoma, a rare but treatable cause of hypertension, can masquerade as a classical hypertensive or as an occult clinical mystery.
- Clinical suspicion of pheochromocytoma can be confirmed by measures of urinary nometanephrine or metanephrine or plasma or urinary catecholamines.
- Localization of the chromaffin tumor is performed with complimentary magnetic resonance imaging and octreotide or metaiodobenzylguanidine imaging or via computed tomography scan.
- Preoperative therapy with α-blockade, usually phenoxybenzamine and often with the addition of β-blockade, should be of sufficient duration to achieve euvolemia and stable left ventricular function.
- Operative resection requires invasive monitoring, selective anesthesia, careful dissection, and adequate supplies of α-antagonists, β-blockers, nitroprusside, colloid replacement, and autologous transfusion.

No stereotype exists for the patient with pheochromocytoma; he or she may present as an emergency room arrival with a transient ischemic attack, completed stroke, congestive heart failure, myocardial infarction, hypercalcemia, or malignant hypertension. Alternatively, the patient may present with the reverse: shock, adult respiratory distress syndrome, and lactic acidosis. The patient may present at an office visit with classic attacks of diaphoresis, headache, or feelings of impending doom, or he or she may have the symptoms and physical findings of primary hypertension.

Some of the facts pertaining to the incidence of pheochromocytoma seem irreconcilable: it is found in 0.5% to 0.8% of autopsies; there are an estimated one to two patients with pheochromocytoma per million persons; and there are between one and five patients with pheochromocytoma per thousand patients with hypertension [1•]. Investigators who conducted a 30-year surveillance of the population of Rochester, Minnesota found an average annual incidence of pheochromocytoma of 0.95 per 100,000 person-years [2]. In five of the 11 patients, pheochromocytoma was diagnosed at autopsy. Unfortunately, pheochromocytoma often remains an occult disease ending the life of the patient abruptly or gradually, but almost always prematurely. Seventy percent of patients who had an autopsy diagnosis of pheochromocytoma were undiagnosed while alive [1•]. Patients in whom symptoms were present for over three months (61%) had the typical symptoms of palpitations, sweating, dyspnea, and headaches. Of these, 10% had hypertension only. The pattern of symptoms was different for those patients who had them for less than three months—almost all had abdominal pain, vomiting, and dyspnea. In addition, one-half had sweating and chest pain.

The tumor occurs with equal frequency in both sexes and at any age, although it is most common in the third and fourth decades. Familial tumors are less common and manifest multiplicity, especially bilateral masses, and are often associated with medullary carcinoma of the thyroid [3]. These tumors occur in patients with multiple endocrine neoplasia type II or Sipple syndrome, which is associated with

TABLE 1 PRESUMPTIVE DIAGNOSIS OF PHEOCHROMOCYTOMA

Symptoms (in order of frequency)*
- Headache
- Palpitation or tachycardia
- Excessive perspiration
- Anxiety, nervousness
- Weight loss
- Tremor
- Pallor
- Chest or abdominal pains
- Nausea, vomiting
- Malaise

Signs (in order of frequency)
- Hyperhidrosis
- Paroxysmal changes in BP
- Postural hypotension
- Hypertension induced by palpation or positioning
- Hypertensive retinotherapy
- Hypermetabolism

Neurofibromatosis
- Cafe-au-lait spots
- Absence of hand veins
- Axillary freckling
- Palpable mass (rare)
- Acrocyanosis, shock, ARDS

Clinical syndromes
- Hypertension (character)
  - Paroxysmal (50%)
  - Malignant accelerated (5%–10%)
  - Paradoxical response to:
    - β-blockers
    - Imipramine, desipramine
    - Guanethidine, hydralazine
    - Induction of anesthesia
- In pregnancy (1st, 3rd trimester)
- Diabetes mellitus (50%)
- Cardiomyopathy (30%)
- In children

Familial
- MEN II (Sipple's syndrome)
  - Familial pheochromocytoma
  - Medullary carcinoma
  - Parathyroid adenoma
- MEN III
  - Thickened corneal nerves
  - Ganglioneuromatosis
  - Marfanoid features
    - Mucosal neuronomas
  - von Reckinghausen's neurofibramotosis
  - von Hippel–Lindau disease

*Absence of all makes diagnoses unlikely with > 90% specificity.
ARDS—adult-respiratory distress syndrome; BP— blood pressure; MEN—multiple endocrine neoplasia.

---

medullary carcinoma of the thyroid, parathyroid adenoma, and bilateral pheochromocytoma (Table 1) [4].

Pheochromocytoma may be associated with other neuroectodermal syndromes, such as neurofibromatosis (approximately 5% of individuals with neurofibromatosis may develop pheochromocytoma), von Hippel–Lindau disease, Sturge-Weber disease, and tuberous sclerosis [5,6]. Pheochromocytoma may occur in association with other endocrine neoplasms. The cells of pheochromocytoma have similar cytochemical and ultrastructural features and a presumed common embryologic origin from the neuroectoderm, sharing amine precursor uptake and decarboxylation [7]. Isolated tumors may arise from these tissues, or they may occur in association with other amine precursor uptake and decarboxylation cell neoplasms as part of a multiple endocrine neoplasia syndrome. The screening of unselected patients with pheochromocytoma discovered 19% with von Hippel-Lindau disease and 4% with multiple endocrine neoplasia type 2 (MEN-II) [7]. When family members with von Hippel-Lindau disease or MEN-II were screened for pheochromocytoma, unsuspected pheochromocytoma was found in 46% [6]. Molecular genetic testing in kindred of patients with familial pheochromocytoma allows for detection of those with RET and VHL protooncogenes to offer presymptomatic diagnosis of renal cell carcinoma [8•], medullary thyroid carcinoma [9••,10], and parathyroid adenoma [9••,10].

Pheochromocytomas arising outside the chromaffin cells of the adrenal medulla are called *functional paragangliomas* [11]. These tumors occur in the posterior mediastinum; in the sympathetic chain in the neck; in the organ of Zuckerkandl, which is ventral to the aorta at the origin of the inferior mesenteric artery; in the pelvis; and in the urinary bladder [12].

ADRENAL MEDULLARY HYPERPLASIA

Whether or not this entity exists has been a topic of controversy since it was first described more than 50 years ago [13]. The normal adrenal has a weight of 6 to 6.5 g and a medullary:cortical ratio of 1:10, (thus, a medullary weight of approximately 0.6 to 0.7 g). Some investigators have reported, however, that medullary weight has approached 1.25 to 2.0 g in patients who had hypertensive crises and attacks similar to pheochromocytoma, but without chromaffin tumors [14,15].

Symptoms

The complaints of patients with pheochromocytoma may resemble those with primary hypertension (Table 1). Symptoms generally have two patterns, persistent or paroxysmal, which are related to a constant or pulsatile release of catecholamines [16]. Attacks occur from once every 2 months to 25 per day and last from 30 seconds to 1 week, with an average time of approximately 15 minutes. Paroxysmal attacks are rarely associated with malignancy [16].

Acute episodes with a constellation of symptoms may occur in patients with pheochromocytoma. Most commonly, these consist of sweating, palpitations, and anxiety with hypertension. Of course, most hypertensive patients with symptoms of pheochromocytoma do not have a chromaffin tumor but instead seem to have spontaneous adrenergic discharge without apparent reasons. Sometimes, the masquerade results from an identifiable cause, such as phenylpropanolamine ingestion or a Munchausen syndrome resulting from self-administration of vasoactive amines, like isoproterenol [17,18]. Kuchel, however, described patients who appear to have episodic dopamine surges that flood phenol sulfotransferase mechanisms that inactivate norepinephrine and epinephrine [19]. Some of our hypertensive patients have had excessive adrenergic tone and appeared to be "caricatures of pheochromocytoma," with surges of free norepinephrine and plasma concomitant with blood pressure elevation. The blood pressure rise in these patients responded to α- and β-receptor blockade [20].

Chromaffin tumors of the adrenal medulla commonly secrete only norepinephrine; less often, a mixture of norepinephrine and epinephrine; and rarely, epinephrine alone. Extra adrenal pheochromocytomas secrete only norepinephrine, which is less potent than epinephrine in causing hypermetabolism and glycogenolysis. Rarely, epinephrine-like effects are seen in patients with tumors excreting only norepinephrine. The history of attacks occurring when the patient bends to one side, wears a tight girdle, or has a full bladder may help to localize or lead to the diagnosis of the tumors.

Physical Findings

Patients with pheochromocytoma often are thin from weight loss, but some remain obese (Table 1). Sweating may be subtle or severe, with drenching night sweats and even dehydration. Facial or digital flushing may also occur, and the extremities may be pale. Vasospasm may be so severe that peripheral pulses are undetectable, and even gangrene may be present. Intense arterial constriction may result in falsely low brachial arterial pressure. The veins on the dorsum of the hands may not be seen because of intense vasoconstriction. Therefore, the clinician must determine whether central pulsations are present, and if they are strong, interarterial monitoring from the femoral region is indicated. Central nervous system findings are diverse and range from anxiety to frank psychosis and from transient ischemic attacks to completed strokes resulting from cerebral hemorrhage. The tumor is rarely palpable, and although such palpation may aid in diagnosis, it may cause a dangerous crisis. Careful quadrant-by-quadrant abdominal massage with intravenous phentolamine available may be useful in localizing the 10% to 20% of tumors in patients who harbor abdominal tumors. Patients with paroxysms related to phcochromocytoma, however, may have a completely normal physical examination during a quiescent period.

Postural hypotension is common in pheochromocytoma, perhaps because of the reduced plasma volume [21]. The hypotension or shock that occurs after removal of a pheochromocytoma results from discontinuation of the catecholamine infusion and reexpansion of the vascular compartment. This phenomenon can be minimized by the preoperative administration of oral α-blockers, such as phenoxybenzamine, and by expansion of the blood volume rapidly after removal of the pheochromocytoma with albumin or autologous blood immediately after the tumor vessels are ligated.

ADULT RESPIRATORY DISTRESS SYNDROME

We have encountered two patients with acrocyanosis and hypertension rapidly proceeding to hypotension that was associated with marked plasma volume contraction, lactic acidosis, bilateral pulmonary infiltrates, and subsequently

at autopsy or surgery, a recent hemorrhage was found in the adrenal tumor. It is exceedingly important to consider the possibility of underlying chromaffin tumor in such patients.

Myocardial Sequelae

Twenty percent to 30% of patients have specific cardiac complications of pheochromocytoma, such as left ventricular hypertrophy, catecholamine myocarditis, and dilated or obstructive cardiomyopathy [22–24]. They often exhibit the ECG abnormalities of sinus tachycardia, junctional rhythm, ventricular tachyarrhythmias, and ST-T changes of left ventricular hypertrophy and ischemia. Recovery can occur rapidly, often within 14 days of beginning therapy with α-blockade [22]. Heart rate variability measured using ambulatory 24-hour electrocardiography is reduced in patients with pheochromocytoma compared to that of patients with hypertension, and may be related in part to enhanced sympathetic as well as increased vagal tone [25].

Myocardial necrosis and fibrosis are related to the arteriolar constriction [26] and hypoxia mediated by adrenergic receptors [27] and enhanced permeability of the cell membrane to calcium [28]. There is also evidence that oxidized catecholamine products are toxic. Pheochromocytoma should be considered in patients with congestive heart failure without other obvious cause, even in normotensives. Normotensive patients may be more likely to die as a result of cardiac injury and lung edema because the diagnosis may not be suspected and the required specific α-blockade may not be given [28–30]. Thus, α-blockade must be used for a sufficient period preoperatively for repair of this cardiac dysfunction. Echocardiography can document or detect global or segmental akinesis or hypokinesis, which usually reverts over a period of days to normal after α-blocking therapy. In one series of necropsies of patients with pheochromocytoma and sudden death, five of 10 had acute myocardial infarction. Several of the young patients had far-advanced atherosclerosis, and two of our own patients in their sixth decade required coronary revascularization. One patient with pheochromocytoma, 35 years of age, sustained an acute myocardial infarction after angiography. Thus, this complication, although relatively rare, must be considered during planning for surgical correction of these tumors. In our experience, surgical excision of the pheochromocytoma in patients with stable angina, coronary artery disease, and pheochromocytoma can be performed successfully prior to eventual coronary artery bypass grafting, although there is a report of combined CABG and pheochromocytoma resection in a patient with unstable angina on maximal antiangial therapy [31]. Rarely, pheochromocytoma occurs in the intraatrial groove or travels to the heart by extension inside the great veins.

Biochemical Assays
Urine
Urinary metanephrines remain the most reliable tests for pheochromocytoma using 24-hour values or the expression of the microgram per creatinine ratio. The sensitivity is 95/100%

TABLE 2 EXCRETION RATES OF CATECHOLAMINES AND CATECHOLAMINE METABOLITES IN NORMAL SUBJECTS AND IN PATIENTS WITH PHEOCHROMOCYTOMA

	Normal*, μg/h	Pheochromocytoma†, μg/h
Catecholamines (free epinephrine plus norepinephrine)	2.5±0.8	10–120
Metanephrine plus normetanephrine (free plus conjugated)	16±5	30–420
Normetanephrine (free and conjugated)	10±5	30–720
Vanillylmandelic acid	240±120	500–3500

*Mean ± standard deviation.
†Presumptive until proved otherwise.

and the specificity 96/98%; positive and negative predictive values are, respectively, 46/47% and 100/100% for the two methods [32]. Patients should avoid stress and activities causing nonspecific elevations of catecholamines during urine collection (Table 2). We prefer to use free catecholamines for screening and use "timed urine" or express the result as μg/h, "per milligram of creatinine" (Table 2).

For patients with labile hypertension, urine should be collected during exacerbations, and this timed specimen can be compared with baseline. When the pattern of catecholamine excretion includes 20% or more as epinephrine, the tumor is usually found in the adrenals or in the organs of Zuckerkandl. Low levels of vanillylmandelic acid excretion do not exclude the diagnosis of pheochromocytoma. In our studies, the levels were normal in 10% to 15% of patients with known pheochromocytoma [33]. Further, false-positive results occurring in 10% to 15% can be caused by beverages high in vanillin and food, such as bananas, coffee, nuts, and other fruits.

Plasma norepinephrine

Plasma catecholamine measurements are of value in episodic crises and before and after clonidine suppression or histamine challenge. To minimize false-positive results, blood obtained 20 to 30 minutes after supine rest avoids the effect of stress and posture on catecholamine levels. The total catecholamine value in normotensive patients ranges from 100 to 500 ng/L [34]. Patients with pheochromocytoma usually have values 10 to 15 times normal. The high predictive value of a plasma catecholamine value that is greater than 2000 ng/L is offset by the low specificity when only mild-to-moderate elevations are found (Table 3). Catecholamine values of less than 2000 ng/L in various stressful states may be considered equivocal because some patients with primary hypertension have elevations ranging from 800 to 1000 g/L. Plasma catecholamine value may be normal during normotensive or asymptomatic intervals. From our unreported experience, a fivefold or greater increase in plasma catecholamines after histamine suggests pheochromocytoma. Assay of plasma normetanephrine in pheochromocytoma is as sensitive as that of plasma norepinephrine and offers the advantage of not requiring plasma preservation [35]. We have encountered patients who have had normal plasma levels of norepinephrine and epinephrine, but elevated levels of normetanephrine that were greater than

500 ng/L [36]. Some of these patients have had metastatic pheochromocytoma. O'Connor and Bernstein [37] demonstrated elevated chromogranin A levels in the plasma of patients with pheochromocytoma. This substance may prove helpful in the diagnosis of patients with pheochromocytoma and in excluding its diagnosis in pseudopheochromocytoma.

Clonidine Suppression Test

The clonidine suppression test has practical clinical value in patients with pseudopheochromocytoma, as described previously. Because of the clinical symptoms and borderline values present in patients with pseudopheochromocytoma, the diagnosis of pheochromocytoma is entertained, and frequently the elevations of the plasma catecholamines are two SD above

TABLE 3 AFTER URINARY SCREENING: DIAGNOSTIC TESTS FOR PHEOCHROMOCYTOMA

Plasma

Norepinephrine and epinephrine, supine (30–60 min)
  700–1000 pg/mL (repeat, especially if urine results positive)
  1000–2000 pg/mL (use clonidine suppression test; should fall to < 50%)
  > 2000 pg/mL (usually diagnostic for pheochromocytoma)

Imaging

CT, 77% sensitivity overall

MRI

Scintigraphy:
  131I MIBG (if CT results are negative or more than one tumor suspected)
  Octreotide scan

Iodocholesterol: nonfunctional tumors in region of clips

Vena caval and regional vein sampling for catecholamine step-up

Ultrasound: pregnancy, screening, near clips

Intravenous pyelography: hypertension screening, urinary bladder

Angiography: to localize and to establish vascular connections

CT—computed tomography; MRI—magnetic resonance imaging; MIBG—metaiodobenzylguanidine.

normal. Oral clonidine, an α_2-agonist, reduces plasma norepinephrine levels in hypertensive patients consonant with its effects in lowering central and thus peripheral sympathetic tone and blood pressure [36,38]. Bravo and coworkers [39,40] applied the method of clonidine suppression of plasma norepinephrine to a population of hypertensive patients and they found no suppression in patients with pheochromocytoma, compared with a 60% to 70% reduction of plasma norepinephrine 3 hours after an oral dose of 0.3 mg of clonidine in patients without pheochromocytoma (Fig. 1). Blood pressure was equally reduced in both groups. We do not know of any patients with pheochromocytoma in whom clonidine lowered the plasma norepinephrine level. Some of our patients have had marginally elevated plasma norepinephrine levels for many years without documentation of pheochromocytoma and have had no suppression of plasma norepinephrine level after clonidine. Thus, a positive test result, that is, suppression of norepinephrine, is strongly predictive of nonpheochromocytoma, but a negative result in the presence of marginally increased catecholamines cannot be considered presumptive evidence for the presence of a chromaffin tumor.

Pharmacologic Diagnosis

The provocative tests for diagnosis of pheochromocytoma may be dangerous. These drugs have caused hypertensive crises, cardiovascular accidents, and fatalities. These tests should be carried out by experienced endocrinologists when indicated.

Localization of the tumor before surgery is required to decrease operative time and the incidence of cardiovascular accidents and to avert unnecessary adrenalectomy. Ninety-eight percent of pheochromocytomas are found below the diaphragm, with most sporadic cases occurring (90%) in the adrenal medulla (Fig. 2). Fifteen percent are multiple. Most of the remainder are found in the posterior mediastinum, middle ear, carotid body, and urinary bladder. Ultrasound, computed tomography, octreotide and/or metaiodobenzylguanidine (MIBG) scintigraphy, and magnetic resonance imaging have supplanted older methods of localization. They should be carried out by experienced radiologists using the most state-of-the-art equipment.

Computed Tomography, Magnetic Resonance Imaging, and Scintigraphy

Computed tomography correctly localized 89% of tumors, including single, intraadrenal, bilateral adrenal, ectopic, and malignant tumors, on initial presentation in 52 patients seen over a 7-year period at the Mayo Clinic [41]. Current state-of-the-art scanners may localize as many as 95%. The Mayo Clinic study noted a localization rate of 73% for recurrent tumors; failures were attributable to small tumor size (8 mm) and artifacts resulting from surgical clips.

Scintigraphic visualization of adrenergic tissues has been made possible by the development of an analogue of guanethi-

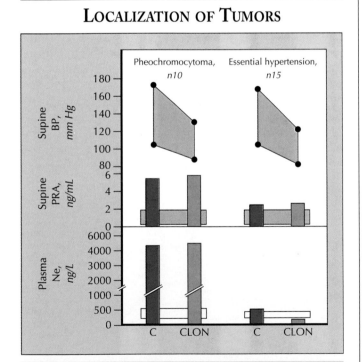

LOCALIZATION OF TUMORS

FIGURE 1 Cardiovascular and humoral responses of 10 patients with proven pheochromocytoma and 15 patients with essential hypertension who underwent the clonidine suppression test. For plasma renin activity (PRA) and plasma norepinephrine (Ne), the cross-hatched areas indicate the mean (±2 SD) of values obtained from healthy adult subjects of similar age. BP—blood pressure; C—control group; CLON—clonidine suppression test group. (*From* Bravo *et al.* [39]; with permission.)

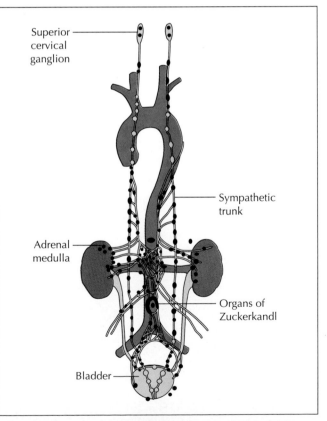

FIGURE 2 Sites of aorticosympathetic paraganglia (extramedullary chromaffin tissue) in a newborn child. Most functional paragangliomas occur below the diaphragm. (*Adapted from* Glenner and Grimbley [66]; with permission.)

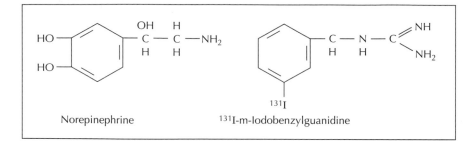

FIGURE 3 Chemical structure of metaiodobenzylguanidine.

Norepinephrine

^{131}I-m-Iodobenzylguanidine

dine, ^{131}I-MIBG (Fig. 3) [42]. ^{131}I-MIBG is concentrated in adrenergic neurons and chromaffin tissue by uptake into norepinephrine-containing storage sites. Discrete images after 48 hours usually represent pheochromocytomas that are rich in adrenergic storage vesicles. The method delivers 0.11 total body cGy and 17.5 cGy to the normal adrenal medullas [43]. Imaging is performed 48 and 72 hours after administration of the tracer. The method is safe, reproducible, and highly specific (Fig. 4). It provides unique functional information that may be of great value when multiple tumors are expected, as in multiple endocrine neoplasia [44]. False-negative results may occur in 4% to 10% of patients, often those with malignancy [45]. Medications known to inhibit norepinephrine uptake, such as labetalol and tricyclic antidepressants, should be discontinued 2 weeks before the study. Because ^{131}I MIBG is excreted by the bladder, imaging of this region with other methods may be necessary in some patients.

Pheochromocytomas contain a high content of somatostatin receptors. Thus, the radiologic somatostatin analog octreotide can be used to localize the primary tumor, as well as any metastases [46]. The scintigraphy with octreotide is not specific for pheochromocytoma; other neuroendocrine (*ie*, carcinoid) and some nonendocrine (*ie*, astrocytoma) tumors, granulomas (*ie*, sarcoid), and some autoimmune processes (*ie*, Graves' disease) can be visualized using this technique. The small size of this peptide allows for rapid clearance and low background activity. In a sample of 1000 patients, 12 of the 14 patients with pheochromocytoma were somatostatin-receptor positive. Perhaps MIBG is more useful in localization of tumors in the

adrenal and renal regions because of the relatively high accumulation of ligand in the kidney. A comparison study with MIBG of patients with 17 tumors yielded the following findings: 12 tumors were pheochromocytoma or paraganglioma, octreotide scans visualized 5 tumors that were not found by MIBG, MIBC localized 2 not found by octreotide scan, and both scans localized 5 tumors. The authors found that 86% of scans were positive for pheochromocytoma (compared with 88% for MIBG in the literature) and that 100% of the paragangliomas were visualized with octreotide (compared with 52% for MIBG in the literature) [46].

Computed tomography can be focused on the region likely to yield a tumor. Presently, both tests are considered complementary [47]. The presence of a mass on computed tomography does not necessarily mean a chromaffin tumor. On the other hand, some chromaffin tumors do not function or absorb MIBG [47]. If the evaluation of patients with hypertension proceeds from clinical suspicion to computed tomography without biochemical confirmation, a small number of incidental asymptomatic adrenal masses will be uncovered, most of which will not be pheochromocytoma. Autopsy data and imaging studies suggest that finding an "incidentaloma" of the adrenal gland rarely yields a functional tumor. Out of 100,000 tumors, 6500, 7000, and 35 will be pheochromocytoma, aldosteronoma, and glucocorticoid adenoma, respectively [48]. Although only 58 of 100,000 tumors will be adrenocortical carcinoma, rapid growth (or growth above 4 to 6 cm) may require excision or biopsy once pheochromocytoma is excluded [48].

Ansari and his colleagues [49] have found a sensitivity of

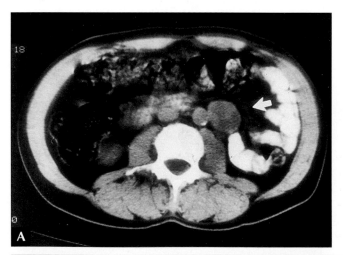

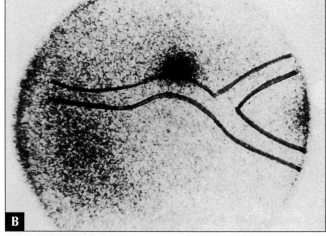

FIGURE 4 **A**, Computed tomographic scan of patient with paraganglioma. Tumor is seen at tip of arrow. **B**, Complementary role of the metaiodobenzylguanidine scan. The functional tumor is seen adjacent to the aorta. There was a plasma norepinephrine step-up increase in the left adrenal vein as well.

77% and a specificity of 92% with MIBG scanning. Their accuracy rate was 96% and 90% for MIBG and computed tomography, respectively.

Magnetic resonance imaging has demonstrated considerable promise in adrenal tissue characterization for both adrenal cortical adenoma and medullary pheochromocytoma and may be able to distinguish adrenal adenoma from adrenal medullary neoplasm on the basis of intensity difference. Patients with pheochromocytoma have demonstrated marked hyperintensity compared with normal liver on T2-weighted pulse sequences [50,51].

In 14 patients with malignant pheochromocytoma encompassing 40 tumor sites, 3 patients with more than 20 sites on MIBG scan had only 1 to 9 sites visualized on 111 indium-ocreotide scintigraphy; 2 patients had no MIBG uptake, but one of these had lung uptake with octreotide; and in 9 patients with a total of 41 MIBG foci there were 33 sites of 111 indium-ocreotide [52••]. Of all these sites, 26 were positive for both, 15 by MIBG only, and 7 were positive only on octreotide scan. In 6 of the latter, the foci were not found by either MRI, CT, or ultrasound [52••].

THERAPY

Medical Control

Advances in perioperative preparation and intraoperative patient management have had a major impact on mortality associated with pheochromocytoma surgery (Table 4). Surgical mortality was approximately 15% before 1950, and many deaths were attributable to hypovolemic shock, hypertensive hemorrhage, and anesthesia-related arrhythmias [53]. Since that time, preoperative therapy with α-blocking drugs, usually phenoxybenzamine as well as propanolol for at least 2 weeks, to allow reexpansion of blood volume, intraoperative anesthesia with improved anesthetic agents, and intraoperative or postresection volume replacement have made surgical mortality an exceptional occurrence (Table 4) [54,55]. Patients are usually prepared for surgery.

Phenoxybenzamine is a noncompetitive adrenergic blocking agent with greater selectivity for α_1 than α_2 receptors (100 to 1 compared with 3–5 to 1 for phentolamine). Therapy is initiated with one or two divided daily doses of 10 mg each. Most patients with pheochromocytoma require 20 to 40 mg per day. However, we have encountered patients who failed to respond adequately to oral phenoxybenzamine, and each has subsequently responded to intravenous phentolamine.

Prazosin hydrochloride, doxazosin mesylate, and terazosin are even more exclusive α_1-receptor blockers that have also been used with mixed success in patients with pheochromocytoma as preoperative therapy [56,57]. I do not believe that these should be relied on as the sole α-blocking agent during surgery because they only block α_1 receptors or they are "competitive" blockers [57]. The main role of alpha-blocker therapy in pheochromocytoma is to prevent vasoconstriction and to provide normalization of blood pressure. However, adverse alpha agonist effects on the myocardium are

also lessened, and congestive heart failure due to catecholamine myocarditis is reversed or prevented. Recent studies suggest that nonselective alpha blockade with agents such as phenoxybenzamine diminish both sympathomimetic stimulation and vagal inhibition of the myocardium, as well as reduce the incidence and frequency of repetitive ventricular dysrhythmia [58]. The addition of β-receptor blockade may be indicated when tachycardia or catecholamine-induced arrhythmias are present, or when epinephrine constitutes 15% to 20% or more of total neurohormone secretion. Propranolol is added in low doses, 10 to 20 mg three to four times per day, only after α-blocking therapy has begun. Propranolol may cause paradoxical hypertension in pheochromocytoma in the absence of prior α-receptor blockade. The combined α- and β-receptor blocker labetalol has been effective in preoperative and intraoperative management [59].

Calcium channel blockade, which is useful in pheochromocytoma both preoperatively and intraoperatively, reduces smooth muscle contractility and also impairs exocytosis release of norepinephrine from storage vesicles and blocks α_2-receptors.

The 5-year survival of patients with benign pheochromocytoma is approximately 96%, and that small fraction of patients (< 10%) with malignant pheochromocytoma have only a 44% survival rate [60]. Therapy for these patients with malignancies and for those who cannot tolerate surgical procedures with α- and β-blocking agents is not entirely satisfactory. For these patients, methylparatyrosine in doses of 1 to 2 g per day can reduce tumor synthesis from active sites and can normalize blood pressure for long periods, more than 15 years in some patients [61]. However, symptoms of parkin-

---

TABLE 4 THERAPY FOR PATIENTS WITH PHEOCHROMOCYTOMA

α-blockade
  Phentolamine: 1–5 mg IV drug of choice for surgery for rapid control of hypertension (many choose nitroprusside)
  Phenoxybenzamide: 20–80 mg/d preoperative and long-term treatment
  Specific α_1 blockade: prazosin, doxazosin, terazosin (less complete control that with phenoxybenzamine)
β-blockade
  Propranolol: 10–40 mg PO qid after α-blockade
α- and β-receptor blockade
  Labetalol: 300 mg/d or more
Vasodilator
  Nonspecific nitroprusside, magnesium sulfate
  Calcium channel blockade: nifedipine, diltiazem
  Converting enzyme inhibitor: captopril enalapril
Malignant or inoperable
  Methylparatyrosine (1–2 g/d)
  Vincristine, cyclophosphamide, dacarbazine (as a regimen)
  Tumoricidal ^{131}I MIBG

IV—intravenous; MIBG—metaiodobenzyguanidine; PO—by mouth; qid—four times a day.

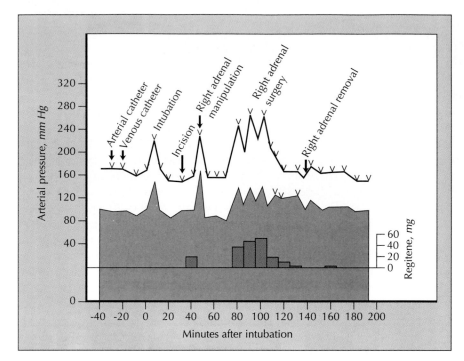

FIGURE 5 Pressor responses during operative removal of adrenal chromaffin tumor. Pressor responses were managed by bolus injections of phentolamine. Time and amount administered are given by arrows and hatched columns, respectively.

sonism, perhaps related to reduction of basal ganglia dopamine content, have been reported [62].

Phentolamine has been the drug of choice for obtaining rapid control of hypertension during crisis, provocative testing, and surgery (Fig. 5). Doses of 1 to 5 mg are given as boluses, and side effects include nausea and tachycardia. Most recently, we have used esmolol hydrochloride (50–100 μg/kg/min) and/or sodium nitroprusside (1 μg/kg/min) infusion during induction and intraoperatively.

Chemotherapy of patients with malignant pheochromocytoma has been ineffective. However, patients treated with cyclophosphamide, vincristine, and dacarbazine have shown regression of tumor size, reduction in catecholamine excretion, and improved quality of life, at least temporarily [63]. Systematically administered or targeted radiopharmaceuticals such as I[131]-labeled MIBG can be used in the therapy of metastatic pheochromocytoma. This therapy can be enhanced with consideration for tumor dosing, concomitant chemotherapy, radiosensitizers, surgical debulking, and external beam radiotherapy [64].

PHEOCHROMOCYTOMA IN PREGNANCY

Pregnant women with undiagnosed pheochromocytoma may die from cerebral vascular accidents, acute pulmonary edema, cardiac arrhythmias, shock, or malignancy. If pheochromocytoma is diagnosed before term, the maternal mortality is reduced to 17% or less. However, fetal mortality may remain high because of spontaneous abortion, with most deaths occurring during or, just after, labor. Increased catecholamine levels in maternal blood may cause fetal anoxia as a result of constriction of uterine arteries and also by heightened uterine contractions.

Maternal pheochromocytoma is extremely uncommon (only 180 patients were described in the world's literature through 1989). It is, however, often fatal (50% for the mother and 20% for the fetus) when undiagnosed (66% to 87% during

pregnancy) [65]. It is then perhaps a reasonable course to perform urinary screening tests for pheochromocytoma on all pregnant patients with hypertension, and to consider diagnostic testing for those with normal blood pressure but classical signs and symptoms of pheochromocytoma. In rare cases, nausea and vomiting and epigastric distress of an occult pheochromocytoma will mimic hyperemesis gravidarum.

KEY REFERENCES

Recently published papers of outstanding interest, as identified in *References and Recommended Reading*, have been annotated.

•• Skinner MA, DeBenedetti MK, Moley JF, *et al.*: Medullary thyroid carcinoma in children with multiple endocrine neoplasia types 2A and 2B. *J Pediatr Surg* 1996, 31:177–182.
The genetic diagnosis of patients with these syndromes may allow for prophylactic surgery before the development of biochemical or clinical evidence of medullary thyroid carcinoma.

•• Tenebaum F, Lumbroso J, Schlumberger M, *et al.*: Comparison of radiolabeled ocreotide and meta-iodobenzylguanidine (MIBG) scintigraphy in malignant pheochromocytoma. *J Nucl Med* 1995, 36:1–6.
Use of octreotide to identify somatostatin receptors seems promising, especially when results from MIBG scans are negative. Moreover, octreotide images could aid in determining a treatment regimen, as well as establishing the extent of disease and prognosis.

REFERENCES AND RECOMMENDED READING

Recently published papers of particular interest have been highlighted as:

• Of interest

•• Of outstanding interest

1.• Platts, JK, Drew PJT, Harvey JN. Death from phaeochromocytoma: lessons from a post-mortem survey. *J Royal Coll Physicians of London* 1995, 29:299–306.

2. Beard C, Sheps SG, Kurland LT, *et al.*: Occurrence of pheochromocytoma in Rochester, Minnesota, 1950 through 1979. *Mayo Clin Proc* 1983, 58:802–804.

3. Moorehead EL Jr, Brenner MJ, Caldwell JR, *et al.*: Pheochromocytoma: a familial tumor. A study of 11 families. *Henry Ford Hosp Med J* 1965, 13:467–478.

4. Sipple J: The association of pheochromocytoma with carcinoma of the thyroid gland. *Am J Med* 1961, 31:163–166.

5. Glushien A, Mansuy M, Littman D: Pheochromocytoma: It's relationship to the neurocutaneous syndromes. *Am J Med* 1953, 14:318–327.

6. Mulholland SG, Atuk NO, Walzak MP: Familial pheochromocytoma associated with cerebellar hemangioblastoma: A case history and review of the literature. *JAMA* 1969, 207:1709–1711.

7. Neumann HPH, Berger DP, Sigmund G, *et al.*: Pheochromocytomas, multiple endocrine neoplasia type 2, and Von Hippel-Lindau disease. *N Engl J Med* 1993, 329:1531–1538.

8.• Crossey PA, Eng C, Ginalska-Malinowska M, *et al.*: Molecular genetic diagnosis of von Hippel-Lindau disease in familiar phaeochromocytoma. *J Med Genet* 1995, 32:885–886.

9.•• Skinner MA, DeBenedetti MK, Moley JF, *et al.*: Medullary thyroid carcinoma in children with multiple endocrine neoplasia types 2A and 2B. *J Pediatr Surg* 1996, 31:177–182.

10. Moers AMJ, Landsaeter RM, Schaap C, *et al.*: Familial medullary thyroid carcinoma: not a distinct entity? Genotype-phenotype correlation in a large family. *Am J Med* 1996, 101:635–641.

11. Pearse AG: Common cytochemical and ultrastructural characteristics of cells producing polypeptide hormones (the APUD series) and their relevance to thyroid and ultimobranchial C cells and calcitonin. *Pro R Soc Lond [Biol]* 1968, 170:71–80.

12. Ober WB: Emil Zuckerkandl and his delightful little organ. *Pathol Annu* 1983, 18:103–119.

13. Quinan C, Berger AA: Observations on human adrenals with especial references to the relative weight of the normal medulla. *Ann Intern Med* 1993, 6:1180–1192.

14. Visser JW, Axt R: Bilateral adrenal medullary hyperplasia: A clinicopathological entity. *J Clin Pathol* 1975, 28:298–304.

15. Carney JA, Sizemore GW, Sheps SG: Adrenal medullary disease in multiple endocrine neoplasia, type 2: Pheochromocytoma and its precursors. *Am J Clin Pathol* 1976, 66:270–290.

16. Gifford R, Dvale W, Maher F, *et al.*: Clinical features, diagnosis, and treatment of pheochromocytomas. A review of 76 cases. *Mayo Clin Proc* 1964, 39:281–302.

17. Hyams JS, Leichtner AM, Breiner RG, *et al.*: Pseudopheochromocytoma and cardiac arrest associated with phenyl-propanolamine. *JAMA* 1985, 253:1609–1610.

18. Lurvey A, Yusin A, DeQuattro V: Pseudopheochromocytoma after self-administered isoproterenol. *J Endocrinol Metab* 1973, 36:766–769.

19. Kuchel O: Pseudopheochromocytoma. *Hypertension* 1985, 7:151–158.

20. DeQuattro V, Campese V, Miura Y, Esler M: Sympathotonia in primary hypertension and in a caricature resembling dysautonomia. *Clin Sci* 1976, 51:435–438.

21. Waldman TA, Bradley JE: Polycythemia secondary to a pheochromocytoma with production of an erythropoiesis stimulating factor by the tumor. *Proc Soc Exp Biol Med* 1961, 108:425–427.

22. Nanda AS, Feldman A, Liang CS: Acute reversal of pheochromocytoma-induced catecholamine cardiomyopathy. *Clin Cardiol* 1995, 18:421–423.

23. Huddle KR, Kalliatakis B, Skoularigis J: Pheochromocytoma associated with clinical and echocardiographic features simulating hypertrophic obstructive cardiomyopathy. *Chest* 1996, 109:1394–1397.

24. Scott IU, Gutterman DD: Pheochromocytoma with reversible focal cardiac dysfunction. *Am Heart J* 1995, 130:909–911.

25. Dabrowska B, Dabrowski A, Pruszczyk P, *et al.*: Heart rate variability in pheochromocytoma. *Am J Cardiol* 1995, 76:1201–1204.

26. Kline IK: Myocardial alterations associated with pheochromocytoma. *Am J Pathol* 1961, 38:539–551.

27. Simons M, Downing SE: Coronary vasoconstriction and catecholamine cardiomyopathy. *Am Heart J* 1985, 109:297–304.

28. Sardesai SH, Farrow B, Gibbons DO: Pheochromocytoma and catecholamine-induced cardiomyopathy presenting as heart failure. *Br Heart J* 1990, 63:234–237.

29. Hamada N, Akamatsu A, Joh T: A case of pheochromocytoma complicated with acute renal failure and cardiomyopathy. *Jpn J Circulation* 1993, 57:84–90.

30. Suga K, Tsukamoto K, Nishigauchi K, *et al.*: Iodine-123-MIBG imaging in pheochromocytoma with cardiomyopathy and pulmonary edema. *J Nucl Med* 1996, 37:1361–1364.

31. Seah PW, Costa R, Wolfenden H: Combined coronary artery bypass grafting and excision of adrenal pheochromocytoma. *J Thorac Cardiovasc Surg* 1995, 110:559–560.

32. Heron E, Chatellier G, Billaud E, *et al.*: The urinary metanephrine-to-tocreatinie ratio for the diagnosis of pheochromocytoma. *Ann Intern Med* 1996, 125:300–303.

33. Bray GA, DeQuattro V, Fisher DA, *et al.*: Catecholamines: a symposium–teaching conference. University of California, Los Angeles and Harbor General Hospital (specialty conference). *California Med* 1972, 117:32–62.

34. DeQuattro V, Chan S: Raised plasma catecholamines in some patients with primary hypertension. *Lancet* 1972, i:806–809.

35. Kobayashi R, DeQuattro V, Kolloch R, Miano L: A radioenzymatic assay for plasma normetanephrine in man and patients with pheochromocytoma. *Life Sci* 1980, 26:567–573.

36. Foti A, Adachi M, DeQuattro V: The relationships of free to conjugated metanephrine in plasma and spinal fluid of hypertensive patients. *J Clin Endocrinol Metab* 1982, 55:81–85.

37. O'Connor DT, Bernstein KN: Radioimmunoassay of chromogranin A in plasma as a measure of exocytotic sympathoadrenal activity in normal subjects and patients with pheochromocytoma. *N Engl J Med* 1984, 311:764–770.

38. Goldstein DS, Levinson PD, Zimlichman R, *et al.*: Clonidine suppression testing in essential hypertension. *Ann Intern Med* 1985, 102:42–48.

39. Bravo EL, Tarazi RC, Fouad FM, *et al.*: Clonidine suppression test: a useful aid in the diagnosis of pheochromocytoma. *N Engl J Med* 1981, 305:623–626.

40. Bravo E: Clonidine-suppression test for diagnosis of pheochromocytoma. *N Engl J Med* 1982, 306:49–50.

41. Welch TJ, Sheedy PF, Heerden JA, *et al.*: Pheochromocytoma: value of computed tomography. *Radiology* 1983, 148:501–503.

42. Wieland DM, Wu J, Brown LE, *et al.*: Radiolabeled adrenergic neuron-blocking agents: adrenomedullary imaging with (131-I) iodobenzylguanidine. *J Nucl Med* 1980, 21:349–353.

43. Sisson JC, Frager MS, Valk TW, *et al.*: Scintigraphic localization of pheochromocytoma. *N Engl J Med* 1981, 305:12–17.

44. Valk TW, Frager MS, Gross MD, *et al.*: Spectrum of pheochromocytoma in multiple endocrine neoplasia: a scintigraphic portrayal using 131-I metaiodobenzylguanidine. *Ann Intern Med* 1981, 94:762–767.

45. Shapiro B, Copp JE, Sisson JE, *et al.*: Iodine-131 metaiodobenzylguanidine for the locating of suspected pheochromocytoma: experience in 400 cases. *J Nucl Med* 1985, 26:576–585.

46. Krenning EP, Kwekkeboom DJ, Bakker WH, *et al.*: Somatostatin receptor scintigraphy with [111In-DPTA-D-Phe1 and 123I-Tyr3]-octreotide: the Rotterdam experience with more than 1000 patients. *Eur J Nucl Med* 1993, 20:716–731.

47. Francis IR, Glazer GM, Shapiro B, *et al.*: Complementary roles of CT and I-MIBG scintigraphy in diagnosing pheochromocytoma. *AJR Am J Roentgenol* 1983, 141:719–725.

48. Gross MD, Shapiro B: Clinical review 50: clinically silent adrenal masses. *J Clin Endocrinol Metab* 1993, 77(4):885.

49. Ansari AN, Siegel ME, DeQuattro V, Gazarian LH: Imaging of medullary thyroid carcinoma and hyperfunctioning adrenal medulla using iodine-131 metaiodobenzylguanidine. *J Nucl Med* 1986, 27:1858–1860.

50. Glazer GM, Woolsey EJ, Borrello J, *et al.*: Adrenal tissue characterization using MR imaging. *Radiology* 1986, 158:73–79.

51. Fink IJ, Reinig JW, Dwyer AK, *et al.*: MR imaging of pheochromocytomas. *J Comput Assist Tomogr* 1985, 9:454–458.

52.•• Tenebaum F, Lumbroso J, Schlumberger M, *et al.*: Comparison of radiolabeled ocreotide and meta-iodobenzylguanidine (MIBG) scintigraphy in malignant pheochromocytoma. *J Nucl Med* 1995, 36:1–6.

53. Apgar V, Papper EM: Pheochromocytoma: anesthetic management during surgical treatment. *Arch Surg* 1951, 62:634–648.

54. Brunjes S, Johns V, Crane M: Pheochromocytoma: Postoperative shock and blood volume. *N Engl J Med* 1960, 262:393–396.

55. Deoreo GA Jr, Stewart BH, Tarazi RC, Gifford RW: Preoperative blood transfusion in the safe surgical management of pheochromocytoma. *J Urol* 1974, 111:715–721.

56. Wallace J, Gill DP: Prazosin in the diagnosis and treatment of pheochromocytoma. *JAMA* 1978, 240:2752–2753.

57. Nicholson JP, Vaughn ED, Pickering TG, *et al.*: Pheochromocytoma and prazosin. *Ann Intern Med* 1983, 99:477–479.

58. Dabrowska B, Pruszczyk P, Dabrowski A, *et al.*: Influence of alpha adrenergic blockade on ventricular arrhythmias, QTc interval and heart rate variability in phaeochromocytoma. *J Human Hypertns* 1995, 9:925–929.

59. Rosca EA, Brown JT, Tever AF, *et al.*: Treatment of pheochromocytoma and clonidine withdrawal hypertension with labetalol. *Br J Clin Pharmacol* 1976, 3:809–815.

60. Manger WM, Gifford RW: Hypertension secondary to pheochromocytoma. *Bull N Y Acad Med* 1982, 58:139–158.

61. Sjoerdsma A, Engelman K, Spector S, Undenfriend S: Inhibition of catecholamine synthesis in man with α-methyl-tyrosine, an inhibitor of tyrosine hydroxylase. *Lancet* 1965, ii:1092–1094.

62. Gitlow SE, Pertsemlidis D, Bertani LM: Management of patients with pheochromocytoma. *Am Heart J* 1971, 83:557–567.

63. Keiser HR, Goldstein DS, Wade JL, *et al.*: Treatment of malignant pheochromocytoma with combination chemotherapy. *Hypertension* 1985, 7:18–24.

64. Tristam M, Alaamr AS, Fleming JS, *et al.*: Iodine-131-metaiodobenzylguanidine dosimetry in cancer therapy: risk versus benefit. *J Nucl Med* 1996, 37:1058–1063.

65. Botchan A, Hauser R, Kupfermine M, *et al.*: Pheochromocytoma in pregnancy: case report and review of the literature. *Obstet Gyn Survey* 1995, 50:321–327.

66. Glenner G, Grimbley P: Tumors of the extra-adrenal paraganglion system. *Ann Tumor Pathol* 1974, Ser 2, fasc 9.

SELECT BIBLIOGRAPHY

Aravot DJ, Banner NR, Cantor AM, *et al.*: Location, localization and surgical treatment of cardiac pheochromocytoma. *Am J Cardiol* 1992, 69:283–285.

Ledger GA, Khosla S, Lindor NM, *et al.*: Genetic testing in the diagnosis and management of multiple endocrine neoplasia type II. *Ann Intern Med* 1995, 122:118–124.

Neumann HPH, Weistler OD: Clustering of features of von Hippel-Lindau syndrome: evidence for a complex genetic locus. *Lancet* 1991, 337:1052–1154.

Orchard T, Grant CS, van Heerden JA, Weaver A: Pheochromocytoma: continuing evolution of surgical therapy. *Surgery* 1993, 116 (6):1153–1159.

Schulumberger C, Gicquel C, Lumbroso J, *et al.*: Malignant pheochromocytoma: clinical, biological, histologic and therapeutic data in a series of 20 patients with distant metastases. *J Endocrinol Invest* 1992, 15:631–642.

Chronic Ischemic Heart Disease 18

Susan Simandl
Peter F. Cohn

Key Points
- The pathophysiology of myocardial ischemia is related to a mismatch between coronary blood flow and myocardial oxygen requirements.
- In most patients with coronary artery disease, the angina threshold is not fixed but varies throughout the day.
- The exercise test is probably still the most important noninvasive diagnostic test.
- Patients with chronic ischemia may or may not demonstrate painful symptoms during ischemic episodes.
- Prognosis in patients with chronic ischemia relates to the severity of coronary artery disease and the degree of left ventricular dysfunction plus objective documentation of ischemia.
- Major therapeutic agents for patients with chronic ischemia are antianginal drugs (nitrates, β-blockers, calcium blockers), antiplatelet drugs (aspirin), and revascularization procedures (coronary angioplasty, coronary artery surgery).

Myocardial ischemia occurs when the coronary blood supply cannot meet the myocardial demands. This discrepancy is termed a supply–demand mismatch. Coronary blood supply is determined by the oxygen-carrying capacity and the coronary blood flow, which is regulated by numerous interacting factors. Myocardial demands are affected by changes in heart rate, contractility, and systolic wall tension; increasing heart rate is believed to be the single most important determinant of increased myocardial oxygen consumption.

In the normal heart, the coronary blood supply increases to match increasing myocardial demands. In the patient with significant coronary atherosclerotic disease, however, myocardial oxygen consumption may exceed the coronary blood supply, resulting in myocardial ischemia. Because it is at the end of the arterial blood supply, the subendocardium is the most vulnerable to ischemia.

CLINICAL PRESENTATION

The clinical presentation of myocardial ischemia resulting from coronary artery disease ranges from asymptomatic silent ischemia to atypical angina to classic angina pectoris. Classic angina has been defined as transient precordial discomfort provoked by exertion and relieved by rest or nitroglycerin. The discomfort can be heaviness, pressure, or tightness in the chest. It also can radiate to the arm, neck, jaw, or back and may be provoked by exercise; cold, hot, or humid weather; heavy meals; or emotional stress. The discomfort begins gradually and reaches maximal intensity over several minutes before resolving. Classic angina eases after rest or 2 to 3 minutes after nitroglycerin is taken. Most importantly, angina is *not* described as a brief, sharp, pleuritic, stabbing, localized, or migratory discomfort.

Atypical angina is a syndrome that has some similar symptoms, but lacks one or more of the criteria for classic angina. Angina equivalents are symptoms of myocar-

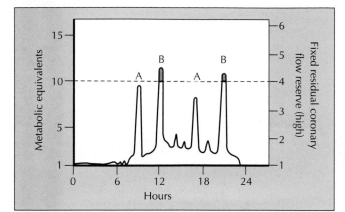

FIGURE 1 Fixed coronary artery obstructions not adequately compensated by collateral flow may reduce coronary flow reserve. In this diagram, it is reduced to only four times the resting values. The patient can exercise up to approximately 10 metabolic equivalents without having ischemia (A); however, if the patient exercises above approximately 10 metabolic equivalents, he or she will consistently develop ischemia (B). (*From* Maseri *et al.* [18]; with permission.)

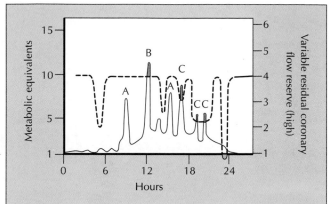

FIGURE 2 Residual coronary flow reserve may have an upper limit that is indeed fixed, but it can decrease because of mechanisms that transiently interfere with coronary blood flow. Thus, residual coronary flow reserve can vary throughout the day. Under these conditions, if the patient exercises beyond the maximal residual coronary flow reserve, the patient will always develop ischemia (B). However, the patient may also develop ischemia on other occasions after smaller degrees of exercise when residual coronary flow reserve is decreased by these functional factors (C). Occasionally, coronary flow reserve can decrease so that resting flow is impaired and ischemia occurs at rest. At other times of the day, this patient can exercise below the level of maximal residual coronary flow reserve without experiencing ischemia (A). In this case, the coronary flow reserve is fixed at approximately four times resting levels, so that the patient can exercise to approximately 10 metabolic equivalents in the absence of transient impairment of coronary flow. This level of work is compatible with most activities of daily life; hence, if the episodes of transient impairment of coronary flow reserve could be prevented, the patient would develop angina only after efforts of unusual intensity. (*From* Maseri *et al.* [18]; with permission.)

dial ischemia other than angina. Exertional dyspnea is often referred to as an anginal equivalent. Others use the term to describe pain in a referred location, such as isolated exertional arm or neck discomfort not accompanied by discomfort in the chest. Variant angina is chest discomfort occurring at rest secondary to coronary vasospasm and associated with ST-segment elevation (rather than depression) on electrocardiography (ECG).

The angina threshold is the level of metabolic activity (physical or emotional) at which myocardial ischemia ensues. If this threshold is fixed, the same amount of exertion, often expressed in metabolic equivalents or as a rate–pressure product (heart rate multiplied by systolic blood pressure), provokes the patient's angina (Fig. 1). In other patients, the threshold varies throughout the day. These patients sometimes have angina at rest or with minimal exertion; at other times, they are able to exercise more vigorously (Fig. 2). Many patients have both fixed- and variable-threshold angina, which is described as mixed angina pectoris.

The clinical history may give clues to the mechanism of a patient's angina (increasing myocardial demands as seen in exertional angina and decreasing coronary blood supply in patients with angina without precipitant). This information may help to guide the physician in choosing a medication (Fig. 3).

DIAGNOSIS

The diagnosis of coronary artery disease cannot be made on physical examination; however, some findings may increase clinical suspicion of coronary artery disease. One such example is systemic hypertension. Skin xanthomas are found in patients with familial hypercholesterolemia who have an increased incidence of premature coronary artery disease. Arcus cornealis (an opaque, grayish ring at the periphery of

the cornea found in young white patients) is a predictor of subsequent coronary events. The presence of carotid or femoral bruits, which is suggestive of peripheral vascular disease, increases the likelihood that the patient also has atherosclerotic heart disease. Cardiac examination may give clues to underlying organic heart disease (*eg*, if pathologic murmurs or gallops are noted) but it is by no means sensitive or specific for the diagnosis of coronary artery disease.

Noninvasive tests include exercise ECG, ambulatory ECG monitoring, nuclear imaging, and echocardiography. The exercise stress test is best used in patients who have normal findings on resting ECG. The patient exercises, commonly with either a treadmill or a stationary bicycle, and the patient's exercise duration, symptoms, blood pressure, heart rate, heart rhythm, physical examination findings, and ECG findings are analyzed. In the context of the clinical history, these parameters are evaluated to formulate a diagnostic impression.

The pretest risk (the probability of disease in the patient having the test) can be ascertained on clinical examination. Pryor and coworkers [1] concluded that the type of chest pain (typical, atypical, or nonanginal) was the most important predictor of significant coronary artery disease, followed by evidence of a prior myocardial infarction, gender, age, tobacco use, hyperlipidemia, ST-T segment changes on ECG, and a history of diabetes. Figures 4 and 5 are nomograms for estimating the likelihood of significant coronary artery disease. The posttest risk (the probability of disease in a patient with a positive test result) is assessed in light of the pretest risk and the test results (Table 1).

Exercise radionuclide ventriculography, thallium-201 stress testing, and stress echocardiography have increased the sensitivity for detecting coronary artery disease [2]. These specialized tests are commonly used in patients with abnormal baseline ECG results that make the exercise ECG findings difficult to interpret. Radionuclide and echocardiographic studies are also commonly used in patients with poor exercise capacity and those who are unable to exercise. In these circumstances, pharmacologic stress agents such as dipyridamole, dobutamine, or adenosine have been employed. The sensitivity and specificity of dipyridamole-thallium stress testing are nearly comparable to those of exercise thallium stress testing [3]. Because of their increased cost and time of performance as well as the marginal benefit for improved detection in some patients, however, nuclear and echocardiographic stress tests are not routinely recommended as screening procedures.

In patients with chronic stable angina, the stress test has been said to provide little diagnostic information after clinical parameters are taken into account. However, the stress test can be used to monitor disease progression and the patient's response to medication. It also can assess the functional significance of a lesion detected angiographically, assess the benefits of revascularization via surgery or angioplasty, and perhaps most importantly, provide a prognostic assessment (aid in risk stratification).

PROGNOSIS

The prognosis in patients with chronic stable angina can be determined by the patient history, physical examination, noninvasive data, and coronary angiographic results. Some investigators believe that severe angina is consistent with a poorer outlook. Thus, the angina score, which takes into account the severity and frequency of the angina as well as the results of resting ECG, has been shown to be an independent predictor of prognosis [4]. Clinical findings suggestive of poor left ventricular function are also associated with a worse prospect.

With information obtained from the clinical examination, the clinician decides if the patient is in a low- or high-risk group. In high-risk patients (those with frequent episodes of angina and evidence of left ventricular dysfunction on clinical examination), coronary angiography with an eye toward revascularization should be performed. In low-risk patients or those in a poorly defined risk category on clinical examination, stress data have helped to delineate high- and low-risk groups. The specific criteria vary from report to report, but the conclusion remains the same: patients with poor exercise capacity and those with severe ischemia by ST response at a low workload compose a high-risk cohort (Table 2).

Radionuclide stress tests (either with ventriculography demonstrating poor resting left ventricular function or failure of the left ventricular ejection fraction to increase with exercise [5] or with perfusion imaging showing severe ischemia as evidenced by multiple reversible thallium defects), thallium uptake in the lungs, and transient postexercise left ventricular dilatation identify patients at higher risk for cardiac events [6,7]. Although left ventricular function

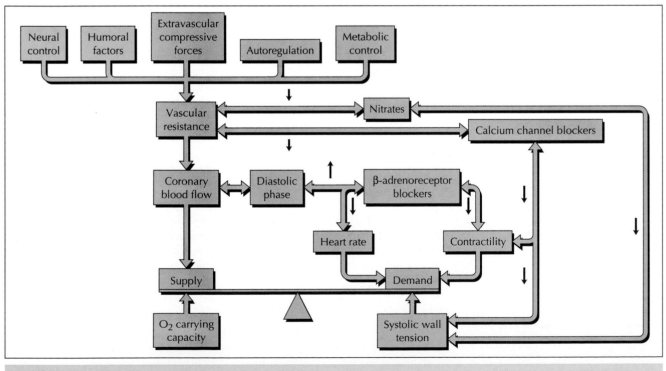

FIGURE 3 Effect of nitrates, beta-adrenoreceptor blockers, and calcium channel blockers on myocardial oxygen supply and demand. Reflex effects are not shown. (*From* Ardehali and Ports [19]; with permission.)

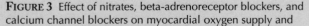

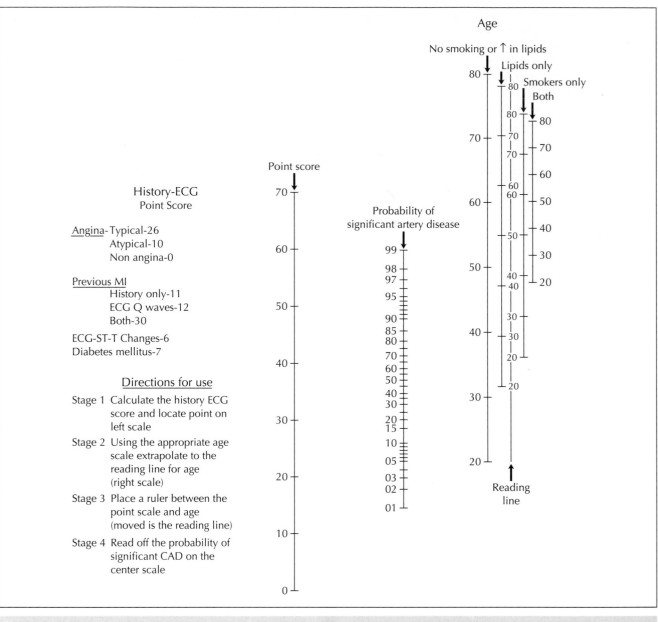

FIGURE 4 Nomogram for estimating the likelihood of significant coronary artery disease (CAD) in men. ECG—electrocardio- graphic; MI—myocardial infarction. (*From* Pryor *et al.* [1]; with permission.)

is probably the strongest predictor of prognosis [8], the severity of the coronary artery disease has significant implications. Both the number of diseased vessels and the severity of the stenosis [8,9] correlate with survival. Left ventricular function and the severity of the coronary artery disease act synergistically in determining survival [8], and patients with left main coronary artery disease have been shown to have the worst prognosis, followed by those with severe three-vessel coronary artery disease [10].

THERAPY

The goals of therapy in managing chronic stable angina are to prolong survival, reduce the incidence of disease progression, alleviate symptoms, and improve exercise capacity. Nitrates, β-blockers, and calcium antagonists are the three classes of agents available to treat chronic stable angina. They can be used alone or in combination [11•,12].

Nitrates dilate coronary arteries and decrease cardiac preload. Their use is associated with reflex tachycardia, an effect that may increase myocardial demands and can be blunted by concomitant use of a β-blocker. Short-acting nitrates, which are most often administered in sublingual or buccal mucosa spray form, are often used to treat an acute episode of angina. Patients should be told to sit down when they take this type of agent, because the vasodilatation may be associated with transient hypotension and dizziness. This effect is especially prominent when there is preexistent vasodilatation, as in very hot, humid weather or after a hot shower. Most patients with chronic stable angina have a short-acting nitrate preparation prescribed for them to take on an "as-needed" basis. They also may be on a daily regimen of a

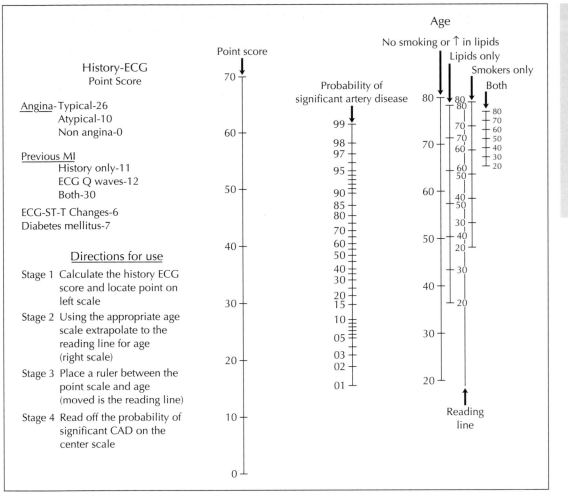

FIGURE 5
Nomogram for estimating the likelihood of significant coronary artery disease (CAD) in women. ECG—electrocardiographic; MI—myocardial infarction. (*From* Pryor *et al.* [2]; with permission.)

longer-acting nitrate. At present, a multitude of preparations are available in different forms and with different half-lives. The most important aspect of long-term nitrate therapy is to ensure an adequate nitrate-free interval, which will prevent nitrate tolerance.

β-Blockers decrease heart rate and contractility. They must be used with caution in patients who have significant bradyarrhythmias, asthma, congestive heart failure, or hypotension. They also must be used prudently in patients with diabetes mellitus and peripheral vascular disease. Because they blunt the tachycardia associated with exercise, these agents are well suited for patients with exertional or effort-induced angina. In addition, they are effective therapy for patients with angina who also have coexisting hypertension.

Calcium channel antagonists are a diverse group of agents, all of which act as vasodilators. Like β-blockers, many can be used as antianginal and antihypertensive agents. Diltiazem and verapamil can be used in patients with coexistent supraventricular arrhythmias, but unlike nifedipine and newer related compounds, they must be used cautiously in patients with bradyarrhythmias. Verapamil is a potent negative inotrope and is not recommended in patients with poor left

TABLE 1 POSTTEST RISK OF OBSTRUCTIVE CORONARY DISEASE AFTER A SYMPTOM-LIMITED EXERCISE TEST*

Clinical presentation	Men, %		Women, %	
	ECG abnormal[†]	ECG normal[‡]	ECG abnormal	ECG normal
Typical angina	95	50	80	30
Probable angina	85	25	55	15
Nonspecific chest pain	40	10	10	5
Asymptomatic	30	5	5	< 1

From Chaitman [20]; with permission.
*Patients without myocardial infarction.
[†]Horizontal or downsloping ST-segment depression of 1 mm or more.
[‡]Heart rate that is 85% or more of the age-predicted maximum.
ECG—electrocardiogram.

TABLE 2 RISK STRATIFICATION BY EXERCISE TESTING

		Risk classification		
Study	**Patients, n**	**Low**	**Intermediate**	**High**
McNeer et al. [22]	1472	< 1 mm ST ↓ FS ≥ IV Peak HR ≥ 160 bpm		≥ 1 mm ST ↓ FS I or II
Bruce et al. [23] (Seattle Heart Watch)	2001	< 1 mm ST ↓ No LV dysfunction	≥ 1 mm ST ↓ No LV dysfunction	FS ≤ I Peak SBP < 130 mm Hg Cardiomegaly
Dagenais et al. [24]	107	≤ 2 mm ST ↓ FS ≥ IV	≤ 2 mm ST ↓ FS ≥ III	≥ 2 mm ST ↓ FS ≤ I
Schneider et al. [25]	80			> 1 mm ST ↓ FS I or II
Weiner et al. [26]	292	≤ 2 mm ST ↓ No LV dysfunction		LV dysfunction or ≥ 2 mm ST ↓ beginning in stage I
Weiner et al. [27] Coronary Artery Surgery Study	4083	< 1 mm ST ↓ FS ≥ III	≥ 1 mm ST ↓ FS ≥ III	≥ 1 mm ST ↓ FS ≤ I

From Deering and Weiner [21]; with permission.

FS—final exercise stage (Bruce protocol); HR— heart rate; LV—left ventricular; SBP—systolic blood pressure; ST ↓—ST-segment depression.

ventricular systolic function. Several recent reports [13•] have called attention to possible harmful effects from the shorter-acting calcium blockers (especially nifedipine), and the Food and Drug administration is now discouraging their use in cardiovascular medicine. However, as Messerli [14] has pointed out, these reports may be unnecessarily anxiety-provoking for many patients, since these conclusions do <u>not</u> apply to the longer-acting agents (such as amlodipine), which have largely replaced the older agents in clinical practice.

All three classes of antianginal drugs decrease the incidence of ischemia and improve exercise performance. These agents can be used as the sole therapy for patients stratified by noninvasive methods to a low-risk group for cardiac events or who are good candidates for revascularization. They are also often used as adjuncts to revascularization. In addition, because of its proven benefit in post–myocardial infarction, unstable angina, and post–coronary bypass patients, daily aspirin use is often recommended. Finally, risk modification with diet counseling, antilipemic therapy, smoking cessation, and exercise programs is strongly advised. All of these measures can be initiated by the generalist; when revascularization is indicated by refractory symptoms or markedly abnormal stress test results, referral to a specialist is appropriate.

Coronary artery bypass graft surgery is performed to improve quality of life and prolong survival. Coronary artery bypass grafting has been shown to relieve angina more effectively than medical therapy [15] and is effective when angina is refractory to medical therapy. The poorer the prognosis (*ie*, severe ischemia combined with poor left ventricular function), the greater the benefits of revascularization (albeit possibly at a higher operative risk).

The role of coronary angioplasty in the treatment of chronic stable angina is evolving. A randomized trial comparing angioplasty with medical therapy in patients with single-vessel coronary artery disease reported a statistically significant improvement in exercise tolerance and anginal symptoms among the angioplasty group [16]. The angioplasty patients had a greater number of hospital days, however, as well as a higher incidence of repeated angioplasty (with its associated risks) and a higher cost than the medically treated patients. Another randomized study, which compared angioplasty with coronary artery bypass surgery, showed no difference in the rate of death or nonfatal myocardial infarction between the two groups 2.5 years after enrollment. However, the angioplasty group had a statistically significant increase in subsequent revascularization procedures (repeated angioplasty, bypass surgery, or both) and the need for repeated coronary arteriography [17]. Surgical patients had less angina and required less antianginal therapy in this study.

REFERENCES AND RECOMMENDED READING

Recently published papers of particular interest have been highlighted as:

- Of interest
- •• Of outstanding interest

1. Pryor DB, Harrell FE Jr, Lee KL, *et al.*: Estimating the likelihood of significant coronary artery disease. *Am J Med* 1983, 75:771–780.

2. Armstrong WF, O'Donnell J, Dillon JC, *et al.*: Complementary value of two-dimensional exercise echocardiography to routine treadmill exercise testing. *Ann Intern Med* 1986, 105:829–835.

3. Francisco DA, Collins SM, Go RT, *et al.*: Tomographic thallium-201 myocardial perfusion scintigrams after maximal coronary artery vasodilation with intravenous dipyridamole: comparison of qualitative and quantitative approaches. *Circulation* 1982, 66:370–379.

4. Califf RM, Mark DB, Harrell FE Jr, *et al.*: Importance of clinical measures of ischemia in the prognosis of patients with documented coronary artery disease. *J Am Coll Cardiol* 1988, 11:20–26.

5. Taliercio CP, Clements IP, Zinsmeister AR, Gibbons RJ: Prognostic value and limitations of exercise radionuclide angiography in medically treated coronary artery disease. *Mayo Clin Proc* 1988, 63:573–582.

6. Ladenheim ML, Pollock BH, Rozanski A, *et al.*: Extent and severity of myocardial reperfusion as predictors of prognosis in patients with suspected coronary artery disease. *J Am Coll Cardiol* 1986, 7:464–471.

7. Weiss AT, Berman DS, Lew AS, *et al.*: Transient ischemic dilatation of the left ventricle on stress thallium-201 scintigraphy: a marker of severe and extensive coronary artery disease. *J Am Coll Cardiol* 1987, 9:752–759.

8. Mock MB, Ringqvist I, Fisher LD, *et al.*: Survival of medically treated patients in the Coronary Artery Surgery Study (CASS) Registry. *Circulation* 1982, 66:562–568.

9. Harris PJ, Behar VS, Conley MJ, *et al.*: The prognostic significance of 50 percent stenosis in medically treated patients with coronary artery disease. *Circulation* 1980, 62:240–248.

10. Proudfit WJ, Bruschke AV, MacMillan JP, *et al.*: Fifteen year survival study of patients with obstructive coronary artery disease. *Circulation* 1983, 68:986–997.

11.• Savonito S, Ardissino D, Egstrup F, *et al.*: Combination therapy with metoprolol and nifedipine versus monotherapy in patients with stable angina pectoris. Results of the International Multicenter Angina Exercise (IMAGE) Study. *J Am Coll Cardiol* 1996, 27:311–316.

12. Dargie HJ, Ford I, Fox KM, *et al.*: Total Ischemic Burden European Trial (TIBET). Effects of ischemia and treatment with atenolol, nifedipine SR and their combination and outcome in patients with chronic stable angina *Eur Heart J* 1996, 17:104–112.

13.• Furberg CD, Psaty BM, Meyer JV: Nifedipine. Dose-related increase in mortality in patients with coronary heart disease. *Circulation* 1995, 92:1326–1331.

14. Messerli FH: Case-controlled study, meta-analysis, and bouillabaisse: Putting the calcium antagonist scare into context. *Annals of Int Med* 1995, 123:888–889.

15. CASS Principal Investigators and Their Associates: Coronary Artery Surgery Study (CASS): A randomized trial of coronary artery bypass surgery. Quality of life in patients randomly assigned to treatment groups. *Circulation* 1983, 68:951–960.

16. Parisi AF, Folland ED, Hartigan P: A comparison of angioplasty with medical therapy in the treatment of single-vessel coronary artery disease. *N Engl J Med* 1992, 326:10–16.

17. Coronary angioplasty versus coronary artery bypass surgery: the Randomized Interaction Treatment of Anginal (RITA) Trial. *Lancet* 1993, 341:573–580.

18. Maseri A, Chierchia S, Kaski JC: Mixed angina pectoris. *Am J Cardiol* 1985, 56:30E–33E.

19. Ardehali A, Ports TA: Myocardial oxygen supply and demand. *Chest* 1990, 90:699–705.

20. Chaitman BR: The changing role of the exercise electrocardiogram as a diagnostic and prognostic test for chronic ischemic heart disease. *J Am Coll Cardiol* 1986, 1195–1210.

21. Deering TF, Weiner DA: Prognosis of patients with CAD. *J Cardiopulmonary Rehabil* 1985, 5:352–331.

22. McNeer JF, Margolis JR, Lee KL, *et al.*: The role of the exercise test in the evaluation of patients for ischemic heart disease. *Circulation* 1979, 57:64–70.

23. Bruce RA, DeRouen TA, Hammermeister KE: Noninvasive screening criteria for enhanced 4-year survival after aortocoronary bypass surgery. *Circulation* 1979, 60:638–646.

24. Dagenais GR, Rouleau JR, Christen A, Fabia J: Survival of patients with a strongly positive exercise electrogram. *Circulation* 1982, 65:452–456.

25. Schneider RM, Seaworth JF, Dohnman ML, *et al.*: Anatomic and prognostic implications of an early positive treadmill exercise test. *Am J Cardiol* 1982, 50:682–688.

26. Weiner DA, McCabe CH, Ryan TJ: Prognostic assessment of patients with coronary artery disease by exercise testing. *Am Heart J* 1983, 105:749–755.

27. Weiner DA, Ryan TJ, McCabe CH, *et al.*: The prognostic importance of a clinical profile and exercise test in medically treated patients with coronary heart disease. *J Am Coll Cardiol* 1984, 3:772–779.

SELECT BIBLIOGRAPHY

Braunwald E, ed: *Heart Disease: A Textbook of Cardiovascular Medicine*, edn 5. Philadelphia: WB Saunders; 1997.

Detrano R, *et al.*: The diagnostic accuracy of exercise electrocardiogram: a meta-analysis of 22 years of research. *Prog Cardiovasc Dis* 1989, 31:173–206.

Unstable Angina and Non–Q-Wave Myocardial Infarction

John Speer Schroeder

Key Points

- Unstable angina and non-Q-wave myocardial infarction are important diagnoses to establish because of a high infarction/death rate that occurs over the next few months.

- These acute coronary syndromes are caused by atherosclerosis plaque rupture with varying degrees of occlusion because of platelet thrombus at the rupture site.

- Diagnosis is established by a history of prolonged angina chest pain, electrocardiographic changes, and serial creatine kinase and creatine kinase MB enzyme testing.

- Therapy is directed at the platelet thrombus (aspirin and heparin), prevention of coronary spasm (intravenous or topical nitroglycerin, rate-lowering calcium blockers), and treatment of contributing factors such as hypertension and tachycardia with beta blockers.

- Sublingual nifedipine is contraindicated for chest pain or hypertension.

The syndromes of unstable angina pectoris (UAP) and non–Q-wave myocardial infarction (NQMI) are referred to as intermediate coronary syndromes, because they sit between predictable exertional angina on the one hand and an acute transmural myocardial infarction (MI) on the other. The diagnosis is important [1,2]. These syndromes frequently precede a more serious cardiovascular event that can now be prevented with aggressive medical therapy and, in many instances, coronary interventional procedures or coronary bypass surgery.

Unstable angina has had many clinical terms through the years, including impending MI, rest angina, angina decubitus, crescendo angina, preinfarction angina, and acute coronary syndrome. It is important for the physician to recognize the diagnosis, rapidly initiate aggressive treatment, and in most instances, obtain a cardiology consultation to assist with the patient's care.

PATHOPHYSIOLOGY

This change from an asymptomatic to an unstable state is thought to result from a rupture of an atherosclerotic plaque in the coronary artery [3,4]. As shown in Figure 1, once the plaque ruptures, exposure of the plaque contents to the blood stream results in platelet thrombosis as part of a "repair process." Platelet aggregation releases vasoactive substances that can cause local vasoconstriction, which can further reduce the coronary lumen diameter. This complex combination of platelet thrombosis, threatening to close off the coronary artery, coronary vasospasm, and counteractive natural lytic mechanisms, attempting to lyse the platelet thrombus combine to cause dynamic, changing degrees of coronary occlusion that lead to the unstable angina syndrome. If this process is not reversed, complete occlusion may occur, leading to a transmural Q-wave MI.

DIAGNOSIS

Unstable angina pectoris should be suspected or included in the differential diagnosis when a patient relates a changing or crescendo pattern of chest pain consistent with myocardial ischemia. The character of the chest pain is typical for angina pectoris, (*ie*, squeezing or pressure), usually in the substernal area that may radiate into the neck, jaw, or inner aspect of either arm. Relief of the pain within 5 minutes by sublingual nitroglycerin assists in the diagnosis. NQMI should be suspected when the patient has a more prolonged episode of ischemic chest pain (> 15–30 min) that resolves spontaneously or with subsequent therapy.

Examples include the following:

1. A patient with known, stable, five-block exertional angina being treated with β-blockers and isosorbide dinitrate reports that pain suddenly began with simply walking across the room.

2. A patient calls and reports that her angina has been occurring at 3 AM the past two nights instead of just during marked exertion.

3. A patient reports that his exertional angina attacks are much more severe and may take three or four nitroglycerin tablets to relieve.

4. A woman with coronary artery disease risk factors calls at 5 AM and reports a 30-minute episode of severe substernal chest pain radiating into her left elbow.

5. A 59-year-old man who has smoked for the past 40 years comes to your office at 9 AM to get treatment for "heartburn." He relates recurring neck pain that has occurred off and on for the past 3 hours.

6. A 65-year-old man who had coronary artery bypass surgery 10 years ago reports sudden onset of "that old chest pain."

7. A patient with known hypertension reports trouble breathing and "maybe a little chest pressure" whenever she climbed three or four steps for the past week.

8. A 72-year-old woman reports two episodes of heaviness in her chest, each lasting approximately 1 hour and associated with mild diaphoresis.

These simple examples reflect the fact that UAP or NQMI can occur in the setting of known coronary artery disease or *de novo* disease, but the characteristics are frequently similar.

Initial Assessment

The initial assessment of a patient presenting with symptoms that may represent UAP or NQMI should include a thorough history, physical examination, laboratory studies, and electrocardiography.

History

The physician should obtain a thorough patient history. Is the chest pain from myocardial ischemia? Is it typical versus atypical pain? Are there known coronary artery disease risk factors? Is there known coronary artery disease? Does nitroglycerin (TNG) relieve or reduce the chest pain?

Physical examination and laboratory studies

Physical examination and laboratory studies should concentrate on whether other factors contributed to the myocardial ischemia. Is there decreased oxygen delivery (*eg*, anemia)? Is there increased oxygen demand, such as tachycardia secondary to new arrhythmia (*eg*, atrial fibrillation with rapid ventricular rate), increased heart rate, increased blood pressure, or hyperthyroidism?

Electrocardiography

Electrocardiography should establish whether ST segment elevation is present. This would be an indication for consideration of immediate thrombolytic therapy.

Diagnostic Testing

If the patient is having acute chest pain during your interview, a trial of sublingual nitroglycerin can be helpful.

Electrocardiography

The electrocardiogram (ECG) is an essential tool in evaluating not only the cause of the patient's chest pain but also its severity. The finding of the ST-segment elevation or T-wave peaking suggests acute transmural ischemia, and the patient generally would be considered for thrombolytic therapy. If

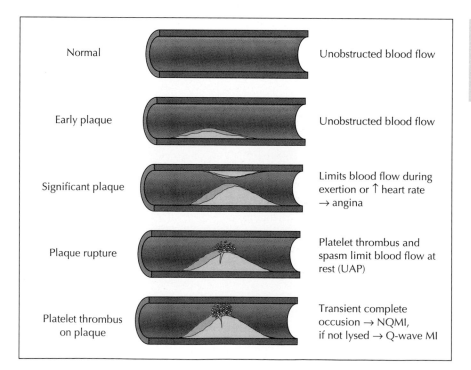

Normal	Unobstructed blood flow
Early plaque	Unobstructed blood flow
Significant plaque	Limits blood flow during exertion or ↑ heart rate → angina
Plaque rupture	Platelet thrombus and spasm limit blood flow at rest (UAP)
Platelet thrombus on plaque	Transient complete occusion → NQMI, if not lysed → Q-wave MI

FIGURE 1 Atherosclerotic plaque in a coronary artery as it relates to clinical syndromes. NQMI—non–Q-wave myocardial infarction; MI—myocardial infarction.

the ST elevation resolves with sublingual nitroglycerin, this suggests that coronary spasm was playing a significant role, but that the setting likely is still a ruptured, unstable atherosclerotic plaque. ST depression and abnormal T waves are consistent with myocardial ischemia, particularly if it is a change from previous ECGs or disappears with relief of chest pain after nitroglycerin. T-wave inversion suggests a recent subendocardial ischemic event that would be consistent with UAP or NQMI (Fig. 2). Serial ECGs are valuable in making the diagnosis of UAP or NQMI, because a

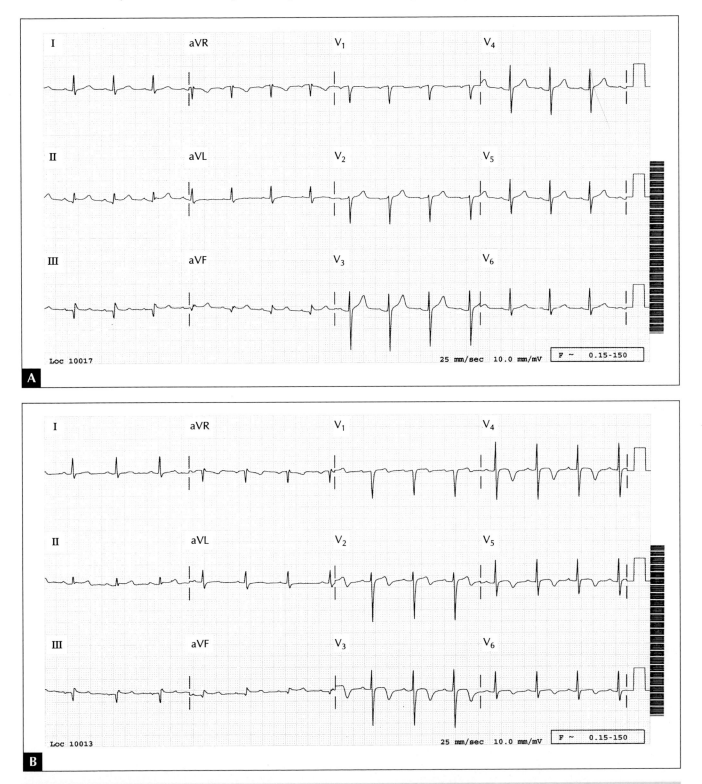

FIGURE 2 **A,** Twelve-lead electrocardiogram (ECG) in a patient complaining of crescendo angina chest pain. Leads qIII and AVG as well as ST-segment elevation in leads II, III, and AVF suggest an acute or recent inferior myocardial infarction. **B,** Twelve-lead ECG of the same patient taken 24 hours later. There is no change in the inferior leads. However, there is new T-wave inversion in anterior leads V_2 through V_6 consistent with severe anterior ischemia and/or a non–Q-wave myocardial infarction if serial creatine kinase or creatine kinase–myocardial band enzyme levels become elevated.

rapidly changing pattern of ST-T waves suggests a dynamic ongoing process.

A normal ECG can be useful to rule out myocardial ischemia, but it also can be misleading. A normal ECG can be consistent with a noncardiac cause for the chest pain in approximately 10% of the patients presenting with a history consistent for unstable angina. However, a normal ECG also may reflect true posterior ischemia or be associated with a dissecting thoracic aneurysm. Exercise testing may be useful if the diagnosis at this point is still not clear. It is best to review the findings with a cardiologist before initiating exercise testing, however, because stress testing in the setting of UAP or NQMI may be hazardous to the patient.

Creatine kinase enzymes

Serial creatine kinase enzyme levels are most useful in differentiating UAP from NQMI (Table 1). Generally, total and myocardial band creatine kinase (MB-CK) are drawn at the time of patient encounter and 8 and 24 hours after the initial patient encounter if the patient had a prolonged (> 15 minute) episode of chest pain that may have resulted in myocardial necrosis. Some patients may not have an elevated total CK, but still show evidence of NQMI based an abnormal increase in the MB fraction that reflects death of myocardial tissue. Tropinin T, a regulatory protein located in the myocyte, has recently been found to be an additional monitor for adverse events in the unstable angina patient [5•,6•].

If the episode of prolonged pain occurred more than 24 hours previously, a creatine kinase elevation may have already returned to normal. In this instance, the MB fraction may still be elevated, or LDH isoenzyme levels can help to establish a diagnosis of NQMI. Other laboratory testing should be used to rule out extracardiac causes of excess oxygen use that have caused the heart to increase its oxygen demand and need for increased coronary blood flow.

TREATMENT

Initial therapy should be directed toward preventing progressive thrombus formation that could completely occlude the vessel and lead to transmural myocardial infarction. Aspirin (325 mg, non–enteric coated) should be given immediately whether the initial contact is by telephone, in the office, or in the emergency room. The basis for this therapy is a 12-week study of 1266 veterans given Alka-Seltzer (Miles Inc, West Haven, CT) containing aspirin (325 mg) or placebo for 12 weeks following diagnosis of UAP [7]. The 12-week death rate was 3.3% in the placebo group and 1.6% in the aspirin group—a 51% reduction. Similar decreases occurred in fatal and nonfatal myocardial infarctions.

Nitroglycerin (usually one tablet sublingually every 5 minutes three times or until dizziness or severe headache occurs) should be used if the patient has it available and has not used it at the time of initial contact. If not available at home, this therapy should be used early during assessment of the patient in the office or the emergency department. The basis for TNG therapy includes reversal of any local coronary vasoconstriction related to the platelet thrombus as well as causing preload and afterload reduction, resulting in lessened myocardial oxygen demand by the heart.

In the Emergency Department

Once the initial assessment has established a probable diagnosis of UAP or NQMI, therapy should be directed toward treating the three ongoing processes: platelet thrombus formation, coronary vasoconstriction, and myocardial oxygen demand exceeding coronary blood supply (Fig. 3). Give TNG sublingually and aspirin if not previously administered. Thrombolytic therapy has not been shown to be therapeutic for the UAP and NQMI syndromes despite the fact that early platelet thrombus formation plays a pathogenic role [8,9]. Heparin therapy has been shown to improve outcome with a further 33% decrease in risk of MI or death [10•]. It is likely that low-molecular-weight heparin will have similar additional benefits.

After initial emergency room therapy, the patient should be reassessed if there is continued diffuse ST-segment depression on ECG, consider emergency coronary angiography. If there is continued ischemic chest pain, add intravenous beta blockers, increase intravenous TNG to blood pressure tolerance, and consider emergency coronary angiography. In the past sublingual nifedipine was frequently given for ongoing chest pain or hypertension in the unstable angina patient. This is now contraindicated because of the reflex tachycardia and hypotension that may occur and because of reports of progression to acute MI or even stroke [11•]. IV diltiazem has been shown to be more effective than IV TNG for reduction in subsequent ischemic events; however, both are appropriate

---

TABLE 1 SERUM ENZYME CHANGES IN UNSTABLE ANGINA AND NON–Q WAVE MYOCARDIAL INFARCTION

Time, h	Unstable angina CK	MB, %	NQMI CK rise CK	MB, %	NQMI MB rise only CK	MB, %
Normal value	< 160	< 5	< 160	< 5	< 160	< 5
0	100	3	100	3	100	3
8	120	4	260	8	160	9
24	110	3	150	7	150	7

CK—creatine kinase; MB—myocardial band; NQMI—non-Q-wave myocardial infarction.

Cardiology for the Primary Care Physician

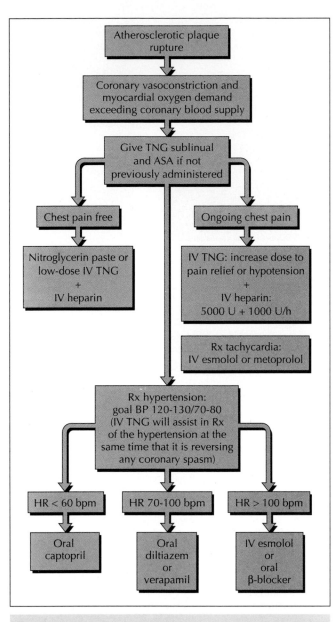

FIGURE 3 Approach to patients presenting with unstable angina or non–Q-wave myocardial infarction. ASA—aspirin; BP—blood pressure; HR—heart rate; IV—intravenous; TNG—nitroglycerin.

heparin until the patient is pain-free for 24 to 48 hours or the decision to proceed with angiography has been made.

Cardiology Consultation

Depending on whether it is immediately available, cardiology consultation will always be necessary to assist in the initial care of the patient, particularly if myocardial ischemic chest pain is persistent. Decision points are usually based on:

- Serial ECGs and enzyme tests;
- Ongoing pain—reassessment after maximizing intravenous TNG and/or β-blocker;
- Severe pain or progressive ECGs change—urgent assessment by coronary angiography.

Initiate additional antiischemic therapy if the patient has not been on antianginal therapy. Consider oral diltiazem if the heart rate is over 70 bpm; the PR interval is less than 0.20, blood pressure is over 110/70 mm Hg, and there is no congestive heart failure. Oral diltiazem has been shown to reduce the frequency of recurrent myocardial infarction and ischemia events in NQMI patients [13–16].

Subsequent Therapy

The great majority of patients with UAP or NQMI "cool down" on hospitalization and initial medical therapy. Further therapeutic decisions are based on response to initial therapy and laboratory assessment. Generally, a decision will be made on whether the patient is a candidate for coronary intervention based on functional status, personal desires, and availability of results.

Long-term medical therapy is directed toward maintaining good blood pressure control in addition to antiplatelet and antiischemic therapy. Typical regimens include the following:

1. Enteric-coated aspirin, 80 mg qd;
2. Long-acting diltiazem, 120–360 mg qd;
3. Angiotensin-converting enzyme inhibitor if additional antihypertensive prescription is required;
4. Lipid lowering with an HMG CoA reductase inhibitor (statin); and
5. Hygienic measures such as low saturated fat diet, walking program, and antioxidants.

Coronary Arteriography and Intervention

Because the patient with UAP or NQMI is at increased risk for a major cardiovascular event over the next 12 months, assessment of the coronary anatomy is usually performed. Decisions regarding subsequent therapy are based on coronary anatomy, suitability for interventional techniques, left ventricular function, and suitability of patient for functional restoration. Figure 4 shows a tight stenosis detected by coronary angiography and treated with coronary angioplasty. Revascularization with coronary angiography is usually highly successful, with low morbidity and mortality associated with the procedure [17].

therapies [12]. If there is a progression to ST-segment elevation, consider thrombolytic therapy.

Hospitalization

Generally, all patients with UAP or NQMI should be hospitalized for initiation of medical therapy and to monitor their course over the next 24 hours. An electrocardiographically monitored bed is useful for assessing heart rate response to therapy and to watch for ischemia-related arrhythmias.

On the first day of hospitalization, continue daily aspirin (plain or enteric-coated). Also, initiate diltiazem therapy if not already started for NQMI. Continue intravenous

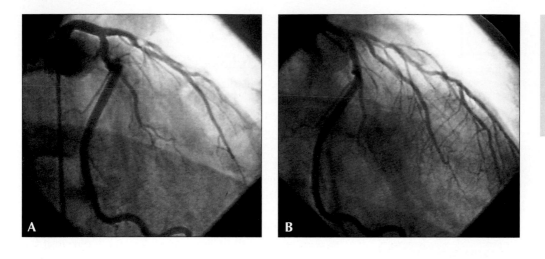

FIGURE 4 Coronary angiogram in the right anterior oblique position showing a tight proximal stenosis of the left anterior descending coronary artery before (**A**) and after (**B**) angioplasty.

REFERENCES AND RECOMMENDED READING

Recently published papers of particular interest have been highlighted as:
* Of interest
** Of outstanding interest

1. Braunwald E: Unstable angina. *Circulation* 1989, 80:410–414.

2. Theroux P: A pathophysiologic basis for the clinical classification and management of unstable angina. *Circulation* 1987, 75(suppl V):V103–V109.

3. Fuster V, Badimon L, Badimon JJ, *et al.*: Mechanisms of disease: the pathogenesis of coronary artery disease and the acute coronary syndromes (first of two parts). *N Engl J Med* 1992, 326:242–250.

4. Fuster V, Badimon L, Badimon JJ, *et al.*: Mechanisms of disease: the pathogenesis of coronary artery disease and the acute coronary syndromes (second of two parts). *N Engl J Med* 1992, 326:310–318.

5.• Ohman EM, Armstrong PW, Christenson RH, *et al.*: Cardiac troponin T levels for risk stratification in acute myocardial ischemia. *N Engl J Med* 1996, 335:1333–1341.

6.• Lindahl B, Venge P, Wallentin L: Troponin T identifies patients with unstable coronary artery disease who benefit from long-term antithrombotic protection. *J Am Coll Cardiol* 1997, 29:43–48.

7. Lewis HD Jr, Davis JW, Archibald JD, *et al.*: Protective effects of aspirin against acute myocardial infarction and death in men with unstable angina: results of a veterans cooperative study. *N Engl J Med* 1983, 309:396–403.

8. Freeman MB, Langer A, Wilson RF, *et al.*: Thrombolysis in unstable angina: randomized double-blind trial of t-PA and placebo. *Circulation* 1992, 85:150–157.

9. Ambrose JA, Hjemdahl-Monsen C, Borrico S, *et al.*: Quantitative and qualitative effects of intracoronary streptokinase in unstable angina and non–Q-wave infarction. *J Am Coll Cardiol* 1987, 9:1156–1165.

10.• Oler A, Whooley MA, Oler J, Grady D: Adding heparin to aspirin reduces the incidence of myocardial infarction and death in patients with unstable angina. *JAMA* 1996, 276:811–815.

11.• Grossman E, Messerli FH, Grodzicki T, Kowey P: Should a moratorium be placed on sublingual nifedipine capsules given for hypertensive emergencies and pseudoemergencies? *JAMA* 1996, 276:1328–1331.

12. Gobel E, Hautvast RWM, vanGilst WH, *et al.*: Randomised, double-blind trial of intravenous diltiazem versus glyceryl trinitrate for unstable angina pectoris. *Lancet* 1995, XX:1653–1657.

13. Gibson RS: Non-Q wave myocardial infarction: diagnosis, prognosis and management. *Curr Probl Cardiol* 1988, 13:1–72.

14. Boden WE, Roberts R: Prognosis and management of patients with non–Q-wave myocardial infarction. *Prog Cardiol* 1991:143–160.

15. The Multicenter Diltiazem Postinfarction Trial Research Group: The effect of diltiazem on mortality and reinfarction after myocardial infarction. *N Engl J Med* 1988, 318:385–392.

16. Gibson RS, Young PM, Boden WE, *et al.*: Prognostic significance and beneficial effect of diltiazem: results from the Multicenter Diltiazem Reinfarction Study. *Am J Cardiol* 1987, 60:203–209.

17. Williams DO, Braunwald E, Thompson B, *et al.*: Results of percutaneous transluminal coronary angioplasty in unstable angina and non-Q-wave myocardial infarction. *Circulation* 1996, 94:2749–2755.

SELECT BIBLIOGRAPHY

Clinical Practice Guidelines, Unstable Angina: Diagnosis and Management AH CPR Publication #94-0602. Available from Unstable Angina Guidelines AHCPR Clearinghouse, PO Box 8547, Silver Spring, MD 20907.

Quick Reference Guide for Clinicians. AH CPR, Publication #94-0603. Available from Unstable Angina Guidelines AHCPR Clearinghouse, PO Box 8547, Silver Spring, MD 20907.

Q-Wave Myocardial Infarction 20

Ernst R. Schwarz
Haim Hammerman
Robert A. Kloner

Key Points

- Myocardial infarction is defined as cardiomyocyte necrosis due to lack of oxygen supply in relationship to oxygen demand. The underlying cause in most cases is rupture of an intracoronary atherosclerotic plaque with subsequent thrombotic occlusion.

- Q-wave myocardial infarction is defined as myocardial cell necrosis with development and maintenance of Q waves on the electrocardiogram.

- The key symptom occurring with acute coronary artery occlusion is severe retrosternal chest pain, but symptoms may vary.

- Early hospitalization and intensive monitoring is required.

- Worldwide mortality of myocardial infarction is 30% to 40%; one third die within the first hours.

- Treatment of choice is early recanalization by thrombolytic or interventional therapy, treatment of complications, and secondary prevention.

- The main prospective goal is public education, early identification, and urgent therapy.

Of the cardiovascular diseases, acute myocardial infarction is the most common cause of death. The incidence of acute myocardial infarction (MI) reaches 900,000/year in the US, and 150,000/year in a representative state in Europe (Germany), with a mortality rate of 30% to 40%, including a 15% mortality rate before reaching the hospital. The underlying cause in most cases is atherosclerotic coronary artery disease. Acute MI can be identified by typical chest pain, electrocardiographic (ECG) changes, and subsequent characteristic elevation of cardiac enzymes. Q-wave MI in some, but not all, cases [1] correlates with transmural cell necrosis, whereas non—Q-wave infarction is often pathologically nontransmural or subendocardial. Q-wave MI tends to be larger in size and has a higher in-hospital mortality.

ETIOLOGY

The underlying disease in most patients who develop MI is coronary artery disease, with atherosclerotic narrowing leading to a reduction of vessel lumen diameter and concomitant alterations of coronary blood flow. Atherosclerotic plaques are known to exist over long periods, but also may rupture suddenly for unknown reasons. Theories regarding rupture of atherosclerotic plaques include alterations of shear stress, as occurs with catecholamine or sympathetic stimulation, as well as infiltration of plaques with monocytes and release of various cytokines. The rough intimal surface attracts platelets, leading to adhesion and finally development of thrombotic occlusion of the coronary vessel. If complete coronary artery occlusion develops quickly, the patient may suffer acute chest pain as a result of myocardial ischemia. If the ischemia is severe and prolonged, MI may develop. With gradual coronary artery occlusion, the patient may be relatively asymptomatic or exhibit only exercise-induced angina. Slow coronary lumen reduction may induce the development of coronary collateral circulation, sufficient to supply oxygen to the myocardial tissue even in the setting of total occlusion. However, the development of new collaterals occurs slowly. Therefore, the management of acute coronary occlusion with MI involves shortening the time of hypoperfusion to avoid cell death.

The risk factors for development of coronary artery disease are multifactorial and include smoking, diabetes, hypertension, hyperlipoproteinemia, age, and male sex. Other risk factors include family history, hyperuricemia, lack of physical exercise, obesity, hyperhomocysteinemia, and a type A personality. The aim for primary and secondary prevention of MI is to minimize exogenous and treat endogenous risk factors.

DIAGNOSIS

The diagnosis of acute MI can be accurately detected by clinical symptoms, ECG findings, and enzyme analysis. However, the decision to institute thrombolytic therapy usually can be based on clinical findings and ECG, because laboratory confirmation of the clinical diagnosis of acute MI caused by chest pain and ST-segment elevation in ECG has been reported in 90% to 100% of cases.

Clinical Findings

Typically, patients suffer acute chest pain that is more severe and longer lasting than angina. The pain may be described as pressure, compression, constriction, squeezing, boring, or burning in the chest [2•]. Prodromal symptoms such as angina pectoris during or after exercise or at rest with increasing frequency are often reported. The pain of myocardial infarction characteristically radiates to the left arm, but also may involve the neck, jaw, epigastrium, right arm, or back. The chest pain is not relieved by rest or nitroglycerin administration, lasts for over 30 minutes, and is often accompanied by anxiety, apprehension, restlessness, hypotension, nausea, paleness ("pale and gray appearance"), and sweating. Between 20% and 30% of patients with acute myocardial infarctions are completely asymptomatic at the onset of coronary occlusion ("silent infarcts"). In particular in the elderly or patients with diabetes, chest pain might be less severe and other symptoms may be present such as syncope, faintness, or dyspnea. Interestingly, only 10% to 20% of patients with acute chest pain admitted to emergency wards are diagnosed with acute MI [3], indicating similarity of symptoms due to other causes.

The acute symptoms of MI are frequently associated with stress such as anger or upsetting life events, or physical exertion [2•]. Factors that increase oxygen demand or decrease oxygen supply may lead to myocardial ischemia, but the additional mechanisms that trigger plaque rupture are not fully understood.

Physical Examination

Findings on physical examination are variable. Patients may appear diaphoretic and unable to find a comfortable position. The heart rate may be rapid due to sinus tachycardia, or atrial or ventricular arrhythmia. Irregular pulse may be a result of premature atrial or ventricular beats, atrial fibrillation, heart block, or other arrhythmia. Hypotension and cool cyanotic extremities typically are present in patients with evolving cardiogenic shock or severe heart failure. Lung examination may or may not reveal rales or wheezes. Cardiac examination often demonstrates a fourth heart sound. A third heart sound and a new systolic murmur or palpable thrill may be recognized with heart failure or volume overload caused by mechanical complications such as acquired ventricular septal defect, papillary muscle rupture, or dysfunction with mitral regurgitation. Low-grade fever and pericardial friction rub may be present within the first days of MI. A diagnostic physical sign of acute MI does not exist. Thus, the clinical appearance is variable (from the healthy-looking athlete carrying his own suitcase to the somnolent patient in cardiogenic shock). However, to detect complications of acute MI, physical examination—in particular, auscultation of the lungs and the heart—should be practiced repeatedly every day in all patients.

Electrocardiographic Findings

The electrocardiogram serves as the hallmark for diagnosis of acute MI because characteristic ST, T, and Q-wave changes are detectable in most of the patients [4•]. In the early stage of acute coronary occlusion (phase 1 or *hyperacute* phase) giant positive T waves appear with taller than normal R waves (Fig. 1). In phase 2 (*acute phase*, more commonly seen at hospital

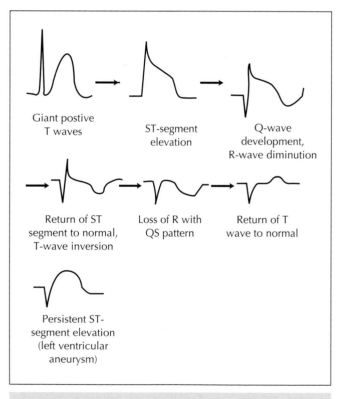

FIGURE 1 Electrocardiographic findings in myocardial infarction. Giant positive T waves are shown in hyperacute phase, followed by ST-segment elevation, then Q-wave development and R-wave diminution. Over time, the ST segment returns to normal, with loss of R wave, T-wave inversion, and sometimes T-wave pseudonormalization. There is persistent ST elevation in left ventricular aneurysm.

admission), ST-segment elevation is evident with a decrease in amplitude of the R wave, followed by pathologic Q-wave development that lasts 0.04 seconds or more and reaches 25% of the amplitude of the R wave (pathologic Q- wave, phase 3, when cell necrosis occurs over hours to days). Over time, the ST segment returns to normal with T wave inversion (terminal negative T wave); the R wave may be lost as a result of transmural necrosis and may be replaced by a QS wave (phase 4, *chronic phase*). The Q wave or QS wave persists, whereas the T wave may return to being positive. ST-wave elevation may persist in cases of left ventricular dyskinesis or aneurysm. The electrocardiographic leads not representing the infarcted area may show inverse ST-segment alterations. A new left bundle branch block may be present and, if it persists, usually indicates large anterior wall infarction. In patients with acute chest pain who present with left bundle branch block, ST-segment elevation of 1 mm or more concordant with the QRS complex, ST-segment depression of 1 mm or more in lead V1, V2, or V3, and ST-segment elevation of 5 mm or more discordant to the QRS complex can be used for the diagnosis of acute MI [5•]. In 20% of patients with acute MI, the ECG at hospital admission is normal without characteristic ST-segment changes. When possible, the current ECG tracing should be compared with previous records. Determination of myocardial infarct localization according to ECG leads is listed in Table 1.

Laboratory Findings

After myocardial injury and cell death, cellular enzymes are released into the bloodstream. The typical time course of enzyme alterations that occur can help to determine the phase of MI. The levels of the following enzymes can be routinely measured: creatine kinase (CK), creatine kinase isoenzyme MB (CK-MB), aspartate aminotransferase (AST), lactate dehydrogenase (LDH), and troponin T or troponin I. CK activity increases 4 to 8 hours after permanent coronary occlusion. With early spontaneous or therapeutically induced reperfusion, there is a peak in the level of CK as early as 8 hours after the onset of chest pain, with a quick recovery to normal values. In nonreperfused infarcts, the mean peak is reached at 24 hours and declines to normal within 72 hours. CK is highly sensitive for MI, but not specific, whereas CK-MB is more specific (if reaching >10% of CK) and thus can help rule out noncardiac causes of CK elevation (such as muscle trauma, hypothermia, diabetic ketoacidosis, rhabdomyolysis, strenuous exercise, seizures, intramuscular injection, surgery, myxedema, and cerebrovascular accident).

For clinical use, it is recommended that the CK-MB level be measured if there is CK elevation in combination with chest pain [6]. Determination of CK isoforms (MM1 to 3, MB1 and MB2) and particularly the ratio of MB2 to MB1 provide earlier information than elevation in CK-MB activity, with reliable diagnostic sensitivity [7]. Cardiac troponin T or troponin I are highly specific myofibrillar proteins and their elevation is an early marker for cardiomyocyte damage; in patients with acute MI, their levels rise as early as 3.5 hours after the onset of chest pain. Immuno-strip assays for bedside measurements provide results within 20 to 30 minutes of application of blood [8–10]. Their maximum is reached after 6 to 8 hours, and is detectable for 5 to 6 days. Even small amounts of myocardial injury without CK elevation can be specifically and sensitively detected with elevated troponin T or troponin I levels. Also, minor cellular damage may be easily and quickly detected in patients presenting with unstable angina who have elevations in troponin T [11]. LDH is elevated from 24 hours, peaks at days 4 to 5, and declines to normal within 10 days. It is therefore useful to measure LDH in patients with chest pain occurring days before admission. LDH has a high sensitivity but poor specificity. As long as other noncardiac causes are excluded (which might be difficult in some cases), enzyme elevation and its typical time course help to determine the age, course, and possible re-occurrence of MI. Therefore, CK-MB and troponin T (or troponin I) values should be determined frequently in the acute phase, *ie*, once every 3 to 4 hours for the first 9 to 12 hours, then once every 8 hours and once daily until levels are normalized. If chest pain is recurrent, intermittent analyses of CK-MB and troponin T are recommended for detection of reinfarction.

TABLE 1 LOCATION OF MYOCARDIAL INFARCTION ACCORDING TO ELECTROCARDIOGRAPHIC LEADS AND INVOLVED CORONARY ARTERY		
ST-segment elevation in ECG leads	**Ventricular location**	**Probable coronary artery involved**
V1 through V3	Anteroseptal	Proximal LAD, septal perforators
V2 through V4	Anteroapical	LAD, diagonal branches
I, aVL, V6	Lateral	LAD, diagonal branch, or circumflex
I, aVL	High lateral	1st diagonal branch or circumflex
I, aVL, V3 through V6	Anterolateral	Mid LAD or circumflex
I, aVL, V1 through V6	Extensive anterior	Proximal LAD
II, III, aVF	Inferior	RCA or circumflex, distal LAD
V1 through V2 (ST depression)	Posterior	Posterior descending of RCA, circumflex
II, III, aVF, V5 through V6	Posterolateral	RCA or circumflex
V1, V3R, V4R	Right ventricular	RCA

ECG—electrocardiogram; LAD—left anterior descending RCA; —right coronary artery.

Other enzymes such as myosin light chains or myoglobin are not routinely used in clinical situations to detect MI.

Imaging Techniques

Echocardiography is not required to make the diagnosis of acute MI in the setting of typical symptoms and ST elevation, but may help in unclear cases. Echocardiographic examination is relatively easy to perform in the emergency ward and may be helpful for detecting regional wall motion abnormalities in patients with acute chest pain, enabling the physician to diagnose acute ischemia or evolving myocardial infarction with a sensitivity of 94% to 100% and a specificity of 84% [12]. Regional wall motion abnormalities alone cannot differentiate acute ischemia from acute infarction. The location of wall motion abnormalities provides insight into which coronary arteries are involved. Regional wall motion abnormalities favor the diagnosis of coronary artery disease, whereas global and diffuse left ventricular dysfunction favor cardiomyopathy. Global ventricular function and mechanical and hemodynamic complications such as papillary muscle rupture, septal rupture, pericardial effusion, mitral regurgitation, intraventricular thrombi, and their follow-up all can be assessed accurately by echocardiography. Stress echocardiography with low-dose dobutamine is a useful technique for differentiating dysfunctional myocardium, and viable ventricular areas from necrotic ventricular areas in the chronic phase after MI [13]. Radionuclide studies are not required in the acute phase of myocardial infarction, although they may help distinguish necrotic myocardium from ischemic but viable myocardium. The potassium analogue thallium201 is widely used to assess myocardial perfusion as well as to test the integrity of cell membranes to distinguish viable tissue from necrotic myocardium [14]. Technetium-99m isonitril (Tc-99m sestamibi) is used for myocardial perfusion imaging and may identify myocardium at risk and residual ischemia, as well as help quantify infarct size [15•,16]. However, in the acute phase, nuclear imaging is not routinely recommended, if the diagnosis is clear [17••].

TREATMENT

Acute management

Because acute MI always represents a life-threatening event, the patient with suspected acute myocardial infarction should be hospitalized immediately to minimize delay in appropriate therapy. The patient should have continuous monitoring of heart rhythm and vital signs and be observed within a coronary care or intensive care unit. An intravenous line should be placed. Once the patient arrives at the hospital, initial evaluation of the patient's history, coronary risk factors, physical signs, 12-lead ECG tracing, possible contraindications for reperfusion therapy, and steps for treatment should be initiated within 20 to 30 minutes ("door-to-needle time"). In the emergency ward the patient should immediately receive aspirin in chewable form, oxygen by nasal prongs (blood gases may be checked, especially in patients with chronic pulmonary diseases), and sublingual nitrates (unless systolic arterial pres-

sure is less than 90 mmHg or heart rate is less than 50 or greater than 100 beats per minute). In many hospitals, thrombolytic therapy can be initiated in the emergency ward. Therapy for acute MI should consist of the following six steps: 1) relief of pain, 2) relief of anxiety and restlessness, and sedation, 3) reperfusion, 4) anticoagulation, 5) therapy for complications, 6) secondary prevention (Fig. 2). For steps 1 and 2, repeated administration of opioids, ie, intravenous morphine (2 to 10 mg or more), is the treatment of choice, which can be combined with antiemetics to reduce side effects.

The patient should be monitored and have bed rest for 12 to 24 hours: ie, the patient's physical activities should be reduced for at least 12 to 24 hours because life-threatening arrhythmias, reinfarction, mechanical complications, and death occur most frequently within the first 24 hours after acute MI. Sedatives, anxiolytics, and stool softeners may be prescribed. When the patient is without pain, clear liquids can be administered prior to a heart-healthy diet with 50% of kilocalories consisting of complex carbohydrates and less than 30% of monounsaturated or unsaturated fats and including foods with high amounts of potassium, magnesium, and fibers, ie, fresh fruits, vegetables, and whole grains [17••].

Reperfusion Therapy

The main goal in the treatment of patients with acute MI is to reduce the extent of irreversible myocardial tissue damage and necrosis. Because acute thrombotic coronary occlusion is found in the majority of cases of acute myocardial infarction [18], the acutely occluded coronary artery must be opened to reperfuse the myocardium within the shortest time interval. Early reperfusion has been convincingly shown to preserve left ventricular function and reduce morbidity and acute and long-term mortality by approximately 50%. Reopening of an acutely occluded coronary artery can be achieved, either by fibrinolytic agents, which are widely available, or by angioplasty, which requires adequate catheterization equipment and well-trained personnel. Fibrinolytic therapy should be initiated as early as possible, because overall benefit correlates inversely with time (the maximum benefit is derived if it is administered within the first 3 hours after onset of persistent chest pain, but some benefit may still be derived if administered up to at least 12 hours) [17••,19]. Even prehospital thrombolysis has been shown to be feasible and effective if an adequate infrastructure with appropriate paramedic patient selection, cardiac monitoring, and therapy for complications is available [19,20]

Thrombolytic therapy should be initiated within 60 to 90 minutes of the patient's calling for medical therapy ("call-to-needle time"). Because fibrinolytic agents increase the risk of hemorrhage, including intracerebral hemorrhage, several cautions and contraindications must be considered before treatment can be initiated (Table 2). Patients with ST-segment elevation or new left bundle branch block substantially benefit from lytic therapy, with a mortality reduction of 35%. Plasminogen activators are the preferred therapeutic approach to achieve rapid thrombolysis. US Food and Drug Administration (FDA)–approved agents for intravenous application are streptokinase, anisoylated plasminogen strep-

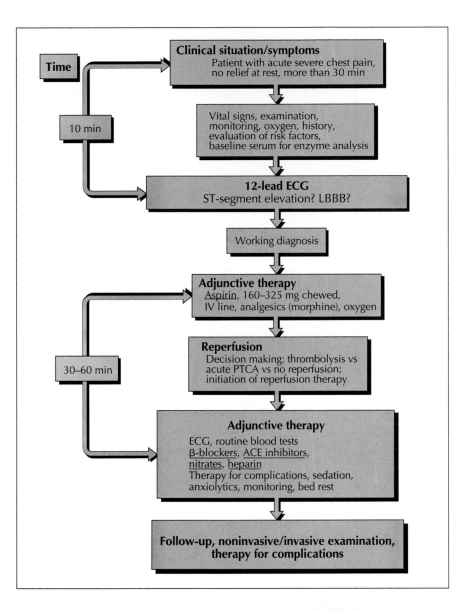

FIGURE 2 In-hospital management of acute myocardial infarction. ACE—angiotensin converting enzyme; ECG—electrocardiograph; LBBB—left bundle branch block.

The flowchart contains the following boxes connected by arrows:

Time (with timing markers: 10 min, 30–60 min)

Clinical situation/symptoms
Patient with acute severe chest pain, no relief at rest, more than 30 min

Vital signs, examination, monitoring, oxygen, history, evaluation of risk factors, baseline serum for enzyme analysis (10 min)

12-lead ECG
ST-segment elevation? LBBB?

Working diagnosis

Adjunctive therapy
Aspirin, 160–325 mg chewed, IV line, analgesics (morphine), oxygen

Reperfusion
Decision making: thrombolysis vs acute PTCA vs no reperfusion; initiation of reperfusion therapy (30–60 min)

Adjunctive therapy
ECG, routine blood tests
β-blockers, ACE inhibitors, nitrates, heparin
Therapy for complications, sedation, anxiolytics, monitoring, bed rest

Follow-up, noninvasive/invasive examination, therapy for complications

---

TABLE 2 CONTRAINDICATIONS FOR THROMBOLYTIC THERAPY

Absolute contraindications	Relative contraindications
Major surgery or trauma or head injury within 3 weeks	Pregnancy
Active internal bleeding (except menses)	Severe hypertension
Gastrointestinal bleeding within last month	Noncompressible vascular punctures
Suspected aortic dissection	Current use of anticoagulants in therapeutic doses
Acute pericarditis	Active peptic ulcer
Known bleeding disorder	For streptokinase/anistreplase: prior exposure within 2 years or prior allergic reaction
Intracranial neoplasm	History of recent transient ischemic attacks
Hemorrhagic stroke	Hemorrhagic diabetic retinopathy, recent retinal laser therapy
Cerebrovascular accident within 6 months	Prolonged cardiopulmonary resuscitation
Endstage neoplasm	

Adapted from Antman and Braunwald [2•]; Ryan *et al.* [17••]; and the Task Force on the Management of Acute Myocardial Infarction of the European Society of Cardiology [54••].

TABLE 3 COMMONLY USED THROMBOLYTIC AGENTS IN ACUTE MYOCARDIAL INFARCTION

Drug	Dose, IV	Characteristics	Half-life, min	Reperfusion rate, %*	Antigenicity	Intracerebral hemorrhage, %*	Additional heparin	US FDA-approved	Approximate cost per dose, US $*
Streptokinase	1.5 million units in 30–60 min	produced by β-hemolytic streptococci	14–20	50–60	Yes	0.3	No	IV use	300
Anistreplase (APSAC)	30 mg/5 min IV	Complex of streptokinase and plasminogen	70–120	60–70	Yes	0.6	No	IV use	1700
rt-PA	15-mg bolus, then 0.75 mg/kg over 30 min (max, 50 mg/30 min), then 0.5 mg/kg over 60 min (max, 35 mg/h); total 100 mg in 90 min	Recombinant single-chain alteplase	6	75–85	No	0.6	Yes	IV use	2200
Reteplase	10 U bolus over 2 min; repeat 10 U bolus at 30 min	Depletion of finger, epidermal growth factor, and kringle-1 from t-PA	13–16	82–88	No	0.77	Yes	IV use	2200

*Numbers obtained from references [2•], [17••], [31], [32], [54••].

IV—intravenous; rt-PA—recombinant tissue-type plasminogen activator; t-PA—tissue-type plasminogen activator.

tokinase activator complex (APSAC, anistreplase), tissue plasminogen activator (tPA, alteplase), and the "third generation" thrombolytic agent recombinant plasminogen activator (reteplase). Intracoronary application (approved for urokinase and streptokinase) is virtually obsolete. Dose regimens and characteristics of these agents are given in Table 3.

Many trials have demonstrated the efficacy of thrombolytic therapy. Most notably, the GISSI (Gruppo Italiano per lo Studio della Streptochinasi nell'Infarto Miocardico, 11,712 patients) trial in 1986 demonstrated the safety and efficacy of streptokinase if administered within 6 hours of onset of symptoms in patients with acute MI with a reduction in acute and 1-year mortality compared with that in placebo-treated controls [21,22]. Debate still exists regarding which thrombolytic agent is superior in acute MI. The TIMI-1 (Thrombolysis in Myocardial Infarction [290 patients]) study in 1987 showed a more rapid reperfusion after rt-PA compared with streptokinase (after 30 minutes and 90 minutes of initiation, 24% and 62% in rt-PA- and 8% and 31% in streptokinase-treated patients achieved TIMI flow 2 or 3, respectively) [23]. In 1990, the GISSI-2 (Gruppo Italiano per lo Studio della Sopravvivenza nell'Infarto Miocardio [12,490 patients]) trial demonstrated equal safety and efficacy of streptokinase and alteplase (24,25). In 1992, ISIS-3 (Third International Study of Infarct Survival [41,299 patients] trial) revealed less reinfarction but higher rates of stroke and noncerebral bleeding as a result of t-PA adminstration, whereas 35-day mortality and 6-month survival were similar in those treated with t-PA, streptokinase, or APSAC [26]. The GUSTO-1 (Global Utilization of Streptokinase and Tissue Plasminogen Activator for Occluded Coronary arteries [41,021 patients]) trial in 1993 demonstrated a lower 30-day mortality rate after the accelerated administration of t-PA plus heparin (6.3%) compared with streptokinase plus subcutaneously or intravenously administered heparin (7.2% or 7.4%, respectively) and a combination of t-PA and streptokinase plus heparin (7.0%) [27]. Moreover, an angiographic substudy in 2431 patients demonstrated that t-PA caused faster and more complete reperfusion and better regional wall motion [28]. However, there was a significant excess of hemorrhagic strokes with the use of t-PA compared with streptokinase (0.72 vs 0.54%, p = 0.03). The TIMI-4 trial in 1994 [382 patients] showed that front-loaded rt-PA is associated with higher rates of early reperfusion and trends toward better clinical outcome and survival compared with APSAC or a combination of both agents [29]. Results of the INJECT (International Joint Efficacy Comparison of Thrombolytics [6010 patients] trial in 1995 compared the effects of streptokinase and the recombinant plasminogen activator (reteplase), showing similar 35-day mortality rates of 9.53% and 9.02%, and 6-month mortality rates of 12.05% and 11.02%, with similar bleeding events of 15.3% and 15.0%, respectively [30]. Additionally, the RAPID trials (Rapid-1: Reteplase Angiographic Phase II International Dose Finding Study; Rapid-2: Reteplase vs. Alteplase Patency Investigation During Acute Myocardial Infarction [606 patients] in 1995 demonstrated a more rapid and complete reperfusion following double-bolus reteplase (10 MU r-PA bolus followed by 10 MU r-PA after

30 min) compared with standard-dose alteplase [31]. Although t-PA is associated with a significantly lower incidence of allergic reactions and severe hypotension compared with streptokinase, because of the higher costs of t-PA, there is still debate concerning which thrombolytic agent is the most cost-effective one in different countries. The choice of thrombolytic therapy strategy therefore depends on experience, individual risk assessment, availability, and cost-benefit analysis rather than on scientific and practical priorities, at least when choosing among streptokinase, t-PA, and the newly available reteplase.

Primary Percutaneous Transluminal Coronary Angioplasty

The American College of Cardiology/American Heart Association Guidelines for the management of patients with acute MI, published in 1996, suggested that primary percutaneous transluminal coronary angioplasty (PTCA) can serve as an alternative to thrombolysis only if performed in a timely fashion by individuals skilled in the procedure and supported by experienced personnel in high-volume centers [17••]. Indications include patients with contraindications to thrombolysis, patients at risk for bleeding, and patients with cardiogenic shock. Studies comparing immediate angioplasty to thrombolytic therapy, such as the PAMI-1 (Primary Angioplasty in Myocardial Infarction) trial in 1993 and 1995, and others demonstrated a successful antegrade coronary flow in approximately 90% of patients receiving PTCA. These patients had a lower incidence of reocclusion, reinfarction, recurrent ischemia, death, coronary artery bypass grafting, and intracranial hemorrhage [32,33••,34–36]. With the advantage of early knowledge of the coronary anatomy and number and degree of additional stenoses, left ventricular function, and the possibility of PTCA with acute stenting, these studies suggest that patients with large anterior infarcts benefit from direct angioplasty, which might be superior to thrombolytic therapy [32,36].

Adjunctive Therapy

Early adjunctive therapy with thrombolysis consists of aspirin, which quickly prevents thromboxane A2 production in platelets and prostacyclin in endothelial cells. Aspirin administration resulted in a 23% reduction in the 35-day mortality rate in patients with MI; if combined with streptokinase, there was a reduction of 42% in the ISIS-2 study [37]. The ACCP guidelines (Fourth American College of Chest Physicians Consensus Conference on Antithrombotic Therapy) and the ACC/AHA guidelines recommend that aspirin be administered at the time of admission to the emergency ward at a dose of 160 to 325 mg, preferably in a chewable form because of its faster absorption, followed by a daily administration indefinitely thereafter [38,39]. In case of true aspirin allergy, dipyridamole or ticlopidine may be used.

Heparin (which forms a complex with antithrombin III, thus inactivating thrombin) is recommended with use of fibrin-specific thrombolytics such as alteplase and reteplase (70 U/kg as a bolus, followed by 15 µg/kg/hr to keep the activated partial thromboplastin time [aPTT, a coagulation parameter] at 1.5 to 2.0 times control for 48 hours). Heparin also should be given for primary PTCA (the activated clotting time [ACT], which can be instantaneously measured in the catheter lab, should be 300 to 350 seconds) and in patients with large or anterior MI, known left ventricular thrombus, or previous embolic events. In patients not treated with thrombolytic therapy or with nonselected thrombolytics (streptokinase, anistreplase, urokinase), and in patients without increased risk for systemic emboli, subcutaneous administration of 7500 U twice daily may be administered [17••]. Prolonged intravenous heparin therapy has not been shown to decrease the rate of reocclusion. Dose regimens leading to an aPTT of more than 90 seconds for hours or days correlate with an unacceptable high risk for bleeding complications. Effects of the direct antithrombin agent hirudin are similar to those of heparin.

β-Adrenergic blockers are known to reduce myocardial oxygen consumption, as well as acute and long-term mortality and morbidity, and should be administered intravenously as early as possible (on day 1 within 12 hours) followed by oral therapy if contraindications are excluded [40]. Furthermore, β-blockers may reduce infarct size and the incidence of ventricular fibrillation and reinfarction [41]. Mortality after MI has also been shown to be reduced in several trials comparing the use of ACE inhibitors with placebo. In the SAVE (Survival and Ventricular Enlargement [2231 patients]) trial, long-term captopril therapy in patients with asymptomatic left ventricular dysfunction following acute MI was associated with a reduction in mortality and morbidity [42]. Several studies confirmed the reduction of mortality as a result of ACE inhibitor administration compared with placebo, which was augmented with early administration [43,44••,45,46••,47,48]. However, in the CONSENSUS II trial enalapril did not improve survival during a 180-day follow-up after acute MI [49]. According to the ACC/AHA guidelines, however, ACE inhibitors should be initiated on day 1 within hours of hospitalization in patients with evolving acute MI with ST-segment elevation or left bundle branch block and continued indefinitely in case of impaired left ventricular function (the lower the ejection fraction, the greater the benefit). The use of intravenous nitroglycerin is recommended during the first 48 hours and beyond this time frame in patients with recurrent angina, large infarction, and pulmonary congestion. Calcium antagonists, predominantly short-acting nifedipine, may be harmful and should be avoided in patients with acute MI. If β-blockers are ineffective, verapamil or diltiazem might be used in patients with ischemia or tachycardia in the absence of left ventricular dysfunction or AV block [17••]. Uncertainty exists concerning the use of magnesium, because a reduction in mortality has been reported in some studies (24% in the LIMIT-2 trial) [50–52], but the ISIS-4 trial could not demonstrate beneficial effects of magnesium treatment in acute MI [43]. In the ACC/AHA guidelines, magnesium administration is recommended only to correct documented magnesium deficits, especially in patients receiving diuretics, in the case of torsades de pointes with a prolonged QT interval, and in high-risk patients not receiving reperfusion therapy [17••].

COMPLICATIONS OF ACUTE MYOCARDIAL INFARCTION

Arrhythmia

The incidence of arrhythmia may be as high as 100% in patients with acute MI, and manifests predominantly as premature ventricular beats. The most serious and life-threatening arrhythmias are ventricular fibrillation and sustained polymorphic ventricular tachycardia requiring early electrical defibrillation (200 J), which is repeated if unsuccessful (up to 360 J). Monomorphic ventricular tachycardia not associated with angina or acute heart failure may be treated with the antiarrhythmic agents lidocaine (1 to 1.5 mg/kg as a bolus, followed by 2 to 4 mg/min intravenously), procainamide, amiodarone, or synchronized electrical cardioversion. A meta-analysis of 14 randomized trials demonstrated a higher mortality rate in patients treated with lidocaine, probably as a result of

TABLE 4 MECHANICAL COMPLICATIONS OF ACUTE MYOCARDIAL INFARCTION	
Complications	**Management**
Severe left ventricular dysfunction, left-sided heart failure *Diagnosis*: low output syndrome; tachycardia, dyspnea, orthopnea, pulmonary congestion, cyanotic limbs, oliguria, cardiac index > 2.5 L/min/m²; auscultation, chest radiography, 2-dimensional echocardiography, invasive hemodynamics.	Invasive hemodynamic monitoring (Swan-Ganz catheter, intraarterial pressure monitoring). If wedge pressure is high and blood pressure stable: diuretics (furosemide), vasodilators (nitrates, reduction of pre- and afterload), ACE inhibitors (afterload reduction); if wedge pressure is high and blood pressure low (hemodynamically unstable): dobutamine, dopamine; consider phosphodiesterase inhibitors, reperfusion, acute coronary angiography and PTCA, intra-aortic balloon pump
Right-sided heart failure/dysfunction due to right ventricular infarction/ischemia *Diagnosis*: prominent jugular veins, distention on inspiration, elevated venous pressure, clear lung fields, tachycardia associated with inferior myocardial infarction, echocardiography, increased right atrial pressure	Invasive hemodynamic monitoring, volume loading, maintenance of AV synchrony; avoid nitrates and diuretics; inotropic support (dobutamine); consider arterial vasodilators (sodium nitroprusside), ACE inhibitors, intra-aortic balloon pump, reperfusion, acute PTCA, emergency CABG
Cardiogenic shock *Diagnosis*: tachycardia, low pressure (cardiac index < 1.8 L/min/m²), dyspnea, tachypnea, cyanosis, shock, low urine output	Invasive hemodynamic monitoring, positive inotropic agents (dobutamine, dopamine, norepinephrine), reperfusion, acute PTCA or emergency CABG; anesthesia, artificial ventilation, intra-aortic balloon pump
Ventricular septal defect, papillary muscle rupture, acute mitral regurgitation *Diagnosis*: heart failure (dyspnea, orthopnea, tachycardia), systolic murmur, chest radiography, echocardiography, Doppler	Hemodynamic monitoring, afterload reduction, intra-aortic balloon pump, surgery
Cardiac rupture, pericardial effusion, and tamponade *Diagnosis*: low output, elevated venous pressure, tachycardia, dyspnea, shock, electrical-mechanical dissociation, echocardiography	Emergency pericardiocentesis, emergency surgery
Pericarditis, Dressler syndrome (late pericarditis) *Diagnosis*: pleuritic chest pain, pericardial friction rub	Aspirin, analgesics, follow-up echocardiography; avoid steroids and nonsteroidal inflammatory agents, if possible
Infarct extension *Diagnosis*: reappearance of CK-MB enzyme activity, chest pain, new ECG changes, left ventricular dysfunction, cardiogenic shock	Angiography and acute recanalization, revascularization, or reperfusion therapy; antiischemic medication (nitrates), anticoagulation; if possible, beta-blockers, ACE inhibitors
Infarct expansion and left ventricular remodeling *Diagnosis*: echocardiography (thinning and dilation of infarct and left ventricle)	Afterload reduction, treatment of heart failure, anticoagulation, ACE inhibitors
Postinfarction angina, re-infarction *Diagnosis*: chest pain, ECG changes, heart failure, CK re-elevation if re-infarction	Nitrates, beta-blockers, anticoagulation, reperfusion, early angiography and PTCA or CABG
Left ventricular aneurysm and mural thrombus *Diagnosis*: embolic events, echocardiography, ventriculography	Anticoagulation: acutely heparin and chronically warfarin recommended for 3–6 months; consider surgical resection of aneurysm

ACE—angiotension converting enzyme; CABG—coronary artery bypass grafting; ECG—electrocardiography; PTCA—percutaneous transluminal coronary angioplasty.

bradycardia and asystole [53]. Therefore, prophylactic use of antiarrhythmic agents (except β-receptor blockers) is not recommended [54••]. For bradyarrhythmia and heart block, either intravenous atropine or temporary transvenous (or, in some cases, transcutaneous) pacing is recommended. Indications for pacing are symptomatic bradycardia (less than 50 beats per minute) with symptoms of hypotension not responding to atropine; asystole; bilateral bundle branch block; newly developed or indeterminate bifascial block with first-degree AV block; second-degree symptomatic or Mobitz type II AV block, advanced (complete) AV-block; and incessant ventricular tachycardia, which requires atrial or ventricular overdrive pacing [17••]. Atrial fibrillation is often transient and may be associated with heart failure, atrial ischemia, or pericarditis. It should be treated by either electric cardioversion in patients with hemodynamic instability or ischemia; or by rapid digitalization, β-blockade in patients without contraindications, diltiazem or verapamil, and heparin to avoid embolic events.

Hemodynamic and Mechanical Complications

Congestive heart failure may result from systolic contractile dysfunction due to large necrotic areas or to postischemic contractile wall motion abnormalities (stunned myocardium). Mechanical complications that worsen cardiac function include myocardial infarct expansion and aneurysm formation, ruptured ventricle, ventricular septal defect, papillary muscle dysfunction, and rupture (Table 4). The primary symptom is dyspnea, caused by pulmonary congestion and tachycardia. Therapy for congestive heart failure should be initiated with diuretics (furosemide, 20 mg intravenously, which may be repeated), nitrates, and oxygen, followed by positive inotropic agents (dobutamine, 2 to 20 μg/kg/min; dopamine 2 to 10 μg/kg/min intravenously). In case of severe ventricular dysfunction or cardiogenic shock, a Swan-Ganz pulmonary artery catheter for measurements of cardiac output, pulmonary artery capillary wedge pressure pulmonary and systemic resis-

tances, and intra-aortic balloon counterpulsation should be considered. The therapeutic approaches to cardiogenic shock (with a high mortality rate), papillary muscle rupture with mitral regurgitation, cardiac rupture, postinfarction pericarditis and other complications are summarized in Table 4.

Postinfarction Evaluation and Secondary Prevention

Coronary angiography and subsequent revascularization, either by PTCA or bypass grafting, ultimately should be performed in patients with recurrent angina or evidence of large areas of reversible ischemia on stress testing, and might be considered selectively in all survivors of acute MI. Before interventional therapy is initiated, recurrent angina should be treated with intravenous nitroglycerin, aspirin, heparin, analgesics, and β-blockers. In all patients following myocardial infarction without contraindications, long-term treatment with aspirin and β-adrenergic blockers is recommended [55•] (Table 5). ACE inhibitors should be a part of secondary prevention in patients with left ventricular dysfunction. Calcium antagonists are not routinely recommended after infarction but may be selectively prescribed in patients with specific indications such as hypertension or angina in the presence of preserved left ventricular function [56,57].

The prognosis after acute myocardial infarction is related to four main factors:

1. Extent of left ventricular dysfunction, including degree of left ventricular dilation
2. Presence of residual ischemia
3. Degree of electrical instability of the myocardium
4. Progression of coronary atherosclerosis

A risk stratification should be evaluated in each patient. Noninvasive evaluation of low-risk patients includes submaximal or symptom-limited stress ECG at 4 to 6 days or 10 to 14 days, respectively. For prognostic assessment, after mobilization, *ie* after 1 week, standard exercise testing should be

TABLE 5 LONG-TERM THERAPY AND SECONDARY PREVENTION AFTER MYOCARDIAL INFARCTION	
Treatment	**Comments**
Drug therapy	
Aspirin	In all patients without contraindications
β-Blockers	In all patients without contraindications
ACE inhibitors	In patients with left ventricular dysfunction
Dietary therapy	
Low saturated fats and cholesterol	Weight-reduction and exercise in overweight patients
Lipid-lowering drugs	If LDL cholesterol > 100 mg/dL, HDL cholesterol < 35 mg/dL, triglycerides > 400 mg/dL
Rehabilitation	Risk factor evaluation, education, return to work (if feasible), self-control,
Physical	knowledge of limitations
Psychological	
Socioeconomic	
Life-style changes	
Physical activity/exercising	
Smoking cessation	

ACE—angiotensin-converting enzyme; HDL—high-density lipoprotein; LDL—low-density lipoprotein.

performed to assess potential exercise-induced angina or left ventricular dysfunction and functional capacity. Stress ECG should be repeated early after hospital discharge and after 4 to 6 weeks. Perfusion imaging with vasodilators (dipyridamole or adenosine) or dobutamine echocardiography should be performed in patients with recurrent ischemic symptoms who are unable to exercise. Patients with evidence of reversible ischemia should be considered for coronary angiography. Knowledge of cardiac function and the coronary artery status is essential for a decision of early or delayed revascularization procedures. The post-infarction strategies for exercise testing are presented in Figure 3. Patients should be educated about

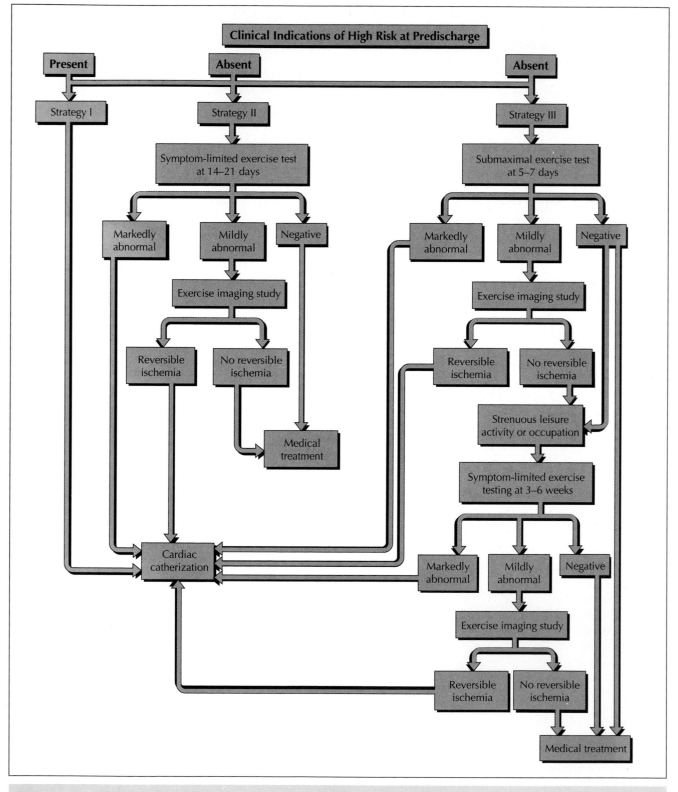

FIGURE 3 Strategies for exercise test evaluation at hospital discharge after myocardial infarction. (*From* Ryan *et al.* [17••]; with permission of the American College of Cardiology.)

risk factor modification, *ie*, cessation of smoking, necessity of physical exercise, and effective lifestyle intervention. Diet recommendations from the American Heart Association consist of low saturated fat and cholesterol for all patients following acute MI.

Several studies like the Scandinavian Simvastatin Survival Study (4S) showed a reduction in mortality with the use of blood cholesterol-lowering agents in patients with MI [58]. Data from the CARE trial demonstrated that patients with average plasma cholesterol levels, *ie*, cholesterol below 240 mg/dL and low density lipoprotein (LDL) cholesterol levels between 115 and 174 mg/dL, receiving pravastatin, 40 mg/d, had a reduction in risk for fatal coronary events or recurrent MI of 24% when compared with placebo-treated patients [59••]. According to the ACC/AHA guidelines, lipid-lowering drugs are recommended in patients after MI if LDL cholesterol levels are greater than 125 mg/dL (or greater than 100 mg/dL despite diet), triglyceride levels are greater than 400 mg/dL, and high-density lipoprotein (HDL) cholesterol levels are less than 35 mg/dL despite dietary therapy. However, according to results from the CARE trial, additional lipid-lowering drug therapy may be considered even in patients with lower (average) cholesterol levels. Social and professional rehabilitation with prescriptive exercise training and patient education is encouraged [17,60].

The recommendations given here are in accordance with the guidelines of the Task Force of the European Society of Cardiology on the Management of Acute Myocardial Infarction, published in January 1996 [54••] and the guidelines of the American College of Cardiology/American Heart Association (ACC/AHA) for the Management of Patients with Acute Myocardial Infarction, published in November 1996 [17••].

KEY REFERENCES

Recently published papers of outstanding interest, as identified in *References and Recommended Reading*, have been annotated.

•• Ryan TJ, Anderson JL, Antman EM, *et al.*: ACC/AHA guidelines for the management of patients with acute myocardial infarction. A report of the American College of Cardiology/American Heart Association Task Force on Practice Guidelines (Committee on management of acute myocardial infarction). *J Am Coll Cardiol* 1996, 28:1328–1428.

This report of the American College of Cardiology/American Heart Association Task Force on practice guidelines for the management of patients with acute myocardial infarction is a revision of the original guidelines from 1990. This update is based on current knowledge from clinical trials and contains 787 references.

•• Stone GW, Grines CL, Browne KF, *et al.*: Predictors of in-hospital and 6-month outcome after acute myocardial infarction in the reperfusion era: the primary angioplasty in myocardial infarction (PAMI) trial. *J Am Coll Cardiol* 1995, 25:370–377.

The 6-month follow-up of the comparison of primary coronary angioplasty with intravenous tissue plasminogen activator in patients with acute myocardial infarction demonstrated that advanced age, prior heart failure, and treatment with t-PA versus angioplasty were independently associated with increased in-hospital mortality, supporting the concept of primary angioplasty in patients with acute myocardial infarction.

•• Latini R, Maggioni AP, Flather M, *et al.*: ACE-inhibitor use in patients with myocardial infarction: summary of evidence from clinical trials. *Circulation* 1995, 92:3132–3137.

This meeting report summarizes the data from clinical trials on ACE-inhibition in patients with myocardial infarction and provides statements for the use of ACE-inhibitors.

•• Ambrosioni E, Borghi C, Magnani B: The effect of the angiotensin-converting-enzyme inhibitor zofenopril on mortality and morbidity after anterior myocardial infarction: the Survival of Myocardial Infarction: Long-Term Evaluation (SMILE) Study Investigators. *N Engl J Med* 1995, 332:80–85.

Patients with acute myocardial infarction not receiving reperfusion therapy were randomized to either zofenopril or placebo, starting 24 hours after the onset of myocardial infarction. Six-week treatment with the ACE-inhibitor zofenopril reduced mortality and the risk of severe heart failure at six weeks and 1 year.

•• The Task Force on the Management of Acute Myocardial Infarction of the European Society of Cardiology: Acute myocardial infarction: pre-hospital and in-hospital management. *Eur Heart J* 1996, 17:43–63.

The guidelines are provided by the European Society of Cardiology for the management and therapy for patients with acute myocardial infarction, as extrapolated from the results of clinical trials.

•• Sacks FM, Pfeffer MA, Moye, LA, *et al.*:Effect of pravastatin on coronary events after myocardial infarction in patients with average cholesterol levels. *N Engl J Med* 1996, 335:1001–1009.

This double-blind trial, which was conducted over a period of 5 years, showed that cholesterol-lowering therapy with pravastatin in patients with myocardial infarction but normal cholesterol levels (below 240 mg/dL) resulted in a significant reduction in fatal coronary events, myocardial infarction, and stroke as well as a reduction in coronary angioplasty and bypass grafting.

REFERENCES AND RECOMMENDED READING

Recently published papers of particular interest have been highlighted as:
• Of interest
•• Of outstanding interest

1. Raunio H, Rissanen V, Roppanen T, *et al*: Changes in the QRS complex and ST segment in transmural and subendocardial myocardial infarctions. A clinico-pathologic study.*Am Heart J* 1979, 98:176–184.

2.• Antman EM, Braunwald E.: Acute myocardial infarction. In Braunwald E, ed. Heart Disease. *A Textbook of Cardiovascular Medicine.*edn. 5. Philadelphia: WB Saunders; 1997:1184–1288.

3. Goldman L, Cook EF, Brand DA, *et al.*: A computer protocol to predict myocardial infarction in emergency department patients with chest pain. *N Engl J Med* 1988, 318:797–803.

4.• Parker AB, Waller BF, Gering LE: Usefulness of the 12-lead electrocardiogram in detection of myocardial infarction: electro-cardiographic-anatomic correlations.*Clin Cardiol* 1996, 19:55.

5.• Sgarbossa EB, Pinski A, Barbagelata DA, *et al.*: Electrocardiographic diagnosis of evolving acute myocardial infarction in the presence of left bundle-branch block. *N Engl J Med* 1996, 334:481–487.

6. Puelo PR, Meyer D, Walthen C, *et al.*: Use of rapid assay of subforms of creatine kinase MB to diagnose or rule out acute myocardial infarction. *N Engl J Med* 1994, 331:561–566.

7. Roberts R, Kleinman NS: Earlier diagnosis and treatment of acute myocardial infarction necessitates the need for a 'new diagnostic mind-set'. *Circulation* 1994, 89:872–881.

8. Katus HA, Rempiss A, Neumann FJ, *et al.*: Diagnostic efficiency of troponin T measurements in acute myocardial infarction. *Circulation* 1991, 83:902–912.

9. Müller-Bardoff M, Freitag H, Scheffold T, *et al.*: Development and characterization of a rapid assay for bedside determinations of cardiac troponin T. *Circulation* 1995, 92:2869–2875.

10. Larue C, Calzolari C, Bertinchant JP, *et al.*: Cardiac-specific immunoenzymometric assay of troponin I in the early phase of acute myocardial infarction. *Clinical Chemistry* 1993, 39:972–979.

11. Seino Y, Tomita Y, Takano T, *et al.*: Early identification of cardiac events with serum Troponin T in patients with unstable angina. *Lancet* 1993, 342:1236–1237.

12. Feigenbaum H: Coronary artery disease. In: Feigenbaum H, ed. *Echocardiography* edn. 5. Philadelphia: Lea and Febiger, 1994:447–510.

13. Pierard LA, DeLandsheere CM, Berthe C, *et al.*: Identification of viable myocardium during dobutamine infusion in patients with myocardial infarction after thrombolytic therapy. *J Am Coll Cardiol* 1990, 15:1021–1031.

14. Dilsizian V, Bonow RO: Current diagnostic techniques of assessing myocardial viability in patients with hibernating and stunned myocardium. *Circulation* 1993, 87:1–20.

15•. Miller GL, Herman SD, Heller GV, *et al.*: Relation between perfusion defects on stress technetium-99m sestamibi SPECT scintigraphy and the location of a subsequent acute myocardial infarction. *Am J Cardiol* 1996, 78:26–30.

16. Marcassa C, Galli M, Temporelli PL, *et al.*: Technetium-99m sestamibi tomographic evaluation of residual ischemia after anterior myocardial infarction. *J Am Coll Cardiol* 1995, 25:590–596.

17.•• Ryan TJ, Anderson JL, Antman EM, *et al.*: ACC/AHA guidelines for the management of patients with acute myocardial infarction. A report of the American College of Cardiology/American Heart Association Task Force on Practice Guidelines (Committee on management of acute myocardial infarction). *J Am Coll Cardiol* 1996, 28:1328–1428.

18. De Wood MA, Spores J, Notske RN, *et al.*: Prevalence of total coronary artery occlusion during the early hours of transmural myocardial infarction. *N Engl J Med* 1980, 303:897.

19. Weaver WD, Cerqueira M, Hallstrom AP, *et al.*: Prehospital-initiated versus hospital-initiated thrombolytic therapy: the myocardial infarction triage and intervention trial. *JAMA* 1993, 270:1211–1216.

20. Weaver WD, Eisenberg MS, Martin JS, *et al.*: Myocardial infarction triage and intervention project-phase I: patient characteristics and feasibility of prehospital initiation of thrombolytic therapy. *J Am Coll Cardiol* 1990, 15:925–931.

21. GISSI (Gruppo Italiano per lo Studio della Streptochinasi nell'Infarto miocardico): Effectiveness of intravenous thrombolytic treatment in acute myocardial infarction. *Lancet* 1986, I:397–401.

22. GISSI (Gruppo Italiano per lo Studio della Streptochinasi nell'Infarto miocardico): Long-term effects of intravenous thrombolysis in acute myocardial infarction: final report of the GISSI study. *Lancet* 1987, II:871–874.

23. Chesbero JH, Knatterud G, Roberts R, *et al.*: Thrombolysis in myocardial infarction (TIMI) trial, phase I: a comparison between intravenous tissue plasminogen activator and intravenous streptokinase. Clinical findings through hospital discharge. *Circulation* 1987, 76:142–154.

24. GISSI (Gruppo Italiano per lo Studio della Streptochinasi nell'Infarto miocardico): GISSI-2: A factorial randomized trial of alteplase versus streptokinase and heparin versus no heparin among 12,490 patients with acute myocardial infarction. *Lancet* 1990, 336:65–71.

25. GISSI (Gruppo Italiano per lo Studio della Streptochinasi nell'Infarto miocardico), The International Study Group: In-hospital mortality and clinical course of 20,891 patients with suspected acute myocardial infarction randomized between alteplase and streptokinase with or without heparin. *Lancet* 1990, 336:71–75.

26. ISIS-3 Collaborative Group: ISIS-3: a randomized comparison of streptokinase versus tissue plasminogen activator versus anistreplase and of aspirin plus heparin versus aspirin alone among 41,299 cases of suspected acute myocardial infarction. *Lancet* 1992, 339:753–770.

27. The GUSTO Investigators: An international randomized trial comparing four thrombolytic strategies for acute myocardial infarction. GUSTO-1 (Global utilization of streptokinase and tissue plasminogen activator for occluded coronary arteries). *N Engl J Med* 1993, 329:673–682.

28. The GUSTO Angiographic Investigators: The effects of tissue plasminogen activator, streptokinase, or both on coronary-artery patency, ventricular function, and survival after acute myocardial infarction. *N Engl J Med* 1993, 329:1615–1622.

29. Cannon CP, McCabe CH, Diver DJ, *et al.*: Comparison of front-loaded recombinant tissue-type plasminogen activator, anistreplase and combination thrombolytic therapy for acute myocardial infarction: results of the Thrombolysis in Myocardial Infarction (TIMI) 4 trial. *J Am Coll Cardiol* 1994, 24:1602–1610.

30. International Joint Efficacy Comparison of Thrombolytics: Randomized, double-blind comparison of reteplase double-bolus administration with streptokinase in acute myocardial infarction (INJECT): trial to investigate equivalence. *Lancet* 1995, 346:329–336.

31. Smalling RW, Bode C, Kalbfleisch J, *et al.*: More rapid, complete, and stable coronary thrombolysis with bolus administration of reteplase compared with alteplase infusion in acute myocardial infarction. *Circulation* 1995, 91:2725–2732.

32. Grines CL, Browne KF, Marco J, *et al.*: A comparison of immediate angioplasty with thrombolytic therapy for acute myocardial infarction. *N Engl J Med* 1993, 328:673–679.

33.•• Stone GW, Grines CL, Browne KF, *et al.*: Predictors of in-hospital and 6-month outcome after acute myocardial infarction in the reperfusion era: the primary angioplasty in myocardial infarction (PAMI) trial. *J Am Coll Cardiol* 1995, 25:370–377.

34. Weaver WD, Litwin PE, Martin JS: Use of direct angioplasty for treatment of patients with acute myocardial infarction in hospitals with and without on-site cardiac surgery: The Myocardial Infarction, Triage, and Intervention Project Investigators. *Circulation* 1993, 88:2067–2075.

35. Zijlstra F, de Boer MJ, Hoorntje JCA, *et al.*: A comparison of immediate coronary angioplasty with intravenous streptokinase in acute myocardial infarction. *N Engl J Med* 1993, 328:680–684.

36. de Boer MJ, Hoorntje JCA, Ottervanger JP, *et al.*: Immediate coronary angioplasty versus intravenous streptokinase in acute myocardial infarction: left ventricular ejection fraction, hospital mortality and reinfarction. *J Am Coll Cardiol* 1994, 23:1004–1008.

37. ISIS-2 Collaborative Group: Randomized trial of intravenous streptokinase, oral aspirin, both, or neither among 17,187 cases of suspected acute myocardial infarction: ISIS-2. *Lancet* 1988, II:349–360.

38. Fourth American College of Chest Physicians Consensus Conference on Antithrombotic Therapy. *Chest* 1995, 108 (suppl.):225S–522S.

39. Fuster V, Dyken ML, Vokonas PS, *et al.*: Aspirin as a therapeutic agent in cardiovascular disease. *Circulation* 1993, 87:659–675.

40. First International Study of Infarct Survival Collaborative Group: Randomised trial of intravenous atenolol among 16,027 cases of suspected acute myocardial infarction: ISIS-1. *Lancet* 1986, 2:57–66.

41. Yusuf S, Peto R, Lewis J, *et al.*: Beta blockade during and after myocardial infarction: an overview of the randomized trials. *Prog Cardiovasc Dis* 1985, 27:335–371.

42. Pfeffer MA, Braunwald E, Moyé LA, *et al.*: Effect of captopril on mortality and morbidity in patients with left ventricular dysfunction after myocardial infarction. Results of the Survival and Ventricular Enlargement trial. *N Engl J Med* 1992, 327:669–677.

43. ISIS-4 (Fourth International Study of Infarct Survival) Collaborative Group: ISIS-4: a randomised factorial trial assessing early oral captopril, oral mononitrate, and intravenous magnesium sulphate in 58,050 patients with suspected acute myocardial infarction. *Lancet* 1995, 345:669–685.

44.•• Latini R, Maggioni AP, Flather M, *et al.*: ACE-inhibitor use in patients with myocardial infarction: summary of evidence from clinical trials. *Circulation* 1995, 92:3132–3137.

45. GISSI (Gruppo Italiano per lo Studio della Sopravvivenza nell'Infarto miocardico). GISSI-3: effects of lisinopril and transdermal glyceryl trinitrate singly and together on 6-week mortality and ventricular function after acute myocardial infarction. *Lancet* 1994, 343:1115–1122.

46.•• Ambrosioni E, Borghi C, Magnani B: The effect of the angiotensin-converting-enzyme inhibitor zofenopril on mortality and morbidity after anterior myocardial infarction: the Survival of Myocardial Infarction: Long-Term Evaluation (SMILE) Study Investigators. *N Engl J Med* 1995, 332:80–85.

47. The AIRE Study Investigators: Effect of ramipril on mortality and morbidity of survivors of acute myocardial infarction with clinical evidence of heart failure. *Lancet* 1993, 342:821–828.

48. Kober L, Torp-Pedersen C, Clarsen JE, *et al.*: A clinical trial of the angiotensin-converting enzyme inhibitor trandolapril in patients with left ventricular dysfunction after myocardial infarction. *N Engl J Med* 1995, 333:1670–1676.

49. Swedberg K, Held P, Kjekhus J, *et al.*:Effects of the early administration of enalapril on mortality in patients with acute myocardial infarction: results of the Cooperative New Scandinavian Enalapril Survival Study II (CONSENSUS -II). *N Engl J Med* 1992, 327:678–684.

50. Antman EM, Lau J, Kupelnick B, *et al.*: A comparison of results of meta-analyses of randomized control trials and recommendations of clinical experts: treatments for myocardial infarction. *JAMA* 1992, 268:240–248.

51. Woods KL, Fletcher S: Long-term outcome after intravenous magnesium sulphate in suspected acute myocardial infarction: the second Leicester Intravenous Magnesium Intervention Trial (LIMIT-2). *Lancet* 1994, 343:816–819.

52. Antman EM: Magnesium in acute MI: timing is critical. *Circulation* 1995, 92:2367–2372.

53. MacMahon S, Collins R, Peto R, *et al.*: Effects of prophylactic lidocaine in suspected myocardial infarction. *JAMA* 1988, 260:1910–1916.

54.•• The Task Force on the Management of Acute Myocardial Infarction of the European Society of Cardiology: Acute myocardial infarction: pre-hospital and in-hospital management. *Eur Heart J* 1996, 17:43–63.

55.• Goldstein RE, Andrews M, Hall WJ, *et al.*: Marked reduction in long-term cardiac deaths with aspirin after a coronary event: Multicenter Myocardial Ischemia Research Group. *J Am Coll Cardiol* 1996, 28:326–330.

56. Kloner RA: Nifidipine in ischemic heart disease. *Circulation* 1995, 92:1074–1078.

57. Psaty BM, Heckbert SR, Koepsell TD, *et al.*:The risk of myocardial infarction associated with antihypertensive drug therapies. *JAMA* 1995, 274:620–625.

58. The Scandinavian Simvastatin Survival Study Group: Randomized trial of cholesterol lowering in 4444 patients with coronary heart disease: the Scandinavian Simvastatin Survival Study (4S). *Lancet* 1994, 344:1383–1389.

59.•• Sacks FM, Pfeffer MA, Moye, LA, *et al.*:Effect of pravastatin on coronary events after myocardial infarction in patients with average cholesterol levels. *N Engl J Med* 1996, 335:1001–1009.

60. American Heart Association: Cardiac rehabilitation programs: a statement for healthcare professionals from the American Heart Association. *Circulation* 1994, 90:1602–1610.

Mitral Stenosis and Regurgitation 21

Sidney C. Smith, Jr.
Park W. Willis IV

Key Points

- Advanced diagnostic techniques such as color flow Doppler echocardiography, and new therapeutic approaches, such as balloon mitral valvuloplasty, left ventricular unloading therapy, and direct mitral valve repair offer improved care for patients with mitral valve disease.

- Rheumatic heart disease remains the major cause of mitral stenosis, and outbreaks of rheumatic fever have been recently reported in the United States.

- An echocardiographic scoring system identifies patients most likely to benefit from balloon mitral valvuloplasty.

- Physicians should make patients with mitral valve disease familiar with the new American Heart Association guidelines for and prevention of infective endocarditis.

- Resting ejection fraction remains preserved late in the course of mitral regurgitation, and exercise radionuclide ejection fractions may assist in selecting patients who are candidates for mitral valve surgery.

Over the past 20 years our understanding of the pathophysiology of mitral valve disease has increased substantially. Advanced echocardiographic methods have expanded our diagnostic capability. New therapeutic approaches such as balloon mitral valvuloplasty, left ventricular unloading therapy, and direct mitral valve repair have improved the treatment and prognosis for patients with mitral valve disease. This chapter details current trends in the diagnosis and therapy of mitral stenosis and regurgitation from the standpoint of the clinician.

MITRAL STENOSIS

Etiology and Pathophysiology

Most cases of mitral stenosis are caused by rheumatic heart disease (Table 1) [1•]. Less frequently, severe mitral annular calcification, malignant carcinoid, or rheumatoid arthritis may be the underlying cause. The clinical presentation and physical findings of left atrial myxoma can mimic rheumatic mitral stenosis. Congenital forms of mitral stenosis are rare and usually present in childhood, associated with other congenital lesions. Two thirds of patients with rheumatic mitral stenosis are female.

Because of the strong association of rheumatic heart disease with mitral stenosis, the practicing physician should be familiar with current diagnostic criteria for acute rheumatic fever. The American Heart Association has recently published updated Jones criteria for the diagnosis of acute rheumatic fever (Table 2) [2]. These changes emphasize the importance of establishing the initial attack of rheumatic fever and expand on the available tools to diagnose streptococcal pharyngitis with clarification of available antibody tests. Echocardiographic abnormalities without accompanying auscultatory findings are considered insufficient to be the sole criteria for valvulitis in acute rheumatic fever.

Patients with mitral valve stenosis often have no definite history of rheumatic fever in childhood or as a young adult and are usually asymptomatic until the third or fourth decade. Multiple episodes of rheumatic fever during childhood may result in an accelerated disease course causing the patient to present with mitral stenosis at an earlier age. This is especially common in patients living in underdeveloped areas and temperate zones where the disease often presents during adolescence. In general, approximately 10 years will elapse between an episode of acute rheumatic fever and the first appearance of the murmur of mitral stenosis.

The rheumatic process, presumably through an autoimmune mechanism, results in fibrosis and scarring, especially at the margins of the mitral valve leaflets. This results in fusion of the valve leaflets and shortening and thickening of the chordae tendineae. The result is progressive narrowing of the mitral valve orifice with increasing left atrial and pulmonary venous pressures. Left atrial enlargement and progressive calcification of the mitral valve follow as this process progresses. The normal valve area of 4 to 6 cm^2 is reduced to less than 2 cm^2. Severe hemodynamic changes occur at valve areas less than 1 cm^2.

Clinical Presentation

The most common presenting symptom of mitral stenosis is exertional dyspnea secondary to pulmonary venous hypertension. The majority of patients with mitral stenosis are women, symptoms often appear initially during the second trimester of pregnancy, when blood volume and cardiac output peak. Patients also may experience orthopnea, paroxysmal nocturnal dyspnea, and progressive fatigue and weakness. Pulmonary hypertension may be associated with chest pain and hemoptysis. Approximately 50% of patients with mitral stenosis are older than 30 years of age and may have significant coronary artery disease. Therefore, it is important to consider multiple causes for chest pain. Hoarseness (Ortner's syndrome) may occur because of compression of the left recurrent laryngeal nerve between the enlarged pulmonary artery, aorta, and ligamentum arteriosum. Unfortunately, systemic embolism may be the first symptom of mitral stenosis, especially in association with the development of atrial fibrillation. Although infective endocarditis is uncommon, it can complicate the clinical course of mitral stenosis [3].

The classic physical findings of mitral stenosis are a loud first heart sound (S$_1$) associated with a low-pitched diastolic rumble best heard at the apex, with the bell of the stethoscope, in the left lateral decubitus position. Positional variation in the

intensity of the diastolic rumble may indicate that left atrial myxoma is present. A high-pitched opening snap (OS) may be heard just after the second heart sound (S$_2$). The S$_2$-OS interval narrows as the severity of mitral stenosis increases. When pulmonary hypertension develops, the amplitude of the pulmonic component of S$_2$ increases and a right ventricular heave may be detected. Pulmonary rales, jugular venous distention, hepatic enlargement, and peripheral edema may be present, representing generalized findings for congestive heart failure. With severe pulmonary hypertension, pulmonary regurgitation may be present (Graham Steell murmur), which should be distinguished from aortic regurgitation. Atrial fibrillation is often present as mitral stenosis progresses in severity, and characteristic ruddy cheeks (mitral facies) may be noted.

Laboratory Findings

Echocardiography is the most valuable clinical test in the management of mitral stenosis. It is useful in gauging the severity of mitral stenosis, distinguishing left atrial myxomas, and identifying coexisting atrial septal defects, thrombi, and valvular vegetations (Fig. 1). In addition, associated valvular lesions such as mitral regurgitation, aortic stenosis or regurgitation, and pulmonary and tricuspid valvular disease, which are also associated with rheumatic heart disease, may be identified. Color flow Doppler echocardiography is useful in assessing the extent of associated mitral regurgitation. Transesophageal echocardiography may help to detect left atrial thrombi (Fig. 2).

Recently, a scoring system based on the results of echocardiography has been devised to assist in identifying patients who may best benefit from balloon mitral valvuloplasty. The scoring system grades from 0 to 4+ the following four echocardiographic factors: valvular rigidity, valvular calcification, valvular thickening, and the amount of subvalvular disease; a score of 4+ represents a severely abnormal finding. Thus, a valve with severe rigidity, extensive calcification, severe thickening, and substantial subvalvular thickening would receive a score of 4 for each category, for a total score

---

TABLE 1 MITRAL STENOSIS

Etiology
Rheumatic heart disease (most common)
Congenital
Mitral annular calcification
Malignant carcinoid
Rheumatoid arthritis
Exclude
Left atrial tumor (usually myxoma)
Cor triatriatum
Associated atrial septal defect

TABLE 2 GUIDELINES FOR DIAGNOSIS OF RHEUMATIC FEVER (JONES CRITERIA, UPDATED 1992)

Major manifestations
Carditis
Polyarthritis
Chorea
Erythema marginatum
Subcutaneous nodules

Minor manifestations
Arthralgia
Fever
Elevated erythrocyte sedimentation rate
Elevated C-reactive protein
Prolonged PR interval
Evidence of antecedent group A streptococcal infection
Positive throat culture or rapid streptococcal antigen test
Elevated or increasing streptococcal antibody titer

Note: When supported by evidence of antecedent group A streptococcal infection, two major or one major and two minor manifestations indicate a high probability of rheumatic fever.
From Dajani et al. [2]; with permission.

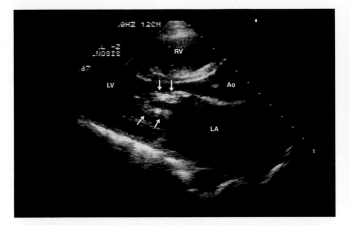

FIGURE 1 Mitral stenosis. Mid-diastolic frame from a transthoracic two-dimensional echocardiogram, in the parasternal long-axis plane, showing a thickened mitral valve with limited leaflet excursion and left atrial enlargement. Note that leaflet calcification and marked subvalvular thickening (*arrows*) would predict a suboptimal outcome after balloon dilatation. Ao—aorta; LA—left atrium; LV—left ventricle; RV—right ventricle.

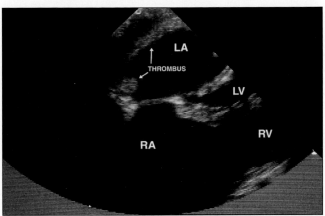

FIGURE 2 Mitral stenosis. Late diastolic frame from an intraoperative transesophageal echocardiogram, in the short-axis plane, showing left atrial mural thrombus. The finding of left atrial thrombus in a patient with mitral stenosis is a contraindication to balloon valvuloplasty. LA—left atrium; LV—left ventricle; RA—right atrium; RV—right ventricle.

of 16. Patients with mitral valve scores of 8 or less generally have the best results from balloon mitral valvuloplasty.

The electrocardiogram is useful in identifying left atrial enlargement with terminal negative P waves in V_1 and the presence of right ventricular hypertrophy pattern with increased R wave in V_1 and a rightward axis. Both of these findings reflect increasing severity of mitral stenosis. It is important to identify the presence of atrial fibrillation, because these patients will require anticoagulation therapy.

Chest x-ray may be useful in identifying left atrial enlargement with elevation of the left mainstem bronchus, pulmonary venous hypertension, and the presence of mitral calcification. In general, and especially during pregnancy, the echocardiogram provides more precise and clinically valuable information for the management of patients with mitral stenosis than other noninvasive tests.

Other adjuncts to the echocardiogram in the diagnosis and management of patients with mitral stenosis include exercise testing and cardiac catheterization. Exercise testing either in association with cardiac catheterization or separately is sometimes valuable in developing management strategies for those patients with mitral stenosis of borderline severity. Cardiac catheterization before surgical intervention for mitral stenosis is generally required to identify coronary artery disease in older patients and to assess the severity of mitral stenosis using hemodynamic parameters [4]. Many patients will be identified as candidates for balloon mitral valvuloplasty and undergo cardiac catheterization for this reason.

Management

Medical therapy for mitral stenosis includes 1) antibiotic prophylaxis for infective endocarditis and recurrent rheumatic fever; 2) management of pulmonary venous hypertension and right heart failure; 3) control of atrial fibrillation; and 4) anticoagulation for prevention of thromboembolism.

The recently published American Heart Association guidelines for antibiotic prophylaxis for infective endocarditis at the time of dental and surgical procedures should be carefully reviewed with the patient (Table 3) [5]. Wallet-sized summary

cards are available from the American Heart Association to assist the patient in this regard. The guidelines for duration of long-term antibiotic therapy using 1.2 million units benzathine penicillin G monthly as prophylaxis against recurrent rheumatic fever are not well established. Generally, continuation to age 40 or later is advisable if the patient is in an occupation such as teaching, where frequent exposure to younger children with streptococcal infection may occur.

Diuretic therapy is useful in managing the symptoms of pulmonary venous congestion and right heart failure; however,

TABLE 3 ANTIBIOTIC PROPHYLAXIS FOR PREVENTION OF ENDOCARDITIS
Regimens for dental, oral, or upper respiratory tract procedures
Amoxicillin 3 g PO 1 h before procedure, then 1.5 g PO 6 h after initial dose
*Erythromycin ethylsuccinate 800 mg or erythromycin stearate 1 g PO 2 h before procedure, then one half the dose 6 h after initial dose
*Clindamycin 300 mg PO 1 h before procedure and 150 mg 6 h after initial dose
Regimens for genitourinary and gastrointestinal procedures
Ampicillin 2 g IV (or IM) plus gentamicin 1.5 mg/kg IV (or IM) (not to exceed 80 mg) 30 minutes before procedure, followed by amoxicillin 1.5 g PO 6 h after the initial dose. Alternatively repeat parenteral regimen may be repeated once 8 hours after initial dose
*Vancomycin 1 g IV over 1 h plus gentamicin 1.5 mg/kg IV (or IM) (not to exceed 80 mg) 1 h before procedure. May be repeated once 8 hours after initial dose
†Amoxicillin 3 g PO 1 h before procedure; then 1.5 g PO 6 hours after initial dose
*For patients allergic to amoxicillin, ampicillin, and/or penicillin.   †Alternate oral regimen for low-risk patients.   *From* Dajani *et al.* [5]; with permission.

vigorous diuresis in the presence of significant mitral stenosis may markedly decrease cardiac output.

It is important to control the heart rate when atrial fibrillation occurs, because rapid ventricular response may increase pulmonary congestion due to shortened diastolic filling time. Thus, prompt therapy should be instituted with digoxin to control ventricular response when atrial fibrillation develops. Digoxin is not helpful in treating patients with mitral stenosis who remain in normal sinus rhythm without atrial fibrillation. β-blockers or calcium channel antagonists may be added to digoxin therapy when the ventricular rate remains poorly controlled. In patients who require prompt control of ventricular rate because of hemodynamic deterioration, intravenous diltiazem or esmolol will provide a more rapid reduction in the ventricular response than digoxin. Anticoagulation therapy should be initiated promptly when atrial fibrillation or a documented thromboembolic event has occurred. Once the ventricular rate is controlled and the patient has completed 3 weeks of anticoagulation therapy, elective pharmacologic or electrical cardioversion may be attempted.

When to Refer

Because the natural history of mitral stenosis is related to symptomatic status, the patient should be evaluated for mechanical intervention such as balloon valvuloplasty, open commissurotomy, or valve replacement as the symptoms progress beyond New York Heart Association (NYHA) Class II. In patients with NYHA Class II symptoms, valve area is usually less than 1.0 cm$_2$/m$_2$ body surface area. Balloon valvuloplasty provides an acceptable alternative to open commissurotomy, with the best results occurring in patients with pliable leaflets, minimal calcification, mild leaflet thickening, and mild subvalvular fibrosis as demonstrated on echocardiography [6,7]. In patients in whom such findings are absent, mitral valve replacement or open commissurotomy should be considered [8]. Because anticoagulation with coumadin is required after valve replacement, valvuloplasty or commissurotomy are the procedures of choice for women of child-bearing age. Findings of significant mitral regurgitation or a heavily calcified valve argue for mitral valve replacement. Bioprostheses in the mitral position can carry a significant risk for embolic events in

TABLE 4 MITRAL REGURGITATION: ETIOLOGY
Acute
Ruptured chordae tendineae
Papillary muscle rupture
Endocarditis
Trauma
Prosthetic valve dysfunction
Chronic
Rheumatic heart disease
Papillary muscle dysfunction
Severe left ventricular dilatation
Endocarditis
Mitral valve prolapse
Associated with hypertrophic obstructive cardiomyopathy
Congenital abnormalities
Marfan's syndrome
Prosthetic valve dysfunction

the absence of anticoagulation, particularly if atrial fibrillation of left atrial dilatation is present.

Because the volume of procedures performed and the operating physician's experience have a significant impact on the outcome for both surgical and cardiac interventional procedures, physicians and patients should base the final decision regarding the choice of mechanical procedure on the results at their local institution. Published mortality rates for mitral valve replacement or open commissurotomy are generally 1% to 4%, whereas the reported mortality for balloon mitral valvuloplasty has ranged from 0% to 4%. Approximately 35% of patients undergoing balloon mitral valvuloplasty will be left with a small residual atrial septal defect which, in the majority of cases, will decrease in size or close. Ten percent of patients undergoing balloon mitral valvuloplasty will develop restenosis after 1 to 2 years. At present, balloon mitral valvuloplasty appears to be the treatment of choice for carefully selected patients with mitral stenosis [9], yielding an 84% 4-year survival rate in the largest multiceuter registry [10].

MITRAL REGURGITATION
Etiology and Pathophysiology

Mitral regurgitation may result from a disorder of any of the components of the mitral valve, which include the annulus, anterior and posterior leaflets, chordae tendineae, and papillary muscles (Table 4). Mitral regurgitation may also be caused by mitral valve prolapse. Mitral regurgitation due to involvement of the leaflets is common secondary to rheumatic heart disease and occurs more often in men than in women. With acute rheumatic fever, severe mitral regurgitation is more likely to involve the anterior leaflet, whereas chordal rupture, either primary or myxomatous in etiology, and papillary muscle ischemia generally involve the posterior leaflet. Endocarditis and Marfan's syndrome are important causes of mitral regurgitation. Degenerative annular calcification, more common in women, may also result in mitral regurgitation. Annular dilatation secondary to cardiomyopathy is an increasingly frequent cause of mitral regurgitation and varying degrees of mitral regurgitation are found in up to 30% of patients undergoing coronary artery bypass surgery [11]. Finally, prosthetic mitral valve dysfunction is becoming a more frequent cause of clinically encountered mitral regurgitation.

Mitral regurgitation results in significant backflow during systole from the left ventricle into the left atrium. The result is chronic progressive enlargement of both chambers to accommodate the regurgitant volume, which may be four to five times the forward flow when severe. Because regurgitant flow occurs at relatively low impedance into the left atrium, the left ventricular ejection fraction may be preserved late into the course of mitral regurgitation. The ejection fraction in mitral regurgitation may not serve as an accurate index of left ventricular function, and thus, may lead to an erroneously favorable estimate of myocardial performance.

The sudden increase in left atrial volume and pressure associated with acute mitral regurgitation may result in severe pulmonary congestion, often in the presence of preserved left ventricular ejection fraction. Atrial fibrillation may cause significant hemodynamic compromise when it occurs in the course of either acute or chronic mitral regurgitation.

Clinical Presentation

Patients with chronic mitral regurgitation may enjoy a relatively asymptomatic course for 20 to 30 years, but finally present with symptoms of progressive weakness and fatigue. Orthopnea and systemic embolism are uncommon presenting symptoms in mitral regurgitation [1]. In contrast with mitral stenosis, the S_1 in mitral regurgitation is usually diminished. The S_2 may be widely split and an apical third heart sound (S_3) may be present. With left ventricular enlargement, the apical impulse becomes diffuse and is displaced laterally. The most prominent finding in mitral regurgitation is a holosystolic murmur beginning with S_1 and extending into the aortic component of S_2. The murmur radiates from the apex to the axilla, but may be heard at the left external edge and at the aortic area when there is marked posterior leaflet prolapse. With marked anterior leaflet prolapse, the murmur may be directed to the posterior wall of the left atrium and may be more prominent over the spine. There is little correlation between the intensity of the murmur and the severity of mitral regurgitation. The murmur may be increased in intensity by isometric exercise, which serves to distinguish it from that of aortic stenosis and hypertrophic obstructive cardiomyopathy. The location of the murmur distinguishes it from the murmur of a ventricular septal defect, which is loudest along the left sternal border and is often associated with parasternal thrill. With pulmonary hypertension, the pulmonic component of S_2 is increased and the systolic murmur of tricuspid regurgitation may be present along the left sternal border.

Laboratory Findings

As with mitral stenosis, color flow Doppler echocardiography has contributed greatly to the management of patients with mitral regurgitation (Fig. 3). It usually aids in establishing the diagnosis and helps to quantify the severity of mitral regurgitation, thereby assisting with patient management. With acute mitral regurgitation, left ventricular and left atrial chamber size may be normal. The left ventricular ejection fraction is usually preserved unless the regurgitation occurs in the setting of acute myocardial infarction, in which case regional wall motion abnormalities and impaired ejection fraction may occur. Echocardiography may be particularly valuable in confirming the presence of flail mitral leaflet or endocarditis. In chronic mitral regurgitation, both left ventricular and left atrial chamber sizes are increased. Assessment of left ventricular wall stress and systolic volume may be more valuable in predicting the patient's suitability for valve replacement than the ejection fraction. Left ventricular dimensions can be followed serially in association with the regurgitant mitral jet volume to assess the results of unloading therapy. Transesophageal echocardiography is especially valuable in assessing patients undergoing mitral valve surgery as possible candidates for direct reconstructive repair rather than mitral replacement.

No electrocardiographic abnormalities are diagnostic for mitral regurgitation. Progressive left ventricular hypertrophy and left atrial enlargement are observed as the mitral regurgitation worsens. Atrial fibrillation generally occurs late in the course of mitral regurgitation. In patients with suspected acute mitral regurgitation, the electrocardiogram results may be normal, except for sinus tachycardia and evidence of acute infarction or ischemia, if that is the underlying etiology.

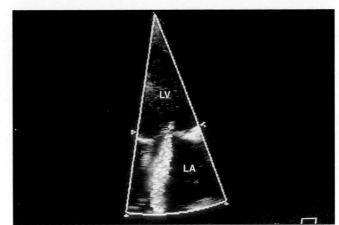

FIGURE 3 Mitral regurgitation. Late systolic frame from a transthoracic color flow Doppler study, in the apical four-chamber plane, showing turbulent flow in the left atrium caused by a high velocity jet of mitral regurgitation. LA—left atrium; LV—left ventricle. (*See* Color Plate.)

The chest radiograph generally demonstrates left ventricular and left atrial enlargement as chronic mitral regurgitation increases in severity. Pulmonary venous congestion may be seen as the clinical course worsens. In patients with acute mitral regurgitation, pulmonary venous hypertension may be the only finding, while left atrial and left ventricular size are normal.

Cardiac catheterization is useful in evaluating older patients with mitral regurgitation to rule out coronary artery disease, before proceeding with mitral valve surgery. In much younger patients with isolated mitral regurgitation, sufficient data may be obtained from echocardiography such that cardiac catheterization is usually unnecessary. In those with acute mitral regurgitation, marked elevation of pulmonary capillary wedge pressure may be noted with prominent regurgitant V waves. As previously mentioned, it is not unusual to find normal or above-normal ejection fractions in patients with acute regurgitation unless myocardial infarction with papillary muscle rupture is the cause, in which case regional wall-motion abnormalities usually are present. Angiographic assessment of mitral regurgitation is the most reliable system for grading mild and severe degrees of mitral regurgitation. However, angiography may not be accurate in assessing moderate regurgitation due to variation in techniques of angiographic injection or left-ventricular-loading conditions. This makes decisions regarding surgery more difficult when moderate regurgitation is noted and other factors previously mentioned should be carefully considered. The V wave amplitude may also be misleading as a guide to severity of mitral regurgitation and should not be used as a reference for surgical decisions.

In patients with moderate mitral regurgitation in whom resting left ventricular ejection fraction appears preserved, exercise radionuclide ejection fractions may help to assess possible candidacy for mitral valve surgery. The inability to elevate ejection fraction with exercise may signal left ventricular dysfunction and a need for surgical intervention.

Management

Patients with acute severe mitral regurgitation should be stabilized with diuretics and afterload reduction. Nitroprusside, which acts as an arteriolar and venous dilator, should be instituted promptly and titrated to optimize systemic vascular resistance, forward cardiac output, and pulmonary capillary wedge pressures. Digoxin and inotropic agents generally are not useful, because ventricular function is usually preserved with acute mitral regurgitation.

Patients with chronic mitral regurgitation who are asymptomatic should be given antibiotic prophylaxis for infective endocarditis as outlined in the discussion for patients with mitral stenosis [5]. The incidence of embolic events is lower than that for mitral stenosis, but anticoagulation should be initiated for those patients in atrial fibrillation and patients with previous embolic events. Patients with minimal or no symptoms should receive follow-up echocardiography on a yearly basis to assess left ventricular size and function unless the mitral regurgitation is mild and ventricular dimensions are normal, in which case follow-up at longer intervals is indicated. Follow-up echo studies may not be required in patients with mild mitral regurgitation. Patients who develop symptoms should be considered for therapy with vasodilators, especially the angiotensin-converting-enzyme (ACE) inhibitors and diuretics. Digoxin should be instituted for atrial fibrillation to control ventricular rate and in patients with progressive left ventricular dysfunction who are not candidates for mitral valve replacement. Symptomatic patients with left ventricular dysfunction and mitral regurgitation who are not candidates for mitral valve surgery should be considered for combined diuretic, ACE inhibitor, and digoxin therapy.

Intraaortic balloon counterpulsation is indicated when severe hemodynamic instability is present. Surgical therapy with mitral valve replacement or repair is pursued promptly when patients cannot be stabilized hemodynamically. In cases of endocarditis, if patients can be stabilized, antibiotic therapy is started before proceeding with mitral valve replacement for acute mitral regurgitation.

When to Refer

Surgery for mitral regurgitation has evolved over the past 10 years such that reconstructive repair is performed as frequently as mitral valve replacement. The advantages of repair include lower operative mortality; preservation of the annular-chordal-papillary muscle continuity, which maintains left ventricular function; elimination of thromboembolic risk, thus obviating the need for anticoagulation; and a lower risk of late failure than might be encountered with the bioprostheses. Transesophageal echocardiography is necessary preoperatively to assess candidates for reconstructive surgery, and intraoperative Doppler color flow mapping is extremely useful in assessing the adequacy of reconstruction.

Both bioprosthetic and mechanical valves have an embolic risk and require anticoagulation in the mitral position, although the risk of emboli with a bioprosthetic valve is lower when normal sinus rhythm is present. Bioprosthetic valves generally calcify and become dysfunctional after 7 to 10 years; thus, mechanical valve replacement is preferred if reconstructive surgery is not feasible. The operative mortality in active centers for isolated mitral valve replacement ranges from 2% to 7% in patients with NYHA Class II or III symptoms undergoing elective valve replacement and 1% to 4% for similar patients undergoing reconstructive surgery. Mortality is higher for

patients with NYHA Class IV symptoms as well as patients undergoing surgery for acute mitral regurgitation or those with concomitant coronary bypass surgery. Because of the improved outcome with earlier surgery, surgery is recommended for most patients with isolated severe mitral regurgitation who remain symptomatic NYHA Class II in association with medical therapy and have elevated end-systolic volumes of greater than 50 mL/m^2. End-systolic volume should be monitored carefully in asymptomatic patients with severe mitral regurgitation and ejection fractions between 55 and 70. Surgical intervention should be performed in these patients as left ventricular function deteriorates. Specifically, elective mitral valve surgery should be considered in this group of patients before ejection fraction is less than 0.50 and the end-systolic volume index greater than 50 mL/m^2.

REFERENCES AND RECOMMENDED READING

Recently published paper of particular interest have been highlighted as:

- Of interest
- •• Of outstanding interest

1.• Braunwald E: Valvular heart disease. In *Heart Disease*, edn 5. Philadelphia: WB Saunders; 1997:1007–1035.

2. Dajani AS, Ayoub E, Bierman FZ, et al.: Guidelines for the diagnosis of rheumatic fever: Jones Criteria, updated 1992. *Circulation* 1993, 87:302–307.

3. McHenry MM: Systemic arterial embolism in patients with mitral stenosis and minimal dyspnea. *Am J Cardiol* 1966, 18:169–174.

4. Reis R, Roberts W: Amounts of coronary arterial narrowing by atherosclerotic plaques in clinically isolated mitral valve stenosis: analysis of 76 necropsy patients older than 30 years. *Am J Cardiol* 1986, 57:1119.

5. Dajani AS, Bisno AL, Chung KJ, et al.: Prevention of bacterial endocarditis. *Circulation* 1991, 83:1174–1178.

6. Wilkins GY, Weyman AE, Abascal VM, et al.: Percutaneous balloon dilatation of the mitral valve: an analysis of echocardiographic variables related to outcome and the mechanism of dilatation. *Br Heart J* 1988, 60:299–308.

7. Abascal VM, Wilkins GT, O'Shea JP, et al.: Prediction of successful outcome in 130 patients undergoing percutaneous balloon mitral valvotomy. *Circulation* 1990, 82:448–456.

8. Cosgrove DM, Stewart WJ: Mitral valvuloplasty. *Curr Prob Cardiol* 1989, 14:359–415.

9. Kirklin JW: Percutaneous balloon versus surgical closed commissurotomy for mitral stenosis. *Circulation* 1991, 83:1450–1451.

10. Dean LS, Mickel M, Bonan R, et al.: Four year follow-up of patients undergoing percutaneous balloon mitral commissurotomy. *J Am Coll Cardiol* 1996, 28:1452–1457.

11. Olson LJ, Subramanian R, Ackerman DM: Surgical pathology of the mitral valve: a study of 712 cases spanning 21 years. *Mayo Clin Proc* 1987, 62:22.

SELECT BIBLIOGRAPHY

Crawford MD, Souchek J, Oprian CA, et al.: Determinants of survival and left ventricular performance after mitral valve replacement. *Circulation* 1990, 81:1173–1181.

Fenster MS, Feldman MD: Mitral regurgitation: an overview. *Curr Probl in Cardiol* 1995, 20:195–280.

Lee EM, Shapiro LM, Wells FC: Importance of subralvular preservation and early operation in mutral valve surgery. *Circulation* 1996, 94:2117–2123.

Reyes VP, Rasju BS, Wynne J, et al.: Percutaneous balloon valvuloplasty compared with open surgical commissurotomy for mitral stenosis. *N Engl J Med* 1994, 331:961–967.

Mitral Valve Prolapse 22
Richard B. Devereux

Key Points

- Mitral valve prolapse is usually a primary, dominantly inherited condition with more consistent gene expression in women than in men or children.
- Diagnosis is by midsystolic click/late systolic murmur; echocardiography confirms and documents severity.
- True mitral valve prolapse syndrome is characterized by low body weight and blood pressure, minor skeletal abnormalities, orthostatic hypotension, palpitations, and mitral regurgitation of variable degree.
- Complications are progressive mitral regurgitation, infective endocarditis, and possible risk of arrhythmic sudden death and orthostatic syncope.
- Risk factors for complications include older age, male gender, mitral regurgitant murmur, and possibly greater weight and higher blood pressure.
- Presence and severity of mitral regurgitation govern frequency and intensiveness of follow-up.

Mitral valve prolapse (MVP) is the most common abnormality of the heart in industrialized nations, affecting 3% to 4% of adults. By definition, MVP reflects abnormal systolic displacement of the mitral valve leaflets superiorly and posteriorly from the left ventricle into the left atrium. That may occur because the mitral leaflets, anulus, and chordae tendineae are enlarged in relation to left ventricular size (Fig. 1) or because they are abnormally distensible.

Although MVP has been reported to have many causes, most cases occur as a primary condition. Primary MVP is passed from affected mothers and fathers to children of both genders in a pattern indicative of autosomal dominant inheritance [1,2]. Familial MVP has an age of onset between 10 and 16 years, is more consistently expressed in women than men, and may become undetectable after middle age in mildly affected women [2]. As a result of the gender difference in the expression of primary MVP, nearly two thirds of adults with this condition are women. A small percentage of cases occur secondarily to other inheritable connective tissue diseases such as Marfan syndrome or Ehlers-Danlos syndrome. Mitral valve prolapse also may be produced by conditions, including anorexia nervosa or atrial septal defect, that make the left ventricle abnormally small.

DIAGNOSIS

In clinical practice, MVP is most commonly first recognized by auscultation. Typical auscultatory features are a midsystolic click and late systolic murmur, which is separated from the first heart sound by a silent interval but continues until the second heart sound. These sounds are best heard by listening over the left ventricular impulse and medial to it, with the patient in the supine, left decubitus, and sitting positions. Because systolic clicks may have other causes and mitral annular calcification may produce a late systolic murmur in older persons, it is important to perform physical maneuvers during auscultation that take advantage of the key role of valvular-ventricular disproportion in producing the manifestations of MVP [2].

As Figure 2 shows, maneuvers that reduce left ventricular chamber size will cause the click and onset of the murmur to move closer to the first heart sound, whereas the loudness of the click and murmur are affected by changes in blood pressure independent of changes in timing. Figure 3 shows how standard maneuvers during physical examination affect the click and murmur. It is especially important to time the

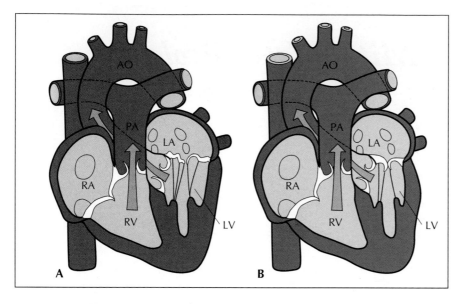

FIGURE 1 Diagram showing enlargement of mitral leaflets, annulus, and chordae **A**, in patients with mitral valve prolapse compared with **B**, findings in healthy persons. AO—aorta; LA—left atrium; LV—left ventricle; PA—pulmonary artery; RA—right atrium; RV—right ventricle.

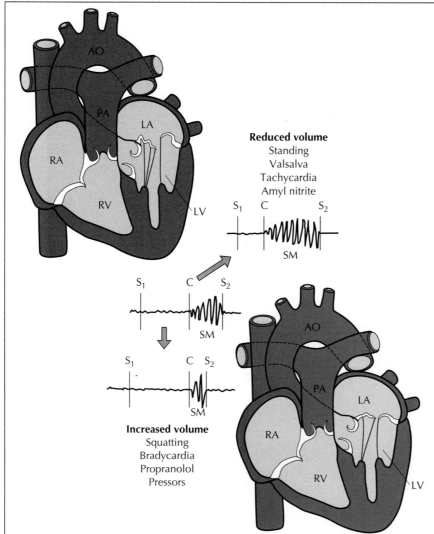

Reduced volume
Standing
Valsalva
Tachycardia
Amyl nitrite

Increased volume
Squatting
Bradycardia
Propranolol
Pressors

FIGURE 2 Effect of maneuvers that change left ventricular (LV) volume on the timing of the click (C) and murmur (SM) of mitral valve prolapse. The onset of the murmur and occurrence of the click move closer to the first heart sound (S_1) when LV volume is reduced and farther from it when LV volume is increased. AO—aorta; LA—left atrium; PA—pulmonary artery; RA—right atrium; RV—right ventricle; S_2—second heart sound. (*From* Devereux *et al.* [21]; with permission.)

Cardiology for the Primary Care Physician

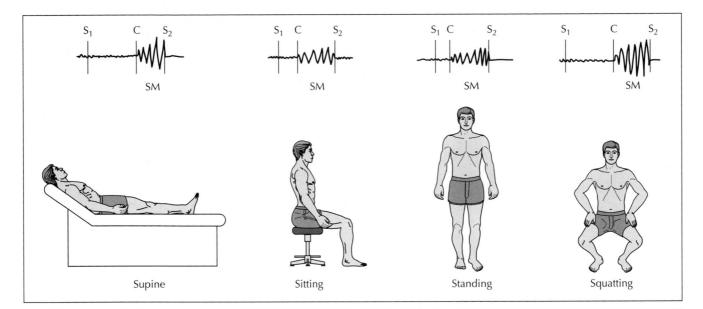

Supine   Sitting   Standing   Squatting

FIGURE 3 Effect of maneuvers during physical examination that change left ventricular chamber volume on the timing of the click (C) and murmur (SM) of mitral valve prolapse. (*From Devereux et al.* [21]; with permission.)

onset after the first sound and continuation until the second sound of the late systolic murmur, as miscategorization of midsystolic murmurs caused by normal blood flow in thin-chested persons or aortic sclerosis in older patients is a common cause of false-positive diagnoses of MVP (Fig. 4). When both a midsystolic click and late systolic murmur are present and respond appropriately to these maneuvers, the diagnosis of MVP can be made confidently by physical examination.

Late-systolic buckling of mitral leaflets on M-mode echocardiographic tracings occurs simultaneously with the midsystolic click and onset of the late systolic murmur (Fig. 5).

An accurate diagnosis can be made on M-mode recordings when continuous mitral leaflet interfaces "turn around" and

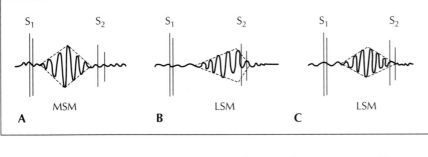

FIGURE 4 Timing of a midsystolic murmur (MSM, **A**), which begins after the first heart sound.(S$_1$) and ends before the second heart sound (S$_2$); and of late systolic murmurs (LSM, **B** and **C**), which begin after S$_1$ but continue to or through S$_2$. Note that both types of murmur may have a crescendo-decrescendo configuration.

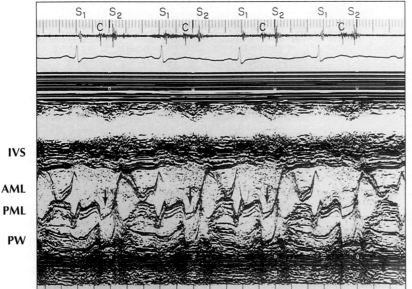

FIGURE 5 M-mode echocardiographic recording of the mitral valve demonstrating late systolic prolapse (*arrows*) and simultaneous phonocardiogram showing a midsystolic click (C) and late systolic murmur. AML—anterior mitral leaflet; IVS—interventricular septum; PML—posterior mitral leaflet; PW—posterior wall; S$_1$—first heart sound; S$_2$—second heart sound.

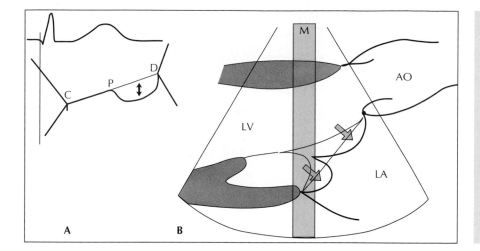

FIGURE 6 **A**, M-mode and **B**, two-dimensional echocardiographic diagnostic criteria of mitral valve prolapse. The condition is diagnosed when there is at least 2 mm of posterior displacement of continuous mitral leaflet interfaces behind the valve's C-D line in late systole on high-quality M-mode recordings (Figure 5) or protrusion of one or both mitral leaflets across the line connecting the hinging points of the mitral leaflets in two-dimensional long-axis views (Figure 7). AO—aorta; LA—left atrium; LV—left ventricle; M—course of M-mode beam. (*From* Devereux *et al.* [3]; with permission.)

move at least 2 mm posterior to the valve's C-D line in late systole (Fig. 6) [2,3]. Holosystolic posterior motion of mitral leaflets on M-mode recordings is no longer used to diagnose MVP because it may be produced artifactually by errors in ultrasound beam angulation.

Two-dimensional (2-D) and Doppler echocardiography is the mainstay of diagnosis of MVP and assessment of its severity. The condition can be accurately diagnosed by two-dimensional echocardiography when one or both mitral leaflets are seen to protrude or "billow" into the left atrium in systole in the parasternal or apical long-axis view (Figs. 6 and 7) [2,4]. It is important *not* to diagnose MVP based on apparent protrusion of the mitral leaflets into the left atrium that is seen only in the apical, four-chamber, two-dimensional view; this is a common normal consequence of the "saddle" shape of the mitral anulus (Fig. 8) [4]. Although conventional and color-flow Doppler echocardiography are not useful in diagnosing MVP, because there are many etiologies of the mitral regurgitation, they are of great value in grading the severity of

regurgitation, which is in turn the most important factor in determining the risk for major complications of MVP.

Two-dimensional echocardiography is especially useful for identifying mitral valve abnormalities associated with more severe forms of MVP. These include enlargement of the mitral leaflets and anulus [5] and prominent leaflet thickening [6], both of which are associated with severe mitral regurgitation. Billowing of one mitral leaflet segment that is so prominent it loses apposition with the appropriate segment of the other mitral leaflet is an anatomic cause of severe mitral regurgitation that can be readily visualized on two-dimensional echocardiography (Fig. 9) [7].

CLINICAL FEATURES

The typical auscultatory features of MVP are useful in making a diagnosis, but these features may vary considerably from one careful examination to another. Consequently, up to one fifth of patients with clinically recognized MVP confirmed by echocardiography and one third of unselected persons with this condition may have "silent" MVP on a single examination (Table 1) [8]. As a result, it is important to examine a patient several times to determine whether a murmur is intermittently present.

Extracardiac features of primary MVP have been shown in both family studies (Table 1) and clinical series. These include a tendency to have low body weight and low blood pressure [9], which may constitute the "selective advantage" that accounts for the high population prevalence of this inherited condition. Also, thoracic bony abnormalities (including pectus excavatum, mild scoliosis, and a straight thoracic spine) occur several times more commonly among adults with MVP than among members of the general population.

A variety of symptoms were associated with the condition often enough in initial clinical reports to suggest a distinct MVP syndrome that included chest pain, dyspnea, palpitations, anxiety, and panic attacks. Carefully controlled studies have found little or no evidence, however, that these symptoms—with the exception of palpitations—are truly linked to MVP (Table 2). The erroneous conclusion of previous studies appears to have resulted from selection bias, which causes more symptomatic patients to seek experts who perform clini-

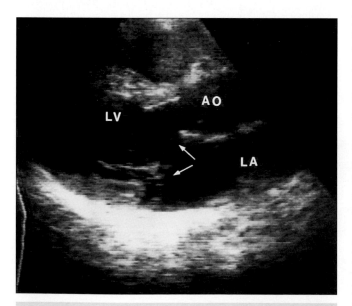

FIGURE 7 Two-dimensional echocardiogram in parasternal long-axis view showing late-systolic billowing of both mitral leaflets (*arrows*) into the left atrium (LA). AO—aorta; LV—left ventricle.

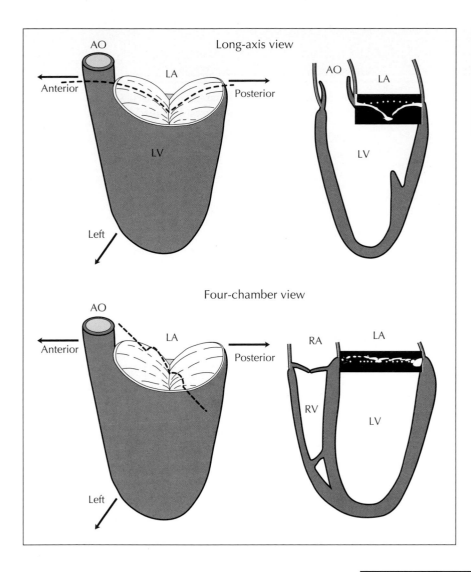

FIGURE 8 Artifactual mitral valve prolapse in the apical four-chamber view resulting from the saddle shape of the mitral anulus. AO—aorta; LA—left atrium; LV—left ventricle; RA—right atrium; RV—right ventricle. (*From* Levine *et al.* [4]; with permission.)

cal studies, and from a true tendency of women to report more of these symptoms than men regardless of whether they have MVP (Table 3).

Another set of symptoms that appears to be truly associated with MVP in controlled studies is syncope or presyncope caused by orthostatic hypotension [10]. The mechanism of this phenomenon is uncertain, but it may relate to the low resting blood pressure found in some patients with MVP.

COMPLICATIONS

In general, MVP is a benign condition, and most patients will never have an important complication. A minority of affected persons develop severe mitral regurgitation, infective endocarditis, neurologic ischemic episodes, or sudden death. Because of the high population prevalence of MVP, however, an appreciable number of adults have these complications (Table 4) [3]. In

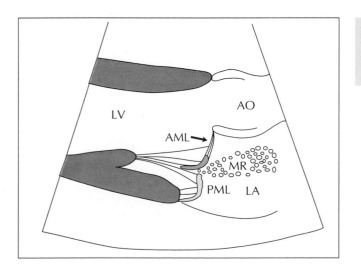

FIGURE 9 Severe posterior mitral leaflet (PML) prolapse into the left atrium (LA) producing loss of coaptation with the anterior mitral leaflet (AML) and allowing severe mitral regurgitation (MR). AO—aorta; LV—left ventricle.

TABLE 1 PREVALENCE OF AUSCULTATORY FEATURES AND EXTRACARDIAC MANIFESTATIONS OF MITRAL VALVE PROLAPSE IN INDEX CASES AND AFFECTED FAMILY MEMBERS

	First-degree relatives with MVP		First-degree relatives and spouses without MVP	
	n	(%)*	n	(%)§
Midsystolic click only	27	(33)†	7	(3)
Late systolic murmur only	14	(17)‡	8	(4)
Click and late systolic murmur	13	(16)†	1	(< 1)
Holosystolic murmur only	1	(1)†	0	(0)
Thoracic bony abnormalities	33	(41)†	34	(15)†
Body weight < 90% of ideal	26	(32)†	29	(13)†
Systolic blood pressure < 120 mm Hg	43	(53)†	65	(28)†

*n=81.
†P < 0.01;
‡P < 0.001.
§n=232.
MVP—mitral valve prolapse.

TABLE 2 PREVALENCE OF SYMPTOMS IN ADULT FAMILY MEMBERS WITH AND WITHOUT MITRAL VALVE PROLAPSE

	First-degree adult relatives with MVP		First-degree adult relatives and spouses without MVP	
	n	(%)*	n	(%)†
Palpitations	32	(40)‡	53	(23)
Atypical chest pain	14	(17)	37	(16)
Dyspnea	5	(6)	21	(9)
Panic attacks	6	(7)	11	(5)
Trait anxiety score > 50	5	(6)	14	(6)
Inferior lead electrocardiogram repolarization abnormalities	9	(11)	23	(10)

*n=81.
†n=232.
‡P < 0.01

TABLE 3 RELATIONSHIP OF GENDER TO CLINICAL FEATURES OF MITRAL VALVE PROLAPSE

	Women		Men		
	n	(%)*	n	(%)	P
Nonanginal chest pain	63	(29)	24	(13)	< 0.001
Dyspnea	50	(23)	15	(8)	< 0.001
Panic attacks	29	(13)	4	(2)	< 0.001
High trait anxiety	23	(11)	6	(3)	< 0.01
Inferior lead ST-T abnormalities	44	(20)	12	(6)	< 0.001

*n=216.
‡=185.

TABLE 4 ANNUAL OCCURRENCE IN THE UNITED STATES OF COMPLICATIONS ASSOCIATED WITH MITRAL VALVE PROLAPSE			
Complication	Patients per year, *n*	Patients with mitral valve prolapse, *n*	Annual events attributable to mitral valve prolapse, *n*
Mitral valve surgery	16,000	25	4000
Infective endocarditis	9000	13	1150
Sudden death*	400,000	1	4000

*Figures for sudden death are less stable than for other complications, because they are based on a single study.

our long-term experience, the rate of complications in relatively unselected patients with MVP is 1% per year or even less [11].

Severe mitral regurgitation is the most common major complication of MVP; conversely, MVP is now the most common valvular cause of severe mitral regurgitation in industrialized nations. Severe mitral regurgitation in a patient with MVP can be suspected on physical examination by a holosystolic or nearly holosystolic mitral regurgitant murmur associated with an audible third heart sound and leftward displacement of an enlarged, dynamic, left ventricular impulse (Fig. 10). Objective confirmation of this complication can be obtained by demonstrating a large mitral regurgitant jet by pulsed or color-flow Doppler echocardiography (Fig. 11). Imaging echocardiography usually reveals left ventricular and left atrial enlargement, and it also demonstrates a spectrum of morphologic valvular abnormalities, including leaflet and annular enlargement, distortion and thickening of leaflet segments, and redundancy or rupture of chordae tendineae.

The likelihood of developing severe mitral regurgitation increases with age and is greater for men than for women [11–13]. By the age of 75 years, approximately 1.5% to 2.0% of women with MVP and 5.5% of affected men will develop regurgitation of sufficient severity to require surgical valve

repair or replacement. Initially, mild regurgitation may become severe during prolonged follow-up of these patients [14]. In addition to the irreversible risk factors of age and gender, some evidence exists that high blood pressure or increased body weight may promote the progression of regurgitation.

Infective endocarditis occurs in approximately 25% as many patients with MVP as develop severe regurgitation (Table 4), implying a cumulative risk of less than 1% by age 75. The risk of endocarditis is increased about threefold in men compared with women, in persons older than 45 years of age compared with younger persons, and in patients with a mitral regurgitant murmur (Table 5) [15]. Whether mitral leaflet thickening or other specific morphologic abnormalities increase the risk of endocarditis independent of their role in causing mitral regurgitation has not yet been established. About one third of endocarditis cases are of dental origin, which is similar to the experience with other predisposing valvular lesions.

Neurologic ischemic events have been suggested to occur more commonly in individuals with MVP, but this association has recently been questioned [16].

Sudden death is the most feared, least understood, and perhaps the rarest major complication of MVP. An

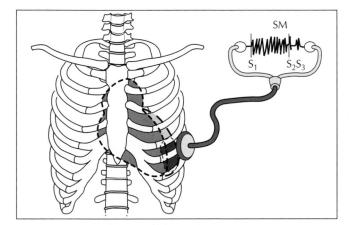

FIGURE 10 Schematic diagram of a nearly holosystolic mitral regurgitant murmur with a third heart sound and leftward displacement of an enlarged left ventricular impulse, which is felt to the left of the midclavicular line in the fifth and sixth intercostal spaces, instead of being smaller than a quarter in diameter and being limited to one interspace in normal persons. S_1—first heart sound; S_2—second heart sound; SM—systolic murmur.

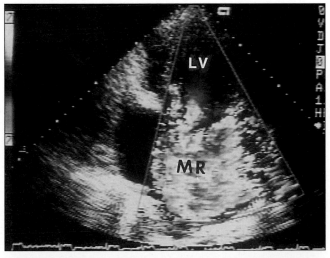

FIGURE 11 Severe mitral regurgitation (MR) demonstrated by color flow Doppler echocardiography. The multicolored MR jet fills almost the entire left atrium, which is nearly 10 cm in diameter. (*See* Color Plate.)

TABLE 5 RELATIVE RISK OF INFECTIVE ENDOCARDITIS IN PERSONS WITH MITRAL VALVE PROLAPSE BY GENDER, AGE, AND HISTORY OF MURMUR

	Total, n	Male	> 45 y, n	History of murmur, n
Cases	21	13	13	15*
Controls	102	36	31	41

	Male vs. female	≥ 45 y vs. < 45 y	Present vs. absent
Odds ratio	2.98	3.72	3.72
P	0.023	0.006	0.009
95% CI	1.35, 7.86	1.40, 9.88	1.33, 10.38

Adapted from MacMahon *et al.* [15]; with permission.
*History of a murmur before development of endocarditis.
CI—confidence interval.

TABLE 6 MATCHING RISK AND MANAGEMENT IN MITRAL VALVE PROLAPSE

Low risk

Subjects without mitral regurgitant murmurs or Doppler regurgitation, especially women younger than 45 years.

Management: reassurance; no clear need for antibiotics; reevaluation and echocardiography at moderate intervals (5 years).

Moderate risk

Subjects with intermittent or persistent mitral murmurs and mild Doppler regurgitation.

Management: antibiotic prophylaxis with amoxicillin or erythromycin; treat even mild established hypertension; reevaluation and echocardiography more frequently (2 to 3 years).

High risk

Subjects with moderate or severe mitral regurgitation.

Management: antibiotic prophylaxis with amoxicillin (unless allergic); optimize afterload (arterial pressure); reevaluate with Doppler echocardiography and other tests if needed annually.

Consider valve repair or replacement for exertional dyspnea or decline of left ventricular function into low-normal range.

increased risk of sudden death is well established in patients with severe mitral regurgitation, but this appears to relate to the degree of regurgitation rather than MVP [17]. Instances of sudden death in patients without known severe mitral regurgitation are often associated with severe valvular deformity but also increased heart weight, suggesting that unrecognized regurgitation or some other hemodynamic overload may have been present [18,19]. To date, neither specific arrhythmias nor other electrocardiographic features such as repolarization abnormalities have been documented to identify the patient with MVP who is at increased risk of sudden death.

MANAGEMENT

The proper starting point of management for most patients with MVP is reassurance by the patient's primary physician that they have a condition that is generally benign and may even be marginally beneficial if they have inherited the common tendency to low body weight and low blood pressure. For a person with only a midsystolic click and no mitral regurgitant murmur on several examinations, and no evidence of mitral regurgitation by Doppler echocardiography if it is performed, no clear evidence exists that peridental endocarditis prophylaxis or other specific medication is needed. It is reasonable to reevaluate such patients at 5-year intervals.

The presence and severity of mitral regurgitation are the best indicators of the need for active treatment and more frequent follow-up (Table 6) [3]. This may be assessed directly by Doppler echocardiography or indirectly by auscultation. Persons with intermittent or persistent mitral murmurs and mild regurgitation need oral antibiotic prophylaxis [20], treatment of mild hypertension, and reevaluation and echocardiography every 2 to 3 years. A person with severe regurgitation requires antibiotic prophylaxis with amoxicillin in the absence of penicillin allergy and annual reevaluation by a cardiologist or experienced internist with Doppler echocardiography and

perhaps other tests (24-hour electrocardiography or exercise test) depending on the clinical circumstances. It is also logical, although not yet proven to be beneficial, to avoid overweight and lower even borderline elevated arterial pressure by antihypertensive drugs in patients with MVP and moderate or severe mitral regurgitation.

Patients with other manifestations of MVP may need other forms of specific management. When distressing palpitation is from frequent, single premature ventricular contractions or self-terminating paroxysms of supraventricular tachycardia at rates that do not cause hemodynamic embarrassment, treatment with a long-acting β-adrenoreceptor blocker or digoxin may give symptomatic relief. Sustained, re-entrant, supraventricular tachycardias now often can be caused by radiofrequency ablation of accessory pathways in the electrophysiology laboratory. Rate-control with β-blockers, digoxin, or both, and anticoagulation with sodium warfarin to prevent stroke is needed if sustained atrial fibrillation develops, usually with hemodynamically important mitral regurgitation or after mitral valve surgery. Patients with MVP and orthostatic hypotension may benefit from stopping low-salt diets, adding sodium chloride in tablet form, or if the above are not successful, taking fluorine 0.05 to 0.10 mg/d to induce expansion of the blood volume.

ACKNOWLEDGMENT

The author thanks Virginia Burns for her assistance in preparing this manuscript.

REFERENCES

1. Devereux RB, Brown WT, Kramer-Fox R, *et al.*: Inheritance of mitral valve prolapse: effect of age and sex on gene expression. *Ann Intern Med* 1982, 97:826–832.

2. Devereux RB, Kramer-Fox R, Shear MK, *et al.*: Diagnosis and classification of severity of mitral valve prolapse: methodologic, biologic and prognostic considerations. *Am Heart J* 1987, 113:1265–1280.

3. Devereux RB, Kramer-Fox R, Kligfield P: Mitral valve prolapse: etiology, clinical manifestations and management. *Ann Intern Med* 1989, 111:305–317.

4. Levine RA, Triulzi MO, Harrigan P, *et al.*: The relationship of mitral annular shape to the diagnosis of mitral valve prolapse. *Circulation* 1987, 75:756–767.

5. Pini R, Devereux RB, Greppi B, *et al.*: Comparison of mitral valve dimension and motion in mitral valve prolapse with severe mitral regurgitation to uncomplicated mitral valve prolapse and to mitral regurgitation without mitral valve prolapse. *Am J Cardiol* 1988, 62:257–263.

6. Levine RA, Stathogiannis E, Newell JB, *et al.*: Reconsideration of echocardiographic standards for mitral valve prolapse: lack of association between leaflet displacement isolated to the apical four chamber view and independent echocardiographic evidence of abnormality. *J Am Coll Cardiol* 1988, 11:1010–1019.

7. Grayburn PA, Berk MR, Spain MG, *et al.*: Relation of echocardiographic morphology of the mitral apparatus to mitral regurgitation in mitral valve prolapse: assessment by Doppler color flow imaging. *Am Heart J* 1990, 119:1095–1102.

8. Devereux RB, Kramer-Fox R, Brown WT, *et al.*: Relation between clinical features of the "mitral prolapse syndrome" and echocardiographically documented mitral valve prolapse. *J Am Coll Cardiol* 1986, 8:763–772.

9. Devereux RB, Brown WT, Lutas EM, *et al.*: Association of mitral valve prolapse with low body-weight and low blood pressure. *Lancet* 1982, ii:792–795.

10. Weissman NJ, Shear MK, Kramer-Fox R, Devereux RB: Contrasting patterns of autonomic dysfunction in patients with mitral valve prolapse and panic attacks. *Am J Med* 1987, 82:880–888.

11. Zuppiroli A, Rinaldi M, Kramer-Fox R, *et al.*: Natural history of mitral valve prolapse. *Am J Cardiol* 1995,75:1028-1032.

12. Devereux RB, Hawkins I, Kramer-Fox R, *et al.*: Complications of mitral valve prolapse: disproportionate occurrence in men and older patients. *Am J Med* 1986, 81:751–758.

13. Wilcken DE, Hickey AJ: Lifetime risk for patients with mitral prolapse of developing severe valve regurgitation requiring surgery. *Circulation* 1988, 78:10–14.

14. Kolibash AJ Jr, Kilman JW, Bush CA, *et al.*: Evidence for progression from mild to severe mitral regurgitation in mitral valve prolapse. *Am J Cardiol* 1986, 58:762–767.

15. MacMahon SW, Roberts JK, Kramer-Fox R, *et al.*: Mitral valve prolapse and infective endocarditis. *Am Heart J* 1987, 113:1291–1298.

16. Orencia AJ, Petty GW, Khanderia BK, *et al.*: Risk of stroke in a population-based cohort study. *Stroke* 1995, 26:7-13.

17. Kligfield P, Hochreiter C, Niles N, *et al.*: Relation of sudden death in pure mitral regurgitation with and without mitral valve prolapse, to repetitive ventricular arrhythmias and right and left ventricular ejection fraction. *Am J Cardiol* 1987, 60:397–399.

18. Farb A, Tang AL, Atkinson JB, *et al.*: Comparison of cardiac findings in patients with mitral valve prolapse who die suddenly to those who have congestive heart failure from mitral regurgitation and to those with fatal noncardiac conditions. *Am J Cardiol* 1992, 70:234–239.

19. Morales AR, Remanelli R, Boncek RJ, *et al.*: Myxoid heart disease: an assessment of extraordinary cardiac pathology in severe mitral valve prolapse. *Hum Pathol* 1992, 23:129–137.

20. Devereux RB, Frary CJ, Kramer-Fox R, *et al.*: Cost-effectiveness of infective endocarditis prophylaxis for mitral valve prolapse with our without a regurgitant murmur. *Am J Cardiol* 1994, 74:1024–1029.

21. Devereux RB, Perloff JK, Reichek N, *et al.*: Mitral valve prolapse. *Circulation* 1976, 54:3–14.

SELECT BIBLIOGRAPHY

Barlow JE, Pocock WA, Marchand P, *et al.*: The significance of late systolic murmurs. *Am Heart J* 1963, 66:443–452.

Leatham A, Brigden W: Mild mitral regurgitation and the mitral prolapse fiasco. *Am Heart J* 1980, 99:659–664.

Nishimura RA, McGoon MD, Shub C, *et al.*: Echocardiographically documented mitral-valve prolapse: long-term follow-up of 237 patients. *N Engl J Med* 1985, 313:1305–1309.

Wooley CF, Boudoulas H, eds.: *Mitral Valve Prolapse and the Mitral Valve Prolapse Syndrome.* Mt. Kisco, NY: Futura; 1988.

Aortic Stenosis and Regurgitation 23
Michael A. Fifer

> ### *Key Points*
> - Aortic stenosis and, less often, aortic regurgitation may cause angina in the absence of coronary artery disease.
> - Sudden death is rare among truly asymptomatic patients with aortic stenosis or regurgitation.
> - The "classic" physical examination findings of aortic regurgitation may be absent when regurgitation develops acutely.
> - Doppler echo examination for aortic regurgitation is so sensitive that many false-positive findings occur.
> - Aortic valve replacement for aortic stenosis is generally reserved for symptomatic patients, whereas surgery for aortic regurgitation may be indicated for low or decreasing left ventricular ejection fraction, even for patients without symptoms.

The clinical manifestations of aortic valve disease are heart failure, angina, syncope, and death. Aortic stenosis is particularly prevalent in the elderly population [1]. It has been increasingly appreciated that aortic regurgitation may result from diseases of the aorta rather than of the aortic valve per se [2]. Clinical recognition of aortic valve disease is critical because properly timed valve replacement may dramatically improve symptoms and prolong life.

AORTIC STENOSIS

Etiology and Pathophysiology

There are three causes of valvular aortic stenosis in adults [3]; these causes are illustrated, along with a normal valve, in Figure 1. The prevalence of congenitally bicuspid aortic valves is approximately 1%, with a male preponderance. Stenosis resulting from fibrosis, calcification, and stiffening of a bicuspid valve is the usual cause of isolated aortic stenosis in patients younger than 60 years of age. Less commonly, bicuspid aortic valves cause aortic regurgitation. A substantial fraction of bicuspid valves cause no hemodynamic abnormality throughout life [4]. Rheumatic aortic stenosis is characterized by thickening of the valve cusps, fusion of the commissures, and calcification. Usually, the central orifice is relatively fixed, so that some degree of regurgitation is present as well. The majority of patients with rheumatic aortic valve disease also have clinically evident mitral valve disease. Senile calcific aortic stenosis is the most common type occurring in patients older than 70 years of age, and results from progressive scarring, calcification, and stiffening of the valve without fusion of the commissures. The consequences of aortic stenosis for systole are a gradient across the aortic valve, high intraventricular pressure, a compensatory increase in ventricular wall thickness and, for a minority of patients, a decrease in ejection fraction (systolic dysfunction). The consequences of aortic stenosis for diastole are diminished distensibility of the ventricle (diastolic dysfunction) caused by the increase in wall thickness,

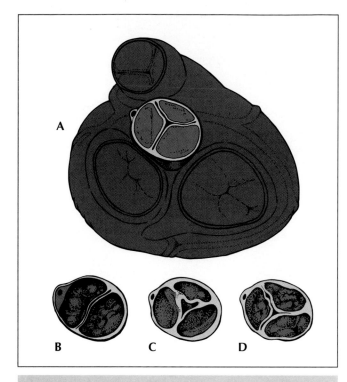

FIGURE 1 Schematic drawings showing **A**, a normal aortic valve; **B**, a calcified bicuspid valve with calcific deposits on the cusps; **C**, a rheumatic valve with commissural fusion; and **D**, a calcific tricuspid "senile" valve with calcific deposits on the cusps without commissural fusion. (*Adapted from* Sutton and Fox [27]; with permission.)

capacity to augment flow at times of stress is correspondingly diminished, which may lead to angina, subendocardial infarction (even with no coronary artery disease), and fibrosis. Angina is induced by exertion or emotion, and may be relieved by nitroglycerin whether or not coronary artery disease is present; rest angina generally indicates concomitant coronary artery disease. Lightheadedness and syncope typically occur during or immediately after exertion and may result from an exercise-induced decrease in systemic vascular resistance without a proportionate increase in cardiac output or from bradyarrhythmias caused by extension of aortic valve calcification into the conduction system. Clinically apparent embolization from the aortic valve and endocarditis are both rare [5]. There is an association between aortic stenosis and gastrointestinal bleeding originating from angiodysplasia, usually of the ascending colon [6].

Hypertension may coexist with severe aortic stenosis. The pulse pressure is usually normal but may be wide, especially in older patients [7,8]. The carotid upstroke is usually weak and delayed but may be normal or nearly so in patients with hypertension and in elderly patients with atherosclerotic, noncompliant arteries. In low-output states, the carotid volume is diminished, so that it is difficult to judge the rate of increase of the upstroke. A thrill is often felt over the carotid arteries, in the suprasternal notch, or in the second right intercostal space.

The left ventricular impulse is forceful and sustained; it is displaced leftward and downward when the ejection fraction is low. The second heart sound (S_2) is single or narrowly or paradoxically split; normal splitting suggests that severe aortic stenosis is not present. A fourth heart sound (S_4) is common and reflects left ventricular diastolic dysfunction. A third heart sound (S_3) is less common and indicates systolic dysfunction [9]. An ejection click is caused by checking of the upward movement of a domed aortic valve and is best heard after the first heard sound (S_1) at the lower left sternal border or apex in the young patient with a mobile valve. It is rare in adults older than 30 years of age, who have calcified, immobile valves. The crescendo-decrescendo (diamond-shaped) systolic murmur of

enhanced importance of the atrial kick for ventricular filling, and the potential for sudden decompensation if the atrial kick is lost, as with atrial fibrillation.

Evaluation

Symptoms of left-side heart failure resulting from aortic stenosis may be caused by systolic or diastolic dysfunction, or both. Whereas resting myocardial blood flow is increased, the

	Aortic stenosis	Hypertrophic cardiomyopathy	Mitral regurgitation
Carotid upstroke	Delayed	Brisk or bisferiens, or both	Brisk
S_2	Single	Split	Split
Ejection click	Sometimes present	Absent	Absent
Murmur location	Right upper sternal border, left sternal border, apex, carotids	Left lower sternal border, apex	Apex, axilla, left sternal border
Murmur during Valsalva maneuver	Softer	Louder	Louder
Murmur of aortic regurgitation	Common	Rare	Unusual
Aortic valve calcification on chest roentgenography	Usual	Absent	Absent
Dilation of ascending aorta on chest roentgenography	Usual	Absent	Absent

TABLE 1 DIFFERENTIAL DIAGNOSIS OF AORTIC STENOSIS

Cardiology for the Primary Care Physician

aortic stenosis is typically described as harsh, rough, or grunting. It is usually best heard in the second right intercostal space and may radiate widely to the neck, left sternal border, and apex. In elderly patients, it is often heard best at the apex, so that mitral regurgitation is erroneously suspected. The intensity of the murmur does not correlate with the severity of stenosis; it may be soft with severe stenosis and low cardiac output. A prolonged crescendo phase with a late peak suggests significant stenosis. The murmur of aortic stenosis must be distinguished from that of other cardiac lesions (Table 1). A diastolic murmur of aortic insufficiency is useful in establishing valvular aortic stenosis as opposed to hypertrophic cardiomyopathy as the cause of a systolic murmur.

The cardinal finding on the electrocardiogram (Fig. 2) is left ventricular hypertrophy, often with a "strain" pattern: ST-segment depression and T-wave inversion, usually in leads I, aV_L, and V_{4-6}. The absence of hypertrophy by electrocardiographic criteria, however, does not exclude hemodynamically significant stenosis. Other, more variable findings are left atrial abnormality, left axis deviation, and left bundle branch block. The chest roentgenogram may show calcification in the region of the aortic valve, although the technique is insensitive; on the other hand, no calcification of the valve seen by fluoroscopy in a patient older than 40 years of age virtually excludes severe aortic stenosis [7]. Poststenotic dilation of the ascending aorta is often seen. A "left ventricular configuration" (ie, rounding of the left ventricular border and apex), indicates left ventricular hypertrophy, whereas left ventricular enlargement suggests systolic dysfunction.

There is considerable variation among physicians in the use of exercise testing to evaluate aortic stenosis. Because of the possibility of inducing angina, severe dyspnea, hypotension, or syncope, some have considered severe aortic stenosis to be a contraindication to exercise testing. Others have suggested that exercise testing is useful to establish safe levels of physical activity in asymptomatic patients with aortic stenosis. Exercise may produce ST-segment and T-wave abnormalities and even thallium defects in the absence of coronary artery disease.

Echocardiography (Fig. 3) is the mainstay of the noninvasive evaluation of aortic stenosis. The valve is seen to be thickened and calcified, and leaflet excursion is reduced. In younger patients, the valve leaflets may be mobile, but tethering of their tips results in "doming" of the valve. In some patients, the valve is bicuspid, although this finding is often obscured by thickening and calcification. The echocardiogram is more sensitive than the electrocardiogram for detecting left ventricular hypertrophy. Left ventricular ejection fraction may be calculated from a technically adequate echocardiogram. The echocardiogram is also useful for distinguishing between valvular aortic stenosis and other causes of outflow gradients, such as hypertrophic cardiomyopathy.

The noninvasive assessment of the severity of aortic stenosis has been revolutionized by Doppler echocardiography. The peak and mean aortic valve gradients are calculated from the simplified Bernoulli equation as $4v^2$, for which v is the velocity of blood flow across the valve in m/sec. The gradient may be underestimated if the Doppler beam is not aligned correctly to measure the maximum blood flow velocity. It should be

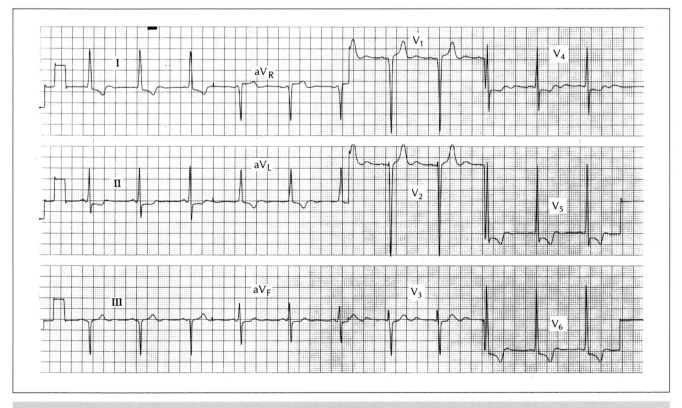

FIGURE 2 Electrocardiogram of a 77-year-old woman with senile calcific aortic stenosis reveals left ventricular hypertrophy, with a "strain" pattern (ST-segment depression and T-wave inversion) in leads I, aV_L, and V_{4-6}.

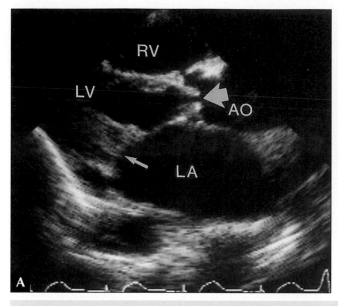

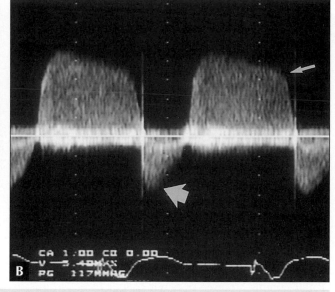

FIGURE 3 A, Two-dimensional echocardiogram and **B**, Doppler velocity tracing in a 70-year-old woman with rheumatic heart disease. The two-dimensional long-axis view in **A** shows the right ventricle (RV), left atrium (LA), left ventricle (LV), and aorta (AO). Two of the aortic valve leaflets (*thick arrow*) are thickened and have restricted openings. The mitral valve (*thin arrow*) is thickened and stenotic. The Doppler tracing in **B**, recorded from the left ventricular outflow tract, shows a peak velocity of 2.9 m/s and mean velocity of 2.1 m/s (*thick arrow*), corresponding to peak and mean gradients of 33 and 18 mm Hg, respectively. The Doppler signal in the opposite direction (*thin arrow*) demonstrates aortic regurgitation. (*Courtesy of* Michael H. Picard, MD.)

recognized that the peak gradient measured by Doppler differs from (and is greater than) the peak-to-peak gradient measured during cardiac catheterization; the mean gradient may be measured by either technique and is the most useful. Doppler echocardiography may also be used to estimate aortic valve area. A technically optimal echocardiogram in a young patient who does not have risk factors for coronary artery disease may preclude the need for cardiac catheterization before aortic valve replacement.

Management

Although patients with aortic stenosis may be asymptomatic for many years, the prognosis for symptomatic patients with significant stenosis is poor, with death usually occurring within 5 years of symptom onset [10–12]. Symptoms of heart failure are the most ominous, followed by syncope and then angina (Fig. 4). Although sudden death may occur, it is almost always preceded by other symptoms in adults with aortic stenosis; the risk of sudden death in truly asymptomatic patients is low [10,13].

Patients with aortic stenosis should be questioned closely at 3- to 6-month intervals for the occurrence of angina, light-headedness, syncope, or symptoms of heart failure and instructed to contact the physician if symptoms appear between visits. Although careful physical examination usually distinguishes aortic stenosis from other conditions and indicates its severity, the work-up usually includes echocardiography for confirmation. Once the presence of severe aortic

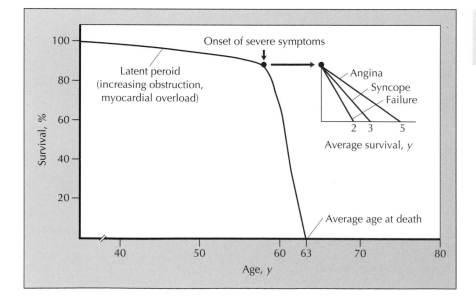

FIGURE 4 The natural history of aortic stenosis. (*From* Ross and Braunwald [28]; with permission.)

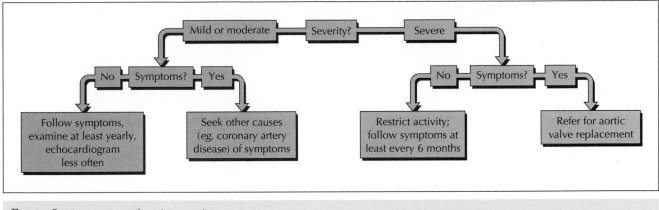

FIGURE 5 Management of aortic stenosis.

stenosis is established, repeat echocardiography is generally not necessary because the indication for surgery is usually the appearance of symptoms (see the following paragraphs). The management of aortic stenosis is diagrammed in Figure 5.

Endocarditis prophylaxis should be administered according to the guidelines of the American Heart Association; this recommendation also applies to patients with bicuspid aortic valves without significant stenosis or regurgitation. Asymptomatic patients with hemodynamically significant stenosis should be prohibited from occupations and sports that require heavy exertion. Most patients with asymptomatic aortic stenosis tolerate noncardiac surgery without complications [14]. Digoxin should be used for rapid supraventricular tachyarrhythmias. If nitrates are needed for concomitant coronary artery disease, they must be used cautiously for fear of inducing hypotension. Drugs with negative inotropic effects, such as β-blockers and calcium channel blockers, should be avoided. Treatment with digoxin and the careful use of diuretics may be indicated to stabilize a patient with heart failure before valve replacement. Vasodilators are relatively contraindicated. Cardiogenic shock caused by aortic stenosis should be managed with dobutamine for inotropic support, intraaortic balloon counterpulsation if necessary, and urgent mechanical relief of aortic stenosis.

When to Refer

The patient should be referred to a cardiologist for consideration of cardiac catheterization if cardiac symptoms are present and there is clinical or echocardiographic evidence of at least moderately severe aortic stenosis. In patients with cardiac symptoms and only mild aortic stenosis, cardiology consultation may be helpful for diagnosing concomitant cardiac conditions, such as coronary artery disease or excessive left ventricular hypertrophy. Cardiology referral should also be considered, even in the absence of symptoms, if aortic stenosis is severe, so that the cardiologist may participate in the decision regarding the timing of surgery.

At cardiac catheterization, the peak-to-peak and mean aortic valve gradients are usually estimated from a catheter advanced in retrograde fashion across the stenotic valve and another in a peripheral (*eg*, femoral) artery. Valve area is calculated from the mean gradient and cardiac output by means of the Gorlin equation. The normal aortic valve area is 3 to 4

cm^2; symptoms do not occur until the valve area decreases to less than 1.0 cm^2. Surgery for aortic stenosis is generally indicated for symptomatic patients with a mean gradient of 40 mm Hg or greater and an aortic valve area of 0.8 cm^2 or less. Patients with low cardiac output, low gradient, and low calculated valve area present a thorny management problem that is beyond the scope of this chapter [15]. Right-side heart catheterization and—if indicated and considered safe—left ventriculography are also performed. If it is necessary to assess the severity of coexisting aortic regurgitation, supravalvular aortography is performed. Because much information may be obtained from a technically optimal echocardiogram, the principal indication for cardiac catheterization in adults is to assess the severity of coexisting coronary artery disease by coronary arteriography; this approach is generally deemed necessary in patients older than the age of 40 years and in younger patients with risk factors for atherosclerosis.

Aortic valve replacement is indicated for patients with even mildly symptomatic severe aortic stenosis if they have no major concomitant noncardiac conditions. Coronary bypass grafting is a generally accepted, if unproven, adjunct to valve replacement in patients with coronary artery disease. Advanced age is not in itself a contraindication to surgery because otherwise healthy octogenarians undergo valve replacement with acceptable mortality and morbidity (Fig. 6) [16]. Similarly, even severe left ventricular systolic dysfunction is not a contraindication to valve replacement if the depression of ejection fraction is caused by severe aortic stenosis and not by another condition, such as coronary artery disease, because clinical outcome is almost invariably good and the ejection fraction improves postoperatively in such cases (Fig. 7) [17]. Surgery is sometimes advocated for asymptomatic patients with aortic stenosis if 1) they are young and have very vigorous lifestyles; 2) they have a markedly abnormal response to exercise during formal testing; 3) they have progressive cardiac enlargement or depression of left ventricular ejection fraction; or 4) they have left heart filling pressures that are markedly elevated at rest or with exercise. These indications for valve replacement are not established [18].

Whereas mechanical valves require life-long anticoagulation therapy with warfarin, bioprosthetic valves degenerate more quickly than mechanical valves, especially in younger patients. For these reasons, young and middle-aged patients usually receive mechanical valves, whereas elderly patients and

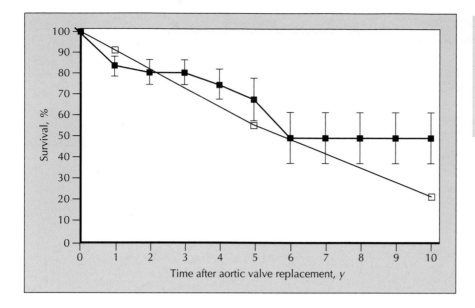

FIGURE 6 Actuarial survival curve for octogenarians undergoing aortic valve replacement for aortic stenosis (*closed squares*). For comparison, actuarial survival curve for unselected 80-year-old persons (*open squares*) *from US census data is also shown. (From* Levinson *et al.* [16]; with permission).

patients with contraindications to anticoagulation usually receive bioprosthetic valves.

In patients with absolute contraindications to aortic valve replacement (*eg*, metastatic cancer or severe emphysema),

percutaneous balloon aortic valvuloplasty may be offered as palliative therapy. Although this technique may provide lasting benefit for young patients with congenital aortic stenosis, it provides only temporary relief for adults with calcific aortic stenosis; restenosis of the valve within 1 year is the rule. Percutaneous aortic valvuloplasty may also have a role as a "bridge" to valve replacement in moribund patients with severe aortic stenosis.

AORTIC REGURGITATION

Etiology and Pathogenesis

Aortic regurgitation may result from diseases causing deformity of the valve leaflets or, alternatively, from diseases causing dilation or distortion of the aortic root, with resultant failure of the leaflets to coapt. This distinction is vital because the causes of aortic regurgitation associated with the two mechanisms differ substantially (Table 2) [2,19]. Like rheumatic aortic stenosis, rheumatic aortic regurgitation is usually accompanied by clinically important rheumatic mitral stenosis or regurgitation, or both. The manifestations of chronic and acute aortic regurgitation are disparate (Table 3) [20]. With chronic aortic regurgitation, there is a gradual and marked increase in left ventricular end-diastolic volume. Left ventricular distensibility is increased, such that there is only a modest increase in end-diastolic pressure. Total left ventricular stroke volume increases, forward stroke volume (total stroke volume minus the volume regurgitated across the aortic valve back into the ventricle) is maintained, ejection fraction is initially normal, and heart rate does not increase markedly. Aortic systolic pressure is high, diastolic pressure is low, and pulse pressure is wide. With long-standing volume overload of the ventricle, there is an eventual loss of myocardial contractility, with consequent increase in end-systolic volume and decrease in ejection fraction. The loss of myocardial contractility may be irreversible. In acute aortic regurgitation (as caused by endocarditis or aortic dissection), regurgitation into an unprepared left ventricle results in a marked increase in end-diastolic pressure, which is transmitted backward to the left

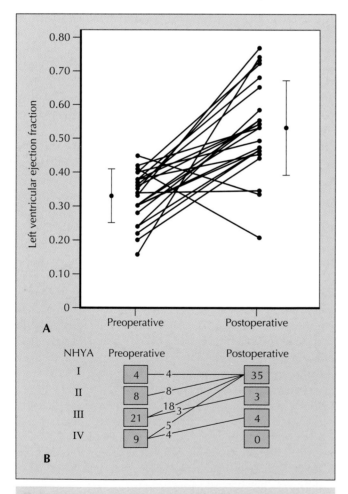

A

B

FIGURE 7 Change in **A**, New York Heart Association (NYHA) class and **B**, left ventricular ejection fraction after aortic valve replacement for aortic stenosis in patients with low preoperative ejection fraction and no significant associated cardiac abnormalities. (*From* Rediker *et al.* [17]; with permission.)

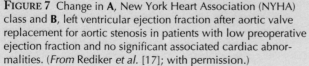

TABLE 2 CAUSES OF AORTIC REGURGITATION

Conditions causing deformity of aortic valve leaflets	Conditions causing dilation or dissection of aortic root
Congenitally bicuspid valve	Idiopathic (annuloaortic ectasia)
Rheumatic fever	Aortic dissection
Endocarditis	Chronic, severe hypertension
Trauma	Inflammatory diseases (*eg*, ankylosing spondylitis)
Myxomatous ("floppy") valve with prolapse	Connective tissue diseases (*eg*, Marfan syndrome)
Inflammatory diseases (*eg*, systemic lupus erythematosus)	Syphilitic aortitis
Radiation	Nonspecific aortitis

atrium and pulmonary circulation, resulting in pulmonary congestion. Total left ventricular stroke volume increases minimally, forward stroke volume falls, and there is compensatory tachycardia in an attempt to maintain cardiac output. Prominent widening of the pulse pressure (and the corresponding physical signs of chronic aortic regurgitation; see the following paragraphs) is absent. The manifestations of aortic regurgitation described in the following paragraphs are of the chronic form unless otherwise noted.

Evaluation

Patients with chronic aortic regurgitation may have no symptoms until left ventricular contractile dysfunction and marked cardiomegaly are apparent. The most common symptoms are those of left-side heart failure: dyspnea on exertion, orthopnea, paroxysmal nocturnal dyspnea, and fatigue. Angina is much less common than that in aortic stenosis but may be caused by increased myocardial oxygen demand associated with hypertrophy in the face of a decreased supply associated with low perfusion (aortic diastolic) pressure. Syncope is rare. Prominent neck pulsations may be noted by the patient, and the high stroke volume may be experienced as uncomfortable palpitations, especially when the patient lies down. Patients with acute aortic regurgitation may have severe dyspnea, weakness, hypotension, and cardiovascular collapse.

In cases of severe chronic aortic regurgitation, the aortic diastolic pressure is usually 60 mm Hg or less. The pulse pressure (which should be measured by the physician) is wide, with muffled sounds continuing to a pressure as low as 0 mm Hg; in such cases, the aortic diastolic pressure correlates best with the onset of muffled (phase IV) Korotkoff sounds. The wide pulse pressure manifests as various peripheral signs, such as Corrigan's pulse (rapid rise and collapse), Quincke's pulse (flushing and blanching of the capillary bed in the fingertips, seen by transmitting a light through the fingers), Duroziez's sign (systolic and diastolic murmurs over a femoral artery lightly compressed by the stethoscope), and "pistol shot" systolic sounds over the femoral artery. The peripheral arterial pulsation may be bisferiens.

The left ventricular impulse is displaced downward and leftward. An S_3 may indicate left ventricular systolic dysfunction [21] or merely left ventricular dilation [9]. A systolic murmur is usually present and reflects the increased total stroke volume traversing the left ventricular outflow tract. A relatively soft, high-pitched, blowing decrescendo diastolic murmur is best heard with the diaphragm of the stethoscope in held expiration with the patient sitting up and leaning forward. It is typically heard at the mid or lower left sternal border in primary valve disease; auscultation predominantly at the right upper sternal border suggests root disease. The

TABLE 3 CHRONIC VERSUS ACUTE AORTIC REGURGITATION

	Chronic	Acute
Symptoms	Often none; exertional dyspnea, orthopnea, paroxysmal nocturnal dyspnea	Dyspnea, often severe and at rest; weakness
Appearance	Often normal	Dyspneic, pale, diaphoretic
Heart rate	Normal	Fast
Pulse pressure	Wide	Normal or slightly widened
Peripheral signs of aortic regurgitation	Present	Absent
Left ventricular impulse	Heaving, displaced laterally and inferiorly	Normal
Murmur	Long	Short
Left ventricular hypertrophy on electrocardiogram	Present	Absent
Cardiomegaly on chest roentgenography	Present	Absent
Pulmonary congestion on chest roentgenography	Absent	Present
Pulmonary capillary wedge pressure	Normal or mildly elevated	Markedly elevated

length and intensity [22] of the murmur correlate with the severity of regurgitation, except in acute aortic regurgitation. Aortic regurgitation may cause a mid and late diastolic rumble at the apex (Austin-Flint murmur), which is distinguished from the murmur of mitral stenosis by the absence of an opening snap and of a loud S_1. In acute aortic regurgitation, there is tachycardia, peripheral vasoconstriction, normal pulse pressure without the peripheral signs of chronic aortic regurgitation, a normal left ventricular impulse, and a short, relatively soft diastolic murmur.

The electrocardiogram shows left ventricular hypertrophy in most patients with chronic aortic regurgitation but not in patients with acute aortic regurgitation. ST-segment and T-wave abnormalities, left atrial abnormality, left axis deviation, or left bundle branch block may be present. Chest roentgenogram shows left ventricular enlargement. The ascending aorta is dilated, markedly so if root disease is the cause of regurgitation. Acute aortic regurgitation produces a roentgenogram characterized by pulmonary edema with normal heart size.

The echocardiogram (Figs. 3 and 8) images both the valve leaflets and the aortic root and is the most useful test, invasive or noninvasive, for determining the cause of regurgitation. Valve abnormalities that may be detected include thickening of cusps, prolapsed or flail leaflets, and vegetations. Transthoracic and, in particular, transesophageal echocardiography are useful for detecting proximal aortic dissection. The echocardiogram may be used for serially assessing left ventricular size and systolic function, which are critical for determining the timing of aortic valve replacement in asymptomatic or minimally symptomatic patients. Doppler echocardiography is so sensitive for detecting valvular regurgitation that it generates "false positives"; a useful rule is that if aortic regurgitation is not discernible by careful cardiac auscultation (see the preceding paragraphs), then it is not responsible for symptoms. Doppler echocardiography is moderately useful for grading the severity of regurgitation. Radionuclide ventriculography provides the ratio of stroke volume ejected by the left ventricle to that ejected by the right ventricle, a useful estimate of the severity of aortic regurgitation in the absence of shunts or other regurgitant lesions. Failure of the ejection fraction to increase during exercise has been proposed as a test of left ventricular reserve in patients with aortic regurgitation, but the validity of this criterion for determining the timing of aortic valve surgery has not been established.

Management

Like patients with aortic stenosis, patients with aortic regurgitation may be asymptomatic for many years. Sudden death may occur, but it is rare in asymptomatic patients [10,23]. Although low left ventricular ejection fraction in aortic stenosis is usually reversed with relief of afterload excess by valve replacement, low ejection fraction in aortic regurgitation often reflects irreversible loss of myocardial contractility.

The work-up of aortic regurgitation includes carefully questioning the patient for symptoms of heart failure, inquiring into the cause of regurgitation, and meticulously assessing left ventricular systolic function. When indicated on clinical grounds or by echocardiography, the erythrocyte sedimentation rate for inflammatory disease, serology for syphilis, and blood cultures for endocarditis should be obtained. The patient should be evaluated clinically every 3 to 6 months, and left ventricular systolic function should be assessed by echocardiography or radionuclide ventriculography (one or the other should be performed consistently, rather than switching from one to the other) every 6 to 12 months. The management of chronic aortic regurgitation is shown schematically in Figure 9.

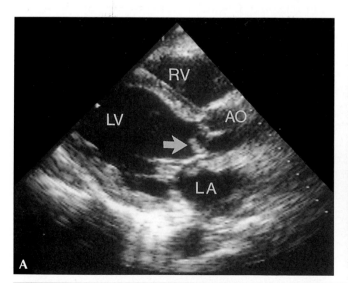

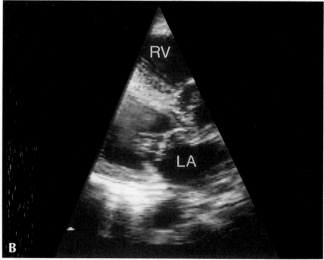

FIGURE 8 Two-dimensional echocardiogram A, without and B, with a superimposed color Doppler signal from a 49-year-old man with severe aortic regurgitation and an aortic root abscess. The right ventricle (RV), left atrium (LA), left ventricle (LV), and aorta (AO) are shown. The left ventricle is dilated. One aortic valve leaflet visualized in end-diastolic frame is in the normal position in the aorta, but the other (*arrow*) has prolapsed into the left ventricular outflow tract. The thickened area between the aorta and the left atrium is the abscess. The light blue color Doppler signal depicts the jet of regurgitation through the aortic valve into the left ventricle. (*see* Color Plate.) (*Courtesy of* Michael H. Picard, MD.)

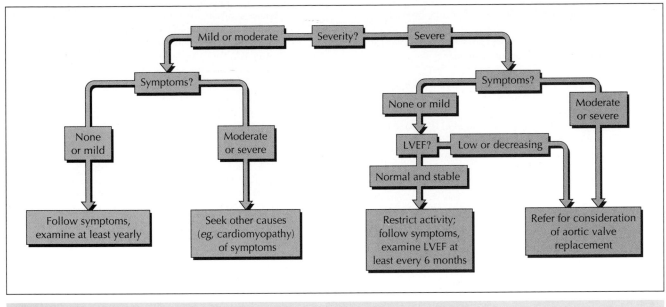

FIGURE 9 Management of aortic regurgitation. Serial left ventricular ejection fraction (LVEF) determinations for an individual patient should be obtained consistently from either echocardiography or radionuclide ventriculography.

Patients with asymptomatic but severe aortic regurgitation should avoid heavy exertion, including competitive sports. Systolic hypertension should be treated, usually with an angiotensin-converting enzyme inhibitor. Long-term therapy with vasodilators (hydralazine, 3 mg/kg/d [24], or enalapril, 20 mg bid [25]) reduces left ventricular volume. It has been reported that treatment with nifedipine, 20 mg bid, delays the need for aortic valve replacement [26]. Endocarditis prophylaxis is necessary. Digoxin, diuretics, and vasodilators are indicated for symptomatic patients with contraindications to cardiac surgery or in preparation for surgery. Drug therapy for acute aortic regurgitation includes diuretics, oral and intravenous vasodilators (in particular, afterload reduction with drugs such as nitroprusside), and, as indicated, inotropic support (usually with dobutamine). Urgent or emergency aortic valve surgery, even with active endocarditis, may be lifesaving. Intra-aortic balloon counterpulsation is not useful because inflation of the balloon in diastole worsens regurgitation across the aortic valve.

When to Refer

Patients should be referred to a cardiologist if they have symptoms or signs of heart failure and aortic regurgitation is evident on physical examination. Asymptomatic patients with aortic regurgitation should be promptly referred if left ventricular ejection fraction is low or in the low-normal range or if serial noninvasive studies indicate that it is decreasing over time.

The definitive test for grading aortic regurgitation is supravalvular aortography performed as part of cardiac catheterization. The regurgitant fraction, derived from a comparison of total (angiographic) and forward (eg, thermodilution) left ventricular stroke volume, is fraught with error and is a less useful index of the severity of regurgitation. Right-side heart catheterization, left ventriculography, and—for patients older than 40 years of age or for younger patients with

atherosclerosis risk factors—coronary arteriography are also performed.

If there is no noncardiac contraindication, surgery is performed if aortic regurgitation is severe and symptoms are more than minimal. Surgery should be strongly considered for asymptomatic or minimally symptomatic patients if left ventricular ejection fraction is mildly or moderately impaired, if there is a decline in left ventricular ejection fraction within the normal range, or if there is very marked left ventricular dilation [23]. Patients with severe depression of ejection fraction may not benefit from valve surgery.

The usual operation for valve disease is aortic valve replacement, although a minority of patients are successfully treated with valve repair. The considerations regarding type of valve prosthesis are similar to those for surgery for aortic stenosis. Patients with root disease require aortic repair, usually accompanied by valve replacement, often with a composite graft.

REFERENCES

1. Lindroos M, Kupari M, Heikkila J: Prevalence of aortic valve abnormalities in the elderly: an echocardiographic study of a random population sample. *J Am Coll Cardiol* 1993, 21:1220–1225.

2. Olson LT, Subramanian R, Edwards WD: Surgical pathology of pure aortic insuffficiency: a study of 225 cases. *Mayo Clin Proc* 1984, 59:835–841.

3. Subramanian R, Olson LJ, Edwards WD: Surgical pathology of pure aortic stenosis: a study of 374 cases. *Mayo Clin Proc* 1984, 59:683–690.

4. Fenoglio JJ, McAllister HA, DeCastro CM, *et al.*: Congenital bicuspid aortic valve after age 20. *Am J Cardiol* 1977, 39:164–169.

5. Selzer A: Changing aspects of the natural history of valvular aortic stenosis. *N Engl J Med* 1987, 317:91–98.

6. King RM, Pluth JR, Giuliani ER: The association of unexplained gastrointestinal bleeding with calcific aortic stenosis. *Ann Thorac Surg* 1987, 44:514–516.

7. Levinson GE: Aortic stenosis. In *Valvular Heart Disease*, edn 2. Edited by Dalen JE, Alpert JS. Boston: Little, Brown and Company; 1987:197–282.

8. Lombard JT, Selzer A: Valvular aortic stenosis: a clinical and hemodynamic profile of patients. *Ann Intern Med* 1987, 106:292–298.

9. Folland ED, Kriegel BJ, Henderson WG, *et al.*: Implications of third heart sounds in patients with valvular heart disease. *N Engl J Med* 1992, 327:458–462.

10. Turina J, Hess O, Sepulci F, Krayenbuehl HP: Spontaneous course of aortic valve disease. *Eur Heart J* 1987, 8:471–483.

11. Horstkotte D, Loogen F: The natural history of aortic valve stenosis. *Eur Heart J* 1988, 9(suppl E):57–64.

12. Aronow WS, Ahn C, Kronzon I, Nanna M: Prognosis of congestive heart failure in patients aged ≥ 62 years with unoperated severe valvular aortic stenosis. *Am J Cardiol* 1993, 72:846–848.

13. Pellikka PA, Nishimura RA, Bailey KR, Tajik AJ: The natural history of adults with asymptomatic, hemodynamically significant aortic stenosis. *J Am Coll Cardiol* 1990, 15:1012–1017.

14. O'Keefe JH, Shub C, Rettke SR: Risk of noncardiac surgical procedures in patients with aortic stenosis. *Mayo Clin Proc* 1989, 64:400–405.

15. Carabello BA: Advances in the hemodynamic assessment of stenotic cardiac valves. *J Am Coll Cardiol* 1987, 10:912–919.

16. Levinson JR, Akins CW, Buckley MJ, *et al.*: Octogenarians with aortic stenosis: outcome following aortic valve replacement. *Circulation* 1989, 80(suppl I):I-49–I-56.

17. Rediker DE, Boucher CA, Block PC, *et al.*: Degree of reversibility of left ventricular systolic dysfunction after aortic valve replacement for isolated aortic stenosis. *Am J Cardiol* 1987, 60:112–118.

18. Braunwald E: On the natural history of severe aortic stenosis. *J Am Coll Cardiol* 1990, 15:1018–1020.

19. Guiney TE, Davies MJ, Leech GJ, Leatham A: The aetiology and course of isolated severe aortic regurgitation: a clinical, pathological, and echocardiographic study. *Br Heart J* 1987, 58:358–368.

20. Morganroth JM, Perloff JK, Zeldis SM, Dunkman WB: Acute severe aortic regurgitation: pathophysiology, clinical recognition, and management. *Ann Intern Med* 1977, 87:223–232.

21. Abdulla AM, Frank MJ, Erdin RAJ, Canedo MI: Clinical significance and hemodynamic correlates of the third heart sound gallop in aortic regurgitation: a guide to optimal timing of cardiac catheterization. *Circulation* 1981, 64:464–471.

22. Desjardins VA, Enriquez-Sarano M, Tajik AJ, *et al.*: Intensity of murmurs correlates with severity of valvular regurgitation. *Am J Med* 1996, 100:149–156.

23. Bonow RO, Lakatos E, Maron BJ, *et al.*: Serial long-term assessment of the natural history of asymptomatic patients with chronic aortic regurgitation and normal left ventricular systolic function. *Circulation* 1991, 84:1625–1635.

24. Greenberg B, Massie B, Bristow JD, *et al.*: Long-term vasodilator therapy of chronic aortic insufficiency: a randomized double-blinded, placebo-controlled clinical trial. *Circulation* 1988, 78:92–103.

25. Lin M, Chiang H, Lin S, *et al.*: Vasodilator therapy in chronic asymptomatic aortic regurgitation: enalapril versus hydralazine therapy. *J Am Coll Cardiol* 1994, 24:1046–1053.

26. Scognamiglio R, Rahimtoola SH, Fasoli G, *et al.*: Nifedipine in asymptomatic patients with severe aortic regurgitation and normal left ventricular function. *N Engl J Med* 1994, 331:689–694.

27. Sutton GC, Fox KM: *A Color Atlas of Heart Disease: Pathological, Clinical and Investigatory Aspects*. London: Current Medical Literature; 1990:136–137.

28. Ross J Jr, Braunwald E: Aortic stenosis. *Circulation* 1968, 37(suppl V):V-61–V-67.

SELECT BIBLIOGRAPHY

Braunwald E: Valvular heart disease. In *Heart Disease*, edn 5. Edited by Braunwald E. Philadelphia: WB Saunders Co.; 1997:1035–1053.

Rahimtoola SH: Perspective on valvular heart disease: an update. *J Am Coll Cardiol* 1989, 14:1–23.

Waller BF, Howard J, Fess S: Pathology of aortic valve stenosis and pure aortic regurgitation: a clinical morphologic assessment—Parts I and II. *Clin Cardiol* 1994, 17:85–92, 150–156.

Tricuspid and Pulmonic Valve Disease 24

William R. Pitts
L. David Hillis

Key Points
- Congenital anomalies of the tricuspid and pulmonic valves constitute 10% to 15% of all congenital heart disease.
- Pulmonic stenosis is the most common congenital right-sided valvular abnormality and is effectively treated by balloon valvuloplasty.
- Pulmonic regurgitation usually results from pulmonary arterial hypertension, and its prognosis is largely determined by the underlying disease process.
- Tricuspid stenosis is nearly always caused by rheumatic disease and is never seen without concomitant mitral or aortic involvement.
- Tricuspid regurgitation (TR) usually results from right ventricular dilatation; patients with TR present with right-sided heart failure.

The tricuspid and pulmonic valves are often overlooked during evaluation of suspected cardiac disease. This is particularly true in the United States, where the incidence of rheumatic valvular disease has declined and other disease processes involving the right-sided valves (*eg*, infective endocarditis in intravenous drug abusers) have increased in frequency.

TRICUSPID VALVE DISEASE

Congenital

Congenital anomalies of the tricuspid valve account for only 1% to 3% of congenital heart disease. Only tricuspid atresia and Ebstein's anomaly are of clinical importance, and almost all patients with the former are diagnosed and surgically corrected in infancy or early childhood.

In Ebstein's anomaly, the septal and inferior tricuspid valve leaflets are displaced away from the tricuspid annulus into the right ventricle. The anterior leaflet retains its normal attachment to the atrioventricular groove and is typically large and redundant. The displacement of the valve apparatus divides the right ventricle into 1) an inlet portion, which is functionally part of the right atrium (the so-called *atrialized* portion) and 2) a distal, functionally small right ventricular chamber. Associated anomalies include an interatrial communication (atrial septal defect or patent foramen ovale) in 50% to 75% of cases, ventricular septal defect, pulmonary stenosis or atresia, and mitral valve prolapse [1]. In addition, as many as 25% of patients with Ebstein's anomaly have ventricular preexcitation, most commonly via a right-sided accessory atrioventricular pathway [2].

Most patients with Ebstein's anomaly survive to adulthood, and an occasional patient lives into the seventh or eighth decade. Early (fetal or neonatal) presentation usually is associated with other cardiac abnormalities and portends a poor prognosis [3]. Most patients remain asymptomatic until the third or fourth decade, when

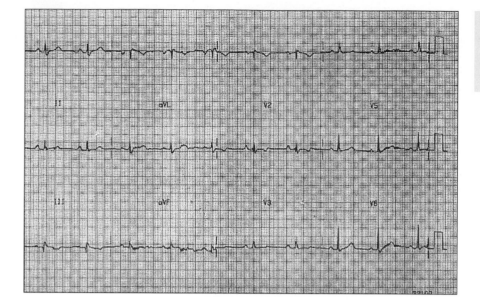

FIGURE 1 Electrocardiogram from a patient with Ebstein's anomaly demonstrating a prolonged PR interval, peaked P waves, and an incomplete right bundle-branch block.

dyspnea, fatigue, or cyanosis appear insidiously. In 15% to 20% of cases, sudden death caused by tachydysrhythmias may be the presenting manifestation. The onset of right heart failure portends a poor prognosis and is the most common cause of death.

On physical examination, the arterial and jugular venous pulses are usually normal. The first heart sound (S_1) is usually loud and widely split, as is the second heart sound (S_2); multiple systolic clicks as well as right-sided gallops may be heard. A murmur of tricuspid regurgitation is almost invariably present at the left lower sternal border and characteristically increases with inspiration.

The electrocardiogram (ECG) usually reveals sinus rhythm, although supraventricular arrhythmias are common. Tall P waves, a prolonged PR interval, and complete or incomplete right bundle-branch block are common (Fig. 1). Chest radiography usually demonstrates globular cardiomegaly and evidence of an enlarged right atrium. Echocardiography is extremely valuable in identifying the anatomic relationship between the tricuspid valve and right heart chambers as well as in assessing right ventricular function, tricuspid regurgitation, and intracardiac shunting [4]. Finally, the diagnosis of Ebstein's anomaly may be made at catheterization by recording a simultaneous intracardiac pressure and electrogram with a single catheter. When this catheter is withdrawn from the

right ventricle to the right atrium, a right ventricular electrical potential continues to be recorded after the pressure contour has changed to a right atrial waveform. Right ventricular angiography is usually diagnostic.

Management of the patient with Ebstein's anomaly is based on the severity of disease. An acyanotic patient with minimal symptoms is managed conservatively, whereas the patient with class III or IV heart failure, a cardiothoracic ratio of 0.65 or higher, severe cyanosis, or paradoxic embolization may benefit from surgical repair [5,6]. Refractory tachydysrhythmias may be treated at the time of surgery.

Acquired

Tricuspid stenosis

Tricuspid stenosis (TS) is uncommon and results almost exclusively from rheumatic scarring; other causes of functional and anatomic TS are listed in Table 1. Isolated rheumatic TS in the absence of concomitant mitral involvement, aortic involvement, or both is rare.

Patients with TS usually have symptoms related to their predominant left-sided valvular abnormality. Indeed, the absence of pulmonary congestion in a patient with severe mitral stenosis should raise the suspicion of concomitant TS. Symptoms that are primarily related to TS result from peripheral venous congestion or a reduced cardiac output (Table 2).

TABLE 1 CAUSES OF FUNCTIONAL OR ANATOMIC TRICUSPID STENOSIS
Tricuspid valve vegetations
Tumor (myxoma, leiomyoma, metastatic melanoma)
Thrombus (ball valve)
Carcinoid syndrome
Löffler's endocarditis
Postsurgical (following tricuspid annuloplasty)
Constrictive pericarditis
Methysergide

TABLE 2 SYMPTOMS OF TRICUSPID STENOSIS
Easy fatigability (because of reduced cardiac output)
Right upper quadrant abdominal discomfort (because of hepatic congestion)
Anorexia, nausea, vomiting, and eructation (because of passive congestion of the gastrointestinal tract)
Syncope/near syncope
Periodic cyanosis (because of right-to-left intracardiac shunting through a patent foramen ovale)
Vague retrosternal chest discomfort

TABLE 3 COMPARISON OF AUSCULTATORY FEATURES IN MITRAL AND TRICUSPID STENOSIS

	Mitral stenosis	Tricuspid stenosis
Location	Apex	Left lower sternal border
Quality	Rumbling	Rumbling
Intensity	Louder	Softer
Pitch	Lower	Higher
Timing	Mid-diastole	Mid-diastole
Duration	Longer	Shorter
Opening snap	Earlier	Later and increases with inspiration

On physical examination, the patient with TS has jugular venous distention with prominent A waves and hepatojugular reflux. Hepatomegaly with presystolic pulsation, ascites, peripheral edema, and pleural effusions are common. The auscultatory findings are usually dominated by concomitant left-sided valvular disease. S_1 is increased in intensity, as is the pulmonic component of S_2 (if pulmonary hypertension is present). The murmur of TS may be confused with that of mitral stenosis, but careful auscultation can usually distinguish them (Table 3).

Both the diastolic murmur and the opening snap of TS are augmented by maneuvers that increase flow across the tricuspid valve (e.g., inspiration).

The electrocardiogram of the patient with TS usually shows right atrial enlargement. The PR interval is often slightly prolonged, and ECG evidence of concomitant mitral stenosis is often present. Atrial dysrhythmias are usually indicative of coexistent mitral valve disease. On chest radiography, the patient has right atrial enlargement with rightward displacement of the right lower cardiac contour. Echocardiography and Doppler ultrasound provide a qualitative assessment of the severity of TS [7]. At catheterization, right atrial and ventricular pressures are recorded simultaneously (Fig. 2). A mean diastolic gradient across the tricuspid valve of 2 to 3 mm Hg is suggestive of TS. Provocative maneuvers during catheterization (*eg*, deep inspiration, exercise, volume infusion) may magnify a small resting gradient.

The patient with isolated TS may be asymptomatic for years. Once symptoms develop, sodium restriction and diuretics are effective in relieving peripheral venous congestion. Once medically refractory symptoms develop, surgical correction via open commissurotomy or valve replacement should be recommended. If valve replacement is required, a bioprosthesis is preferable because of its proven durability in the tricuspid position and the increased risk of a thromboembolic complication with a mechanical prosthesis in this position [8,9].

Tricuspid regurgitation

Tricuspid regurgitation (TR) may be functional or organic. Functional TR (from dilatation of the right ventricle and tricuspid anulus) is far more common than organic TR and results from right ventricular dilatation, which in turn may result from pulmonary hypertension of any cause, right ventricular outflow obstruction (valvar, supravalvar, or infundibular), right ventricular infarction, or dilated cardiomyopathy. Organic TR may result from a variety of disease processes (Table 4). Recently, TR caused by infective endocarditis has appeared with increasing frequency, most commonly in intravenous drug abusers. The causative organism is usually *Staphylococcus aureus*. Fortunately, most of these patients respond to medical therapy and have a better prognosis than those with left-sided endocarditis. Organic TR is generally well tolerated in the absence of elevated right ventricular systolic pressure; indeed, the surgical procedure of choice in the patient with right-sided endocarditis refractory to medical therapy is tricuspid or pulmonic valve excision *without* immediate valve replacement [10].

Symptoms of TR are similar to those of tricuspid stenosis. On physical examination, the patient usually has distended neck veins with prominent V waves, hepatomegaly that may be pulsatile, ascites, and peripheral edema. Cardiac examination may reveal a prominent right ventricular impulse. On

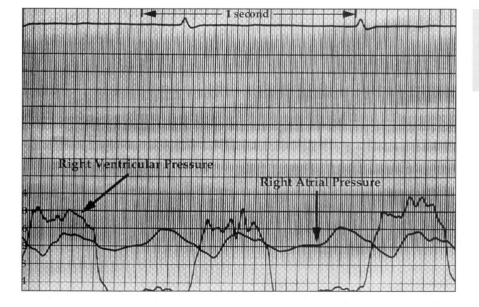

FIGURE 2 Simultaneous right atrial and ventricular pressure tracings in a patient with tricuspid stenosis. There is a gradient of 11 mm Hg across the tricuspid valve during diastole.

auscultation, S_1 is typically diminished, and the pulmonic component of S_2 may be prominent in the presence of pulmonary hypertension. A holosystolic murmur is present at the left lower sternal border and characteristically increases in intensity with inspiration (Carvallo sign). In addition, a right ventricular gallop (S_3) and a diastolic rumble ("relative" tricuspid stenosis) may be audible.

Common ECG features include right-axis deviation, right-atrial enlargement, and right ventricular hypertrophy. Chest radiography reveals right atrial and right ventricular enlargement. Two-dimensional echocardiography with Doppler color-flow mapping is useful for detecting TR and estimating right ventricular peak-systolic pressure. Recent studies have shown a good correlation between proximal regurgitant jet size (measured with transthoracic color flow mapping) and regurgitant fraction in subjects with tricuspid regurgitation [11]. At catheterization, right atrial and right ventricular diastolic pressures are elevated. A right ventricular systolic pressure greater than 60 mm Hg suggests a functional etiology of TR, whereas a systolic pressure less than 40 mm Hg implies organic valvular disease. Although right ventricular angiography will demonstrate regurgitation of contrast material into the right atrium, quantitation of TR by this method is imprecise.

Treatment of functional TR is directed at the underlying disease process. In the absence of pulmonary hypertension, TR usually does not require surgical treatment; when surgical therapy is necessary, tricuspid annuloplasty with (Carpentier) or without (De Vega) a prosthetic ring may be performed [12]. When valve replacement is indicated, a bioprosthesis is preferred. If surgery is not feasible, medical therapy with sodium restriction, digoxin, and diuretics should be employed.

PULMONIC VALVE DISEASE

Congenital

Valvular pulmonic stenosis (PS) is almost always congenital and is present in about 7% of patients with congnital heart disease. Acquired PS is exceedingly rare but may result from rheumatic scarring, infective endocarditis, trauma, malignant carcinoid syndrome, cardiac tumors, or an aneurysm of a sinus of Valsalva [13].

The patient with PS is frequently asymptomatic. He or she eventually may note exertional dyspnea, fatigue, syncope, or chest pain; peripheral edema and other evidence of peripheral venous congestion may develop if right ventricular failure occurs. If the foramen ovale is patent, intermittent or continuous right-to-left intracardiac shunting with resultant clubbing or cyanosis may occur.

On physical examination, the patient may have evidence of right ventricular failure (peripheral edema, hepatomegaly, jugular venous distention), right ventricular lift at the left sternal border, and a systolic thrill over the pulmonic area (second left intercostal space). On auscultation, S_1 is normal, and S_2 is widely split but moves with respiration. The pulmonic component is soft and markedly delayed. A harsh, crescendo–decrescendo systolic murmur is audible along the

TABLE 4 CAUSES OF ORGANIC TRICUSPID REGURGITATION
Rheumatic
Infective endocarditis
Ebstein's anomaly
Right ventricular papillary muscle dysfunction
Myxomatous degeneration
Carcinoid syndrome
Trauma
Tricuspid valve prolapse
Connective tissue disorders (rheumatoid arthritis, systemic lupus erythematosus, Marfan syndrome)
Right atrial myxoma
Methysergide
Endomyocardial fibrosis
Thyrotoxicosis

left sternal border and loudest over the pulmonic area. An ejection click that softens or even disappears with inspiration may be heard at the pulmonic area.

The ECG may reveal right-axis deviation, right ventricular hypertrophy, right atrial enlargement, and complete or incomplete right bundle-branch block (Fig. 3). Chest radiography demonstrates diminished pulmonary vascular markings and a markedly dilated main pulmonary artery. Cardiomegaly may be present. Two-dimensional echocardiography with Doppler ultrasound is useful to visualize the pulmonic valve, to assess the severity of stenosis, and to identify coexisting anomalies [14]. Cardiac catheterization demonstrates a pressure gradient during systole between the right ventricle and pulmonary artery. The severity of PS is quantitated according to the right ventricular peak-systolic pressure (Table 5).

Many adults with mild or moderate PS are asymptomatic and require no treatment. Surgical valvotomy, balloon valvuloplasty, or (rarely) valve replacement is warranted for the indications outlined in Table 6. Balloon valvuloplasty is currently the procedure of choice for relief of valvular PS; its results are excellent and comparable to surgical valvotomy [15,16].

Acquired

Similar to TR, acquired pulmonic regurgitation (PR) may be functional or organic. Functional PR usually results from pulmonary arterial hypertension, regardless of etiology. Rarely, it occurs with idiopathic dilatation of the pulmonary artery [17]. Organic PR is relatively rare; it may occur with infective endocarditis, rheumatic scarring, chest trauma, carcinoid syndrome, syphilis, or following balloon valvuloplasty or surgical valvotomy.

The patient with functional PR presents with symptoms induced by the underlying disease. Organic PR in the absence of pulmonary hypertension may be well tolerated for many years. When severe and long-standing, it may cause symptoms and signs of right ventricular failure.

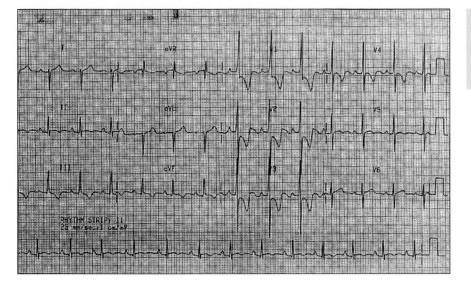

FIGURE 3 Electrocardiogram from a patient with congenital pulmonic stenosis showing right-axis deviation, right atrial enlargement, and right ventricular hypertrophy with strain.

Cardiac examination may reveal a palpable pulsation over the pulmonic area. On auscultation, S_2 is widely split, with an accentuated pulmonic component. A blowing, decrescendo diastolic murmur is audible in the second and third left intercostal spaces and increases in intensity with inspiration. A systolic ejection murmur caused by increased flow across the pulmonic valve is frequently heard. If right ventricular dilatation and decompensation have occurred, a right-sided S_3 and holosystolic murmur of TR may be present.

The ECG demonstrates right-axis deviation, right ventricular hypertrophy, and possibly right bundle-branch block. Chest radiography shows right ventricular enlargement and dilatation of the pulmonary artery. Echocardiography may reveal right ventricular dilatation, paradoxic motion of the interventricular septum during systole, and occasionally, diastolic fluttering of the tricuspid valve. As with TR, a small amount of PR is seen in most normal subjects (93%) with Doppler color-flow mapping. At catheterization, right ventricular systolic and diastolic pressures are similar to pulmonary arterial pressures provided that PS is not present. With pulmonary angiography, there is reflux of contrast material into the right ventricle.

The prognosis of a patient with functional PR is determined by the underlying disease process, and therapeutic measures should be tailored accordingly. Organic PR is usually benign. In the occasional patient in whom severe PR causes right ventricular failure despite medical therapy, surgical intervention is warranted.

TABLE 5 GRADING OF VALVULAR PULMONIC STENOSIS

Right ventricular peak-systolic pressure, *mm Hg**	Grade
30–49	Mild
50–99	Moderate
≥100	Severe

*As determined at cardiac catheterization.

TABLE 6 INDICATIONS FOR BALLOON PULMONIC VALVULOPLASTY OR SURGICAL TREATMENT

Symptoms attributable to the stenosis
Intermittent or continuous cyanosis
Right ventricular peak-systolic pressure >100 mm Hg, even without symptoms

REFERENCES

1. Giuliani ER, Fuster V, Brandenberg RO, Mair DD: Ebstein's anomaly: the clinical features and natural history of Ebstein's anomaly of the tricuspid valve. *Mayo Clin Proc* 1979, 54:163–173.

2. Smith WM, Gallagher JJ, Kerr CR, *et al.*: The electrophysiologic basis and management of symptomatic and recurrent tachycardia in patients with Ebstein's anomaly of the tricuspid valve. *Am J Cardiol* 1982, 49:1223–1234.

3. Celemajer DS, Bull C, Till JA, *et al.*: Ebstein's anomaly: presentation and outcome from fetus to adult. *J Am Coll Cardiol* 1994, 23:170–176.

4. Shiina A, Seward JB, Tajik AJ, *et al.*: Two-dimensional echocardiographic-surgical correlation in Ebstein's anomaly: preoperative determination of patients requiring tricuspid valve plication vs. replacement. *Circulation* 1983, 68:534–544.

5. Driscoll DJ, Mottram CD, Danielson GK: Spectrum of exercise intolerance in 45 patients with Ebstein's anomaly and observations on exercise tolerance in 11 patients after surgical repair. *J Am Coll Cardiol* 1988, 11:831–836.

6. Mair DD, Seward JB, Driscoll DJ, Danielson GK: Surgical repair of Ebstein's anomaly: selection of patients and early and late operative results. *Circulation* 1985, 72(suppl 2):70–76.

7. Pearlman AS: Role of echocardiography in the diagnosis and evaluation of severity of mitral and tricuspid stenosis. *Circulation* 1991, 84(suppl 1):193–197.

8. Guerra F, Bortolotti U, Thiene G, *et al.*: Long-term performance of the Hancock bioprosthesis in the tricuspid position. A review of 45 patients with 14-year follow-up. *J Thorac Cardiovasc Surg* 1990, 99:838–845.

9. Kobayashi Y, Nagata S, Ohmori F, *et al.*: Serial doppler echocardiographic evaluation of bioprosthetic valves in the tricuspid position. *J Am Coll Cardiol* 1996, 27:1693–1697.

10. Arbulu A, Holmes RJ, Asfaw I: Tricuspid valvulectomy without replacement. Twenty years' experience. *J Thorac Cardiovasc Surg* 1991, 102:917–922.

11. Rivera JM, Vandervoort P, Mele D, *et al.*: Value of proximal regurgitant jet size in tricuspid regurgitation. *Am Heart J* 1996, 131:742–747

12. McGrath LB, Gonzalez-Lavin L, Bailey BM, *et al.*: Tricuspid valve operations in 530 patients. Twenty-five year assessment of early and late phase events. *J Thorac Cardiovasc Surg* 1990, 99:124–133.

13. Waller BF, Howard J, Fess S: Pathology of pulmonic valve stenosis and pure regurgitation. *Clin Cardiol* 1995, 18:45–50.

14. Richards KL: Assessment of aortic and pulmonic stenosis by echocardiography. *Circulation* 1991, 84(suppl 1):182–187.

15. Rao PS: Transcatheter treatment of pulmonary outflow tract obstruction: a review. *Prog Cardiovasc Dis* 1992, 35:119–158.

16. Chen CR, Cheng TO, Huang T, *et al.*: Percutaneous balloon valvuloplasty for pulmonic stenosis in adolescents and adults. *N Engl J Med* 1996, 335:21–25.

17. Ansari A: Isolated pulmonary valvular regurgitation: current perspectives. *Prog Cardiovasc Dis* 1991, 33:329–344.

18. Pellikka PA, Tajik AJ, Khandheria BK, *et al.*: Carcinoid heart disease. Clinical and echocardiographic spectrum in 74 patients. *Circulation* 1993, 87:1188–1196.

SELECT BIBLIOGRAPHY

Braunwald E: Valvular Heart Disease. In *Heart Disease. A Textbook of Cardiovascular Medicine*, edn 5. Edited by Braunwald E. Philadelphia: WB Saunders; 1994:1054–1060.

Hypertrophic Cardiomyopathy

Gregg M. Yamada
Joseph S. Alpert

Key Points

- Familial hypertrophic cardiomyopathy (HCM) is a rare autosomal dominant disorder linked to mutations of the cardiac myosin heavy chain genes.

- In obstructive HCM, systolic anterior motion of the mitral valve leaflet creates a subaortic pressure gradient.

- Echocardiography is the most useful study in the diagnosis of HCM, providing both anatomic and physiologic information.

- Sudden death is the most devastating consequence of HCM, associated with a 2% to 3% annual mortality rate in patients younger than 30 years of age.

- Medical therapy, including β-blockers, calcium channel blockers, and antiarrhythmic agents, is the initial treatment for most patients with HCM.

- Surgical therapy is considered for patients refractory to medical therapy.

The most characteristic morphologic feature of hypertrophic cardiomyopathy (HCM) is idiopathic left ventricular hypertrophy. Hypertrophy of the nondilated left ventricle results in abnormal diastolic function and produces a dynamic subaortic pressure gradient. The pattern of left ventricular hypertrophy is typically asymmetrical, primarily involving the anterior and basal septum; however, other segments may be selectively involved.

ETIOLOGY

Hypertrophic cardiomyopathy occurs in less than 0.2% of the population, and approximately 45% of these cases are sporadic [1]. Familial HCM is transmitted in an autosomal dominant pattern, although the anatomic distribution and severity of ventricular hypertrophy may vary within a single family.

The etiology of HCM is unknown; however, familial patterns have been linked genetically to the cardiac myosin heavy chain genes on chromosome 14 band q1. Different mutations within this gene can be identified in approximately 50% of families with HCM [2,3].

PATHOPHYSIOLOGY

Hypertrophic cardiomyopathy may be either obstructive or nonobstructive depending on the presence or absence of a dynamic subaortic pressure gradient (Fig. 1). In obstructive HCM, it is uncertain if forceful ventricular contraction produces this gradient or if a true mechanical obstruction to flow exists. Systolic anterior motion of the mitral valve leaflet is the proposed mechanism of mechanical outflow obstruction. In this hypothesis, hypertrophy of the ventricular septum results in narrowing of the left ventricular outflow tract. Consequently, during ventricular systole, blood is expelled at a higher velocity, creating a Venturi effect near the anterior mitral leaflet. The mitral leaflet is drawn into contact with the ventricular septum, creating

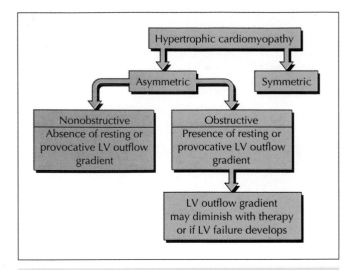

FIGURE 1 Classification of hypertrophic cardiomyopathy (HCM). LV—left ventricular.

a subaortic gradient and resulting in ventricular outflow obstruction (Fig. 2). The severity of the pressure gradient may vary at rest, during exercise, or after pharmacologic therapy.

Nonobstructive HCM is characterized by left ventricular hypertrophy in the absence of a resting pressure gradient. Diastolic dysfunction, due to decreased compliance and incomplete relaxation of the hypertrophied ventricle, leads to impaired early diastolic filling and increased left ventricular end-diastolic pressure (LVEDP). Myocardial ischemia may result from increased myocardial oxygen demand in the absence of coronary artery disease (Fig. 3).

CLINICAL MANIFESTATIONS

The clinical presentation of HCM is variable. Many patients are asymptomatic. The most common symptoms include dyspnea (diastolic dysfunction), exertional angina (myocardial ischemia), fatigue, near syncope, and syncope (decreased cardiac output or arrhythmias). The morphologic and functional severity of the cardiomyopathy are not necessarily correlated with the severity of the clinical symptoms. Patients with minimal hypertrophy may have severe complaints, whereas those with marked hypertrophy may be relatively asymptomatic.

The cardiac examination is abnormal in patients with significant subaortic pressure gradients. The characteristic systolic murmur of HCM is harsh, in character with a crescendo–decrescendo pattern. The murmur is heard best between the left sternal border and the cardiac apex and often radiates to the axilla. In patients with prominent gradients, the murmur tends to be holosystolic at the cardiac apex because of accompanying mitral regurgitation. Abrupt standing and Valsalva's maneuver accentuate the murmur of HCM, whereas squatting and isometric handgrip diminish it. The apical impulse is displaced laterally, and a systolic thrill is often palpable. Additionally, forceful atrial contraction combined with interrupted systolic flow due to left ventricular outflow obstruction may generate a triple apical impulse (Fig. 4).

DIAGNOSIS

Echocardiography is the most useful study in the diagnosis of HCM, providing morphologic and functional information (Fig. 5). The most characteristic finding is asymmetrical septal hypertrophy, which contributes to the narrowing of the left ventricular outflow tract. As previously mentioned, it is unclear if systolic anterior motion of the mitral valve leaflet is solely responsible for the subaortic pressure gradient; however, when present, a high incidence of outflow obstruction is seen. Variable degrees of mitral regurgitation are present in patients with outflow gradients. Diastolic dysfunction occurs in most patients with HCM, even in the absence of a ventricular

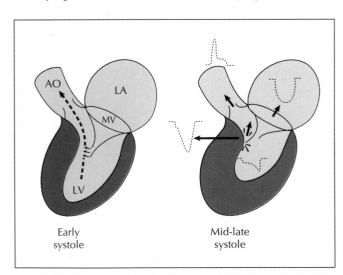

FIGURE 2 Mechanism of systolic anterior motion of the mitral leaflet in obstructive hypertrophic cardiomyopathy. AO—aorta; LA—left atrium; LV—left ventricle; MV—mitral valve. (*From* Wigle [24]; with permission.)

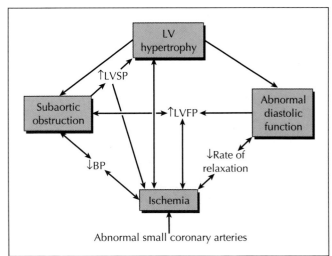

FIGURE 3 Pathophysiologic interrelationships of left ventricular (LV) hypertrophy, subaortic obstruction, diastolic dysfunction, and myocardial ischemia in hypertrophic cardiomyopathy. BP—blood pressure; LVFP—left ventricular filling pressure; LVSP—left ventricular systolic pressure. (*From* Maron *et al.* [25]; with permission.)

	HCM	MR, AS
Decreased LV cavity size Valsalva, standing, excercise, tachycardia, hypovolemia, inhalation of amyl nitrite	↑	↓
Increased LV cavity size Squatting, passive elevation of patient's legs, isometric handgrip, administration of phenylephrine	↓	No change or slight ↑

FIGURE 4 Response of murmurs of hypertrophic cardiomyopathy (HCM), aortic stenosis (AS), and mitral regurgitation (MR) to various maneuvers.

outflow gradient, but the presence of diastolic dysfunction does not always correlate with clinical symptoms [4].

The most characteristic electrocardiographic features include nonspecific ST segment and T wave changes, left ventricular hypertrophy, abnormal Q waves in the anterolateral and inferior leads (pseudoinfarction pattern), and left atrial enlargement. Large amplitude (> 10 mm), inverted T waves in the left precordial leads may identify patients with apical HCM, but the clinical significance of these T-wave inversions is uncertain [5].

The chest radiograph often is unrevealing. The left ventricle may be prominent, but the cardiac silhouette usually is not enlarged. The left atrium and atrial appendage may be prominent secondary to increased pressure and associated mitral regurgitation.

Cardiac catheterization is performed if surgery is contemplated or if the diagnosis remains uncertain despite noninvasive assessment. Typically, a left ventricular outflow gradient is detected, and LVEDP is increased. Variable degrees of atherosclerosis may be present.

Electrophysiologic study is indicated in high-risk patients, including those with a history of previous syncope, cardiac arrest, and symptomatic ventricular tachycardia. Induction of sustained ventricular tachycardia (predominantly polymor-

phic) is associated with cardiac arrest in 77% of patients and syncope in 49% [6]. The role of electrophysiologic testing in other subsets of patients with HCM is unclear. Signal-averaged electrocardiography helps to identify high-risk patients with HCM, but its utility remains uncertain [7].

COURSE AND PROGNOSIS

The clinical course is variable. It is not known why some patients remain clinically stable for years and only mildly symptomatic, whereas others deteriorate more rapidly [8]. Sudden death is the most devastating sequelae of HCM, with an annual mortality rate of 2% to 3% in patients younger than 30 years of age [9]. Much of the published literature, however, has originated from tertiary care centers and may overestimate the actual mortality rate in the general population because of selection bias [10]. Risk factors for sudden death include nonsustained ventricular tachycardia on Holter monitor, age less than 30 years, syncope, and a family history of sudden death.

The predictive value of a large resting outflow gradient is uncertain; however, decreased left ventricular end-diastolic volume is associated with future syncopal events and sudden death [11,12]. Nonsustained ventricular tachycardia on Holter monitor is associated with an 8% annual mortality rate [13]. However, ventricular tachycardia is poorly predictive of sudden death in the absence of presyncope, syncope, or inducible sustained ventricular tachycardia on electrophysiologic study [14]. Although ventricular arrhythmias are the most common cause of sudden death, acute hemodynamic derangements (both physiologic and pharmacologic) that augment the outflow gradient and diminish diastolic filling also may play a role.

Patients with mild hypertrophy without resting outflow gradients, or nonobstructive HCM, have a more favorable prognosis [15]. The prognosis in patients older than 60 years of age is similar to that in younger patients and appears related to cardiac function [16]. Patients with HCM who are symptomatic or who have a family history of sudden death should be referred to a cardiologist. Patients with asymptomatic HCM also should be restricted from competitive athletics; however, noncompetitive athletics are not contraindicated (*eg*, walking, bicycling).

TREATMENT

The clinical spectrum of disease in HCM is variable. Because of the lack of prospective, randomized, controlled trials, therapeutic comparisons are difficult, and treatment must be individualized. Medical therapy is the initial treatment of choice for most patients. Those who remain refractory to therapy or who are unable to tolerate medications are then evaluated for possible surgical correction.

Medical Therapy

The most commonly used drugs, all with proven efficacy in alleviating symptoms, are β-blockers, calcium channel blockers, and antiarrhythmic agents.

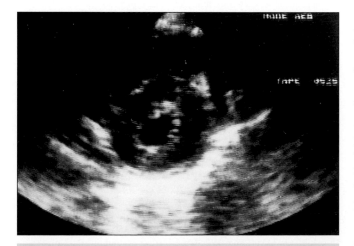

FIGURE 5 Echocardiogram of hypertrophic cardiomyopathy as seen in the short-axis view (*Courtesy of* Linda A. Pape, MD).

β-blockers are effective in alleviating angina, dyspnea, and other symptoms of HCM. Overall clinical improvement, however, may be seen in only one third to one half of all patients treated. Mechanisms of action include a decrease in myocardial oxygen consumption (negative inotropy), increased diastolic filling time (decreased heart rate), and inhibition of sympathetic stimulation during exercise. The effect of β-blockers on the incidence of sudden death has not been determined conclusively.

Verapamil is the most frequently used calcium channel blocker for the treatment of HCM. It alleviates symptoms and improves exercise function in approximately two thirds of patients who have failed β-blocker therapy [17]. A more recent report has corroborated symptomatic improvement observed in patients with HCM taking verapamil, but found no increase in exercise capacity [18]. Mechanisms of action include a decrease in the systolic left ventricular outflow gradient through negative inotropic effects and an improvement in diastolic function. Verapamil should be used with great caution in patients with severe left ventricular outflow gradients and elevated left ventricular end-diastolic pressures [19]. The effect of verapamil on sudden death remains undetermined. Only limited information is available on the use of other calcium channel blockers in the treatment of HCM.

Disopyramide is a type IA antiarrhythmic agent with negative inotropic properties that effectively relieves symptoms of HCM and improves exercise capacity [20]. Although disopyramide is potentially effective in treating supraventricular and ventricular arrhythmias in patients with HCM, a clear survival benefit remains to be proved [21].

In addition to its antiarrhythmic effects, amiodarone may relieve symptoms and improve exercise capacity in patients refractory to β-blockers and calcium channel blockers through an undefined mechanism. Although amiodarone effectively suppresses supraventricular and ventricular tachycardia, its role in preventing sudden death remains unknown.

Surgical Therapy

Patients refractory to medical therapy are considered for ventricular septal myotomy–myectomy with possible mitral valve replacement following cardiac catheterization. The operative mortality rate is approximately 5%, and a majority of patients report long-term symptomatic improvement [22]. Patients refractory to medical therapy are considered for dual-chamber pacing or ventricular septal myotomy-myectomy with possible mitral valve replacement following cardiac catheterization. The operative mortality of ventricular septal myotomy-myectomy is approximately 5%, and a majority of patients report long-term symptomatic improvement [22].

In recent years, dual-chamber pacing has been considered as an alternative method of decreasing left ventricular outflow tract obstruction. Unfortunately, much of the initial success of dual-chamber pacing was subjective, and more recently, objective studies have indicated that the effectiveness of dual-chamber pacing is inconsistent. Due to the high variability of patient response to permanent dual-chamber pacing, this therapy remains controversial. Further studies will be required to define if a particular subset of patients will benefit from this therapy [23•].

REFERENCES AND RECOMMENDED READING

Recenty published papers of particular interest have been highlighted as:

• Of interest

•• Of outstanding interest

1. Maron BJ, Bonow RO, Cannon RO, *et al.*: Hypertrophic cardiomyopathy: interrelations of clinical manifestations, pathophysiology, and therapy. *N Engl J Med* 1987, 316:780–789.

2. Watkins H, Rosenzweig A, Hwang DS, *et al.*: Characteristics and prognostic implications of myosin missense mutations in familial hypertrophic cardiomyopathy. *N Engl J Med* 1992, 326:1108–1114.

3. Garcia JA, McKenna W, Pare P, *et al.*: Mapping a gene for familial hypertrophic cardiomyopathy to chromosome 14q1. *N Engl J Med* 1989, 321:1372–1378.

4. Nihoyannopoulos P, Karatasakis G, Frenneaux M, *et al.*: Diastolic function in hypertrophic cardiomyopathy: relation to exercise capacity. *J Am Coll Cardiol* 1992, 19:536–540.

5. Alfonso F, Nihoyannopoulos P, Stewart J, *et al.*: Clinical significance of giant negative T waves in hypertrophic cardiomyopathy. *J Am Coll Cardiol* 1990, 15:965–971.

6. Fananapazir L, Tracy CM, Leon MB, *et al.*: Electrophysiologic abnormalities in patients with hypertrophic cardiomyopathy: a consecutive analysis in 155 patients. *Circulation* 1989, 80:1259–1268.

7. Cripps TR, Counihan PJ, Frenneaux MP, *et al.*: Signal-averaged electrocardiography in hypertrophic cardiomyopathy. *J Am Coll Cardiol* 1990, 15:956–961.

8. McKenna WJ: The natural history of hypertrophic cardiomyopathy. *Cardiovasc Clin* 1988, 19:135–142.

9. McKenna WJ, England D, Doi YL, *et al.*: Arrhythmia in hypertrophic cardiomyopathy. I: Influence on prognosis. *Br Heart J* 1981, 46:168–172.

10. Spirito P, Chiarella F, Carratino L, *et al.*: Clinical course and prognosis of hypertrophic cardiomyopathy in an outpatient population. *N Engl J Med* 1989, 320:749–755.

11. Maron BJ, Bonow RO, Cannon RO, *et al.*: Hypertrophic cardiomyopathy: Interrelations of clinical manifestations, pathophysiology and therapy. *N Engl J Med* 1987, 316:780–789.

12. Nienaber CA, Hiller S, Spielmann RP, *et al.*: Syncope in hypertrophic cardiomyopathy: multivariate analysis of prognostic determinants. *J Am Coll Cardiol* 1990, 15:948–955.

13. Maron BJ, Savage DD, Wolfson JK, Epstein SE: Prognostic significance of 24 hour ambulatory electrocardiographic monitoring in patients with hypertrophic cardiomyopathy: a prospective study. *Am J Cardiol* 1981, 48:252–257.

14. Fananapazir L, Chang AC, Epstein SE, McAreavey D: Prognostic determinants in hypertrophic cardiomyopathy: prospective evaluation of a therapeutic strategy based on clinical, Holter, hemodynamic and electrophysiological findings. *Circulation* 1992, 86:730–740.

15. Aron LA, Hertzeanu L, Enrique FZ, *et al.*: Prognosis of nonobstructive hypertrophic cardiomyopathy. *Am J Cardiol* 1991, 67:215–216.

16. Pelliccia F, Cianfrocca C, Romeo F, Reale A: Natural history of hypertrophic cardiomyopathy in the elderly. *Cardiology* 1991, 78:329–333.

17. Rosing DR, Idanpaan-Heikkila U, Maron BJ, *et al.*: Use of calcium-channel blocking drugs in hypertrophic cardiomyopathy. *Am J Cardiol* 1985, 55(Suppl):185B–195B.

18. Gilligan DM, Chan WL, Joshi J, *et al.*: A double-blind, placebo-controlled crossover trial of nadolol and verapamil in mild and moderately symptomatic hypertrophic cardiomyopathy. *J Am Coll Cardiol* 1993, 21:1627–1629.

19. Epstein S, Rosing D: Verapamil: Its potential for serious complications in patients with hypertrophic cardiomyopathy. *Circulation* 1981, 64:437–439.

20. Hartmann A, Kuhn J, Hopf R, *et al.*: Effect of propranolol and disopyramide on left ventricular function at rest and during exercise in hypertrophic cardiomyopathy. *Cardiology* 1992, 80:81–88.

21. Blanchard DG, Ross J: Hypertrophic cardiomyopathy: prognosis with medical or surgical therapy. *Clin Cardiol* 1991, 14:11–19.

22. McIntosh CL, Maron BL: Current operative treatment of obstructive hypertrophic cardiomyopathy. *Circulation* 1988, 78:487–494.

23.• Nishimura RA, Hayes DI, Ilstrup DM, *et al.*: Effect of dual-chamber pacing in systolic and diastolic function in patients with hypertrophic cardiomyopathy. Acute Doppler echocardiographic and catheterization hemodynamic study. *J Am Coll Cardiol* 1996, 27:421–430.

24. Wigle ED: Hypertrophic cardiomyopathy: a 1987 viewpoint (editorial). *Circulation* 1987, 73:311–322.

25. Maron BJ, Bonow RO, Cannon RO, *et al.*: Hypertrophic cardiomyopathy: Interrelations of clinical manifestations pathophysiology, and therapy. *N Engl J Med* 1987, 316:844–852.

SELECT BIBLIOGRAPHY

Blanchard DG, Ross J: Hypertrophic cardiomyopathy: Prognosis with medical or surgical therapy. *Clin Cardiol* 1991, 14:11–19.

Fananapazir L, Chang AC, Epstein SE, McAreavey D: Prognostic determinants in hypertrophic cardiomyopathy: Prospective evaluation of a therapeutic strategy based on clinical, Holter, hemodynamic and electrophysiological findings. *Circulation* 1992, 86:730–740.

Maron BJ, Bonow RO, Cannon RO, *et al.*: Hypertrophic cardiomyopathy: Interrelations of clinical manifestations, pathophysiology, and therapy. *N Engl J Med* 1987, 316:780–789.

McKenna WJ: The natural history of hypertrophic cardiomyopathy. *Cardiovasc Clin* 1988, 19:135–142.

Nienaber CA, Hiller S, Spielmann RP, *et al.*: Syncope in hypertrophic cardiomyopathy: Multivariate analysis of prognostic determinants. *J Am Coll Cardiol* 1990, 15:948–955.

Congestive Cardiomyopathy 26

Mohammad Asif

Timothy J. Regan

Key points

- Document borderline heart disease by imaging for size and function.
- Low ejection fraction without symptoms can benefit from treatment.
- ACE inhibitors improve mortality.
- Digoxin improves symptoms but not mortality.
- The diuretic dosage should be carefully adjusted according to patient's circulatory status.
- A selective subset of patients may respond to the use of β-blockers.
- Heart transplantation should be considered in refractory cases.

CLINICAL PRESENTATION

Congestive cardiomyopathy is usually associated with impaired systolic function of the ventricle. In some patients, diastolic function may be the predominant abnormality and require a different therapeutic approach. More often, however, this alteration is combined with systolic dysfunction. Symptoms usually develop gradually after an asymptomatic period with cardiac dysfunction. There are three cardinal symptoms, any of which may predominate: fatigue (caused by low cardiac output), dyspnea (Table 1) [1], and weight gain (often with venous and hepatic congestion). Some patients have noncongestive symptoms including palpitations, chest pains, fainting spells, and lightheadednesss. Orthopnea, paroxysmal nocturnal dyspnea, chronic cough, abdominal distention, right upper quadrant pain, or nausea also may be present. Occasionally, the first symptom to occur is secondary to an embolic event.

CAUSES OF CONGESTIVE CARDIOMYOPATHY

Consideration of the etiologic factor that may precipitate or play a role in the development of the diffuse myocardial disease is crucial to preventing or ameliorating the process (Table 2). More frequent causes include hypertension, alcohol consumption, age, viral infection, and drug toxicity.

Hypertension is a leading cause of heart failure resulting from both systolic and diastolic dysfunction, even without significant coronary atherosclerosis. Early symptoms are often caused by diastolic dysfunction of the left ventricle [2••]. Many patients with hypertension have evidence of abnormal left ventricular relaxation and filling, even without left ventricular hypertrophy [3].

Alcoholism is one of the most common, identifiable causes of cardiomyopathy. Over time, excessive alcohol consumption can lead to heart muscle disease without evident malnutrition. Although no specific cardiovascular markers exist, plasma tests used in the diagnosis of liver injury and urinary ethanol levels may be helpful.

TABLE 1 MECHANISMS OF DYSPNEA IN HEART FAILURE

Decreased pulmonary function
   Decreased compliance
   Increased airway resistance
Increased ventilatory drive
   Hypoxemia—$\uparrow$ PCW
   V/Q mismatching—$\uparrow$ PCW
   $\uparrow$ CO_2 production—$\downarrow$ CO-lactic acidosis
Respiratory muscle dysfunction
   Decreased strength
   Decreased endurance
   Ischemia

CO—cardiac output; PCW—mean pulmonary capillary wedge pressure; V/Q—ventilation\perfusion.
Adapted from Mancini [1].

TABLE 2 ETIOLOGIES OF CONGESTIVE CARDIOMYOPATHY

Frequent incidence
Hypertension
Ethyl alcohol abuse
Viral infection
Age
Idiopathic

Less frequent incidence
Metabolic
   Nutritional–obesity, thiamine
   Endocrinologic–diabetes mellitus, myxedema
   Uremia
   Amyloid
   Electrolyte imbalance
Infectious
   Bacterial
   Mycobacterial
   Parasitic
   Spirochetal
   Rickettsial
   Fungal
Immune
   Transplantation rejection
   Autoimmune disease (collagen diseases)
   Peripartum
Toxic
   Chemotherapeutic agents
   Catecholamines
   Cocaine
   Cobalt
Familial
   Myotonia dystrophica
   Progressive muscular dystrophy
   Neuromyopathic
Hypersensitivity
   Methyldopa
   Penicillin
   Sulfonamides
   Tetracycline
   Phenylbutazone

TABLE 3 SYSTOLIC VS. DIASTOLIC DYSFUNCTION IN HEART FAILURE

Parameters	Systolic	Diastolic
History		
Coronary heart disease	++++	+
Hypertension	++	++++
Diabetes	+++	+
Valvular heart disease	++++	–
Paroxysmal dyspnea	++	+++
Physical examination		
Cardiomegaly	+++	+
Soft heart sounds	++++	+
S_3 gallop	+++	+
S_4 gallop	+	+++
Hypertension	++	++++
Mitral regurgitation	+++	+
Rales	++	++
Edema	+++	+
Jugular venous distention	+++	+

Parameters	Systolic	Diastolic
Chest roentgenogram		
Cardiomegaly	+++	+
Pulmonary congestion	+++	+++
Electrocardiogram		
Low voltage	+++	–
Left ventricular hypertrophy	++	++++
Q waves	++	+
Echocardiograms		
Low ejection fraction	++++	–
Left ventricular dilation	++	–
Left ventricular hypertrophy	++	++++

Plus signs suggestive of dysfunction (the number reflects relative weight); minus signs not very suggestive.
Adapted from Young [5].

Progression of heart disease may be delayed or even reversed in patients who abstain from alcohol.

The normal aging process may be associated with a decline of ventricular diastolic function, whereas ventricular systolic function is unaltered at rest. Elderly persons are more prone to develop diastolic heart failure if they also have hypertension. The prevalence of systolic hypertension attributable to increased arterial stiffness is high among the elderly.

Presentation of patients with heart muscle disease caused by a viral infection is quite varied. Patients may have a distinct viral syndrome with severe cardiovascular compromise that may be fatal or may spontaneously resolve. Acute fulminating myocarditis is usually associated with left ventricular dysfunction, which may progress to dilated cardiomyopathy.

Doxorubicin and other anthracycline antitumor agents are causes of dose-related and irreversible toxic cardiomyopathy. Evidence also supports the concept that a specific diabetic cardiomyopathy without accelerated coronary atherosclerosis

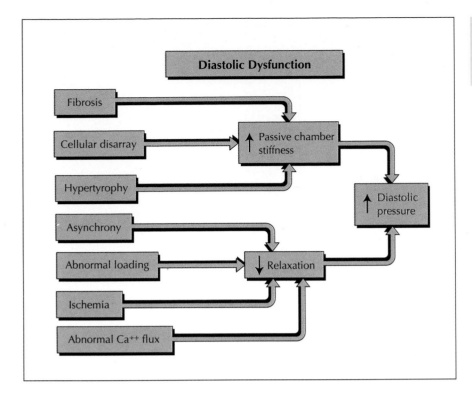

FIGURE 1 Factors responsible for diastolic dysfunction and increased left ventricular diastolic pressure (*From* Gaasch and Izzi [12]; with permission)

or hypertension increases the incidence of heart failure, more so in females than males [4•]. Finally, morbid obesity may cause circulatory congestion associated with increased blood volume and arterial pressure as well as eccentric hypertrophy.

FUNCTIONAL ABNORMALITIES

During the early stages of the disease, stroke volume is maintained despite decreased ejection fraction by increased end-diastolic volume. Increased ventricular wall stress stimulates myocyte hypertrophy, which may normalize wall stress. With further reductions of the ejection fraction, ventricular volume and stress increase and stroke volume decreases (Table 3) [5]. Increased heart rate may sustain normal cardiac output. Fluid retention, which is initially adaptive, may further increase ventricular volume, leading to pulmonary and systemic venous congestion. Multiple neurohumoral mechanisms, including the release of circulating norepinephrine and stimulation of the renin-angiotensin system, are activated. Peripheral circulation undergoes local changes in response to heart failure: fractional distribution of blood flow to the kidneys, limbs, and splanchnic beds decreases, whereas blood flow to the heart and brain is preserved [6,7]. The diminished exercise capacity of limb muscles in patients with heart failure may be due in part to chronically diminished nutritive perfusion [8,9••]. Renal hypoperfusion and altered intrarenal hemodynamics may contribute to sodium and water retention [10••,11••]. Atrial natriuretic factor partly counteracts the undesirable fluid retention promoted by vasopressin. During the advanced stage, these neurohumoral mechanisms override serum osmolarity homeostasis, causing a decrease in serum sodium levels and resistance to medical therapy.

Up to 40% of symptomatic patients have diastolic heart failure. The mechanisms responsible for diastolic dysfunction (Fig. 1) despite normal systolic function are decreased compli-

ance (increased stiffness) and impaired ventricular relaxation [12,13•]. Hence, the left ventricle is unable to fill adequately at normal diastolic pressures (Table 4). Reduced left ventricular filling volume leads to decreased stroke volume and symptoms of low cardiac output, whereas increased filling pressure leads to pulmonary congestion.

Physical Examination

Physical signs vary according to when a patient is seen during the natural history of congestive cardiomyopathy. Commonly, the patient has tachypnea, tachycardia, and usually sinus but occasionally atrial fibrillation. Systolic blood pressure may be normal, high, or low. Pulse pressure is narrow, reflecting a diminished stroke volume; there may be pulsus alternans. Jugular veins are frequently distended with a prominent V wave, a sign of tricuspid regurgitation. The liver may be enlarged and pulsatile, and ascites and peripheral edema may be present. The apical impulse is usually displaced laterally and inferiorly. The most prominent and

TABLE 4 PARAMETERS OF LEFT VENTRICULAR DIASTOLIC FILLING MEASURED BY DOPPLER ECHOCARDIOGRAPHY

Peak E	79 ± 26 cm/sec
Peak A	48 ± 22 cm/sec
E/A	1.7 ± 0.6
E Deceleration time	184 ± 24 msec
E Deceleration rate	5.6 ± 2.7 m/sec
Isovolumetric relaxation time	74 ± 26 msec
Peak pulmonary venous AR wave	19 ± 4 cm/sec

From Little and Downes [33]; with permission.

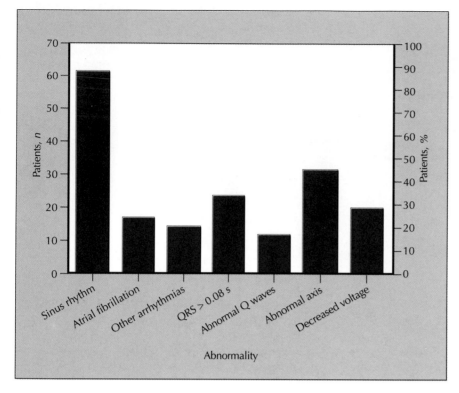

FIGURE 2 Electrocardiographic findings in a series of 74 patients with congestive cardiomyopathy. (*From* Kristinsson [14].)

useful finding on auscultation is a loud third heart sound, best heard with the bell of the stethoscope placed lightly over the cardiac apex with the patient in the left lateral position. During diastolic heart failure, however, a fourth heart sound is most common (Table 4). Systolic murmurs of functional mitral and tricuspid regurgitation may be present. Patients may have physical signs of congested lungs and pleural effusion if seen before treatment.

Laboratory Evaluation

Chest radiography reveals varying degrees of cardiomegaly and pulmonary venous congestion, ranging from pulmonary venous redistribution to frank pulmonary edema in the acutely ill patient. Kerley's B lines and peribronchial cuffing as signs of interstitial edema are common during the acute phase.

Electrocardiography (ECG) commonly reveals sinus tachycardia with nonspecific ST-T wave changes and an intraventricular conduction defect (IVCD). Other ECG abnormalities are shown in Figure 2 [14]. Holter monitoring shows a high incidence of ventricular extrasystoles, which are frequently complex. More than 70% of patients have multiformed ventricular extrasystole or ventricular couplets, and 30% to 70% have episodic nonsustained (≥ 3 beats in series and < 30 seconds) or sustained (> 30 seconds) ventricular tachycardia [15•]. Less common, but by no means infrequent, are atrial extrasystole and supraventricular tachycardia. There is no

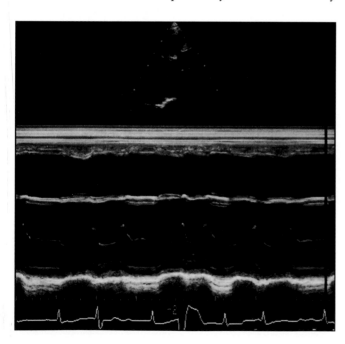

FIGURE 3 M-mode echocardiogram of a patient with congestive cardiomyopathy. The left ventricular (LV) and right ventricular (RV) cavities are dilated, and systolic motion of the interventricular septum and the LV posterior wall is decreased. Note the increased E–to–septal point separation. LV cavity in diastole = 60 mm; RV cavity in diastole = 35 mm.

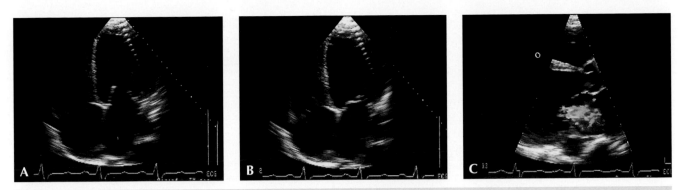

FIGURE 4 Four-chamber view in diastole (**A**), and systole (**B**) of a patient with congestive cardiomyopathy. Note the dilation of all four chambers of the heart. Color Doppler study (**C**) in the parasternal long-axis view shows functional mitral regurgitation (*See* Color Plate.)

consensus that complex or frequent ventricular arrhythmias predict sudden (presumably arrhythmic) death, but they do appear to predict total mortality. At least one annual baseline 24-hour Holter recording with repeat monitoring is recommended. Unfortunately, an unremarkable Holter recording ($\leq$ 1000 ventricular extrasystole per 24 hours) does not exclude the possibility of future sudden death.

Electrophysiologic studies may be helpful for patients with repeated runs of sustained monomorphic tachycardia or arrhythmia-induced syncope or near-syncope who have reliably induced ventricular tachycardia. In these patients, electrophysiologic study can be used to select the optimal antiarrhythmic drugs [6]. If these antiarrhythmic drugs fail to suppress the arrhythmia, the patient should have an automatic cardioverter/defibrillator device implanted.

The echocardiographic features of congestive cardiomyopathy are characteristic (Figs. 3 and 4; Table 5). Echocardiography is very useful for excluding heart failure secondary to a primary valvular disease. It is sometimes difficult to distinguish between this cardiomyopathy and ischemic left ventricular failure, because segmental wall-motion abnormalities characteristic of ischemic disease are also observed in cardiomyopathy. Radionuclide ventriculography is usually not needed unless the echocardiographic study is inadequate.

Cardiac catheterization is not routinely done unless a question exists of ischemic heart disease. Parameters obtained from right- and left-side heart catheterization are listed in Table 6. Endomyocardial biopsy is not useful except when a diagnosis of myocarditis or infiltrative disease is considered.

Assessment of Functional Status

Severity of heart failure is estimated by clinical and radiographic examination, measures of ventricular performance

---

TABLE 5 ECHOCARDIOGRAPHIC FINDINGS IN DILATED CARDIOMYOPATHY

M-mode
Increased diastolic dimensions of left ventricular and possibly right ventricular cavity
Decreased left ventricular fractional shortening
Decreased mitral valve opening in diastole
Increased E–to–septal point separation
Increased left atrial size
Pericardial effusion

Two-dimensional
Four-chamber dilation
Decreased ejection fraction
Possible mural thrombus (any chamber)
Pericardial effusion

Doppler studies (including color Doppler)
Demonstrate tricuspid and mitral regurgitation
Estimate pulmonary hypertension

TABLE 6 HEMODYNAMIC PARAMETERS IN CONGESTIVE CARDIOMYOPATHY

Systolic failure
Right-side heart catheterization
  Increased systemic and pulmonary vascular resistance
  Increased right ventricular end-diastolic pressure
  Increased mean pulmonary artery pressure
  Increased pulmonary capillary wedge pressure (reflects left ventricular filling pressure)
  Decreased cardiac index
Left-side heart catheterization
  Increased left ventricular end-diastolic pressure
  Increased left ventricular systolic and diastolic volume
  Decreased ejection fraction

Diastolic failure
Right-side heart catheterization
  Increased right ventricular end-diastolic pressure
  Increased mean pulmonary artery pressure
  Increased pulmonary capillary wedge pressure
  Decreased cardiac index
Left-side heart catheterization
  Increased left ventricular end-diastolic pressure
  Normal left ventricular systolic volume
  Normal left ventricular diastolic volume
  Normal ejection fraction

(ejection fraction and serial hemodynamic parameters measured with right heart catheterization), and exercise capacity. All these methods have limitations when used independently. In practice, the most frequently used methods are clinical, radiographic, and echocardiographic.

Patients are often classified according to the New York Heart Association (NYHA) scheme (Table 7). This classification is relatively subjective, however, and only assesses functional capacity and the degree of disability. It is not a measure of the severity of left ventricular dysfunction.

Differential Diagnosis

The differential diagnosis includes all causes of congestive heart failure. Organic valvular or congenital heart disease usually can be readily differentiated; principal differential causes include coronary artery disease with ischemic left ventricular failure, restrictive cardiomyopathy, hypertrophic cardiomyopathy, pulmonary disease, rheumatic heart disease, and effusoconstrictive pericardial disease (Table 8). Heart muscle disease secondary to specific etiologies must be recognized early to enhance the potential for reversibility.

In coronary heart disease, there often is a history of angina or myocardial infarction. Electrocardiograms can show evidence of previous myocardial infarction but may be misleading, because Q waves are present in some patients with congestive cardiomyopathy and normal coronary arteries on coronary angiography.

Clinical Course and Prognosis

The clinical course of congestive cardiomyopathy is usually steadily downhill over a period of 3 to 6 years, during which time progressive deterioration in exercise tolerance occurs and the heart size increases. (Data collected from the Framingham Heart study between the years 1948 to 1988 indicate that the median survival was 3.2 years for males and 5.4 years for females.) Patients become increasingly refractory to diuretics, leading to escalating dose requirements and, in turn, progressive electrolyte imbalance and a further increase in plasma catecholamine levels. A sudden, symptomatic deterioration should alert the clinician to look for exacerbating factors (Table 9). The most useful means of following the clinical course of the disease is a careful history and physical examination, including body-weight measurements. Serial chest radiographs, echocardiographs, or both to evaluate increasing heart size are helpful.

The single most powerful prognostic factor is ejection fraction, and in patients with ejection fractions under 20%,

---

TABLE 7 NEW YORK HEART ASSOCIATION FUNCTIONAL CLASSIFICATION

Class I

No limitation during ordinary physical activity. Does not cause undue fatigue, dyspneas, or palpitation.

Class II

Slight limitation of physical activity. Ordinary physical activity results in fatigue, palpitation, dyspnea, or angina.

Class III

Marked limitation of physical activity. Although patients are comfortable at rest, less than ordinary activity will lead to symptoms.

Class IV

Inability to carry on any physical activity without discomfort. Symptoms of congestive failure are present even at rest; with any physical activity, discomfort is increased.

TABLE 8 DIFFERENTIAL CHARACTERISTICS OF THE CARDIOMYOPATHIES

Anatomic feature	Dilated	Hypertrophic	Restrictive
Dilated ventricular cavities	+	–	–
Dilated atrial cavities	+	+	±
Hypertrophied left ventricular walls	±	+	±
Asymmetric septal hypertrophy	–	±	–
Increased heart weight	+	+	+
Abnormally thickened intramural arteries	–	+	±
Intracardiac thrombus	+	–	±
Thickened anterior mitral valve leaflet	–	+	±
Myocardial fiber disarray	–	+	–
Functional			
Systolic function	D	I	N
Diastolic function	N or abnormal	Abnormal	Abnormal
Dynamic left ventricular outflow gradient	–	±	–
Systolic anterior motion of the mitral valve	–	±	–
"Square root sign" in ventricular pressure tracings	–	–	+

D—decreased; I—increased; N—normal.

TABLE 9 PRECIPITATING FACTORS IN CHRONIC HEART FAILURE

Precipitant	Number of Patients
Lack of compliance	64
With diet	22
With drugs	6
With both (diet and drugs)	37
Uncontrolled hypertension	44
Cardiac arrhythmias	29
Atrial fibrillation	
Atrial flutter	7
Multifocal atrial tachycardia	1
Ventricular tachycardia	1
Environmental factors	19
Adequate therapy	17
Pulmonary infection	12
Emotional stress	7
Administration of inappropriate medications	
Fluid overload	4
Myocardial infarction	6
Endocrine disorders (thyrotoxicosis)	1

the 1-year mortality rate is more than 50% (Table 9). Male gender has also been shown to be associated with a high mortality rate. Adequate total body magnesium stores serve as an important prognostic indicator because of an amelioration of arrhythmia, digitalis toxicity, and hemodynamic abnormalities [16•]. When the NYHA class is integrated with maximal oxygen consumption during exercise, the mortality rate is 20% per year in patients in class III with a VO$_2$max of 10 to 15 mL/kg/min and rises to 60% in patients in class IV or VO$_2$max of less than 10 mL/kg/min [17••]. The distance walked in 6 minutes predicted both morbidity and mortality in the SOLVD trial [18•]. Percent of predicted VO$_2$max achieved provides important information that can be used to stratify risk in the ambulating patient with heart failure with ischemic or dilated etiology that exceeds that provided by measurement of VO$_2$max have an excellent short-term prognosis when treated medically and heart transplant can be deferred [19•]. Half of all deaths from severe congestive cardiomyopathy occur suddenly, associated with a tachy- or bradyarrhythmia. Less common (but important) in patients who are subjectively well with less severe ventricular dysfunction is sudden death from a major thromboembolic event.

The treatment of heart failure consists of nonpharmocologic and pharmacologic management. Nonpharmacologic management consists of restrictions of salt intake to 2 to 3 g/d, regular exercise as symptoms permit, and treating a correctible cause of ischemia by revascularization and valvular disease (Fig. 5). Factors that contribute to the survivability of patients with congestive heart failure are outlined in Table 10;

associated causes of sudden death are addressed in Table 11.

Pharmacologic Management
Systolic Dysfunction

Various circulating neurohormonal agents have a very important role in the pathophysiology of heart failure but measurement of their levels is of little value in the routine assessment and management of patients with heart failure [10••]. Myocarditis is a rare cause of rapidly progressive heart failure and requires myocardial biopsy to establish the diagnosis. There is no evidence that immunosupressive therapy is beneficial [10••].

Goals for the management of systolic dysfunction are as follows:

1. Short-term goal: relief of symptoms and improvement of the quality of life; drugs include diuretics, vasodilators, and digoxin.
2. Long-term goal: prolonging life by slowing, halting, or actually reversing the progressive left ventricular dysfunction.
3. Prevention of life-threatening ventricular arrhythmias and systemic emboli.
4. Ultimately, the proper selection of patients for cardiac transplantation.
5. Cardiac rehabilitation.
6. New approaches.

Diuretics in patients with fluid overload can relieve circulatory congestion and the accompanying pulmonary and peripheral edema. Thiazide diuretics administered intermittently two or three times weekly may be adequate to maintain normal intravascular volume in mild states of congestion but the daily administration of a loop diuretic such as furosemide is necessary when the congestion is more severe or when impaired renal function reduces the response to thiazides. In more resistant cases proximal tubular diuretics such as metolozone, 2.5 mg to 5 mg daily or intermittently given 1 hour before furosemide, may be effective while monitoring serum potassium levels [11••].

Vasodilators: Data from the V-HeFT I and II trials [10••] established the role of isosorbide dinitrate (ISN) and hydralazine for patients with functional class II and III heart failure. Although angiotensin-converting enzyme (ACE) inhibitors are the cornerstone of treatment for heart failure, ISN and hydralazine should be considered when ACE inhibitors are not tolerated because of symptomatic hypotension, azotemia, hyperkalemia, cough, rash, or angioedema. Although the target daily dose in clinical trials was 300 mg of hydralazine and 160 mg of ISN, an initial dose of 5 to 10 mg of ISN three times daily and 10 mg of hydralazine four times daily should be gradually increased toward the target level as long as tolerated. A minimal 10-hour nitrate-free period at night should be maintained to avoid nitrate tolerance.

Digoxin: Although the therapeutic efficacy of digoxin in patients with heart failure and normal sinus rhythm has long been controversial, recent evidence indicates that drug therapy withdrawal can adversely affect symptoms of heart failure. The most recently completed trial by the Digitalis Investigation Group (DIG) showed no significant effect of

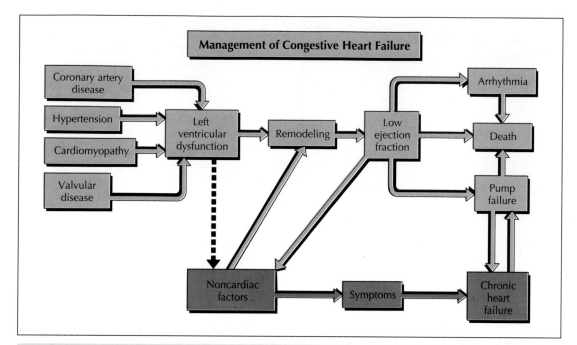

FIGURE 5 Management of congestive heart failure. The treatment of heart failure involves counteracting two related by largely independent processes. Left ventricular dysfunction, regardless of cause (coronary artery diseases, cardiomyopathy, hypertension, or valvular disease), develops through ventricular remodeling that results in a dialted chamber with a low ejection fraction, leading to episodes of arrhythmia, progressive pump failure, and premature death. Noncardiac factors (neurohormonal stimulation, endothelial dysfunction, vasconstriction, and renal sodium retention) may or may not be stimulated by left ventricular dysfunction, vasoconstriction, and renal sodium retention) may or may not be stimulated by left ventricular dysfunction, but ultimately contribute to the same progressive process of cardiac remodeling; the noncardiac factors independently cause the dyspnea, fatigue, and edema that are characteristic of the clinical syndrome of congestive heart failure. (*From* Cohn [20]; with permission.)

TABLE 10 FACTORS AFFECTING SURVIVAL IN PATIENTS WITH CONGESTIVE HEART FAILURE

Clinical

Coronary artery diseases etiology
New York Heart Association Class
Exercise capacity
Heart rate at rest
Systolic arterial pressure
Pulse pressure
S_3

Hemodynamic

LV ejection fraction
RV ejection fraction
LV stroke work index
LV filling pressure
Right atrial pressure
Maximal O_2 uptake
LV systolic pressure
Mean arterial pressure
Cardiac index
Systemic vascular resistance

Biochemical

Plasma norepinephrine
Plasma renin
Plasma vasopressin
Plasma atrial natriuretic peptide
Serum sodium
Serum potassium
Total potassium stores
Serum magnesium

Electrophysiologic

Frequent ventricular asystole
Complex ventricular arrhythmias
Ventricular tachycardia
Atrial fibrillation/flutter

LV—left ventricular; RV—right ventricular.
From Cohn and Rector [34]; with permission.

TABLE 11 CAUSES OF SUDDEN DEATH IN HEART FAILURE

Underlying cause	Rhythm observed
Acute myocardial ischemia or infraction (coronary artery disease or embolus)	VT (usually polymorphic) or VF, bradycardia, EMD
Pulmonary embolism	Bradycardia, EMD
Embolic or hemorrahgic stroke	Bradycardia, polymorphic
Drugs prolonging QT interval	Polymorphic VT
Electrolyte depletion (potassium, magnesium)	Polymorphic VT
Hyperkalemia	Bradycardia
	Apparent VT*
Exaggerated vagal reflexes	Sinus bradycardia
	Complete heart block
Primary arrhythmia	
Ventricular tachyarrhythmias	VT, VF
Conduction system disease	Sinus bradycardia
	Complete heart block

EMD—Electromechanical dissociation; VF—ventricular fibrillation; VT—ventricular tachycardia.

*:Rhythms during hyperkalemia are frequently diagnosed as ventricular tachycardia. These may also be "sinoventricular rhythms" in which the prolopnged conduction causes absence of apparent atrial activity and marked widening of the QRS complex.

Adapted from Stevenson *et al.* [35]; with permission.

digoxin on mortality but reduction in the hospitalization rate in the DIG group as compared with the placebo group [11••]. The dose of digoxin should be calculated according to creatinine clearance and levels should be monitored in patients with renal insufficiency.

Inotropes: The use of dobutamine and phosphodiestase inhibitors to temporarily improve cardiac output and renal blood flow is effective in lessening symptoms and relieving refractory salt and water retention. These drugs improve quality of life and decrease hospital stays, but long-term survival benefit is unclear and warrants further evaluation [21•]. A low dose of dobutamine (2–5 µ/kg/min) or milrinone (0.375–0.75 µg/kg/min) after a loading dose of 50 µg/kg is being used in severely decompensated cases as well as in outpatients for 12 to 24 hours, or continuous outpatient therapy in patients in whom weaning is difficult as an inpatient [10••].

ACE inhibitors have a favorable effect on prevebting the progression of left ventricular dysfunction [11••]. Current recommendations based on the SOLVD, SAVE, GISSI-III, ISIS-IV, V-HeFT-II, and CONSENSUS trials are to use ACE inhibitors for all patients with significant reduction of left ventricular ejection fraction (LV EF%) (< 30%) unless contraindicated. The starting dose may be as low as 6.25 mg or 12.25 mg of capoten three times daily or 2.5 mg of enalapril every day with a goal to gradually increase the dose to a level that has been shown to reduce mortality (*ie*, 150 mg of capoten, 20 mg of enalapril, 20 mg lisinopril, or 10 mg of quinapril). Preliminary evidence from one trial suggests that ACE inhibitors may reduce the risk of coronary ischemic events and improve the endothelial dysfunction [22]. The selective angiotensin II receptor blocker, losartan, has all the benefits of conventional ACE inhibitors

with an advantage in that there is no disruption of prostaglandin and bradykinin biosynthesis [23]. One advantage of the use of ACE inhibitors to relieve symptoms is that they tend to conserve potassium by reducing the secretion of aldosterone. Consequently, hypokalemia induced by diuretics can often be prevented without the need for supplemental potassium or a potassium-sparing diuretic.

β-blockers Several trials using metoprolol have suggested that long-term β-blockade may reduce morbidity and mortality in patients with chronic heart failure [16•]. Carvedilol, a second generation β-blocker with vasodilator (α_1-blocking) and antioxidant properties revealed a 65% reduction in mortality [17••]. Further studies suggest that in addition to its favorable effects on survival, carvedilol produces important benefits in patients with moderate to severe heart failure treated with digoxin, diuretics, and an ACE inhibitor [18••].

Anticoagulants: Because thromboembolism is a potential complication with heart failure, many physicians administer anticoagulation therapy to patients with an ejection fraction of less than 20% or with an intracardiac thrombus [10••].

Antiarrhythmics: With atrial fibrillation of new onset or uncertain duration an attempt should be made to convert to normal sinus rhythym. Failure to convert should then be managed with β-blockers, or in some cases, amiodarone [19•]. Occasionally, catheter ablation or modification of the AV node with a dual-chamber pacemaker is attempted for AV synchrony and improvement of congestive heart failure [24••]. Antiarrhythmic drugs are not recommended for ventricular arrhythmia in dilated cardiomyopathy except for the treatment of ventricular tachycardia. Amiodrone substantially reduces cardiac death and hospitalization in nonischemic patients with congestive heart failure better

TABLE 12 CONTRAINDICATIONS TO HEART TRANSPLANTATION

Advanced age (> 70 years)

Irreversible hepatic, renal, or pulmonary dysfunction

Severe peripheral vascular or cerebrovascular disease

Insulin-requiring diabetes mellitus with end-organ damage

Active infection

Recent cancer with uncertain status

Psychiatric illness, poor medical compliance

Systemic disease that would significantly limit survival or rehabilitation

Pulmonary hypertension with pulmonary vascular resistance

> 6 Wood untis or 8 Wood units after treatment with vasodilators

---

than other antiarrhythmic agents [25]. RF catheter ablation is less effective for ventricular tachycardia in patients with dilated cardiomyopathy. ICD implantation in high-risk patients without symptoms is a feasible approach that may result in benefit in some patients. A large-scale randomized trial currently under way will determine the risk/benefit ratio of this management [26].

Transplantation: Heart transplantation should be considered in patient with heart failure refractory to drug therapy if there are no contraindications to the procedure (Table 12). Before labeling a patient refractory to medical treatment, however, physicians should step back and re-examine the possible patient for possible common errors in the management of heart failure including other underlying medical conditions, infection, neoplasm, inadequate doses of medicine, and the treatment diastolic versus systolic dysfunction. Cardiac transplantation improves the survival rate to about 60% after 6 years.

Cardiac rehabilitation and exercise: Intense physical activity should be discouraged, but moderate exercise to tolerance should be strongly encouraged. Recent studies have shown that exercise is well tolerated in patients with congestive heart failure and yields positive physiologic adaptation [27].

New approaches and future treatment: Drugs that inhibit the sympathetic nervous system or the renin-angiotensin system including ibiopamide, imidazole receptor agents, α_2-adrenergic receptor agents, neural endopeptidase inhibitors, ANP, BNP, angiotensin-II receptor antagonists, modulators of sympathetic activity, OPC-18790, growth hormone, interferon-α_2, thymomodulin, or drugs that manipulate nitrous oxide generation are in various stages of evolution as probable therapies for heart failure. Surgical procedures such as cardiomyoplasty, including the latissimus dorsi patch, and use of a mechanical ventricular assist device are encouraging but long-term benefit has yet to be determined [28•–32•,33].

Diastolic dysfunction

An ideal agent with purely leusitropic properties that selectively enhances myocardial relaxation without affecting left ventricular contractility or peripheral vasculature is not available. The goal of drug therapy in diastolic dysfunction is to reduce symptoms by lowering the elevated filling pressure without significantly reducing cardiac output. This reduction can be accomplished by the judicious use of diuretics and nitrates, avoiding dehydration and hypotension. β-blockers, ACE inhibitors, and calcium channel blockers have been proposed to improve diastolic dysfunction directly by augmenting ventricular relaxation or improving compliance. Agents with pure inotropic actions are not indicated in patients with normal systolic dysfunction. Patients with diastolic dysfunction that is refractory to optimal medical/surgical management should be evaluated for heart transplantation [10••].

KEY REFERENCES

Recently published papers of outstanding interest, as identified in *References and Recommended Reading*, have been annotated.

•• Iriate MM, Olea JP, Sagastagoitia D, *et al*.: Congestive heart failure due to hypertensive ventricular diastolic dysfunction. *Am J Cardiol* 1995, 76:43d–47d.

Very interesting article reviewing the various categories of hypertensive cardiomyopathy; notes that mortality due to heart failure from impair inotropism is higher than mortality due to diastolic dysfunction, but morbidity is lower.

•• S. Tellcan Am, Yonis LT, Jennison SH, *et al*.: Prognostic value of cardiomyopathy exercised testing using percent achieved of predicted peak oxygen uptake for patient with ischemic dilated cardiomyopathy. *J Am Cardiol* 1996, 27:345–352.

Showed that percent achieved of predicted VO$_2$ max is a better predictor for long-term outcome, and that patients with more than 75% predicted VO$_2$ max can be handled medically.

•• ACC/AHA Task Force Report: Guidelines for the evaluation and management of heart failure. *Circulation* 1995, 92:2764–2784.

Reviews in detail the management of heart failure.

•• Cohn JN: The management of chronic heart failure. *N Engl J Med* 1996:490–498.

Recent review article on the management of chronic heart failure clears up controversies in the treatment of heart failure as well as failure in the treatment of CHF.

•• Packer M, Bristow M, Cohn JN, *et al*.: Carvedilol US Heart Failure Study Group: Effect of carvedilol on morbidity and mortality in patient with chronic heart failure. *N Engl J Med* 1996, 334:1349–1355.

Carvedilol reduces the risk of death significantly as well as hospitalization for cardiovascular causes.

•• Doval HC, Nul DR, *et al*.: Randomized trial of low dose amiodarone in severe congestive heart failure (GESICA). *Lancet* 1994, 344:493–498.

The PRECISE Trial indicates that the administration of carvedilol to patients with moderate to severe heart failure can ameliorate symptoms, diminish disabilities and reduce morbidity associated with this disorder.

•• Packer M, Colucci WS, Sackner-Bernstein JD: Double blind placebo controlled study of the effects of carvedilol in patients with moderate to severe heart failure: the PRECISE trial. *Circulation* 1996, 94:2793–2799.

Indicates role of dual-chamber pacemaker in dilated or hypertophic cardiomyopathy.

References and Recommended Reading

Recently published papers of particular interest have been highlighted as:

• Of interest

•• Of outstanding interest

1. Mancini DM: Pulmonary factors limiting exercise capacity in patients with heart failure. *Prog Cardiovasc Dis* 1995, 37:347.

2.•• Iriate MM, Olea JP, Sagastagoitia D, *et al.*: Congestive heart failure due to hypertensive ventricular diastolic dysfunction. *Am J Cardiol* 1995, 76:43d–47d.

3. Cuocola A, Sax FI, Brush JE, *et al.*: Left ventricular hypertrophy and impaired diastolic filling in essential hypertension: diastolic mechanism for systolic dysfunction during exercise. *Circulation* 1990, 81:978.

4.• Shehadeh A , Regan TJ: Cardiac consequences of diabetes mellitus. *Clin Cardiol* 1995, 18:301–305.

5. Young JB: Assessment of heart failure. In *Heart Failure: Cardiac Function and Dysfunction*. Edited by Colucci WS. In *Atlas of Heart Disease*, vol. 4. Edited by Braunwald E. Philadelphia: Current Medicine; 1995:7.1–7.20.

6. Kulic DL, Bhandari AK, Hong R, *et al.*: Effect of acute hemodynamic decompensation on electrical inducibility of ventricular arrhythmia in patient with dilated cardiomyopathy and complex non-sustained ventricular arrhythmia. *Am Heart J* 1990, 119:878.

7. Douban S, Brodsky M, Whong D: Significance of magnesium in CHF. *Am Heart J* 1996, 132:664–671.

8. Bittner V, Weiner DH, Yusuf H, *et al.*: Prediction of mortality and morbidity with a six minute walk test in patient with LV dysfunction. *JAMA* 1993, 270:1702–1707.

9.•• S. Tellcan Am, Yonis LT, Jennison SH, *et al.*: Prognostic value of cardiomyopathy exercised testing using percent achieved of predicted peak oxygen uptake for patient with ischemic dilated cardiomyopathy. *J Am Cardiol* 1996, 27:345–352.

10.•• ACC/AHA Task Force Report: Guidelines for the evaluation and management of heart failure. *Circulation* 1995, 92:2764–2784.

11.•• Cohn JN: The management of chronic heart failure. *N Engl J Med* 1996:490–498.

12. Gaasch WH, Izzi G: Clinical diagnosis and management of left ventricular diastolic dysfunction. In *Cardiac Mechanics and Function in the Normal and Diseased Heart*. Edited by Hori M, Suga H, Baan J, Yellin EL. New York: Springer-Verlag; 1989:296.

13.• Vasan RS, Benjamin EJ, Levy D: Prevalence, clinical features and prognosis of diastolic heart failure. *J Am Cardiol* 1995, 26:1556–1574.

14. Kristinsson A: *Diagnosis, National History, and Treatment of Congestive Cardiomyopathy*. PhD Thesis: University of London, 1969.

15.• Doval HC, Nul DR, Granceli HO, *et al.*: for The GESICA-GEMA Investigation: Nonsustained ventricular tachycardia in severe heart failure: independent marker of increased mortality of sudden death. *Circulation* 1996, 94:3198–3203.

16.• Rhman MA, Daly PA, Hara K, *et al.*: Reduction in muscles sympathetic nerve activity after long term metoprolol for dialated cardiomyopathy. *Br Heart J* 1995, 74:431–436.

17.•• Packer M, Bristow M, Cohn JN, *et al.*: Carvedilol US Heart Failure Study Group: Effect of carvedilol on morbidity and mortality in patient with chronic heart failure. *N Engl J Med* 1996, 334:1349–1355.

18.•• Doval HC, Nul DR, *et al.*: Randomized trial of low dose amiodarone in severe congestive heart failure (GESICA). *Lancet* 1994, 344:493–498.

19.• Nishimura RA, Symanski JD, Hurrell DC, *et al.*: Dual chamber pacing for cardiomyopahty. *Mayo Clin Proc* 1996, 71:1077–1087.

20. Cohn JN: The management of congestive heart failure. *N Engl J Med* 1996, 335:490–498.

21.• Jennison SH, Dhar SC, Derfler MC: Outpatient use of continuous IV milranone in heart failure. *Congestive Heart Failure* 1996, Sept/Oct:15–20.

22. Yousef S, Pepine CJ, Grace C, *et al.*: Effect of cactopril on myocardial infarction and unstable angina in patient with low ejection fraction. *Lancet* 1992, 340:1173–1178.

23. Awan NA, Mason DT: Direct selective blocking of the vascular angiotensin-II receptor in therapy for hypertension and severe CHF. *Am Heart J* 1996, 131:177–185.

24.•• Packer M, Colucci WS, Sackner-Bernstein JD: Double blind placebo controlled study of the effects of carvedilol in patients with moderate to severe heart failure: the PRECISE trial. *Circulation* 1996, 94:2793–2799.

25. Massie BM, Fisher SG, Deedwani PC, *et al.*: Effect of amiodarone on clinical status and LV function with CHF. *Circulation* 1996, 93:2128–2134.

26. Levine JH, Waller T, Hoch D, *et al.*: ICD use in patient with no symptoms and at high risk. *Am Heart J* 1996, 131:59–65.

27. Kokkinos PF, Narayan P, Papdemitriou V, *et al.*: CHF and exercise training. *Congestive Heart Failure* 1996, July/Aug:33–37.

28.• Fazio S, Sabatini D, Capaldo B, *et al.*: A preliminary study of growth hormone in the treatment of dilated cardiomyopathy. *N Engl J Med* 1996, 334:809–814.

29.• Feldman MD, Park PH, Wu CC, *et al.*: Acute cardiovascular effects of OPC-18790 in patient with CHF. *Circulation* 1996, 93:474–483.

30.• Miric M, Vasil J, Bojie M: Long term follow up of patient with dilated heart muscle disease and relation with human lymphocyte interferon alpha. *Heart* 1996, 75:596–601.

31.• Sigurdsson A, Swedberg K: Role of neurohormonal activation in chronic heart failure and post myocardial infarction. *Am Heart J* 1996, 132:229–234.

32.• Moreira LF, Stolf NA, Braile DM, *et al.*: Dynamic cardiomyoplasty in South America. *Ann Thorac Surg* 1996, 61:408–412.

33. Little UC, Downes TR: Clinical evaluation of left ventricular diastolic performance. *Prog Cardiovasc Dis* 1990, 32:273.

34. Cohn JN, Rector TS: Prognosis of congestive heart failure and predictors of mortality. *Am J Cardiol* 1988, 52:25A.

35. Stevenson WG, Stevenson LW, Middlekauff HR, Saxon LA: Sudden death prevention in patients with advanced ventricular dysfunction. *Circulation* 1993, 38:2953.

Restrictive Cardiomyopathy 27

Martin E. Goldman
Edward A. Fisher

Key Points

- The hallmark of restrictive cardiomyopathy is abnormal diastolic filling of the ventricles, which are stiff because of fibrosis, hypertrophy, or secondary infiltration.
- The classic Doppler echocardiographic finding is rapid diastolic ventricular inflow and early cessation of diastolic flow.
- Differential diagnosis includes congenital, valvular, hypertensive, and pericardial disease (especially constrictive pericarditis).
- Endomyocardial biopsy can differentiate restriction from constriction and other causes of heart failure.
- Conventional treatment can temporize by relieving symptoms caused by restricted diastolic ventricular filling and subsequent passive right- and left-sided congestion.

Cardiomyopathies (diseases affecting the myocardium) are categorized as restrictive, hypertrophic, or dilated. Restrictive cardiomyopathy, the least common of these, is manifested by impaired diastolic filling of the ventricles, which are stiff as the result of fibrosis, hypertrophy, or secondary infiltration. Restrictive cardiomyopathies are more common in Africa, the tropics, and subtropics than in North America and Europe. The etiology of restrictive cardiomyopathy may be primary, including idiopathic, or secondary, resulting from a known cause or associated with a disease affecting other organ systems.

Right and left ventricular chamber sizes are usually normal, and systolic function may be preserved until late in the disease course. Wall thickness may be normal or increased, depending on the etiology [1]. Importantly, the diagnosis of restrictive cardiomyopathy is made in the absence of congenital, valvular, hypertensive, or pericardial disease, and it is essential to differentiate it from constrictive pericarditis as the latter may be surgically treated. Clinical presentation and hemodynamic data of the two may be very similar, but echocardiography, cardiac catheterization, endomyocardial biopsy, computed tomography (CT), and magnetic resonance imaging (MRI) may assist in differentiating the two diseases (Table 1).

Idiopathic causes of restrictive cardiomyopathy include "primary restriction," endomyocardial fibrosis, and eosinophilic myocardial disease. Common secondary causes of restrictive physiology include amyloidosis, sarcoidosis, glycogen storage disease (including Fabry's disease), carcinoid, hemochromatosis, and less frequently, fibroelastosis (in infants), tumors, pseudoxanthoma elasticum, and collagen-vascular diseases.

CLINICAL MANIFESTATIONS

As a result of increased myocardial stiffness, intracavitary ventricular pressure increases with minimal increases in volume. Patients may be asymptomatic, but because either ventricle may be involved, they can present with either right heart

TABLE 1 CLASSIFICATION OF RESTRICTIVE CARDIOMYOPATHIES ACCORDING TO CAUSE

Myocardial
Noninfiltrative
  Idiopathic cardiomyopathyfamilial cardiomyopathy
  Hypertrophic cardiomyopathy
  Scleroderma
  Pseudoxanthoma elasticum
  Diabetic cardiomyopathy
Infiltrative
  Amyloidosis
  Sarcoidosis
  Gaucher's disease
  Hurler's disease
  Fatty infiltration
Storage diseases
  Hemachromatosis
  Fabry's disease
  Glycogen storage disease

Endomyocardial
Endomyocardial fibrosis
Hypereosinsophilic syndrome
Carcinoid heart disease
Metastatic cancers
Radiation
Anthracycline toxicity
Drugs-induced fibrous endocarditis (serotonin, methysergide, ergotamine, mercurials, busulfan)

failure (jugular venous distention, peripheral edema, and ascites) or left heart failure (dyspnea, paroxysmal nocturnal dyspnea, or orthopnea). Because of the diastolic filling abnormality and limited ability to increase cardiac output, decreased exercise tolerance and fatigue are common. One-third of patients with idiopathic restrictive cardiomyopathy may present with thromboembolic complications [2].

Presentation is very similar to that of constrictive pericarditis, which must be excluded. The degree of jugular venous distention correlates with the severity of disease. The most prominent jugular venous pulse is the rapid y descent. Jugular venous pressure may paradoxically increase with inspiration (Kussmaul's sign). Peripheral edema, ascites, and hepatomegaly are present late in the disease. A left ventricular apical impulse may be palpable in restrictive cardiomyopathy, but not with constriction. The first and second heart sounds are normal, and there is usually a third, and less commonly, a fourth heart sound. Low output late in the disease may be characterized by sinus tachycardia and weak peripheral pulses.

DIAGNOSIS

The most common and characteristic electrocardiographic (ECG) findings are low voltage, nonspecific ST-segment and T-wave abnormalities, left-axis deviation, and Q waves mimicking infarction. Chest radiography often shows a normal heart size with signs of pulmonary edema, although an enlarged silhouette may be seen, often caused by atrial enlargement, especially in the presence of mitral or tricuspid regurgitation. There is no pericardial calcification.

M-mode and two-dimensional echocardiography generally confirm normal left and right ventricular size and are important in excluding hypertrophic cardiomyopathy and valvular heart disease. Unfortunately, echocardiographic diagnosis of pericardial thickening is technique-dependent (gain, etc.) and does not correlate well with pericardial thickness of pathologic specimens [3,4]. Digitized M-mode echocardiograms analyzing instantaneous rates of change of left ventricular chamber and posterior wall dimensions have been used with some success to study left ventricular filling abnormalities and differentiate restrictive cardiomyopathy from constrictive pericarditis. The rate of maximum left ventricular posterior wall diastolic thinning is significantly slower in restrictive cardiomyopathy than in pericardial constriction [5], and the diastolic filling period and minimal dimension to peak rate of filling interval are prolonged in restrictive cardiomyopathy, but shortened in constriction [6]. Thus, ventricular filling occurs earlier and more completely in constriction than in restriction because of the latter's noncompliant myocardium.

With constriction, the abnormal pericardium impedes normal ventricular filling and elevates end-diastolic pressures, whereas with restriction, the abnormal myocardium elevates diastolic pressures. During inspiration, the right ventricle fills as its free wall bulges out; however, with constriction, this occurs at the expense of left ventricular filling. The rigid pericardial restraint inhibits diastolic expansion of the right ventricular free wall, and the pliant interventricular septum bulges into the left ventricle, limiting its filling. With expiration, the opposite occurs: the left ventricle fills as the septum bulges into the right ventricle. These respiratory variations in ventricular filling can be detected by two-dimensional and Doppler echocardiography.

Two-dimensional echocardiography can image respiratory variations in ventricular dimensions as well as the undulating interventricular septum characteristic of constriction. Other distinctive features of constriction include abnormal diastolic flattening of the left ventricular posterior wall and early pulmonic valve opening. Hatle et al. [7] used pulsed Doppler echocardiography to differentiate constrictive pericarditis from restrictive cardiomyopathy, demonstrating respiratory-dependent changes in inflow velocity filling patterns across the mitral and tricuspid valves in patients with constriction but not with restriction. Patients with constriction showed marked changes in left ventricular isovolumic relaxation time and early mitral and tricuspid velocities at the onset of inspiration and expiration, which were not seen in patients with restriction or in normal controls. Patients with restriction, however, were more likely to have diastolic mitral or tricuspid regurgitation, indicative of marked elevation of ventricular diastolic pressure.

Appleton et al. [8] studied 14 patients with restrictive myocardial filling using pulsed Doppler echocardiography.

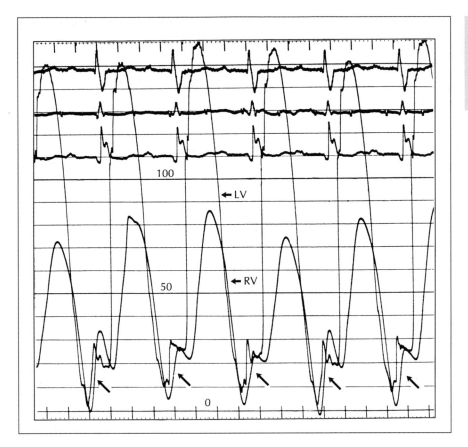

FIGURE 1 Restrictive cardiomyopathy. Hemodynamic tracings demonstrating a sharp pressure increase (*arrows*) in mid-diastole in both the left (LV) and right ventricles (RV). Note that diastolic pressures in the two ventricles are similar.

The most striking abnormalities of patients with restriction were the short periods (<150 ms) of mitral and tricuspid deceleration, indicative of rapid equalization of atrial to ventricular diastolic pressures and an early end to ventricular diastolic filling. In addition, deceleration time across the tricuspid valve was even shorter during inspiration than during apnea. Flow reversal across one of the atrioventricular valves in mid or late diastole (*ie*, diastolic mitral or tricuspid regurgitation) was seen in 11 of 14 patients because at end-diastole ventricular pressures were higher than atrial pressures. Hepatic vein flow velocities demonstrated a reversal of normal systolic (represented by *x*) to diastolic (represented by *y*) predominance. (Normally, both *x* and *y* are positive as they move toward the right atrium). In 8 of 14 patients, systolic forward flow velocity intervals were less than diastolic intervals, and 6 had forward flow only in diastole. The inspiratory increase in venous flow reversal is a sensitive indicator of restriction of right heart filling.

Color-flow Doppler echocardiography has also been used to differentiate restriction from constriction. Mancuso *et al.* [9] studied six patients with restrictive cardiomyopathy and seven with constrictive pericarditis, and found moderate or severe mitral and tricuspid regurgitation in all patients with restrictive cardiomyopathy, but only trivial regurgitation in two controls and one patient with constriction.

Ultrasonic tissue characterization uses quantitative backscatter imaging to detect abnormal cardiac tissues and can identify the soft-tissue acoustic characteristics of the restrictive cardiomyopathies. Sound waves are attenuated and reflected differently by the denser fibrosed and infiltrated myocardium. Backscatter imaging estimates the amount of ultrasound energy reflected from the myocardium back to the transducer [10]. Backscatter varies through the cardiac cycle, with peak levels at end-diastole and lowest levels at end-systole [11]. Perez *et al.* [12] used the magnitude of cyclic variation of integrated backscatter to differentiate abnormal myocardium in diabetic versus normal patients. Similar application in patients with amyloid, sarcoid, and primary restriction may be useful in detecting cardiac involvement before ventricular function has been affected and when treatment of the cardiomyopathy may be possible.

Magnetic resonance imaging also has been used to diagnose restrictive cardiomyopathy. Although MRI demonstrates a thickened pericardium in constriction, suggestive findings of restriction include enlarged atrial chambers, thick ventricular walls, impaired ventricular filling (demonstrated by a prominent signal within the atria at all phases of the cardiac cycle consistent with stasis of blood secondary to elevated ventricular diastolic pressure), and normal pericardial thickness [13]. Computed tomography can detect the pericardial abnormalities of constriction [14].

Hemodynamic and angiographic evaluation during cardiac catheterization shows that both constriction and restriction manifest preserved systolic function, prominent and rapid decline in ventricular pressures at the onset of diastole, and a rapid increase in pressure forming a dip and plateau suggestive of a square-root sign (Fig. 1) [15–17]. In restriction, left atrial pressure may exceed that of the right by 9 mm Hg, and left ventricular filling pressure usually exceeds that of the right by more than 5 mm Hg [16]. Also in restriction, the left ventricle is usually more involved than the right; with constriction, the abnormal pericardium constrains both ventricles equally.

Thus, to differentiate restrictive from constrictive physiology in patients who have elevated end-diastolic pressures in both ventricles, a rapid intravenous infusion of saline will maximize the separation of left from right ventricular end-diastolic pressure only in restriction [19, 20]. Pulmonary artery systolic pressure is usually elevated (> 45 mm Hg) with restriction and lower with constriction [21].

Coronary arteriography has been used to accentuate the pericardial thickening and lack of motion of major epicardial coronary arteries in most patients with constriction but not restriction [22]. In contrast to the major arteries, the septal perforators have an exaggerated motion in constrictive, but limited motion in restrictive cardiomyopathy [23]. Endomyocardial biopsy is the definitive method to differentiate restriction from constriction and other causes of heart failure; a specific etiology of restriction was identified in 15 of 30 patients studied with class III or IV heart failure, with 11 patients with amyloidosis [24]. Myocyte diameter, nuclear area, and severity of fibrosis can be measured on the biopsy specimen. Myocyte hypertrophy and interstitial fibrosis are frequently found in restriction as well as hypertrophic cardiomyopathy, but without the latter's myocardial disarray [25].

TREATMENT AND PROGNOSIS

Conventional treatment of restrictive cardiomyopathy is directed toward relief of symptoms caused by restricted diastolic ventricular filling and subsequent passive right- and left-sided congestion. Diuretics are used to reduce peripheral edema and ascites. Angiotensin-converting enzyme (ACE) inhibitors should be used with caution because they may reduce ventricular filling to an excessive degree, reducing cardiac output [26]. Digoxin should also be avoided because it may be arrhythmogenic, especially in patients with amyloidosis. With the onset of atrial fibrillation and loss of atrial contribution to cardiac output, patients often decompensate. Attempts should be made to maintain sinus rhythm, and amiodarone may be helpful. If patients are at risk for thromboembolic events (atrial fibrillation and low cardiac output) they may benefit from anticoagulation. Calcium blocking agents have been useful in treating diastolic abnormalities in patients with hypertensive or hypertrophic cardiomyopathy, but these agents also must be used with caution in patients with restriction because of their vasodilating effects. Glucocorticoid steroids and cytotoxic agents may play a role in specific causes of restrictive cardiomyopathy.

Patients with primary restrictive cardiomyopathy have a reasonably good 5-year survival rate, which may result from early diagnosis and recognition by noninvasive techniques. Of 26 Japanese patients, only 2 with idiopathic restriction died within 1 year, 2 died within 5 years, and 6 others died after 10 years [27]. Once the onset of heart failure occurs, however, mean survival decreases significantly. Mean survival has been reported to be 9 years after the onset of initial symptoms, but only 5 years following the onset of heart failure [28]. Of eight children studied (age range, 1 to 10 years), those having evidence of heart failure with systemic venous congestion and whose biopsies were consis-

tent with idiopathic restrictive cardiomyopathy had a median survival of only 1.4 years [29].

PRIMARY CAUSES
Idiopathic Restrictive Cardiomyopathy

Idiopathic restrictive cardiomyopathy characteristically produces a modest increase in heart weight. Atria are enlarged and atrial appendage thrombi are often noted. Ventricular chamber size and wall thickness are usually normal, and systolic function may be normal. Patchy endocardial fibrosis is commonly noted. The disease is occasionally familial and may or may not be associated with distal skeletal myopathy [25, 29, 30]. There may be a genetic predisposition to this disease, and, in some patients, a genetic locus assciated with myopathic syndromes [31]. In children, in whom the prognosis appears to be worse than in adults, studies with very small patient populations suggest that idiopathic restrictive cardiomyopathy may be more common in girls [32]. A review of the Mayo Clinic data base found eight children with the disease between 1975 and 1993 [33]. Five of these patients who had pulmonary venous congestion at presentation had a median survival of only 1 year. The clinical course of idiopathic cardiomyopathy in adults is probably better [33].

Endomyocardial Fibrosis

In addition to idiopathic cardiomyopathy, the two other primary causes of restrictive cardiomyopathy are endomyocardial fibrosis and hypereosinophilic syndrome. Endomyocardial fibrosis is a progressive disease most commonly occurring in children and young adults living in Africa, particularly Uganda and Nigeria, as well as in India, Brazil, and other tropical regions, where it may cause up to 25% of deaths from heart disease [34]. Clinically, patients present with pulmonary and venous congestion. Pathologically, ventricular involvement predominates, with extensive fibrous endocardial lesions of the inflow portion of the right and left ventricles and involvement of the mitral and tricuspid valves. Mural thrombi occur in up to 41% of patients [35,36].

Endomyocardial biopsy can confirm the diagnosis. Two-year mortality rate is approximately 50% [37], and medical therapy is not very successful. Surgical excision and stripping of the fibrous endothelial layer of endocardium and valve replacement have been successful, but this carries a high operative mortality (15% to 25%) [38,39].

Hypereosinophilic Syndrome

Hypereosinophilia (> 1500 eosinophils/mL) is seen as a response to parasitic infections, allergies and hypersensitivity, connective tissue diseases, neoplasias, autoimmune disorders, and cutaneous diseases. When no underlying cause is found, it is called idiopathic. The clinical diagnosis of idiopathic hypereosinophilic syndrome connotes end-organ (heart, central nervous system, kidney, lung, gastrointestinal, and skin) dysfunction. Cardiac involvement, occurring in approximately 50% of cases, is the most serious clinical presentation [40]. The disease may be due to local deposition of toxic eosinophillic proteins, including cationic protein and major basic protein, which ultimately cause fibrosis (Fig. 2).

Atrioventricular valves often become regurgitant. Heart failure and restrictive symptoms progress rapidly, and both medical treatment (digitalis, diuretics, afterload-reducing agents, and anticoagulation therapy) and surgical treatment may be beneficial. Glucocorticoid steroids and cytotoxic agents (hydroxyurea) have improved the prognosis of hypereosinophilic syndromes, which has traditionally been poor [40].

SECONDARY CAUSES

Amyloidosis

Amyloidosis is a systemic disease caused by extracellular deposition of insoluble amyloid protein fibrils that accumulate in tissues and cause pressure atrophy and dysfunction of the infiltrated organs. Cardiac involvement is the most common cause of death in primary amyloidosis [41], which is composed of an NH_2-terminal portion of an immunoglobulin light chain or fragment (designated AL amyloid) originating from a monoclonal population of plasma cells,

which may be derived from a malignant clone (Fig. 3). AA amyloid is found in amyloidosis secondary to various chronic inflammatory diseases such as rheumatoid arthritis, Crohn's disease, and suppurative processes such as tuberculosis, osteomyelitis, and bronchiectasis. Six types of familial amyloidosis involve "AF", amyloid-related transthyretin (prealbumin) [41]. Senile systemic amyloidosis ("AS") has been found in the hearts of elderly patients at autopsy, and is usually not of clinical significance (Fig. 4) [42]. Of 153 patients with primary amyloidosis studied by Cohen and coworkers [41], 41% had cardiac involvement and 27% evidence of heart failure. These patients had the worst prognosis: median survival was 7.7 months and 5-year survival 2.4%. In contrast, the 48% of patients who presented with renal symptoms and primary nephrotic syndrome had a 5-year survival rate of 20%. Cardiac involvement is less common in secondary or familial amyloidosis, but cardiac deposition is common in senile amyloidosis (an autosomal dominant disease). It may contribute to diastolic dysfunction, which is commonly seen, or to significant systolic dysfunction, which is rarely seen (Fig. 4) [44]. In patients older than 60 years of age in the United States, isolated cardiac involvement is four times more common in blacks than whites, and 4% of blacks are heterozygous for an

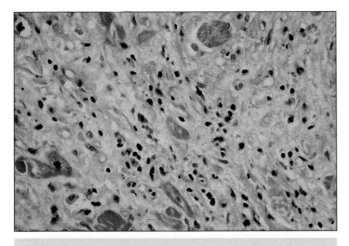

FIGURE 2 Hypereosinophilic syndrome. Endomyocardial biopsy demonstrating areas of scarring with mixed inflammatory infiltrate containing scattered eosinophils.

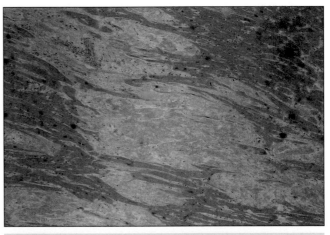

FIGURE 3 Cardiac amyloidosis. Nodular interstitial deposits of amyloid separating myocytes. This pattern is seen with AL amyloid.

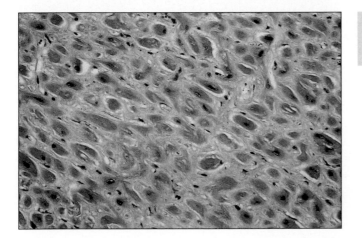

FIGURE 4 Cardiac amyloidosis. Interstitial pattern of amyloid deposition surrounding individual myocytes. This pattern is seen with senile amyloidosis.

amyloidogenic allele of the normal serum carrier protein transthyretin (isoleucine substituted valine at postion 122) [43].

Although distinctive echocardiographic features are adequate evidence for the diagnosis of amyloidosis, definitive diagnosis is made by tissue biopsy (rectal mucosa, gingiva, fat pad, liver, and kidney). Transvenous endomyocardial biopsy confirms cardiac amyloidosis.

Clinical management of amyloidosis is based on treatment of symptoms. Diuretics reduce venous congestion. Calcium blockers are relatively contraindicated because of their negative inotropic effect [45]. Additionally, ACE inhibitors should be used with caution, because they may significantly reduce ventricular filling and cardiac output. Patients may be sensitive to digitalis, which may predispose to significant arrhythmias because of the selective binding of digoxin to amyloid fibers in the heart. Although several regimens have been used to treat amyloidosis, including melphalan, prednisone, and colchicine, none has been effective [46,47]. Of two published cases of heart transplantation for amyloidosis, one patient died postoperatively and one had recurrence of amyloidosis in the allograft [48,49].

Sarcoidosis

Sarcoidosis is a multisystem granulomatous disorder of unknown etiology, with an estimated prevalence of 10 to 70 cases per 100,000 [50]. The disease occurs most commonly in adults and is more common in blacks than in whites. Involvement is manifested by bilateral hilar adenopathy, pulmonary infiltrates, and typical cutaneous and ocular lesions.

Although cardiac involvement is clinically recognizable in only 5% of patients with proven sarcoidosis, pathologic evidence of myocardial granulomas is found in approximately 25% of cases. Antemortem diagnosis is made with endomyocardial biopsy, but a negative biopsy does not rule out the disease because of its patchy involvement. Noncaseating granulomas may infiltrate the myocardium, with the preponderant deposition in the left ventricular free wall and basal intraventricular septum, but also in the right ventricle, papillary

muscles, and atria [63]. These granuloma eventually fibrose, and ventricular aneurysms may occur [63]. The clinical spectrum ranges from asymptomatic to arrhythmias (especially ventricular), conduction abnormalities, heart failure (right and/or left sided), or sudden death. Ventricular tachycardia may occur in 23% of patients with myocardial sarcoidosis [64].

The prognosis is much worse if myocardial involvement exists. The most common cause of death is sudden cardiac arrest, presumably on the basis of ventricular tachycardia and complete heart block. Patients also develop pulmonary fibrosis with respiratory failure and cor pulmonale [51]. Syncope may be common, either because of cardiac arrhythmias or pulmonary dysfunction.

Patients are treated with appropriate conventional therapy, including heart-failure medications, pacemaker implantation, and antiarrhythmic agents. Because the 1-year mortality rate of cardiac sarcoidosis may be 60%, with many patients dying suddenly, aggressive investigation and management of the ventricular arrhythmias may improve the overall mortality [51]. Additionally, steroids may be beneficial in improving pulmonary and cardiac manifestations. Transplantation is probably not a viable alternative because of the risk of recurrence.

Fabry's Disease

Fabry's disease is an X-linked disorder of glycosphingolipid metabolism from an enzyme deficiency (ceramide trihexosidase) leading to lipid deposition in vasculature of various organs, precipitating myocardial, cerebral, and renal dysfunction. Accumulation of glycosphingolipid in the lysosomes of cardiac tissue can cause increased ventricular wall thickness, simulating hypertrophic cardiomyopathy, mitral valve prolapse, ascending aortic dilatation [52], heart failure, hypertension, or mitral regurgitation. Patients usually have noncardiac presentation, including paresthesias and typical skin lesions (angiokeratomas). Patients may develop congestive heart failure related to myocardial involvement, systemic hypertension, mitral regurgitation, or significant ventricular myocardial deposition simulating hypertrophic cardiomyopathy.

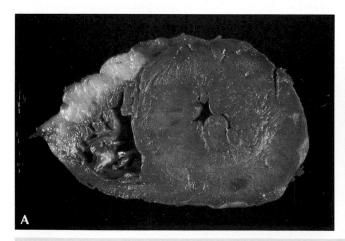

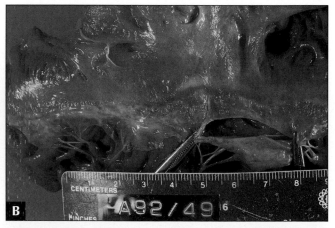

FIGURE 5 Cardiac amyloidosis. **A**, Cross-section through right and left ventricles (LV) demonstrating thickening of LV wall. The myocardium has a somewhat pale and waxy appearance.

B, Endocardial amyloid deposits of right atrium and tricuspid valve. Note the waxy appearance.

Carcinoid Heart Disease

Carcinoid heart disease occurs in 50% to 70% of patients with classic carcinoid syndrome and metastatic tumors [53]. Carcinoid tumor, most commonly originating in the appendix, secretes serotonin, which causes cutaneous flushing and bronchoconstriction. Usually, serotonin is inactivated by the liver, but hepatic metastasis facilitates development of carcinoid heart disease. The right side of the heart is affected more than the left because of pulmonary inactivation of the humeral substances [55]. Grossly visible, focal, fibrous lesions can be seen on the mural endocardium of the right atrium, right ventricle, or left ventricle, and diffuse or focal thickening of the tricuspid and pulmonic valves can be seen with rare involvement of left-sided valves. Histologic examination reveals fibrous tissue devoid of elastic fibrils [55].

Two-dimensional echocardiography may reveal dilated right-sided chambers with a thickened, echodense, tricuspid valve that is severely incompetent because of immobile leaflets. The pulmonic valve is also thickened and may be stenotic [56]. Patients are managed with α-adrenergic receptor and serotonin blockers. Diuretics may be useful in reducing symptoms of severe tricuspid regurgitation. Replacement of the tricuspid and/or pulmonic valve with heterografts has been successful [53]. Interferon treatment has been attempted with some success.

Hemochromatosis

Hemochromatosis results from excessive iron deposition because of increased iron absorption (primary hemochromatosis) or excessive transfusions or oral intake. Clinical manifestations result from deposition in the liver, pancreas, heart, and pituitary, causing fibrosis and organ failure. Hemochromatosis is one of the most common genetic diseases inherited as an autosomal recessive trait, and clinical manifestations include skin hyperpigmentation, diabetes mellitus, cardiac impairment, arthropathy, and hypogonadism.

Endomyocardial biopsy can document cardiac involvement. Patients with hemochromatosis have been successfully treated with venesection [56]; chelation therapy has also been used successfully in the treatment of congestive cardiomyopathy resulting from iron overload [57].

Anthracycline Toxicity, Radiation, and Drug-Induced Fibrous Endocarditis

Anthracyclines cause a dilated cardiomyopathy, but endomyocardial fibrosis can also produce a restrictive cardiomyopathy [58]. These diastolic findings can appear years after treatment and may not be related to dose [84]. Endomyocardial fibrosis can also be caused by drugs, including serotonin, methysergide [85], ergotamine, mercurial agents, and busulfan, and the diagnosis may necessitate the performance of a biopsy [86]. Radiation can also cause myocardial and endocardial interstitial fibrosis and an ensuing restrictive cardiomyopathy.

Conclusions

Restrictive cardiomyopathy is the least common of the major primary cardiomyopathies; however, restriction should be suspected in patients with unexplained diastolic dysfunction. Two-dimensional and Doppler evaluation are frequently diagnostic, but endomyocardial biopsy is definitive. Unfortunately, therapeutic modalities are limited for management of most patients with restrictive heart disease. Because of the similar presentation of constrictive heart disease, however, which is surgically treatable, a full investigation of the underlying disease of a patient presenting with elevated end-diastolic pressure and suspected restrictive disease is warranted.

References

1. Richardson P, McKenna W, Bristow M, *et al.*: Report of the 1995 World Health Organization/International Society and Federation of Cardiology Task Force on the Definition and Classification of Cardiomyopathies. *Circulation* 1996, 93:841–842.

2. Hirota Y, Shimizu G, Kita Y, *et al.*: Spectrum of restrictive cardiomyopathy: report of the national survey in Japan. *Am Heart J* 1990, 120:188–194.

3. Voelkel AG, Pietro DA, Follard ED, *et al.*: Echocardiographic features of constrictive pericarditis. *Circulation* 1978, 58:871–875.

4. Plehn JF, Friedman BJ: Diastolic dysfunction in amyloid heart disease: restrictive cardiomyopathy or not. *J Am Coll Cardiol* 1989, 13:54–56.

5. Morgan JM, Raposo L, Clague JC, *et al.*: Restrictive cardiomyopathy and constrictive pericarditis: Non-invasive distinction by digitized M-mode echocardiography. *Br Heart J* 1989, 61:29.

6. Janos GG, Kalavathy A, Meyer RA, *et al.*: Differentiation of constrictive pericarditis and restrictive cardiomyopathy using digitized echocardiography. *J Am Coll Cardiol* 1983, 1:541–549.

7. Hatle LK, Appleton CP, Popp RL, *et al.*: Differentiation of constrictive pericarditis and restrictive cardiomyopathy by Doppler echocardiography. *Circulation* 1989, 79: 357–370.

8. Appleton CP, Hatle LK, Popp RL, *et al.*: Demonstration of restrictive ventricular physiology by Doppler echocardiography. *J Am Coll Cardiol* 1988, 11:757–768.

9. Mancuso L, D'Agostino A, Pitrolo F, *et al.*: Constrictive pericarditis versus restrictive cardiomyopathy: the role of Doppler echocardiography in differential diagnosis. *Int J Cardiol* 1991, 31:319–328.

10. Skorton DJ, Miller JG, Wickline SA, *et al.*: Ultrasonic characterization of cardiovascular tissue. In *Cardiac Imaging*. Edited By: Marcus ML, Schelbert HR, Skorton DJ, Wolf GL. Philadelphia: WB Saunders; 1991:886–895.

11. Vered Z, Barzilai B, Mohr GA, *et al.*: Quantitative ultrasonic tissue characterization with real-time integrated backscatter imaging in normal human subjects and in patients with dilated cardiomyopathy. *Circulation* 1987, 76:1067–1073.

12. Perez JE, McGill JB, Santiago JV, *et al.*: Abnormal myocardial acoustic properties in diabetic patients and their correlation with the severity of disease. *J Am Coll Cardiol* 1992, 19:1154–1162.

13. Sechtem U, Higgins CB, Sommerhoff BA, *et al.*: Magnetic resonance imaging of restrictive cardiomyopathy. *Am J Cardiol* 1987, 59:480–482.

14. Sutton FJ, Whitley NO, Applefeld MM, *et al.*: The role of echocardiography and computed tomography in the evaluation of constrictive pericarditis. *Am Heart J* 1985, 109:350.

15. Vaitkus PT, Kussmaul WG: Constrictive pericarditic versus restrictive cardiomyopathy: a reappraisal and update of diagnostic criteria. *Am Heart J* 1991, 122:1431–1441.

16. Meaney E, Shabetai R, Bhargava V, *et al.*: Cardiac amyloidosis, constrictive pericarditis and restrictive cardiomyopathy. *Am J Cardiol* 1976, 38:547–556.

17. Shabetai R: Pathophysiology and differential diagnosis of restrictive cardiomyopathy. *Cardiovasc Clin* 1988, 19:123.

18. Benotti JR, Grossman, W: Restrictive cardiomyopathy. *Ann Rev Med* 1984, 35:113.

19. Bush CA, Stang JM, Wooley DF, *et al.*: Occult constrictive pericardial disease: diagnosis by rapid volume expansion and correction by pericardiectomy. *Circulation* 1977, 56:924–930.

20. Pacold I, Hwang MH, Palac RT, *et al.*: The effects of rapid volume expansion on the right and left cardiac filling pressures after coronary artery bypass surgery. *Chest* 1988, 93:1144–1147.

21. Child JS, Perloff JK, *et al.*: The restrictive cardiomyopathies. *Cardiol Clin* 1988, 6:289–316.

22. Alexander J, Kelly MJ, Cohen LS, *et al.*: The angiographic appearance of the coronary arteries in constrictive pericarditis. *Radiology* 1979,131:609.

23. Soto B, Shin MS, Arciniegas J, *et al.*: The septal arteries in the differential diagnosis of constrictive pericarditis. *Am Heart J* 1984, 108:332.

24. Schoenfeld MH, Supple EW, Dec GW Jr, *et al.*: Restrictive cardiomyopathy versus constrictive pericarditis: role of endomyocardial biopsy in avoiding unnecessary thoracotomy. *Circulation* 1987, 75:1012–1017.

25. Katritsis D, Wilmshurst PT, Wendon JA, *et al.*: Primary restrictive cardiomyopathy: clinical and pathologic characteristics. *J Am Coll Cardiol* 1991,18:1230–1235.

26. Bengur AR, Beekman RH, Rocchini AP, *et al.*: Acute hemodynamic effects of captopril in children with a congestive or restrictive cardiomyopathy. *Circulation* 1991, 83:523–527.

27. Hirota Y, Shimizu G, Kita Y, *et al.*: Spectrum of restrictive cardiomyopathy: report of the national survery in Japan. *Am Heart J* 1990, 120:188–194.

28. Siegel RJ, Shan PK, Fishbein MC, *et al.*: Idiopathic restrictive cardiomyopathy. *Circulation* 1984, 70:165–169.

29. Lewis AB: Clinical profile and outcome of restrictive cardiomyopathy in children. *Am Heart J* 1992, 123:6.

30. Fitzpatrick AP, Shapiro LM, Rickards AF, Poole-Wilson PA: Familial restrictive cardiomyopathy with atrioventricular block and skeletal myopathy. *Br Heart J* 1990, 63:114–118.

31. Katritsis D, Wilmshurst PT, Wendon JA, *et al.*: Primary restrictive cardiomyopathy: clinical and pathologic characteristics. *J Am Coll Cardiol* 1991, 18:1230–1235.

32. Aroney C, Bett N, Radford D: Familial restrictive cardiomyopathy. *Aust NZ J Med* 1988,18:877–878.

33. Kushwaha SS, Fallon JT, Fuster V: Restrictive cardiomyopathy. *N Engl J Med* 1997, 336:237–242.

34. Cetta F, O'Leary PW, Seward JB, Driscoll DJ. Idiopathic restrictive cardiomyopathy in childhood: diagnostic features and clinical course. *Mayo Clin Proc* 1995, 70:634–640.

35. Benotti JR, Grossman W, Cohn PF. Clinical profile of restrictive cardiomyopathy. *Circulation* 1980, 61:1206–1212.

36. Valiathan MS, Balakrishnan KG, Kartha CC, et al. A profile of endomyocardial fibrosis. *Indian J Pediatr* 1987, 54:229.

37. Gupta PN, Valiathan MS, Balakrishnan KG, *et al.*: Clinical course of endomyocardial fibrosis. *Br Heart J* 1989, 62:450–454

38. Metras D, Coulibaly AQ, Quattara K, *et al.*: Recent trends in the surgical treatment of endomyocardial fibrosis. *J Thorac Cardiovasc Surg* 1987, 28:607.

39. Martinez EE, Venturi M, Buffolo E, *et al.*: Operative results in endomyocardial fibrosis. *Am J Cardiol* 1989, 63:627–629.

40. Barretto AC, da Luz PL, de Oliveira SA, *et al.*: Determinants of survival in endomyocardial fibrosis. *Circulation* 1989, 80(Suppl 1):177–182.

41. Valiathan MS, Balakrishnan, KG, Sankarkumar R, *et al.*: Surgical treatment of endomyocardial fibrosis. *Ann Thorac Surg* 987, 43:68.

42. Mady C, Pereira Barretto AC, de Oliveira SA, *et al.*: Effectiveness of operative and non-operative therapy in endomyocardial fibrosis. *Am J Cardiol* 1989, 15:1281.

43. Fauci AS, Harley VB, Robert WC, *et al.*: The idiopathic hypereosinophilic syndrome: clinical, pathologic, and therapeutic considerations. *Ann Intern Med* 1982, 97:78–92.

44. Löffler W, *et al.*: Endocarditis parietalis fibroplastica mit bluteosinophile. Ein eigenartiges krankheitsbild. *Schweiz Med Wochenschr* 1936, 66:817–820.

45. Davies JNP, *et al.*: Endocardial fibrosis in Africans. *East Afr Med J* 1948, 25:10.

46. Gerbaux A, de Brux J, Bennaceur M, *et al.*: L'endocardite parietale fibroplastique avec eosinophile sanguine endocardite de Löffler. *Bull et Men Soc Med Hop Paris* 1956, 72:456–465.

47. Cohen AF: Amyloidosis. *N Engl J Med* 1967, 277:522–530.

48. Osserman EF, Takatsuki K, Talal N, *et al.*: The pathogenesis of "amyloidosis": studies on the role of abnormal gamma globulins and gamma globulin fragments of the Bence Jones (L-polypeptide) type in the pathogenesis of "primary" and "secondary" amyloidosis," and the "amyloidosis" associated with plasma cell myeloma. *Semin Hematol* 1964, 1:3–86.

49. Varga J, Wohlgethan JR, *et al.*: The clinical and biochemical spectrum of hereditary amyloidosis. *Semin Arthritis Rheum* 1988,18:14–28.

50. Soyka I, Steiner I, *et al.*: Prvni popis "senilniho" amyloidusrdce-I. Soyka, 1876. (Eng abstr) *Praha Cesk Patol* 1984, 20:11–13.

51. Gertz MA, Kyle RA, *et al.*: Primary systemic amyloidosis — a diagnostic primer. *Mayo Clin Proc* 1989, 64:1505–1519.

52. Pomerance A, *et al.*: Senile cardiac amyloidosis. *Br Heart J* 1965, 27:711–718.

53. Jacobson DR, Pastore RD, Yaghoubian MD, *et al.*: Variant-sequence transthyretin (isoleucine 122) in late-onset cardiac amyloidosis in black Americans. *N Engl J Med* 1997, 336:466–473.

54. Gertz MA, Falk RH, Skinner M, *et al.*: Worsening of congestive heart failure in amyloid heart disease treated by calcium channel-blocking agents. *Am J Cardiol* 1985, 55:1645.

55. Kyle RA, Greipp PR: Primary systemic amyloidosis: comparison of melphalan and prednisone versus placebo. *Blood* 1978, 52:818–827.

56. Cohen AS, Rubinow A, Anderson JJ, *et al.*: Survival of patients with primary (AL) amyloidosis colchicine-treated cases from 1976 to 1983 compared with cases seen in previous years (1961-1973). *Am J Med* 1987, 82:1182–1190.

57. Skinner M, Anderson JJ, Simms R, *et al.*: Treatment of 100 patients with primary amyloidosis: a randomized trial of melphalan, prednisone, and colchicine versus colchicine only. *Am J Med* 1996, 100:290–298.

58. Conner R, Hosenpud JD, Norman DJ, *et al.*: Heart transplantation for cardiac amyloidosis: successful one-year outcome despite recurrence of the disease. *J Heart Transplant* 1988, 7:165–167.

59. Moulin G, Cognat T, Delaye J, *et al.*: Amylose disseminee primitive familiale (nouvelle forme clinique?). *Ann Dermatol Venerol* 1988, 115:565–570.

60. Sharma ONP, *et al.*: *Sarcoidosis, Clinical Management.* Boston: Butterworth; 1978:4 –7.

61. Temple-Camp CR: Sarcoid myocarditis: a report of three cases. *NZ Med J* 1989, 102:501–502.

62. Roberts WC, McAllister HA Jr, Ferrans VJ, *et al.*: Sarcoidosis of the heart. *Am J Med* 1977, 63:86–108.

63. Roberts WC, McAllister HA, Ferrans VJ, *et al.*: Sarcoidosis of

the heart: a clinicopathologic study of 35 patients (Group I) and review of 78 previously described necropsy patients (Group II). *Am J Cardiol* 1977, 63:86.

64. Goldman ME, Cantor R, Schwartz MF, *et al.*: Echocardiographic abnormalities and disease severity in Fabry's disease. *J Am Coll Cardiol* 1986, 7:1157–1161.

65. Smith RL, Hutchins GM, Sack GH Jr, Ridolfi RL: Unusual cardiac, renal and pulmonary involvement in Gaucher's disease: interstitial glucocerbroside accumulation, pulmonary hypertension and fatal bone marrow embolization. *Am J Med* 1978, 65:352–360.

66. Renteria VG, Ferrans VJ, Roberts WC: The heart in the Hurler syndrome: gorss, histologic and ultrastructural observations in five necropsy cases. *Am J Cardiol* 1976, 38:487–501.

67. Lundin L, Hansson HE, Landelius J, *et al.*: Surgical treatment of carcinoid heart disease. *J Thorac Cardiovasc Surg* 1990, 100:552–561.

68. Millward JJ, Blake MP, Byrne MJ, *et al.*: Left heart involvement with cardiac shunt complicating carcinoid heart disease. *Aust NZ J Med* 1989, 19:716.

69. Ross EM, Roberts WC: The carcinoid syndrome: comparison of 21 necropsy subjects with carcinoid heart disease to 15 necropsy subjects without carcinoid heart disease. *Am J Med* 1985, 79:339–354.

70. Lundin L, Landelius J, Andren B, *et al.*: Transesophageal echocardiography improves the value of cardiac ultrasound in patients with carcinoid heart disease. *Br Heart J* 1990, 64:190–194.

71. McLaren GD, Muir WA, Kellermeyer RW, *et al.*: Iron overload disorders: natural history, pathogenesis, diagnosis and therapy. *CRC Crit Rev Clin Lab Sci* 1983,19:205–266.

72. Evans J, *et al.*: Treatment of heart failure in hemochromatosis. *Br Med J* 1979, 1:1075–1078.

73. Easley RM, Schreiner BF, Yu PN, *et al.*: Reversible cardiomyopathy associated with hemochromatosis. *N Engl J Med* 1972, 287:866–867.

74. Rahko PS, Salerni R, Uretsky BF, *et al.*: Successful reversal by chelation therapy of congestive cardiomyopathy due to iron overload. *J Amer Coll Cardiol* 1986 8:436–440.

75. Mortensen SA, Olsen HS, Baandup U: Chronic anthracycline cardiotoxicity: haemodynamic and histopathological manifestatins suggesting a restrictive endomyocardial disease. *Br Heart J* 1986, 55:274–282.

Infectious Myocarditis 28

Martin E. Goldman

> ### Key Points
> - Infectious myocarditis has an acute phase with a clinical spectrum ranging from no symptoms to severe heart failure.
> - The chronic phase of illness may result from autoimmune mechanisms triggered by the initial infection without residual evidence of the inciting agent.
> - Endomyocardial biopsies have limited value in most patients and should be reserved for specific subgroups.
> - The value of immunosuppressive therapy has not been established.
> - Therapy should be directed to the inciting infectious agent if specific therapy is available and to alleviating symptoms of heart failure and treating arrhythmias if life-threatening.

Myocarditis is an inflammation of the heart muscle, primarily associated with an infectious agent, although other substances also may precipitate an inflammatory response by the myocardium. Most episodes of infectious myocarditis are clinically silent and resolve spontaneously, but noninvasive technologies such as cardiac ultrasound facilitate recognition and diagnosis of even mild, asymptomatic cases. The other end of the spectrum is an acute presentation with severe heart failure. Additionally, some patients may develop dilated cardiomyopathy years after their silent episode of myocarditis. Because of its varied presentation, the actual incidence of infectious myocarditis is difficult to assess. The estimated incidence of cardiac involvement in all viral infections is 5% [1]. The mean annual incidence of acute infectious myocarditis in a defined subpopulation (Finnish Military conscripts) was 0.02%, confirmed by myocardial enzyme release and serially evolving electrocardiograph (ECG) changes [2].

DISEASE MECHANISM

In animal models, viral myocarditis is a two-component disease. The initial phase of direct cytopathogenic myocardial damage, viral replication, minimal myocyte necrosis, or cellular infiltrate is an infectious phase and may last 7 to 14 days, usually followed by complete recovery. The second phase, which develops as the virus is cleared, involves a T-lymphocytic response against a myocardial/viral antigen, resulting in myocyte destruction and, ultimately, congestive failure [2].

A cellular mechanism is the principal immune response causing cardiac dysfunction. Recognition of an immunogenic epitope by antigen-specific T lymphocytes leads to macrophage and lymphocyte infiltration. T cells of the CD4 phenotype are responsible for the recognition, activation, proliferation, and differentiation of subgroups of effect or lymphocytes. This immune response leads to a release of inflammatory cytokines, including interferon gamma, tumor necrosis factor, and interleukin-2,3,4,5,6, and 10. These cytokines lead to differentiation of B lymphocytes into antibody-secreting plasma cells and T lymphocytes into CD4 cells and cytotoxic CD8 cells. The latter attach to and lyse target cells by disrupting their plasma membrane and their DNA. Adhesion cell activation is essential for leukocyte activation and lymphocytic endothelial cell interaction, which precedes transendothelial migration. Monocytes are differentiated into activated macrophages, which release damaging proteases and cytokines. Cardiac dendritic cells and macrophages are in the front of the inflammation, and T cells are found at a distance from the necrotic areas. Myocarditis induced by group B coxsackievirus is characterized by scattered foci of myocardial necrosis and infection of myocytes by the virus. At this stage, the virus is undetectable in the myocardium and a mononuclear cell infiltration (macrophages, T lymphocytes and natural killer cells) occurs. In the chronic phase, macrophages and T cells are abundant, but the virus itself is not found. Cardiac dysfunction may be due to the number of damaged and necrosed contractile myocytes, densensitization of cardiac beta-adrenergic receptors and modification of the regulatory protein G_i, uncoupling adrenergic receptors [3]. Sole and Liu [4] propose a multifactoral mechanism of myocarditis, including repetitive cycles of microvascular constriction and spasm and reperfusion, which causes dissolution of the myocardial matrix and diffuse loss of cardiac muscle mass ultimately leading to myocardial failure.

VIRAL INFECTIOUS MYOCARDITIS

Infectious myocarditis can be caused by bacterial, fungal, parasitic, rickettsial, or spirochetal organisms, although viral agents are the most common infectious etiology (Table 1). The enteroviruses appear to be the major pathogens responsible, with more than 50% of human cases attributable to coxsackie B virus [5]. In the 10-year period from 1975 through 1985, the World Health Organization reported that coxsackie B viruses carried the highest incidence of cardiovascular disease (34.6/1000), followed by influenza B (17.4/1000), influenza A (11.7/1000), coxsackie A(9.1/1000), and cytomegalovirus (8/1000) [6]. The spectrum of clinical manifestations ranges from a totally asymptomatic response to severe congestive heart failure or life-threatening arrhythmias. Symptoms may consist of a viral prodrome, myalgia, rhinorrhea, mild fatigue, shortness of breath, palpitations, chest pain, and fever. Importantly, symptoms may mimic an acute myocardial infarction (MI) [7].

Physical examination may be normal or include sinus tachycardia and ventricular gallops and evidence of pulmonary congestion. Chest radiograph may demonstrate normal or enlarged cardiac silhouette with evidence of pulmonary congestion.

Electrocardiography may demonstrate sinus tachycardia, ST-T wave abnormalities, Q waves, atrial abnormalities, or conduction defects. Morgera and coworkers [8] reviewed ECGs from 45 consecutive patients with histologic diagnosis of active myocarditis; the ECG pattern was abnormal in 43 patients. Normal P waves, atrioventricular (AV) block, and repolarization abnormalities were common among patients with cardiac symptoms of short duration (< 1 month). Patients with a longer clinical history, however, had atrial abnormalities (left atrial enlargement and atrial fibrillation), left ventricular hypertrophy, and left bundle-branch block (LBBB). Supraventricular arrhythmias were noted in 20% of patients. Complete and advanced AV block were observed in 15% and was not a reliable marker of

TABLE 1 INFECTIOUS ETIOLOGIES OF MYOCARDITIS		
Viral	**Bacterial**	**Metazoal**
Coxsackievirus	Brucellosis	Cysticercosis
Cytomegalovirus	Diphtheria	*Echinococcus*
Echovirus	Clostridia	Schistosomiasis
Epstein-Barr virus	Endocarditis-associated myocarditis	Trichinosis
Hepatitis	*Gonococcus*	
Human immunodeficiency virus	*Meningococcus*	**Fungal**
Influenza	*Salmonella typhi*	Actinomycosis
Mumps	*Staphylococcus*	Aspergillosis
Mycoplasma pneumoniae	*Streptococcus*	Blastomycosis
Poliomyelitis	Tuberculosis	Candidiasis
Rabies		Histoplasmosis
Retrovirus	**Spirochetal**	
Rubella	Leptospirosis	**Rickettsial**
Rubeola	Lyme disease	Q fever
Varicella	Syphilis	Rocky Mountain spotted fever
		Typhus
	Protozoal	
	Amebiasis	
	Chagas' disease (*Trypanosoma cruzi*)	
	Toxoplasmosis	

myocardial damage [8]. Patients with abnormal QRS complexes had more severe left ventricular impairment and higher frequency of hypertrophy and fibrosis. The ECG abnormality that correlated best with the most severe left ventricular dysfunction was LBBB. Patients with right bundle-branch block had a shorter clinical history and higher right ventricular filling pressures. In the group of 13 patients who died, sudden death occurred in 4 of the 9 patients with abnormal QRS complexes [8]. Thus, presence of an abnormal QRS or LBBB on the ECG of a patient with myocarditis implies more severe myocardial damage and a poorer prognosis. Significant ventricular arrhythmias are another serious complication of myocarditis and may be the initial presentation [9].

Echocardiography facilitates initial diagnosis and frequent noninvasive monitoring of the patient's clinical course [10]. The echocardiogram may be normal or demonstrate varying degrees of left and right ventricular dysfunction, which may be focal or global (Fig. 1). Doppler findings may include mild valvular regurgitation or diastolic dysfunction, which may precede systolic abnormalities. Importantly, diffuse myocardial damage may be documented by involvement of the right and left ventricles and dilation of all four chambers, but some patients may have only minimal or focal left ventricular dysfunction. Echocardiographic tissue characterization and more sensitive indices of systolic and diastolic myocardial performance may detect subtle abnormalities in myocarditis [11]. Radionuclide imaging may confirm biventricular involvement. An abnormal left ventricle response to exercise, by either radionuclear-gated blood pool scanning (multiple-gated acquisition [MUGA]) or exercise echocardiography, may demonstrate abnormal ventricular reserve even with normal resting function.

Monoclonal antimyosin antibody radiolabeled with indium-111 may reveal diffuse uptake, because cellular myosin is released into the extracellular fluid due to myocar-

dial necrosis and cellular disruption [12]. In a study of patients with suspected myocarditis, antimyosin antibody imaging had a sensitivity of 100% and specificity of 58% [13]. Gallium-67 also may demonstrate diffuse uptake but has high sensitivity and low specificity [14]. The potential value of nuclear magnetic resonance imaging and positron-emission tomography in the diagnosis of myocarditis has not yet been defined.

Serologic studies including CK-MB fractions may be abnormal, indicating myocardial damage. Identification of viral particles in throat swabbing, stool, or blood and increased viral antibody titers may be useful but are not specific for the diagnosis of viral myocarditis.

With recent analysis of the genome of cardiotropic viruses, radiolabeled genetic probes can identify a viral signal in biopsy specimens even if no evidence of an inflammatory response exists. Bowles and coworkers [11] using a coxsackie B viral probe, found virus-specific RNA sequences in up to 50% of patients with myocarditis or dilated cardiomyopathy [15]. Sole and Liu used the polymerase chain reaction to rapidly duplicate and amplify specific DNA sequences for analyzing endomyocardial biopsy specimens [4]. Thus genetic probe techniques may elucidate the complex relationship between viral infections and myocarditis.

ENDOMYOCARDIAL BIOPSY

Sutton and coworkers [16] first described the transthoracic needle biopsy technique in human subjects in 1956. Subsequently, Sakakibara and Konno [17] reported the currently used technique of performing endomyocardial biopsy via a fluoroscopically guided transvenous bioptome to sample the apex, free wall, and septum of the right ventricle. Usually, the right internal jugular vein is the preferred entry site, with the subclavian veins as alternatives.

In more than 4000 biopsies performed at Stanford Univer-

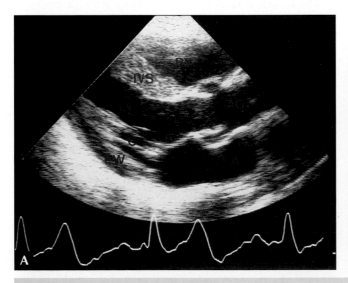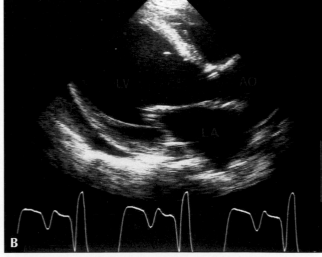

FIGURE 1 Two-dimensional echocardiogram. **A,** Long-axis view, systolic frame: normal wall thickening and cavity size. **B,** Dilated and severely hypocontractile left ventricle. A—anterior leaflet of the mitral valve; Ao—aorta; C—chordae tendonae; EFF—pericardial effusion; IVS—interventricular septum; LA—left atrium; LV—left ventricle; PW—posterior LV wall; RV—right ventricle.

sity in the 1970s, the morbidity rate was less than 1%, and there were no deaths [18]. Rare complications of transvenous endomyocardial biopsy include pneumothorax, ventricular or atrial arrhythmias, bradycardia, hypotension, and perforation of the right ventricular free wall and tricuspid regurgitation because of damaged chordae tendineae [19]. Echocardiographic guidance can substantially reduce the incidence of complications as well as radiation exposure [20]. Usually, more than five small tissue samples (1 to 3 mm) are required to obtain representative samples of the myocardium. Importantly, myocardial tissue more than 5 mm below the endocardial surface is not sampled by the bioptome. Because myocarditis may be a focal disease involving only 5% of the myocardium, sampling error accounts for most false-negative diagnoses and may occur in up to 40% of patients [21]. A larger number of biopsy specimens has a greater diagnostic yield. Histologically defined myocarditis has been diagnosed in only 5% to 30% of patients clinically suspected of having myocarditis, up to 41% of patients with acutely dilated cardiomyopathy, and up to 63% of patients with chronic dilated myopathy [22–24]. In a study of 100 consecutive right ventricular endomyocardial biopsies, a positive biopsy was found in only 11% of patients clinically thought to have myocarditis [25].

Because of differing patient populations, sampling error, and conflicting criteria for defining myocarditis, the Dallas criteria were established to standardize histologic criteria [26] (Table 2). This classification, based on findings of the first biopsy, was defined by the type, distribution, and extent of cellular infiltrate and fibrosis (Fig. 2). Specific lymphocyte counts, formerly considered critical, were no longer recommended; however, this morphologic criterion lacks clinical correlation and is prone to sampling error and interobserver variability. Thus, Lieberman and coworkers [27] introduced a clinicopathologic description of myocarditis combining clinical and histologic findings. Their four categories were fulminant myocarditis, acute, chronic active, and chronic persistent patients.

The fulminant group had acute onset of symptoms with significant left ventricular dysfunction. Their endomyocardial biopsy demonstrated foci of active myocarditis, and patients went on to complete recovery or death. Immunosuppressive therapy was of no benefit. Patients with acute myocarditis had distinct onset of cardiac symptoms with varying degrees of congestive heart failure. Their biopsies demonstrated active or borderline myocarditis according to the Dallas criteria, and they usually had resolution of their myocarditis. Immunosuppressive therapy was sometimes beneficial. The chronic active patients had varying degrees of left ventricular dysfunction, with biopsies demonstrating active or borderline myocarditis. They developed dilated cardiomyopathy, and immunosuppressant therapy was of no benefit. Patient with chronic persistent myocarditis had varying degrees of left ventricular dysfunction and no significant symptoms of congestive heart failure. Their biopsies also demonstrated active or borderline myocarditis. The classification of Lieberman and coworkers is similar to that used for viral hepatitis and attempts to integrate clinical and pathologic findings [28].

NATURAL HISTORY AND TREATMENT OF VIRAL MYOCARDITIS

Myocarditis can result in 1 of 3 outcomes: 1) complete recovery; 2) continued rapid progression to heart failure developing dilated cardiomyopathy; or 3) apparent short-term recovery followed by a latent asymptomatic period of variable duration, which is followed later by congestive heart failure and arrhythmias [29•].

The natural history of myocarditis varies with etiology. The vast majority of patients with viral myocarditis have few or no symptoms and a totally benign course. However, the incidence of viral myocarditis resulting in dilated cardiomyopathy is estimated to be 10 to 20% [4]. Cardiac autoantibodies of the organ-specific type were found in 28/110 (25%) of patients with dilated cardiomyopathy presenting with heart failure and arrhythmias, compared to only 1/160 (1%) in patients with ischemic heart failure, and 7/200 (3%) in healthy controls. At follow-up visit (14±12 months), cardiac autoantibodies were found in only 10% of patients, with a lower antialpha myosin antibody titer than at diagnosis [30•]. Thus, direct evidence of a viral infection may decrease as time elapses from the onset of acute infection. Another study by Marti found antimyosin uptake (with indium-111–labeled monoclonal antimyosin antibodies), which is indicative of sarcolemma disruption; irreversible myocyte damage was found in 16 of 19 (84%) patients with chronic idiopathic dilated cardiomyopathy. RNA viral sequences were detected in endomyocardial biopsies from 4 of these 16 [31].

TABLE 2 DALLAS CRITERIA

Initial biopsy
Myocarditis, with or without fibrosis
Borderline
No myocarditis

Inflammation
Type: eosinophilic, giant cell, granulomatous, lymphocytic, neutrophilic, mixed
Distribution: interstitial, endocardial
Extent: mild, moderate, severe

Fibrosis
Type: pericellular, perivascular, replacement
Distribution: interstitial, endocardial
Extent: mild, moderate, severe

Subsequent biopsies
Ongoing (persistent)
Resolving (healing)
Resolved (healed)

Adapted from Aretz [26]; with permission.

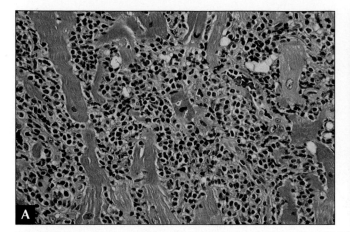
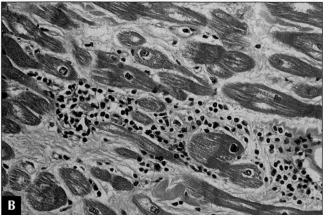

FIGURE 2 Viral myocarditis. **A,** First biopsy showing severe lymphocytic myocarditis with myocyte necrosis. **B,** Follow-up biopsy 6 months later showing resolving myocarditis with fibrosis and residual lymphocytic infiltrate.

Treatment should be geared to manage specific clinical symptoms with the standard regimen for heart failure and arrhythmias. In the early phases of myocarditis, bed rest may be beneficial in limiting myocardial oxygen consumption and ventricular wall stress. Congestive heart failure is treated with diuretics, vasodilators, angiotensin-converting enzyme inhibitors, and digitalis. Patients with myocarditis may be sensitive to digitalis during the acute stages of myocarditis. By blocking replication of certain viruses, inhibition of inter-leukin-2 (IL-2) messenger RNA, and preventing the microvascular spasm, the calcium channel–blocking agent verapamil improved the clinical and pathological course of experimental murine myocarditis [32]. Captopril, which besides being an afterload 3-reducing agent can also neutralize oxygen free radicals, had a similar beneficial effect in another animal model [33]. Human studies have not yet confirmed these findings. If the patient presents with symptomatic brad-yarrhythmias, or atrioventricular block a temporary pacemaker should be inserted. If prolonged and symptomatic, ventricular arrhythmias may require electrophysiological study for selection of appropriate management. Consideration of prolonged observation in a monitored setting to determine if the inflammatory process is transient may obviate treatment with potential proarrhythmic agents or even automatic implantable cardioverting devices.

Because of the varying criteria used and the small number of patients reported from individual centers, the National Institutes of Health (NIH)–sponsored myocarditis treatment trial was established [34•]. Enrollment was initiated in 1986 and completed in 1990. Approximately 10% of the 2200 patients screened with suspected myocarditis had a positive biopsy. The myocarditis treatment trial was designed to evaluate the efficacy of immunosuppression in patients with acute myocarditis. The randomized ill patients with unexplained heart failure and a histologic diagnosis of myocarditis with an ejection fraction of less than 45% were randomized as follows: those in the treatment group received prednisone supplemented with either cyclosporine or azathioprine; controls received no immunosuppressive therapy. The primary outcome was LV ejection fraction (EF) at 28 weeks. The 10%

mean improvement in LVEF in the treated group was not different from the 7% improvement in the control group. There was also no significant difference in mortality between the two groups. The mortality rate for the entire group was 20% at 1 year and 56% at 4.3 years [34•].

Because of the variation in diagnostic yield from biopsies and the controversy regarding appropriate therapeutic response, indications for endomyocardial biopsy for suspected myocarditis should be limited to patients with unexplained heart failure and normal coronary arteries who are experiencing progressive deterioration in their clinical course or present with significant ventricular ectopy. Though immunosuppressive therapy cannot be recommended routinely for patients with acute myocarditis that has been confirmed by biopsy, a two-month treatment trial may be worthwhile for patients with fulminant myocarditis with rapidly progressive heart failure or life-threatening arrhythmias. Unfortunately, based on current data, one cannot predict which patients with myocarditis will respond to such treatment. A meta-analysis of reports on a mixed cohort of biopsied and unbiopsied patients with myocarditis, demonstrated that a mean of 57% of patients improved with standard therapy and restricted physical activity alone. This figure was similar to the spontaneous improvement rate in biopsy-positive patients in the Myocarditis Treatment Trial (53%) [35].

Therapeutic efforts to modify the immune response have had promising results in limited animal and human studies. Antitissue necrosis factor antibody administered to a murine model of myocarditis improved their survival and reduced the myocardial lesions [36]. The immunomodulating effects of the positive inotropic agent veznarinone make it an effective treatment for encephalomyocarditis [36]. Nitrous oxide's (NO) known properties as a radical molecule, vasodilator neurotransmitter, and a cytotoxic effector of the immune system allow it to inhibit viral replication in murine myocarditis [37]. Autoimmune myocarditis in genetically susceptible mice was inhibited by blocking their interleukin-1 receptors [38].

At two-year follow-up, 21 of 26 (81%) patients with idiopathic myocarditis or idiopathic dilated cardiomyopathy with

an LVEF of less than 45% treated with immunotherapy consisting of interferon-alpha and thymomodulin improved their LVEF; only 8 of 12 (66%) of patients given standard therapy made comparable improvement. At two years, 73% of treated patients improved their functional class compared to only 25% of conventionally treated patients [39].

CARDIAC TRANSPLANTATION

Currently, cardiac transplantation is offered to patients with end-stage cardiomyopathy. Early cardiac transplantation may be an alternative for patients with acute myocarditis and a fulminant course who do not respond to conventional therapy or a trial of immunosuppressive agents. However, two studies comprising 38 patients demonstrated a higher rejection rate and lower survivor rates in patients with acute myocarditis treated with transplantation compared with controls [40,41].

SPECIFIC AGENTS OF VIRAL MYOCARDITIS

Coxsackievirus A and B, echovirus, and influenza are the most common viruses causing myocarditis, with coxsackievirus the most frequent [5,6]. Clinical manifestations such as pleurodynia, generalized myalgias, and arthralgic and upper respiratory symptoms should raise suspicion of a viral etiology. Patients may have pleuritic or pericarditic chest pain and diffuse ST-T wave abnormalities on ECG. Elevated antibody titers to cardiotrophic viruses are reported in over 50% of asymptomatic adults (probably from silent viral infection) and are of little value in establishing the diagnosis of myocarditis [43]. Atrioventricular block may require temporary pacemaker implantation. Treatment is geared to specific symptoms.

Immunosuppressive therapy in the acute phase may be deleterious, and its benefit in the second phase of illness is unclear. In most patients, viral myocarditis is a benign illness, and there is complete recovery without sequelae. Approximately 50% of patients with left ventricular dysfunction may stabilize or even demonstrate spontaneous improvement [34,35,42].

Human Immunodeficiency Virus

In 1989, Levy and coworkers [43] reported that 32 of 62 patients (52%) infected with human immunodeficiency virus (HIV) had evidence of cardiac abnormalities either by echocardiogram, ECG, or Holter monitoring. Echocardiography can detect asymptomatic pericardial effusions or biventricular dysfunction. Clinical congestive heart failure may occur in 10% to 25% of patients with AIDS. Cardiomyopathy has become a significant complication of human immunodeficiency virus - 1 infection, occurring in 6.2% of 450 patients studied prospectively [45].

The mechanism of myocardial involvement in AIDS may be related to primary viral infection with HIV or secondary to cytomegalovirus or other cardiotropic viruses, other infectious agents (tuberculosis or toxoplasmosis), ischemic cardiomyopathy, malnutrition, cytokines such as tumor necrosis factor, and in intravenous drug abusers, cocaine-related damage (Table 3). Baroldi and coworkers [46] found evidence of cardiac lymphocytic infiltrate in 20 of 26 patients (77%) with AIDS; although 9 of the 26 met the Dallas criteria for myocarditis, none had cardiac symptoms. In a study by Anderson and Virmani [47] of 71 patients with AIDS, necropsy demonstrated the incidence of fungal, mycobacterial, and protozoal opportunistic pathogens to be 58%, 42%, and 80%, respectively, with no evidence of direct HIV involvement. Kaposi's sarcoma was found in 49% of heart specimens, and 52% of patients had histologic evidence of myocarditis. Clinical characteristics associated with severe symptomatic cardiac dysfunction included low CD4 T cell counts, myocarditis associated with nonpermissive cardiotropic virus infection on endomyocardial biopsy, and persistent elevation of anti-heart antibodies. Virus-related myocarditis and cardiac autoimmunity probably play a role in the pathogenesis of progressive cardiac injury [48].

Mortality secondary to progressive heart failure, lethal ventricular arrhythmias, or pericardial tamponade may be as high as 18%. Symptoms and manifestations of heart failure are treated with digoxin, diuretics, afterload reduction, and vasodilators. Treatment alternatives are limited in patients with AIDS because of their underlying immunodeficiency. However, when the cardiac manifestations are disproportionate to other clinical signs of disease and treatable fungal or mycobacterial involvement is suspected, myocardial biopsy may be worthwhile to direct specific treatment. Pentamidine, which is used to treat *Pneumocystis carinii* pneumonia, may precipitate ventricular arrhythmias and should be used with caution because of the frequency of clinical and subclinical cardiac involvement in AIDS.

Giant Cell Myocarditis

Giant cell myocarditis, identified by the presence of giant cells in the myocardium, aorta, and other major arteries, is part of the spectrum of systemic giant cell arthritis (temporal arthritis). It is occasionally associated with autoimmune diseases such as myasthenia gravis, lupus, and thyrotoxicosis, and has an acute course manifested by chest pain and dyspnea. bradyarrhythmias and tachyrhythmias are common. The disease may respond to corticosteroid therapy adjusted to the erythrocyte sedimentation rate.

TABLE 3 CARDIAC INVOLVEMENT IN ACQUIRED IMMUNODEFICIENCY SYNDROME	
Myocarditis	**Malignant**
Viral	Kaposi's sarcoma
Opportunistic infections	Lymphoma
Autoimmune	**Toxicity**
Pericarditis	Cocaine
Autoimmune	Pentamidine
Infectious	Other drugs

Bacterial Myocarditis

Diphtherial myocarditis may occur in up to 20% of cases of diphtheria infection [49]. Dilated cardiomyopathy with congestive heart failure may develop rapidly and is the most common cause of death in diphtheria. Antitoxin therapy, erythromycin, or penicillin G and diuretics are the mainstays of treatment. Streptococcal myocarditis is a major manifestation of acute rheumatic fever pancarditis following a β-hemolytic streptococcal infection and may be the etiology of left ventricular dysfunction seen many years after the initial infection. Although ECG abnormalities (primarily ST-T and Q-Tc) may be frequent in typhoid fever (*Salmonella typhi*), clinical myocarditis is rare. Bradycardia may be a harbinger of myocarditis. Treatment of typhoid fever includes trimethoprim-sulfamethoxazole or ceftriaxone.

Lyme Carditis

Lyme disease is a nonfatal multiorgan disorder caused by *Borrelia burgodorferi* and may involve the heart, nervous system, skin, and muscles. The spirochete is transmitted by a tick *Ixodes dammini*; *Ixodes pacificus* is found in the western United States. The white-tailed deer is the dominant host for the adult tick. The initial manifestation of Lyme disease is a characteristic skin rash, erythema chronicum migrans (ECM), which occurs in 60% to 80% of cases and may clear without therapy. Additional symptoms include fever, myalgias, arthralgias, headache, lymphadenopathy, and fatigue [50]. Late persistent infection is manifested by arthritis in 40% to 50% of patients and clinical nerve palsies and meningoencephalitis in 7% to 19%. Cardiac involvement may be seen 2 to 6 weeks after the tick bite in 1.6% to 10% of patients [51].

The ECG may demonstrate no abnormality or mild ST-T abnormalities. The most common cardiac manifestation is varying degrees of AV block at the level of the AV node; McAllister and coworkers [52] found an incidence of AV block in 87% of 52 cases of Lyme carditis that they reviewed. The AV block usually resolves without requiring a permanent pacemaker. Gallium-67 or indium-111 antimyosin antibody scanning may be positive. Lyme carditis is usually treated with penicillin G 20 mμ or ceftriaxone 2 gm/d intravenously for 10 to 20 days, or oral tetracycline 250 mg four times a day [51].

Trypanosomiasis (Chagas' Disease)

Chagas' disease is caused by the hemoflagellate protozoan parasite *Trypanosoma cruzi* and is the leading cause of cardiac disease in South and Central America, especially Brazil, Chile, and Argentina [53]. The clinical course is triphasic and includes an acute, an indeterminate or latent, and a chronic stage. Acute disease follows a parasitic infection transmitted to humans through the bite of a blood-sucking insect of the order *Hemiptera* (the reduviid bug), which harbors the parasite in its gastrointestinal tract. At night, while the bug feeds on humans by piercing the skin, the bug may defecate, releasing trypanosomes that may enter the skin after the affected person scratches the bite. Localized swelling of the infected area is called a *chagoma*. The bug may bite around the human eye, leading to a conjunctival infection, unilateral periorbital edema, and swelling of the eyelid called *Romaña's sign* [53]. The acute

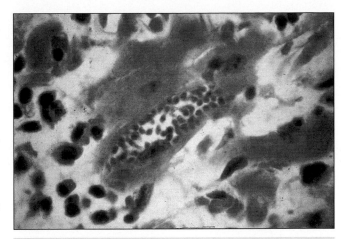

FIGURE 3 Myocarditis in acute Chagas' disease. Parasites forming a pseudocyst are seen within a cardiac myocyte. Note the surrounding inflammatory infiltrate.

phase results from trypanosomal transformation to a flagellate form in which they enter the bloodstream and infect the myocardial and muscle cells and the glia of the nervous system. Acute disease manifestations include fever, myalgias, vomiting, diarrhea, meningeal irritation, lymphadenopathy, hepatosplenomegaly, and myocarditis [54]. During this phase, parasites are seen in the cardiac fibers with a marked lymphocytic infiltrate and contraction band necrosis (Fig. 3) [55].

Acute myocarditis may develop with prolongation of the PR interval, low QRS voltage, and heart failure. Symptoms of the acute phase resolve spontaneously within 3 to 4 months in over 85% of cases. Following a latent period of clinical quiescence that may last for 10 to 50 years after the initial infection (average, 20 years), approximately 30% will develop chronic Chagas' disease. Cardiac manifestations of the chronic phase include congestive heart failure (the most common), arrhythmias, conduction defects, thromboemboli, and sudden death [56]. Megaesophagus or megacolon may develop as well.

Diagnosis is confirmed by parasites in the myocardium (Fig. 4), the complement fixation test (Machado-Guerreiro test), and enzyme-linked immunosorbent assay. Xenodiagnosis, in which the patient suspected of having Chagas' disease is bitten by a reduviid bug sucking parasites into its intestine, may be positive in 30% to 40% of patients with chronic Chagas' disease. Echocardiography may demonstrate dilated cardiomyopathy with the distinctive appearance of preserved ventricular septum function, posterior-wall hypocontractility, and apical aneurysm with possible thrombus [56].

In a recent study, the *T. cruzi* antigen was detected in 11 of 16 patients with chronic Chagas' heart disease, with histological evidence of myocarditis; the antigen was also found in 10 of 14 regions with moderate to severe myocarditis [57].

Chronic Chagas' cardiomyopathy may result from several factors. These include an intense allergic response to the parasite, autoimmune response, microvascular pathology from an infection of endothelial cells and myocytes altering synthetic function, inflammatory response, parasitic-associated fibroblast stimulation, and other factors [53].

The most common ECG changes in patients with chronic

Chagas' disease are right bundle-branch block (30% to 60% of cases) and left anterior hemiblock [58]. Ajmaline, a conduction-depressing antiarrhythmic agent, may evoke fascicular block in an infected patient before the disease is clinically manifest [59]. Atrial fibrillation and ventricular arrhythmias are common, the latter being a major cause of sudden death among patients with chronic Chagas' disease. The overall 10-year mortality is reported to be 36% and the incidence of sudden death 17.6% [60].

Treatment includes management of the clinical symptoms of congestive heart failure with anticoagulation and antiarrhythmic therapy when indicated. Analogues of primaquine may clear parasites from the blood in the early stage of infection but may have no impact on the inexorable development of the chronic phase. Currently recommended antibiotic treatment is nifurtimox, 8 to 10 mg/kg by mouth in four divided doses for 120 days [61]. Amiodarone and mexiletine appear to be useful in treating the ventricular arrhythmias of Chagas' disease. Recently, Giniger reported that electrophysiological studies may be valuable to guide treatment in Chagas' patients with significant ventricular tachycardia [62]. The potential benefit of implantable antitachycardic devices requires further investigation. Future immune therapy may prove beneficial in halting this devastating disease. Interferon-gamma given to mother rats, protected the offspring from acute *T. cruza* infection [63]. Heart transplantation has been surprisingly successful. Long-term follow-up (34±38 months) of 10 patients with Chagas' heart disease with cyclosporine immunosuppression revealed that the 7 who lived were classified in NYHA Class I. There were no signs of recurrence of Chagas' in the allograft [64]. A larger study of 22 patients who underwent orthotopic heart transplantation had a total actuarial survival at of 60% at 24 months. However, Chagas' disease reactivation was seen in 6 patients [65].

Toxoplasmosis

Toxoplasmosis is a parasitic infection caused by *Toxoplasma gondii*. Three patterns of infection are seen: diffuse, miliary type; glandular, involving only the lymph nodes; and organ infiltration. Toxoplasma infection is a potentially severe disease in the immunocompromised patient. Myocyte infection may be of little consequence until a cyst ruptures, causing myocytic necrosis, lymphocytic infiltration, and interstitial fibrosis [66]. Symptoms may include chest pain, arrhythmias, and heart failure. The diagnosis is confirmed by a toxoplasma-antibody titer greater than 1:256. Currently recommended treatment is pyrimethamine 25 mg once a day and sulfadiazine 4 g/d in four divided doses for 3 to 4 weeks [61]. Antibiotic prophylaxis for prevention of donor-acquired *T. gondii* infection in transplant recipient is recommended.

Helminthic Myocarditis

Trichinosis, caused by *Trichinella spiralis*, is fatal in 5% of cases, primarily because of myocardial involvement. Chest pain and heart failure may develop because of lymphocytic and eosinophillic infiltration. Treatment includes mebendazole 200 to 400 mg orally three times a day for 3 days, then 400 to 500 mg three times a day for 10 days, with corticosteroids [61].

Echinococcosis occurs primarily in sheep-raising areas of the world and is caused by *Echinococcus granulosus*. Dogs are the primary host, sheep the intermediate host, and human infection results from accidental ingestion of infected feces. Infestation in the liver, lung, or heart may result in a hydatid cyst. Cysts developing in the left or right ventricle may obstruct flow, rupture and embolize, or cause an anaphylactic reaction. A calcified cyst may be seen on chest radiography or two-dimensional echocardiography. Careful surgical resection is recommended if feasible. Medical therapy is with albendazole 400 mg orally twice a day for 28 days [64].

CONCLUSIONS

Myocarditis remains a challenging dilemma both in its diagnosis and management. Endomyocardial biopsy may prove beneficial in patients with fulminant heart failure unresponsive to conventional therapy or in whom an opportunistic or unusual treatable infection is suspected. Management is supportive to relieve symptoms, and when available, specific treatment is directed to the infectious agent. Research to determine the specific antigens provoking the aggressive immune reaction and new genetic approaches to more accurate diagnosis coupled with new immunomodulating therapeutic approaches may significantly reduce the acute and chronic effects of infectious myocarditis.

REFERENCES AND RECOMMENDED READING

Recently published papers of particular interest have been highlighted as:

• Of interest

•• Of outstanding interest

1. Woodruff JF: Viral myocarditis: a review. *Am J Pathol* 1980, 101:427–484.
2. Karjalainen J, Heikkila J, Nieminen M, *et al.*: Etiology of mild acute infectious myocarditis. *Acta Med Scand* 1983, 213:65–73.
3. Maze SS, Adolph RJ: Myocarditis: unresolved issues in diagnosis and treatment. *Clin Cardiol* 1990, 13:69–79.
4. Sole MJ, Liu P: Viral myocarditis: a paradigm for understanding the pathogenesis and treatment of dilated cardiomyopathy. *J Am Coll Cardiol* 1993, 22(Supplement A):99A–105A.
5. Leslie K, Blay R, Haisch, *et al.*: Clinical and experimental aspects of viral myocarditis. *Clin Microbiol Rev* 1989, 2:191–203.
6. Grist MR, Reid D: Epidemiology of viral infection of the heart. In *Viral Infections of the Heart*. Edited by Bantrala E. Hodder and Stoughton Ltd. 1993:23–31.
7. Dec GW Jr, Waldman H, Southern J, *et al.*: Viral myocarditis mimicking acute myocardial infarction. *J Am Coll Cardiol* 1992, 85–89.
8. Morgera T, Dilenarda A, Dreas L, *et al.*: Electrocardiography of myocarditis revisited. *Am Heart J* 1992, 124:456–467.
9. Wiles HB, Gillette PC, Harley RA, Upshur JK: Cardiomyopathy and myocarditis in children with ventricular ectopic rhythm. *J Am Coll Cardiol* 1992, 20:359–362.
10. Pinamonti B, Alberti E, Cigalotto A, *et al.*: Echocardiographic findings in myocarditis. *Am J Cardiol* 1988, 62:285.
11. Lieback E, Hardouin I, Meyer R, *et al.*: Clinical value of echo tissue characterization in the diagnosis of myocarditis. *Eur Heart J* 1996, 17:135–142.

12. Khaw BA, Gold HK, Yasuda T, *et al.*: Scintigraphic quantification of myocardial necrosis in patients after intravenous injection of myosin-specific antibody. *Circulation* 1986, 74:501–508.

13. Yasuda T, Palacios IF, Dec W, *et al.*: Indium[111] monoclonal antimyosin antibody imaging in the diagnosis of acute myocarditis. *Circulation* 1987, 76:306–310.

14. Wakafugi S, Kajiya S, Hayakawa M, *et al.*: Ga[67] myocardial scintigraphy in patients with acute myocarditis. *Jpn Circ* J 1987, 51:1373.

15. Bowles N, Richardson P, Olsen E, Archard L: Detection of Coxsackie B virus specific RNA sequences in myocardial biopsy samples from patients with myocarditis and dilated cardiomyopathy. *Lancet* 1986, 1:1120–1123.

16. Sutton DC, Sutton GC, Kent G: Needle biopsy of the human ventricular myocardium. *Q Bull Northwest Univ Med Sch* 1956, 30:213.

17. Sakakibara S, Konno S: Endomyocardial biopsy. *Jpn Heart J* 1962, 3:537–543.

18. Mason JW: Techniques for right and left ventricular endomyocardial biopsy. *Am J Cardiol* 1978, 41:887.

19. Fowles RE, Mason JW: Myocardial biopsy. *Mayo Clinic Proc* 1982, 57:459.

20. Miller LW, Labovitz AJ, McBride LA, *et al.*: Echocardiography guided endomyocardial biopsy: A 5 year experience. *Circulation* 1988, 78:99.

21. Chow LH, Radio SJ, Sears TD, McManus BM: Insensitivity of right ventricular endomyocardial biopsy in the diagnoses of myocarditis. *J Am Coll Cardiol* 1989, 14:1915.

22. Mason JW, Billingham ME, Ricci DR: Treatment of acute inflammatory myocarditis assisted by endomyocardial biopsy. *Am J Cardiol* 1989, 45:1037–1044.

23. Dec GW Jr, Palacios IF, Fallon JT, *et al.*: Active myocarditis in the spectrum of acute dilated cardiomyopathies: clinical features, histologic correlates, and clinical outcome. *N Engl J Med* 1985, 312:885–890.

24. Zee-Cheng CS, Tsai CC, Palmer DC, *et al.*: High incidence of myocarditis by endomyocardial biopsy in patients with idiopathic congestive cardiomyopathy. *J Am Coll Cardiol* 1984, 3:63–70.

25. Nippoldt TB, Edwards WD, Holmes DR Jr, *et al.*: Right ventricular endomyocardial biopsy: clinicopathologic correlates in 100 consecutive patients. *Mayo Clin Proc* 1982, 57:407–418.

26. Aretz HT: Myocarditis: the Dallas criteria. *Hum Pathol* 1987, 18:619–624.

27. Lieberman EB, Hutchins GM, Herskowitz A, *et al.*: Clinicopathologic description of myocarditis. *J Am Coll Cardiol* 1991, 18:1617–1626.

28. Waller BF, Slack JD, Orr CD, *et al.*: "Flaming," "Smoldering" and "Burned Out": The fireside saga of myocarditis. *J Am Coll Cardiol* 1991, 18:1627–1630.

29.• Rossen R, Birdsall H, Mann D: The enemy within: immunologic responses to cardiac tissue. *Cardiol Rev* 1996, 4:237–253.

30.• Caforio ALP, Goldman JH, Baig MK, *et al.*: Cardiac autoantibodies in dilated cardiomyopathy become undetectable with disease progression. *Heart* 1997, 77:62–67.

31. Marti V, Coll P, Ballester M, *et al.*: Interovirus persistence and myocardial damage detected by In-monoclonal antimyosin antibodies in patients with dilated cardiomyopathy. *Eur Heart J* 1996, 17:545–549.

32. Dong R, Liu P, Wee I, *et al.*: Verapamil ameliorates the clinical and pathological course of murine myocarditis. *J Clin Invest* 1992, 90:2022–2030.

33. Rezkalla S, Raikar S, Kloner RA: Treatment of viral myocarditis with focus on captopril. *Am J Cardiol* 1996, 77:634–636.

34.• Mason JW, O'Connell JB, Herskowtiz A, *et al.*: Myocarditis Treatment Trial Investigators. A clinical trial of immunosuppive therapy for myocarditis. *N Engl J Med* 1995, 333:269–275.

35. Maisih B, Herzum M, Hufnagel G, *et al.*: Immunosuppressive treatment for myocarditis and dilated cardiomyopathy. *Eur Heart J* 1995, 16(Supplement 0):153–161.

36. Matsumori A, Sasayoma S: Immunomodulating agents for the management of heart failure with myocarditis and cardiomyopathy. *Eur Heart J* 1995, 16(Supplement 0):140–143.

37. Lowenstein C, Hill S, LaFond-Walker A, *et al.*: Nitrous oxide inhibits viral replication in murine myocarditis. *J Clin Invest* 1996, 97:1837–1843.

38. Rose N, Itill S: The pathogenesis of postinfectious myocarditis. *Clin Immunopathology* 1996, 80:S92–S99.

39. Miric M, Vasiljevic J, Milovan B, *et al.*: Long-term follow-up of patients with dilated heart muscle disease treated with human leukocytic inteferon alpha or thymic hormones. *Heart* 1996, 75:596–601.

40. O'Connell JB, Dec GW, *et al.*: Results of heart transplantation for active lymphocytic myocarditis. *J Heart Transplant* 1990, 9:351–356.

41. Pham JM, Kormos RL *et al.*: Cardiac transplantation in patients with active myocarditis. *J Heart Lung Transp* 1993, 12:A146.

42. Weiss MB, Marboe CC, Escala EL, *et al.*: Natural history of untreated chronic myocarditive (active myocarditis with fibrosis). *Eur Heart J* 1987, 8(J):247.

43. Levy WS, Simon GL, Rios JC, Ross AM: Prevalence of cardiac abnormalities in human immunodeficiency virus infection. *Am J Cardiol* 1989, 63:86.

44. Reilly JM, Cunnion RE, *et al*: Frequency of myocarditis, LV dysfunction and ventricular tachycardia in AIDS. *Am J Cardiol* 1988, 62:789–793.

45. Herskowitz A, Willoughby J, Wu T-C, *et al.*: Immunopathogenesis of HIV-1 associated cardiomyopathy. *Clin Immunol Immunopathol* 1993, 68:235–241.

46. Baroldi G, Corallo S, Moroni M, *et al.*: Focal lymphocytic myocarditis in acquired immunodeficiency syndrome (AIDS): a correlative morphologic and clinical study in 26 consecutive fatal cases. *J Am Coll Cardiol* 1988, 12:463.

47. Anderson DW, Virmani R: Emerging patterns of heart disease in human immunodeficiency virus infection. *Hum Pathol* 1990, 21:253.

48. Herskowitz A, Willoughby SB, Vlahov D, *et al.*: Dilated heart muscle disease associated with HIV infection. *Eur Heart J* 1995.

49. Havaldar PV, Patil VD, Siddibhavi BM, *et al.*: Fulminant diphtheritic myocarditis. *Indian Heart J* 1989, 41:265.

50. Steere AC, Batsord WP, Wineberg M: Lyme carditis: cardiac abnormalities of Lyme disease. *Ann Intern Med* 1980, 93:8–16.

51. Steere AC: Lyme disease. *N Engl J Med* 1989, 321:586–596.

52. McAlister HF, Klementowicz PT, Andrews C, *et al.*: Lyme carditis: An importantcause of reversible heart block. *Ann Intern Med* 1989, 110:339–345.

53. Morris SA, Tannowitz HB, Wittner M, Bilezikian JP: Pathological physiological insights into the cardiomyopathy of Chagas' disease. *Circulation* 1990, 82:1900.

54. Hudson L, Britten V: Immune response to South American trypanosomiasis and its relationhship to Chagas' disease. *Br Med Bull* 1985, 41:175.

55. Edwards WD, Holmes DR Jr, Reeder GS: Diagnosis of active lymphocytic myocarditis by endomyocardial biopsy. Quantitative criterial for light microscopy. *Mayo Clin Proc* 1982, 57:419–425.

56. Oliveira JSM, Correa DA *et al.:* Cardiac thrombosis and thromboembolism in chronic Chagas' heart disease. *Am J Cardiol* 1983, 52:147–151.

57. Belloti G, Bocchi E, Moraes A, *et al.:* In vivo detection of Trypanosoma Cruzi antigens in heart of patients with chronic Chagas' heart disease. *Am Heart J* 1996, 131:301–307.

58. Rosenbaum MB, Alvarez AJ: The electrocardiogram in chronic Chagasic myocarditis. *Am Heart J* 1955, 50:492–527.

59. Chiale PA, Przybylski J, Laino RA, *et al.*: Electrocardiographic changes evoked by ajmaline in chronic Chagas' disease without clinical manifestations. *Am J Cardiol* 1982, 49:14–20.

60. McGuire JH, Hoff R, Sherlock I, *et al.*: Cardiac morbidity and mortality due to Chagas' disease: prospective electrocardiographic study of a Brazilian community. *Circulation* 1987, 75:1140–1145.

61. Mandell GL, Douglas RG Jr., Bennet JE: *Principles and Practice of Infectious Diseases: Antimicrobial Therapy 1992.* Churchill Livingstone. New York, 1992.

62. Giniger AG, Ratykeo, Lainora *et al.*: Ventricular tachycardia in Chagas' disease. *Am J Cardiol* 1992, 70:459–462.

63. Davila HD, Revelli S, Didoli G, *et al.*: Protection of young rats from acute T. Cruzi infection by interferon-gamma given to their mothers during pregnancy. *Am J Trop Med Hyg* 1996, 54:660–664.

64. Carvalho V, Sousa E, Vila J, *et al.*: Heart transplantation in Chagas disease. *Circulation* 1996, 94:1815–1817.

65. Bocchi E, Bellotti G, Mocelin A, *et al.*: Heart transplantation in chronic Chagas disease. *Ann Thorac Surg* 1996, 61:1727–1733.

66. Leak D, Meghji M: Toxoplasmic infection in cardiac disease. *Am J Cardiol* 1979, 43:841–849.

Infectious Endocarditis 29
Gordon A. Ewy

> ### *Key Points*
> - The diagnostic criteria for infectious endocarditis now include echocardiographic features.
> - The classic triad of findings in patients with infectious endocarditis is fever, organic heart murmur, and positive blood culture.
> - Cardiac auscultation is important in the prevention, diagnosis, and assessment of severity in patients with infectious endocarditis.
> - Echocardiography is used to identify vegetations or perivalvular abscesses and to determine chamber size and function and condition of the valves.
> - Infectious endocarditis is a potentially lethal disease; patients should be referred when this diagnosis is seriously considered.

DIAGNOSTIC CRITERIA

Although infectious endocarditis is rare, the annual incidence varies from two to four per 100,00 people; failure to diagnose and treat appropriately results in excess mortality and morbidity. The clinical criteria [1••] outlined in Table 1 make the task of diagnosis easier. The diagnosis is definitive when both major criteria, one major and three minor criteria, or five minor criteria are present. [1••].

One of the major criteria is a positive blood culture with typical organisms. Typical organisms include *Streptococcus viridans*, *Streptococcus bovis*, enterococcus, staphylococcus, or the HACEK group (*Haemophilus*, *Actinobacillus*, *Cardiobacterium*, *Eikenella*, and *Kingella* species). A single positive culture positive for any of these organisms fulfills the criterion of positive culture with a typical organism, except that the frequency of short-lived bacteremia in patients without endocarditis requires two positive cultures for *Streptococcus viridans*. If there is another focus of infection (*eg*, skin abscess, pneumonia), a positive blood culture becomes a minor criterion.

Persistently positive blood cultures are two positive cultures at least 12 hours apart. Persistently positive cultures are necessary if the organism is not one typically associated with infectious endocarditis.

The echocardiographic criteria are straightforward but cannot be preexistent if they are to be used as a major criterion. Nonoscillating masses are a minor echocardiographic criterion.

Predisposing conditions include the presence of an organic regurgitant cardiac murmur, prosthetic heart valves, immunologic compromise, intravenous drug use, and previous endocarditis. Vascular phenomena include embolus, Osler's nodes, Janeway lesions, and conjunctival petechiae; splinter hemorrhage or petechiae elsewhere are not specific enough. Immunologic phenomena include glomerulonephritis, positive rheumatoid factor, and C-reactive protein.

CLINICAL PRESENTATION

The classic triad of infectious endocarditis is fever, organic heart murmur, and positive blood culture; however, one, two, or (rarely) all three may be absent. Fever, the most frequent finding, may be absent in debilitated patients, but the most frequent cause of absent fever is previous antibiotic use. A heart murmur may be absent very early in the disease, especially when a normal valve is infected by a virulent organism. Murmurs of tricuspid or pulmonary valve involvement are often soft, low frequency, or atypical, and they can be easily overlooked. Patients who have undergone cardiac transplantation can have an infection at the atrial suture line. Other immunocompromised patients can have endocarditis without organic murmurs, as may occur with infection on a lead of a permanently implanted cardiac pacemaker. These are rarer causes of infectious endocarditis without a heart murmur. As discussed later, blood culture is negative in approximately 5% of patients with infectious endocarditis.

Constitutional symptoms of fatigue, malaise, anorexia, and weight loss are variable and relate to the state of the patient, the infecting organism, and (most importantly) to the duration of the infection. Peripheral manifestations, such as petechiae, splinter hemorrhages, Osler's nodes (vasculitis vs.

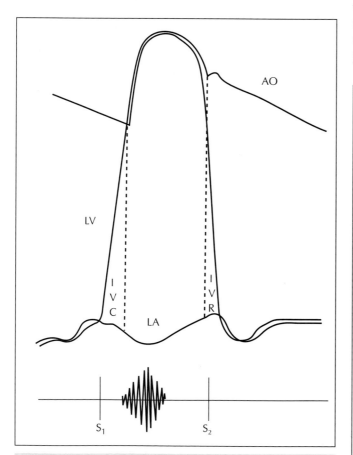

FIGURE 1 Flow murmurs have a distinct period of silence between the heart sounds and the murmur. During the isovolumetric contraction (IVC) period (the time between the closure of the atrioventricular [AV] valve and the opening of the semilunar valve), all valves are closed. Any murmur during this period must result from an abnormality. All valves are also closed during the isovolumetric relaxation (IVR) period (the time between the closure of the semilunar valves and the opening of the AV valves). This produces the silent periods right after the first heart sound (S₁) and right before the second heart sound (S₂). AO—aortic pressure; LA—left atrial pressure; LV—left ventricular pressure.

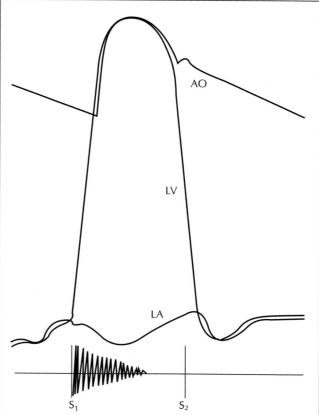

FIGURE 2 Murmurs that begin with the first heart sound (S₁) and therefore involve the isovolumetric contraction period (when all heart valves are closed) are regurgitant and therefore require endocarditis prophylaxis. AO—aortic pressure; LA—left atrial pressure; LV—left ventricular pressure; S₂—second heart sound.

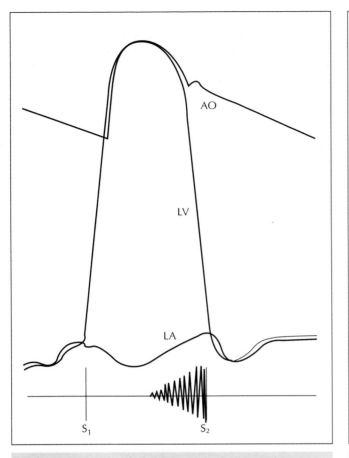

FIGURE 3 Systolic murmurs that are coincident with the second heart sound (S_2), and thus involve the isovolumetric relaxation period (a period when all heart valves are closed) and are regurgitant, require endocarditis prophylaxis. AO—aortic pressure; LA—left atrial pressure; LV—left ventricular pressure; S_1—first heart sound; S_2—second heart sound.

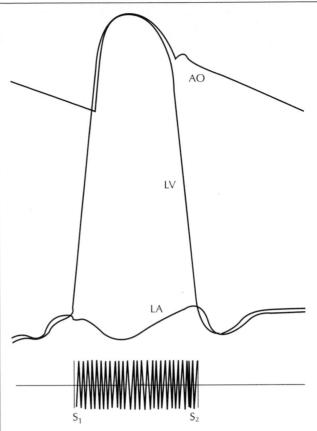

FIGURE 4 Pansystolic or holosystolic murmurs are always regurgitant, because they involve both isovolumetric periods (times when all of the heart valves are closed). AO—aortic pressure; LA—left atrial pressure; LV—left ventricular pressure; S_1—first heart sound; S_2—second heart sound.

bacteremia), Janeway lesions, and Roth spots in the fundi, are directly related to the duration of the infection.

Other findings, such as splenomegaly, anemia, and embolic phenomena, are likewise related in part to the duration of the infection. Thromboembolic phenomena may be pulmonary (from right-sided endocarditis) or systemic (central nervous system, renal, or other peripheral sites) from left-sided endocarditis. Mycotic aneurysms result from peripheral infection of an arterial wall and may rupture.

AUSCULTATION

Cardiac auscultation plays an important role in infectious endocarditis. It not only allows for the identification of patients at increased risk for infectious endocarditis (those with regurgitant valvular lesions) but also identifies organic lesions and changing lesions in patients with endocarditis, helping to identify the state of cardiac function during the course of the illness.

Prevention

Patients with flow or ejection murmurs are not at risk for infectious endocarditis, but patients with regurgitant murmurs should have endocarditis prophylaxis. Therefore, it is important to identify by auscultation the presence of clinically significant regurgitant murmurs. The emphasis is on auscultation, because Doppler echocardiography frequently identifies valvular regurgitation that is not clinically significant, especially in elderly patients. Likewise, "echo-only" mitral valve prolapse without a murmur or a thickened mitral valve is a benign condition. Overdiagnosis of mitral valve prolapse by echocardiography is less frequent since Levine and coworkers [2] pointed out the saddle shape of the normal mitral ring and the fact that, in normal patients, apparent mitral valve prolapse is frequently present in the apical four-chamber view but not in the two-chamber view.

A flow murmur across the aortic or pulmonary valve is confined to the early and midsystolic period. There is a distinct period of silence between the first heart sound and the onset of the murmur, and another between the end of the murmur and the second heart sound (Fig. 1). Flow murmurs during ventricular ejection are early systolic. In patients with normal ventricular function, two thirds of the left ventricular volume is ejected in the first one third of systole. Mild obstruction results in little change. Moderate to severe aortic or pulmonary valve obstruction prolongs the duration of maximal flow, and the duration of the murmur increases.

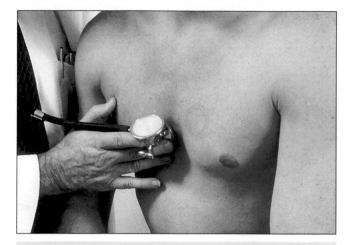

FIGURE 5 The pressure on the stethoscope should be such that an imprint from the stethoscope diaphragm remains on the skin when removed. One listens for a soft diastolic murmur; at times, this murmur is so soft that it simulates the sound of a gentle wind in the trees.

In contrast, regurgitant murmurs involve either the isovolumetric contraction period or the isovolumetric relaxation period, producing a murmur that begins coincident with the first heart sound (Fig. 2), the second heart sound (Fig. 3), or both. In the latter, the murmur is pan- or holosystolic (Fig. 4),

because during the isovolumetric contraction period (the time between the closure of the atrioventricular [AV] valve and the opening of the semilunar valves) all valves are closed. Any murmur during this period must result from an abnormality. The same holds for the isovolumetric relaxation period, thus the silent periods right after the first heart sound and before the second heart sound.

As in systole, not all diastolic murmurs result from an organic abnormality of the heart. Diastolic murmurs include regurgitation of the semilunar (aortic or pulmonic) valves, and obstruction of the AV (mitral or tricuspid) valves. Functional diastolic murmurs result from enhanced flow across the AV valves from another defect.

The technique of cardiac auscultation must be done carefully so as not to overlook murmurs that make the individual susceptible to infectious endocarditis. The room should be quiet, the stethoscope of top quality, and the patient examined in several positions. When listening for the murmur of aortic regurgitation, one must place the diaphragm of the stethoscope firmly against the chest wall in the third left intercostal space (Fig. 5). The patient should be auscultated in the supine, sitting, standing, and squatting (Fig. 6) positions during normal respiration and leaning forward during forced full expiration.

Likewise, when auscultating for mitral regurgitant murmurs, the patient must be examined with the stethoscope

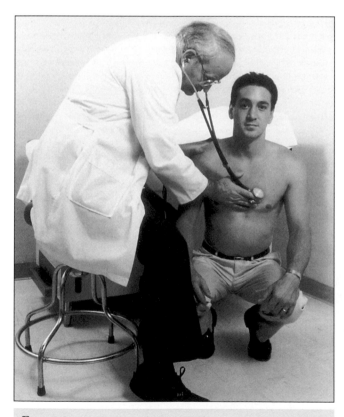

FIGURE 6 Auscultation with patient in the squatting position (note physician sitting on a stool) is an important maneuver, as squatting increases venous return (preload) and blood pressure (afterload), accentuates the murmur of aortic regurgitation, and decreases the murmur of hypertrophic obstructive cardiomyopathy.

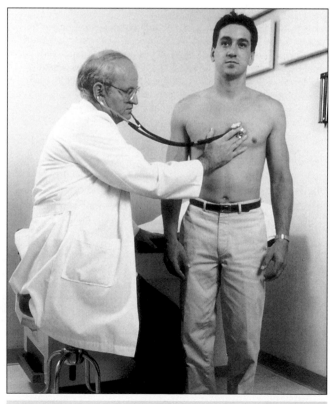

FIGURE 7 Auscultation of the patient standing after squatting is an important provocative maneuver, because this maneuver decreases venous return and thereby results in less filling of the left ventricle (decreased preload). This maneuver also decreases the blood pressure (decreased afterload). The resultant decrease in left ventricular volume increases or unmasks the murmur of mitral valve prolapse and hypertrophic obstructive cardiomyopathy.

placed at the apex with the patient in the supine, left lateral, sitting, standing, squatting, and restanding positions. It is often only on restanding after squatting (Fig. 7) that the murmur of mitral valve prolapse or hypertrophic obstructive cardiomyopathy becomes apparent.

Is the presence of a single systolic click an indication for antibiotic prophylaxis? The opinion of cardiologists is divided. My practice guidelines, and the current American Heart Association (AHA) guidelines [3] are not to recommend antibiotic prophylaxis for clicks only. The caveat is that the patient must be examined carefully and thoroughly in appropriate positions without eliciting a murmur. Although endocarditis has been described in patients with clicks only, these descriptions were from an era when patients were not routinely examined in the standing, squatting, and restanding positions.

In addition, there are a number of sounds that can be mistaken for clicks that do not originate from the mitral valve (Table 2). The characteristic of a systolic click of mitral valve prolapse is its variable position in systole depending on the left ventricular volume. The smaller the left ventricular volume (as with abrupt standing), the earlier the click; the larger the ventricular volume (as with squatting), the later the click. Endocarditis prophylaxis is also recommended for patients at very high risk without regurgitant murmur, such as those with prosthetic heart valves or severely immunocompromised patients.

Diagnosis

Cardiac auscultation is also an important aspect of the diagnosis of infectious endocarditis. Exact interpretation of auscultatory findings is not as critical for diagnosis as it is in prevention, because echocardiography is an essential diagnostic tool in the diagnosis of infectious endocarditis.

Rarely, a murmur will be absent in the early days of endocarditis, especially when endocarditis occurs on a normal valve, such as endocarditis from staphylococci. These virulent organisms soon destroy enough of the valve that a murmur appears.

In the appropriate clinical setting, the sudden appearance of a new regurgitant murmur is nearly diagnostic of infectious endocarditis. Regurgitant apical systolic murmurs in infectious endocarditis may result from AV valve perforation, rupture of chordae tendineae, destruction of the valve, or functional AV incompetence. Regurgitant diastolic murmurs are caused by aortic or pulmonary valve perforation or destruction secondary to aortic-ventricular or aortic-atrial connections resulting from abscess-induced connections.

The auscultatory findings of tricuspid valve incompetence are more subtle. The murmur may not be typically regurgitant. The murmur may increase with inspiration (the Caravallo sign) [4], but these diagnostic features are frequently absent. The jugular venous pulse should be carefully observed for the presence of regurgitant CV waves.

Low-frequency diastolic murmurs can result from inflow obstruction caused by large vegetations or flow from increased AV valve incompetence or nonpulmonary hypertensive pulmonary valve incompetence. Inflow obstructions are rare in infectious endocarditis and most commonly result from fungal vegetation or clot formation on vegetations. The development of an apical diastolic flow murmur in a patient with preexisting mitral regurgitation usually indicates an increased degree of mitral regurgitation. The diastolic murmur of pulmonary artery insufficiency in a patient with normal pulmonary artery pressures is also low frequency but is best heard along the left sternal border.

High-frequency diastolic murmurs from the pulmonary valve occur in patients with preexisting pulmonary hypertension, such as in patients with Eisenmenger syndrome. The usual cause of a high-frequency diastolic murmur in infectious endocarditis is destruction or perforation of the aortic valve. These murmurs likewise are best heard along the left sternal border, but on occasion, perforation may lead to an eccentrically directed jet producing a high-frequency murmur best heard in the third or fourth right intercostal space compared with the third or fourth left intercostal space. Right-sided murmurs of aortic regurgitation suggest unusual causes of aortic regurgitation such as infectious endocarditis.

Determining Severity

Low-frequency third and fourth heart sounds indicate deterioration of ventricular function, usually from increasing severity of the lesions. Third heart sounds are heard with the development of heart failure. They occur at the peak of the rapid filling wave of the left ventricular pressure curve and the peak of the Doppler transmitral velocity wave (E point).

Development of a fourth heart sound suggests acute valvular incompetence, myocarditis, or a hyperkinetic state. This sound occurs at the height of the A wave in the left ventricular pressures trace and the *A* point on the Doppler transmitral velocity tracing. These low-frequency sounds are best heard with the bell of the stethoscope placed lightly on the skin, just

TABLE 2 CLICK-LIKE SOUNDS NOT CAUSED BY MITRAL OR TRICUSPID VALVE PROLAPSE

Early systolic	**Early diastolic**
Pulmonic ejection sound	Opening snap
Aortic ejection sound	**Late diastolic**
Split first heart sound	Pacemaker chest wall sound
Late systolic	**Variable systolic and diastolic**
Wide split second heart sound	Extracardiac (pneumothorax)
Variable systolic	
Atrial septal aneurysm	

TABLE 3 MANIFESTATIONS OF SEVERE AORTIC REGURGITATION

	Acute	**Chronic**
First heart sound	Absent	Present
Diastolic murmur	Short	Long
Pulse pressure	Normal	Increased
Ejection sound	Absent	Present
Heart rate	Fast	Normal

	Acute	Chronic

TABLE 4 MANIFESTATION OF SEVERE MITRAL REGURGITATION

	Acute	Chronic
Rhythm	Sinus	Atrial fibrillation
Left atrial size	Normal	Enlarged
Fourth heart sound	Present	Absent
Third heart sound	Present or absent	Present
Pulmonary component S_2	Increased	Normal
Murmur	Late systolic attenuation	Pansystolic
Pulmonary congestion	Early	Late

TABLE 5 ECHOCARDIOGRAPHY IN INFECTIOUS ENDOCARDITIS

Visualization of vegetations: evaluate valvular anatomy and function

Detect abscess, fistula, or perforation

Evaluate hemodynamic consequences

Negative transesophageal echocardiography, very high probability of not having infectious endocarditis

Bacteremia without endocarditis in patients with valvular heart disease are treated much differently

Transesophageal echocardiography should be repeated in patients; a negative study if the clinical course dictates

making an air seal. Firm pressure stretches the skin, making it a diaphragm and filtering out low-frequency sounds.

The auscultatory findings of acute severe aortic and mitral regurgitation are quite different from those of chronic aortic and mitral regurgitation. These are described in Tables 3 and 4, respectively.

ECHOCARDIOGRAPHY

The sensitivity of echocardiography for identifying vegetations in patients with infectious endocarditis is approximately 55% for M-mode techniques, 70% to 80% for two-dimensional, and over 90% for transesophageal echocardiography [5]. The role of echocardiography is outlined in Table 5. Echocardiography can identify a vegetation or a perivalvular abscess, and it can document chamber size and function as well as the condition of the valves. Identification of a mobile or oscillating mass, an abscess, or dehiscence of a prosthetic valve are components of definite clinical criteria for the diagnosis of infectious endocarditis.

The echocardiographic size of the vegetation in some series has important prognostic significance. In right-sided endo-

carditis, lesions over 20 mm were associated with a 33% 6-month mortality rate, whereas 6-month mortality was only 1% if the mass was smaller [6].

The prognostic implications of vegetation size remain controversial. Some studies of left-sided endocarditis found a worse prognosis with large-sized vegetation. In some studies, emboli are more likely with large vegetation size [5] when they are mobile (*ie*, have a stalk) [6–8]. It appears that the mobility of the vegetation or those with a stalk have a higher risk on systemic emboli.

Emboli may depend on factors other than size and mobility. Some studies have implicated the organism (more common with streptococcus), the antibiotic used, and the response of vegetation size to therapy.

BLOOD CULTURES

Blood cultures are critically important to the diagnosis and management of infectious endocarditis. It is recommended that three blood cultures be taken 1 hour apart with at least 10 mL of blood for each. The reason for drawing the cultures 1 hour apart is that transient bacteremia from *Streptococcus viridans* endocarditis is not uncommon. Bacteremia from endocarditis is relatively constant, so most of the cultures are usually positive. Contamination is less likely if three separate cultures are taken.

TABLE 6 CATEGORIES OF CULTURE-NEGATIVE ENDOCARDITIS

Prior antimicrobial therapy before culture

Infection by fastidious microorganisms

  HACEK group

  Nutritionally deficient streptococci

  Brucella spp.

  Neisseria spp.

  Anaerobes

  Corynebacterium spp.

  Legionella spp.

  Fungi

Q fever (*Coxiella burnetti*)

Chlamydia sp.

Subacute right-sided endocarditis

HACEK—*Haemophilus, Actinobacillus, Cardiobacterium, Eikenella*, and *Kingella* species.

TABLE 7 NONINFECTIOUS ENDOCARDITIS OR MASSES

Myxoma

Papilloma

Acute rheumatic carditis

Lupus nonbacterial verrucous endocarditis

Marantic endocarditis

Endocardial fibroelastosis

Fibroblastic endocarditis (Löffler's endocarditis)

Carcinoid

TABLE 8 PROCEDURES AND CONDITIONS FOR WHICH ENDOCARDITIS PROPHYLAXIS IS RECOMMENDED

Dental procedures likely to cause gingival bleeding
Surgical operations that involve intestinal or respiratory mucosa
Esophageal dilation
Gallbladder surgery
Cystoscopy
Urethral dilation
Prosthetic surgery
Incision and drainage abscess
Vaginal hysterectomy
Vaginal delivery during an infection
Prosthetic cardiac valves
Previous endocarditis
Rheumatic valve dysfunction
Mitral valve prolapse with mitral regurgitation
Hypertrophic cardiomyopathy

TABLE 9 PROCEDURES AND CONDITIONS FOR WHICH INFECTIOUS ENDOCARDITIS PROPHYLAXIS IS NOT RECOMMENDED

Dental procedures not likely to produce gingival bleeding
Bronchoscopy with flexible scope
Endoscopy without biopsy
Cesarean section
Cardiac catheterization
Isolated secundum atrial septal defect
Atrial septal defect, ventricular septal defect, and patent ductus arteriosus repair after 6 months
Coronary artery bypass surgery
Mitral valve prolapse without mitral regurgitation
Functional heart murmurs
Implanted pacemakers

Culture-Negative Endocarditis

Blood cultures are negative in 5% to 10% of patients with the infectious endocarditis. Common causes of culture-negative endocarditis are listed in Table 6. The major cause of negative blood cultures in patients with infectious endocarditis is prior antibiotic therapy. The longer the therapy with effective antibiotics before they are discontinued, the longer it takes for bacteremia to reappear.

Bacteremia Versus Endocarditis

A major diagnostic dilemma may occur in a patient with organic heart disease who presents with fever. The problem is compounded if there are positive blood cultures or the patient has an endocardial mass or endocarditis of noninfectious origin (Table 7).

ANTIBIOTIC PROPHYLAXIS

The AHA recommendations for who should and should not receive prophylactic therapy are outlined in Tables 8 and 9, respectively. Recommendations for antibiotic therapy for endocarditis prophylaxis are outlined in Table 10.

WHEN TO REFER

Infectious endocarditis is a potentially lethal disease. Accordingly, patients should be referred whenever this diagnosis is seriously considered. All patients should be followed up by a team consisting of the patient's primary-care physician, cardi-

TABLE 10 BACTERIAL ENDOCARDITIS PROPHYLAXIS IN ADULTS

Dental/oral/upper respiratory tract procedures for patients at high risk
Amoxicillin 3.0 g orally 1 h before procedure, then 1.5 g six hours after initial dose

For amoxicillin/penicillin allergic patients
Erythromycin ethylsuccinate 800 mg or erythromycin stearate 1.0 g orally 2 hours before procedure, then one half this dose 6 hours after initial dose

Genitourinary/gastrointestinal procedures
Ampicillin 2.0 q IV plus gentamycin 1.5 mg/kg IV (not to exceed 80 mg) 30 minutes before procedure, followed by amoxicillin 1.5 g orally 6 hours after the initial dose

Adapted from Dajani *et al.* [3]; with permission.

TABLE 11 COMPLICATIONS OF INFECTIOUS ENDOCARDITIS

Cardiac
Neurologic
Septic
Associated with medical treatment
Renal
Extracranial systemic emboli
Septic pulmonary emboli
Complications related to surgery
Acute prosthetic heart valve insufficiency

ologist, infectious disease specialist, and cardiovascular surgeon.

INDICATIONS FOR SURGERY

Surgery is indicated when antibiotics fail to control endocarditis. Evidence of failure may be signs of progressive invasion of the myocardium with abscess formation, heart block, or development of fistulas; persistent sepsis; progressive hemodynamic instability; or repeated emboli [9]. Most fungal infections require surgery for cure. Surgery for persistent culture-positive active endocarditis is necessary at times. Although morality is high, averaging about 25% of patients, the long-term outcome of survivors is good [10].

COMPLICATIONS AND PROGNOSIS

Complications are not uncommon in infectious endocarditis. Table 11 lists the more common complications in order of frequency [11]. Although cardiac complications are the most common, fatality rates may be higher from neurologic or septic complications.

KEY REFERENCES

Recently published papers of outstanding interest, as identified in *References and Recommended Reading*, have been annotated.

•• Durack DT, Luke AS, Bright DK, and the Duke Endocarditis Service: New criteria for diagnosis of infective endocarditis: Utilization of specific echocardiographic criteria. *Am J Med* 1994, 96:200–209.
New criteria for the diagnosis of endocarditis. This is a classic.

REFERENCES AND RECOMMENDED READING

Recently published papers of particular interest have been highlighted as:
• Of interest
•• Of outstanding interest

1.•• Durack DT, Luke AS, Bright DK, and the Duke Endocarditis Service: New criteria for diagnosis of infective endocarditis: Utilization of specific echocardiographic criteria. *Am J Med* 1994, 96:200–209.

2. Levine RA, Triulzi MO, Harrigan P, *et al.*: The relationship of mitral annular shape to the diagnosis of mitral valve prolapse. *Circulation* 1987, 75:756–767.

3. Dajani AS, Bisno AL, Chung KJ, *et al.*: Prevention of bacterial endocarditis. Recommendations by the American Heart Association. *JAMA* 1990, 264:2919–2922.

4. Gooch AS, Maranchao V, Scampardonis G, *et al.*: Prolapse of both mitral and tricuspid leaflets in systolic murmur-click syndrome. *N Engl J Med* 1972, 287:1218–1222.

5. Siddiq S, Missri J, Silverma DJ: Endocarditis in an urban hospital in the 1990s. *Arch Intern Med* 1996, 156:2454–2458.

6. Heinle SK, Durack DT, Longabaugh JP, *et al.*: Can echocardiography predict risk of embolic events in infectious endocarditis? *Choices Cardiol* 1992, 7:79–81.

7. Hecht SR, Berger M: Right-sided endocarditis in intravenous drug users. Prognostic features in 102 episodes. *Ann Intern Med* 1992, 117:560–566.

8. Khandheria BK: Suspected bacterial endocarditis: to TEE or not TEE. *J Am Coll Cardiol* 1993, 21:222–224.

9. Jamieson SW: Surgical therapy for infective endocarditis. *Mayo Clin Proc* 1995, 70:598–599.

10. Mullany CL, Chua YL, Schaff HV, *et al.*: Early and late survival after surgical treatment of culture-positive active endocarditis. *Mayo Clin Proc* 1995, 70:517–525.

11. Mansur AJ, Grinberg M, da Luz PL, *et al.*: The complications of infectious endocarditis: a reappraisal in the 1980s. *Arch Intern Med* 1992, 152:2428–2432.

SELECT BIBLIOGRAPHY

Kay D: *Infectious Endocarditis*, edn 2. New York: Raven Press; 1992.

Reid CL, Chandraratna PAN, Rahimtoola SH: Infectious endocarditis: improved diagnosis and treatment. *Curr Probl Cardiol* 1985, 10:1–51.

Pericardial Disease 30

Paul T. Vaitkus
Martin M. LeWinter
Joseph S. Alpert

Key Points

- Pericarditis is a disease of diverse origins; treatment consists of administering a combination of antiinflammatory drugs and therapy directed at the specific underlying disease.

- Purulent pericarditis remains an underdiagnosed medical emergency; tuberculous pericarditis may increase in frequency with the reemergence of multiple drug-resistant strains.

- Cardiac tamponade constitutes an emergency that requires prompt recognition and treatment.

- Constrictive pericarditis is a curable disease that should be considered in patients with unexplained heart failure; evaluation with a combination of noninvasive testing and cardiac catheterization can accurately establish the diagnosis in most patients.

The pericardium is not essential for sustaining life or health, as evidenced by a lack of cardiac dysfunction when it is congenitally absent or surgically opened. Normal functions of the pericardium include maintenance of an optimal cardiac shape, promotion of cardiac chamber interaction, restraint of overfilling of the heart, reduction of friction between the beating heart and adjacent structures, provision of a physical barrier to infection, and limitation of cardiac displacement during the cardiac cycle. Most often the clinical importance of the pericardium is seen through its involvement in a number of disease states.

ACUTE PERICARDITIS

Pathophysiology

Acute pericarditis is an inflammatory condition of the pericardium caused by a variety of agents and disease states (Table 1). The most common etiologic agents are viral and likely account for most cases of "idiopathic" pericarditis. With the recent epidemic of multiple drug–resistant tuberculosis in urban populations, tuberculous pericarditis may very well become an increasing problem after decades of declining incidence [1,2]. Tuberculous pericarditis most commonly occurs in the absence of demonstrable pulmonary or extrapulmonary tuberculosis. Patients with AIDS can develop pericarditis as a result of infection with the virus itself or a large number of opportunistic organisms [3,4]. Pericarditis can be clinically identified in 7% to 23% of patients with transmural myocardial infarction [5,6], and the risk for pericarditis is proportional to the size of the infarction [5,6]. Bacterial pericarditis often develops in the context of significant extracardiac infections, particularly intrathoracic infections [7].

Clinical Manifestations

The cardinal clinical features of acute pericarditis are chest pain, friction rub, and electrocardiographic (ECG) changes. Many patients relate prodromal symptoms

TABLE 1 CAUSES OF PERICARDITIS

Idiopathic

Viral (Coxsackie B5, B6, Echovirus, adenovirus, influenza, AIDs, others)

Purulent (Most common organisms in recent series are *Pneumococcus*, *Streptococcus*, *Staphylococcus*, gram-negative bacilli, and fungi)

Tuberculosis

Sarcoidosis

Amyloidosis

Uremia

Myocardial infarction

    Acute pericarditis

    Dressler's syndrome (postmyocardial infarction syndrome)

    Dissection of the Aorta

Neoplastic disease (lung, breast, melanoma, lymphoma, leukemia)

Radiation therapy

Autoimmune diseases (lupus, rheumatoid arthritis, etc.)

Trauma (cardiac or intravenous catheterization, chest trauma, pacemaker insertion, thoracic surgery)

Drugs (daunorubicin, diphenylhydantoin, hydralazine, isoniazid, methysergide, penicillin, phenylbutazone, procainamide)

Anticoagulants (warfarin, heparin)

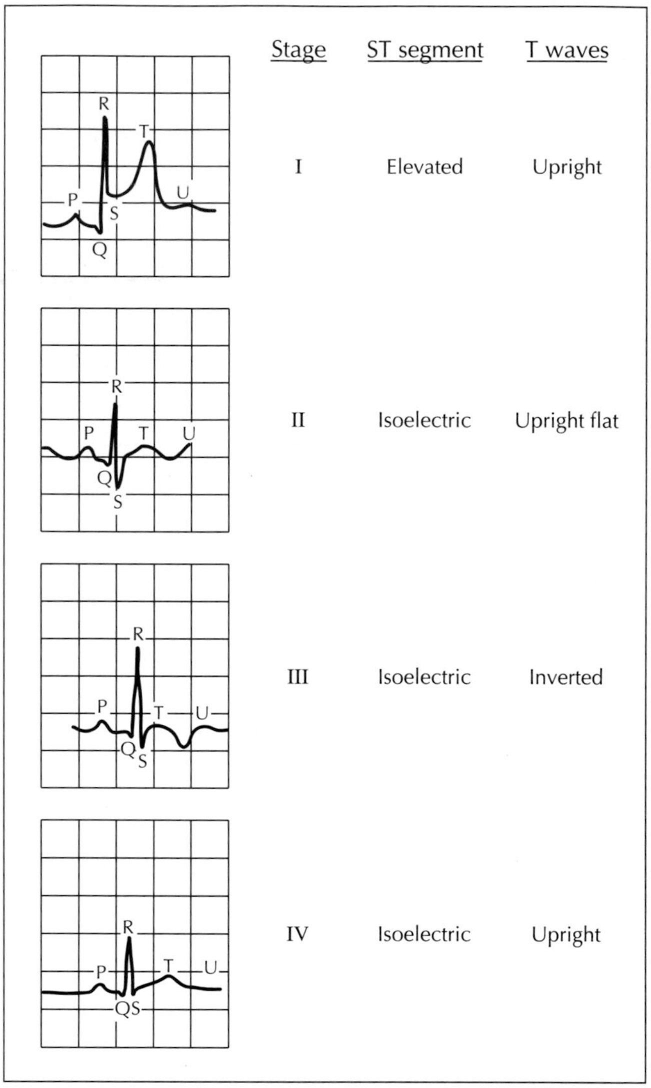

Stage	ST segment	T waves
I	Elevated	Upright
II	Isoelectric	Upright flat
III	Isoelectric	Inverted
IV	Isoelectric	Upright

FIGURE 1 The four stages of electrocardiographic changes in acute pericarditis.

suggestive of a viral infection. The chest pain of pericarditis varies in location, intensity, and character; it may be described as sharp or dull. Most often, it is precordial or retrosternal and may be referred to the trapezius ridge. It is often aggravated by inspiration, coughing, or recumbency, and it is lessened by sitting upright and leaning forward. Although typically taking 1 or 2 hours to develop fully, at times the pain can appear with remarkable abruptness. Patients with pericarditis may be febrile and tachycardic. The pericardial friction rub is the pathognomonic auscultatory finding. It is typically scratchy and characteristically has three components, although it is not unusual for only one or two components to be audible. The systolic component is most consistently present. The friction rub may be evanescent or influenced by the patient's position; thus, repeated auscultation, and auscultation with the patient in several positions, is essential.

Bacterial pericarditis should be suspected in the presence of high fevers, chills, or night sweats. Patients with bacterial pericarditis frequently lack pleuritic chest pain or pericardial friction rubs.

Laboratory Findings

Evaluation of a patient with suspected pericarditis should include ECG, chest radiography, a complete blood count, and echocardiography. Serial ECGs are valuable in establishing or confirming the diagnosis of pericarditis; four stages of ECG evolution have been described (Fig. 1). Although ECG abnormalities occur in 90% of cases, all four stages can be serially identified in approximately 50%

of patients. Early ECG changes of pericarditis must be distinguished from the normal variant of early repolarization and from myocardial ischemia or infarction. In early repolarization, the distribution of the ST-segment elevation may be very similar to that in pericarditis, but the elevation remains unchanged and does not evolve through the serial changes seen in acute pericarditis. The ST:T ratio in lead V_6 can help in differentiating early repolarization from pericarditis. If the ratio of ST-segment elevation to T-wave amplitude is less than 1:4, early repolarization is more likely; if this ratio is greater than 1:4, pericarditis is more likely (Fig. 2). The ST-segment elevation of pericarditis differs from that of myocardial ischemia in that it is typically concave upward and present in all leads except aVR and V_1, where the ST segment frequently will be depressed. Furthermore, ST segments typically return to normal before the T waves become inverted in patients with pericarditis, whereas in those with myocardial infarction, T-wave inversion evolves while the ST segments are still elevated. Finally, the ECG in patients with pericarditis often demonstrates depression of the PR segment in those leads with ST elevation.

Mild leukocytosis and mild elevation of the erythrocyte sedimentation rate are common in viral or idiopathic pericarditis. These findings are less common in the pericarditis of uremia or connective tissue disorders. A significant leukocytosis with a shift to the left raises the possibility of bacterial pericarditis. Cardiac enzyme levels may be slightly elevated in cases where the inflammatory process involves subepicardial myocardium. Chest radiography usually reveals no abnormalities in uncomplicated pericarditis, but it may show an enlarged cardiac silhouette if a significant pericardial effusion is present. Echocardiography may reveal a pericardial effusion, but absence of an effusion by no means excludes the diagnosis.

When the suspicion of bacterial or tuberculous pericarditis is high, a diagnostic pericardiocentesis is indicated. The pericardial fluid should be examined with Gram and acid-fast bacillus stains and cultured for bacteria, mycobacteria, and fungi. Tubercle bacillus is demonstrated by stain or culture in only one third to one half of patients with tuberculous pericarditis. The diagnosis is often based on a history of contact or conversion of a purified protein derivative (PPD) skin test. The presence of reduced levels of adenosine deaminase in pericardial fluid has been proposed as a specific test for tuberculous pericarditis [8].

Management
Idiopathic and viral pericarditis
In most cases of idiopathic acute pericarditis, antiinflammatory treatment with nonsteroidal antiinflammatory agents usually suppresses the clinical manifestations within 24 hours. For patients in whom nonsteroidal agents fail to ameliorate symptoms, steroid therapy can be initiated. In most patients, a single course of antiinflammatory therapy controls the illness, and the pericarditis resolves without sequelae. In some patients, the pericarditis may recur over weeks or months after the initial episode [9]. These episodes can be treated with repeated courses of nonsteroidal or steroidal antiinflammatory agents. Colchicine is promising as prophylaxis for cases of recurrent pericarditis [10], and immunosuppressive drugs (eg, azathioprine) have been used occasionally [9]. In rare cases, frequent and severe recurrences despite aggressive drug therapy have prompted the need for pericardiectomy [9]. Unfortunately, this procedure is often ineffective, either because of

residual pericardial tissue or a shift of the inflammatory process to the pleura [9].

Bacterial and tuberculous pericarditis
Bacterial pericarditis is a medical emergency that must be treated with drainage and antibiotic agents. Mortality rates range from 56% to 77% [7]. The presence of gram-negative organisms indicates a poor prognosis. Untreated tuberculous pericarditis is associated with 80% mortality rates. Management involves administration of three antituberculous drugs for at least 9 months. The role of corticosteroid therapy and early surgical pericardiectomy in patients with tuberculous pericarditis has been a source of controversy [1]. In the only prospective controlled trial addressing this question, prednisolone therapy was associated with a reduction in mortality and the need for emergent repeat pericardiocentesis; the rates of subsequent constrictive pericarditis did not differ between patients receiving prednisolone and placebo [11]. Complete open drainage reduced the need for subsequent urgent pericardiocentesis but did not influence development of subsequent constriction or mortality [11].

Uremia
Uremic pericarditis prior to dialysis almost always responds to the initiation of dialysis. Pericarditis in patients already receiving chronic dialysis is a more complex challenge. The pericarditis may have an identifiable cause with a specific remedy in a significant proportion of these patients. In the majority of cases, however, no specific cause will be identified, and the pericarditis typically responds to intensification of the dialysis regimen [12]. Pericardial effusions, however, will not consistently resolve with intensive dialysis [13]. Lack of response to intensive dialysis may be predicted by several clinical variables (Table 2) [12]. Nonsteroidal antiinflammatory agents can be used in these patients. Also, indomethacin has been successful in alleviating fevers but did not influence the duration of chest pain, pericardial rub, or the subsequent development of tamponade [14].

Transmural myocardial infarction and thrombolytic therapy
Pericarditis can be mistaken for acute myocardial infarction, leading to inappropriate administration of thrombolytic agents with potentially catastrophic results [15]. Indeed, pericarditis

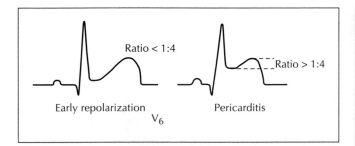

Ratio < 1:4

Ratio > 1:4

Early repolarization   Pericarditis

V₆

FIGURE 2 The ratio of the ST-segment elevation to the T-wave amplitude in lead V_6 is useful in differentiating early repolarization (*left*) from pericarditis (*right*).

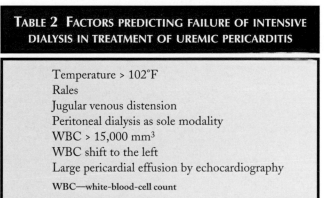

TABLE 2 FACTORS PREDICTING FAILURE OF INTENSIVE DIALYSIS IN TREATMENT OF UREMIC PERICARDITIS

Temperature > 102°F
Rales
Jugular venous distension
Peritoneal dialysis as sole modality
WBC > 15,000 mm³
WBC shift to the left
Large pericardial effusion by echocardiography

WBC—white-blood-cell count

TABLE 3 PHYSICAL FINDINGS IN CARDIAC TAMPONADE

Physical finding	Frequency, %
Jugular venous distention	100
Tachypnea	80–97
Tachycardia	77–100
Pulsus paradoxus	77–89
Arterial pulse pressure < 40 mm Hg	46
Systolic blood pressure < 100 mm Hg	36–42
Diminished heart sounds	34–88
Pericardial friction rub	22–29

TABLE 4 CHEST RADIOGRAPHIC FINDINGS IN PERICARDIAL EFFUSION

Radiographic sign	Size of effusion	
	Moderate and large	Small
Enlarged cardiac silhouette	78%	68%
Pericardial fat stripe	22%	8%
Left-sided pleural effusion	43%	12%
Increase in cardiac diameter since last chest radiograph	27%	54%

is a relative contraindication to both thrombolytic therapy and anticoagulation treatment. Most cases of pericarditis complicating myocardial infarction, however, develop later in the illness and are not a confounding factor in the early hours, when decisions concerning thrombolytic therapy are being made [5,6]. Thrombolytic therapy is associated with a reduced incidence of pericarditis, probably because it reduces the size of the infarction [5]. When pericarditis occurs after infarction, it usually resolves promptly and does not require therapy beyond the use of analgesic drugs. The incidence of Dressler's syndrome (postmyocardial infarction syndrome consisting of fever, malaise, and pleural and pericardial effusions associated with pleuropericardial pain) appears to have decreased, a trend some authorities attribute to decreased use of anticoagulation agents in patients who have had myocardial infarction [16].

PERICARDIAL EFFUSION AND CARDIAC TAMPONADE

Pericardial effusion may develop as a result of pericarditis or as a response to injury to the parietal pericardium [17]. Once the relatively small reserve volume of the pericardium is filled, intrapericardial pressure rises precipitously with the addition of more fluid. Pericardial effusions may be encountered in the absence of pericarditis in many clinical settings, including uremia, cardiac trauma or chamber rupture, malignancy, AIDS, and hypothyroidism. Clinical manifestations relate to the pressure in the pericardium, which in turn depends on the rapidity of accumulation and the absolute volume of the effusion. Rapid accumulation of even modest volumes can be associated with increased intrapericardial pressures and life-threatening hemodynamic compromise. With a slowly accumulating effusion, the pericardium can accommodate 1 to 2 L of fluid without a clinically significant elevation in intrapericardial pressure. Cardiac tamponade ensues when the accumulation of fluid compromises the filling of the heart and, consequently, impairs cardiac output.

Clinical Manifestations

The widespread availability of echocardiography has led to the identification of small effusions in asymptomatic patients in a wide variety of clinical settings. Small, incidentally discovered effusions rarely cause symptoms or complications. Large effu-

sions may become clinically manifest by compressing adjacent structures, and they may cause dysphagia, cough, dyspnea, hiccups, hoarseness, nausea, or a sense of abdominal fullness. Signs of pericardial effusion are absent in patients with small effusions without increased pressure. Large effusions may muffle the heart sounds or cause rales or dullness on auscultation of the chest as a result of compression of the lung parenchyma. The typical signs of cardiac tamponade include high venous pressure, low systemic arterial pressure, diminished pulse pressure, tachycardia, tachypnea, and pulsus paradoxus. The jugular venous pressure is usually markedly elevated, with obliteration of the normal Y-descent. The frequency of these physical findings is somewhat variable (Table 3). A paradoxic pulse may be absent in certain clinical situations (*eg*, tamponade coexisting with atrial septal defect or aortic insufficiency). This absence can be an important confounding variable in cases of proximal aortic dissection, which can cause both acute severe aortic insufficiency and cardiac tamponade.

Laboratory Findings

Chest radiography can demonstrate a number of findings in patients with pericardial effusion (Table 4, Fig. 3) [18]. Because these radiographic signs are inconsistently present, however, chest radiography cannot reliably confirm or exclude the diagnosis [18]. Chest radiography also may offer clues to important coexisting conditions such as aortic dissection or malignancy. The ECG may be entirely normal or include changes typical of pericarditis; large effusions can cause a reduction in QRS voltage and electrical alternans.

Echocardiography is the most rapid and accurate means to diagnose a pericardial effusion. The effusion appears as an echofree space between the moving epicardium and stationary pericardium. Small effusions tend to be imaged only posteriorly; however, a posterior echo-free space in some cases may reflect subepicardial fat rather than pericardial effusion. Larger effusions are distributed anteriorly as well as posteriorly. Large effusions can be associated with a swinging motion of the heart within the fluid-filled pericardium—the mechanism of electrical alternans. Diastolic collapse of the right atrium and right ventricle is a useful echocardiographic sign indicating increased intrapericardial pressure. In a recent analysis, however, the size of the pericardial effusion was the most important predictor of subsequent tamponade or emergent drainage; no echocardiographic sign was uniformly successful in predicting the presence or absence of tamponade [19]. Cardiac catheterization in the setting of tamponade will reveal elevated and equal (or near-equal) filling pressures in all four chambers as well as a depressed cardiac output. Examination of the atrial pressure waveforms reveals the loss of the normal Y-descent. The initial presentation and hemodynamic profile of tamponade may be altered by a concomitant state of intravascular volume depletion, a scenario termed *low-pressure cardiac tamponade*. In most cases of cardiac tamponade, however, cardiac catheterization is not necessary to establish the diagnosis.

Fluid obtained by pericardiocentesis should be sent for culture and cytologic examination except in the case of clear-cut traumatic tamponade. The gross appearance of the fluid is not helpful in establishing the cause, and cell counts and chemistries are of limited value. Fluid cytologic smears will be abnormal in approximately 80% of malignant effusions; the remainder are usually identified via surgical biopsy of the pericardium.

Management

Management of pericardial effusions is largely dictated by the presence or absence of hemodynamic compromise from increased pericardial pressure and the nature of the underlying disorder. In most cases, a small or incidentally discovered effusion warrants no specific intervention. Once an effusion of a certain magnitude is present, however, accumulation of even small additional amounts of fluid may result in a marked increase of intrapericardial pressure and rapid clinical deterioration. Thus, patients with any evidence of increased intrapericardial pressure or rapidly accumulating effusions must be monitored closely.

Drainage of pericardial fluid is the cornerstone of therapy for cardiac tamponade. Administration of fluids and vasopressor agents may be useful temporizing measures, but they are not a substitute for drainage and should never delay prompt removal of the pericardial fluid. Most commonly, drainage is achieved by percutaneous pericardiocentesis performed via the subxiphoid route under echocardiographic guidance. The procedure is effective and safe but may be complicated by laceration or puncture of the heart. Echocardiography can decrease the risk of cardiac puncture. At least 1 cm of an echofree space anterior to the heart should be present before percutaneous pericardiocentesis is undertaken. Pericardiocentesis is ideally carried out in the cardiac catheterization laboratory with echocardiographic or fluoroscopic guidance and concomitant right-heart catheterization. On occasion, emergency pericardiocentesis may need to be performed at the bedside. Rarely are circumstances sufficiently emergent to preclude confirmation of the diagnosis with echocardiography. Evacuation of the pericardial fluid also can be achieved via a subxiphoid surgical pericardiotomy; this procedure permits pericardial biopsy in cases of suspected malignant effusion.

In some cases, a single pericardiocentesis is effective in fully alleviating the effusion, but in most cases, consideration should be given to leaving a catheter temporarily in the pericardium for continued drainage. Subsequent management of the patient is largely dictated by the specific cause of the effusion. For malignant effusions, potential treatment modalities include chemotherapy, radiation therapy, intrapericardial sclerosis, indwelling pericardial drainage catheters, surgery, or percutaneous balloon pericardiotomy [20]. No clinical trials have directly compared these various options, but success rates have been similar in individual reports [20]. The specific tumor type and the severity of hemodynamic compromise caused by the effusion must be taken into account when deciding among the various treatment options [20].

CONSTRICTIVE PERICARDITIS

The major perturbation of constrictive pericarditis is thickening of the pericardium, causing it to encase the heart in a solid, noncompliant envelope, thereby impairing diastolic filling [21]. The rigid pericardium markedly increases intracardiac filling pressures. Effusive-constrictive pericarditis is a syndrome with features of both effusion and constriction. The

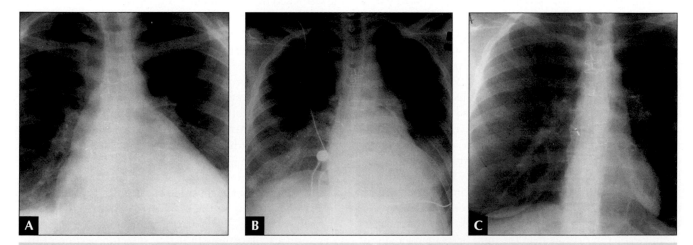

FIGURE 3 Chest radiographs illustrating the characteristic enlarged cardiac silhouette in a large pericardial effusion (**A**), after therapeutic pericardiocentesis (**B**), and several months later, after complete resolution of the pericardial effusion (**C**). The shape of the heart in the patient with a large effusion (**A**) has been likened to a water bottle.

TABLE 5 CAUSES OF CONSTRICTIVE PERICARDITIS

Cause	Frequency %
Idiopathic	42
Radiation therapy	28
Previous open heart surgery	20
Infectious (nontuberculous)	4
Neoplasia	3
Dialysis	2
Tuberculosis	1

patient initially presents with clinical symptoms most consistent with a pericardial effusion, but after the effusion is relieved, clinical and hemodynamic features of coexistent constriction appear. This syndrome may represent an intermediate step in the development of constrictive pericarditis.

Pathophysiology

Constrictive pericarditis may result from virtually any cause of pericardial injury or inflammation; the most common causes are outlined in Table 5 [21]. Tuberculous constriction may again become more common as the incidence of tuberculosis increases [2]. Intervals of many years between the inciting event and clinical manifestations of constriction are common.

Clinical Manifestations

Many symptoms of constrictive pericarditis are nonspecific and relate to chronically elevated cardiac filling pressures and chronically depressed cardiac output. Patients usually develop ascites, peripheral edema, dyspepsia, anorexia, and postprandial fullness. Cardiac cirrhosis may develop. Symptoms of left-sided congestion such as exertional dyspnea, orthopnea, and cough may occur, but these are much less prominent. The chronically low cardiac output results in fatigue and wasting.

Physical examination may reveal a massively swollen abdomen and edematous lower extremities combined with a cachectic, wasted upper torso. The liver is frequently enlarged and pulsatile. The presence of predominant right-sided failure or ascites out of proportion to peripheral edema may be clues to the presence of constriction rather than other causes of heart failure.

Patients with constrictive pericarditis have marked jugular venous distention with prominent X- and Y-descents, typically resulting in an M or W shape of the venous waves. Kussmaul's sign, which consists of the loss of normal inspiratory decrease in the jugular venous pressure with inspiration, may be present. Arterial pulse pressure may be diminished or normal, and a pulsus paradoxus is present in perhaps one third of cases. Auscultation of the heart can reveal a characteristic, early diastolic sound: the pericardial knock. The knock occurs slightly earlier in diastole than the third heart sound and is of a higher acoustic frequency.

Laboratory Findings

The ECG abnormalities seen in patients with constrictive pericarditis include low voltage, T-wave inversions, P mitrale, atrial fibrillation, atrioventricular and intraventricular conduction delays, and the development of Q waves. The cardiac silhouette on a chest radiograph may be small, normal, or enlarged. The presence of pericardial calcification is helpful in confirming the diagnosis and suggests tuberculosis as the cause. Only 50% of patients with constriction will have pericardial calcification, however, and conversely, a calcified pericardium does not automatically connote constriction.

Echocardiography demonstrates pericardial thickening in most cases of constriction, although the presence or absence of echocardiographic pericardial thickening does not establish or exclude the diagnosis with certainty. The suspicion of constrictive pericarditis in a patient with heart failure is sometimes first raised when the echo demonstrates preserved left ventricular systolic function and normal cardiac chamber sizes. Left ventricular systolic function may be impaired; despite signs of right-heart failure. Doppler studies reveal a pattern of restricted ventricular filling. Preserved systolic function is not a prerequisite for diagnosis.

Differentiation of constrictive pericarditis from restrictive cardiomyopathy is a major diagnostic challenge. Constrictive pericarditis is a treatable disease, whereas restriction usually carries a poor prognosis despite therapy. Restriction is most commonly caused by infiltrative diseases of the myocardium such as amyloidosis, sarcoidosis, and hemochromatosis. Both constrictive pericarditis and restrictive cardiomyopathy are characterized by impaired diastolic filling of the ventricles. A number of criteria have been employed to distinguish between constrictive pericarditis and restrictive cardiomyopathy [22]; these indices are based on detecting differences in ventricular diastolic filling patterns in the two conditions. Because they have been evaluated only in small groups of patients, these indices have not been widely adopted [22]. Computed tomography and magnetic resonance imaging are more accurate for detecting pericardial thickening than echocardiography and are therefore important diagnostic modalities in differentiating restriction from constriction (Fig. 4) [23].

Cardiac catheterization demonstrates elevated and virtually equal diastolic pressures in both ventricles. The individual hemodynamic criteria that have been used to differentiate constriction from restriction have varying degrees of accuracy and are capable of providing the correct diagnosis in approximately 75% of patients [22]. Catheterization also provides the opportunity to perform endomyocardial biopsy to search for evidence of infiltrative cardiomyopathy. The finding of amyloid, sarcoid, or hemochromatosis precludes the need for further investigation [22].

With the combined use of these diagnostic tests, it is possible to differentiate constrictive pericarditis from restrictive cardiomyopathy in the majority of cases (Fig. 4) [23]. When the diagnosis remains ambiguous, it may be necessary to perform a thoracotomy to permit direct inspection of the pericardium.

Management

Pericardiectomy is the definitive treatment for constrictive pericarditis. In most cases, patients will exhibit dramatic and sustained improvement, although several months may elapse before complete improvement is noted. The outcome is not uniformly favorable, because hepatic or cardiac failure may be irreversible or the myocardium atrophied because of long-standing compression, leading to a persistent low-cardiac-output state after pericardiectomy. Constrictive physiologic features and symptoms also may recur because of involvement of the epicardial layers by the inflammatory and fibrotic process.

WHEN TO REFER

Because these various pericardial disorders can occur in a wide variety of clinical contexts, patients typically will first undergo evaluation by generalists or noncardiology subspecialists. The history, physical examination, ECG, and radiographic features of acute pericarditis, pericardial effusion, and tamponade should be familiar to all family practitioners, internists, and internal medicine subspecialists. Indeed, the primary-care physician will most often be the one who identifies the possibility of a pericardial emergency (tamponade and bacterial pericarditis). When percutaneous pericardial drainage procedures are contemplated, either for diagnostic or therapeutic reasons, echocardiographic evaluation should precede pericardiocentesis. Echocardiography and subsequent pericardiocentesis should ideally be performed by physicians experienced in these procedures. In hospitals with cardiac catheterization laboratories, pericardiocentesis is best performed in this arena so as to permit the opportunity to obtain confirmatory hemodynamic measurements and any other adjuvant diagnostic information. It is also the setting best equipped to respond to complications.

The patient with suspected constriction should be referred to a cardiologist for evaluation. Although the diagnosis may be firmly established in some cases with radiographic imaging, the patient will often require further diagnostic evaluation in order to confirm the diagnosis and to evaluate the possibility of associated conditions before referral to a cardiothoracic surgeon for thoracotomy.

Management of the patient whose pericardial disease relates to a systemic illness (including uremia, connective tissue disorders, malignancy, or AIDS) will usually necessitate participation of the appropriate subspecialist. In most of these circumstances, treatment of the pericardial disease is but one component of managing a complicated illness, and management will frequently entail use of specialized procedures such as dialysis or antitumor therapy.

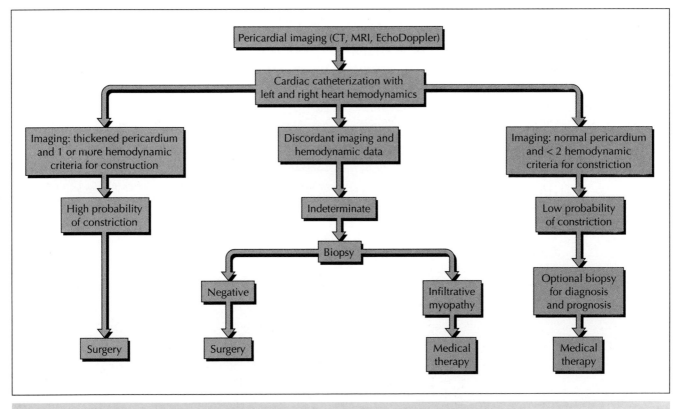

FIGURE 4 An algorithm for distinguishing restriction from constriction. If pericardial calcification is evident on chest radiography, more sophisticated imaging modalities are unnecessary. (*From* Vaitkus and Kussmaul [23]; with permission.)

REFERENCES

1. Fowler NO: Tuberculous pericarditis. *JAMA* 1991, 266:99–103.

2. Bloom BR, Murray CJ: Tuberculosis: commentary on a reemergent killer. *Science* 1992, 257:1055–1064.

3. Acierno LJ: Cardiac complications in acquired immunodeficiency syndrome (AIDS): a review. *J Am Coll Cardiol* 1989, 13:1144–1154.

4. Dacso SS: Pericarditis in AIDS. *Cardiol Clin* 1990, 8:697–699.

5. Correlae E, Maggioni AP, Romano S, *et al.*: Comparison of frequency, diagnostic and prognostic significance of pericardial involvement in acute myocardial infarction treated with and without thrombolytics. *Am J Cardiol* 1993, 71:1377–1381.

6. Tofler GH, Muller JE, Stone PH, *et al.*: Pericarditis in acute myocardial infarction: characterization and clinical significance. *Am Heart J* 1989, 117:86–90.

7. Sagrista-Sauleda J, Barrabes JA, Permanyer-Miralda G, Soler-Soler J: Purulent pericarditis: review of a 20-year experience in a general hospital. *J Am Coll Cardiol* 1993, 22:1661–1665.

8. Sagrista-Sauleda J, Permanyer-Miralda G, Soler-Soler J: Tuberculous pericarditis: ten-year experience with a prospective protocol for diagnosis and treatment. *J Am Coll Cardiol* 1988, 11:724–728.

9. Koh KK, Kim EJ, Cho CH, *et al.*: Adenosine deaminase and carcinoembryonic antigen in pericardial effusion diagnosis, especially in suspected tuberculous pericarditis. *Circulation* 1994, 89:2728–2735.

10. Fowler NO, Harbin AD: Recurrent acute pericarditis: follow-up study of 31 patients. *J Am Coll Cardiol* 1986, 7:300–305.

11. Guindo J, de la Serna AR, Ramio J, *et al.*: Recurrent pericarditis: relief with colchicine. *Circulation* 1990, 82:1117–1120.

12. Strang JI, Gibson DG, Mitchison DA, *et al.*: Controlled clinical trial of complete open surgical drainage and of prednisolone in treatment of tuberculous pericardial effusion in Transkei. *Lancet* 1988, ii:759–764.

13. De Pace NL, Nestico PF, Schwartz AB, *et al.*: Predicting success of intensive dialysis in the treatment of uremic pericarditis. *Am J Med* 1984, 76:38–46.

14. Frommer JP, Young JB, Ayus JC: Asymptomatic pericardial effusion in uremic patients: effect of long-term dialysis. *Nephron* 1985, 39:296–301.

15. Spector D, Alfred H, Siedlecki M, Briefel G: A controlled study of the effect of indomethacin in uremic pericarditis. *Kidney Int* 1983, 24:663–669.

16. Renkin KJ, DeBruyne B, Benit E, *et al.*: Cardiac tamponade early after thrombolysis for acute myocardial infarction: a rare but not reported hemorrhagic complication. *J Am Coll Cardiol* 1991, 17:280–285.

17. Lichstein E, Arsura E, Hollander G, *et al.*: Current incidence of postmyocardial infarction (Dressler's) syndrome. *Am J Cardiol* 1982, 50:1269–1271.

18. Ilan Y, Oren R, Ben-Chetrit E: Etiology, treatment and prognosis of large pericardial effusions. *Chest* 1991, 100:985–987.

19. Eisenberg MJ, Dunn MM, Kanth N, *et al.*: Diagnostic value of chest radiography for pericardial effusion. *J Am Coll Cardiol* 1993, 22:588–593.

20. Eisenberg MJ, Oken K, Guerrero S, *et al.*: Prognostic value of echocardiography in hospitalized patients with pericardial effusion. *Am J Cardiol* 1992, 70:934–939.

21. Vaitkus PT, Herrmann HC, LeWinter MM: Treatment of malignant pericardial effusion. *JAMA* 1994, 272:59–64.

22. Fowler NO: Constrictive pericarditis: Its history and current status. *Clin Cardiol* 1995, 18:341–350.

23. Vaitkus PT, Kussmaul WG: Constrictive pericarditis versus restrictive cardiomyopathy: a reappraisal and update of diagnostic criteria. *Am Heart J* 1991, 122:1431–1441.

SELECT BIBLIOGRAPHY

Cimino JJ, Kogan AD: Constrictive pericarditis after cardiac surgery: report of three cases and review of the literature. *Am Heart J* 1989, 118:1292–1301.

Feigenbaum H: Pericardial disease. In *Echocardiography*, edn 4. Edited by Feigenbaum H. Philadelphia: Lea & Febiger; 1986:548–578.

Fowler NO: *The Pericardium in Health and Disease.* New York: Futura Publishing; 1985.

Gregoratos G: Pericardial involvement in acute myocardial infarction. *Cardiol Clin* 1990, 8:601–608.

Lorell BH, Grossman W: Profiles in constrictive pericarditis, restrictive cardiomyopathy, and cardiac tamponade. In *Cardiac Catheterization, Angiography, and Intervention*, edn 4. Edited by Grossman W. Philadelphia: Lea & Febiger; 1991:633–653.

Rostand SG, Rutsky EA: Pericarditis in end-stage renal disease. *Cardiol Clin* 1990, 8:701–707.

Spodick DH: Pericarditis in systemic diseases. *Cardiol Clin* 1990, 8:709–716.

Congenital Heart Disease, Including Unrepaired Lesions in the Adult 31

Melvin D. Cheitlin

John A. Paraskos

> ### *Key Points*
> - More patients with congenital heart disease will be seen by the internist than ever in the past; patients with congenital heart disease are living to have children with congenital heart disease.
> - In adult patients, congenital heart disease is frequently not recognized and is misdiagnosed.
> - Atrial septal defect is the most common significant congenital heart defect seen in the adult and is unrecognized because the physical findings are subtle.
> - The pregnant patient with Eisenmenger's syndrome has a high maternal and fetal mortality rate.
> - The most common cause of a continuous murmur is a patent ductus arteriosus; clinicians should remember that patent ductus arteriosus is not the *only* cause of continuous murmur.
> - With the exception of the patient with a septal defect or patent ductus arteriosus with pulmonary vascular disease, cyanotic congenital heart disease is very unusual and is unexpected in the adult. However, it can occur and can frequently be corrected if recognized.
> - Doppler echocardiography is the single most important diagnostic tool in congenital heart disease and frequently makes cardiac catheterization unnecessary.

Congenital heart disease is usually the province of the pediatrician and the pediatric cardiologist. Most significant lesions are found in children and are identified or surgically "corrected" by the time the internist sees the patient. However, the conditions of some patients are not discovered in childhood, and the internist sees congenital heart disease most often in the five ways listed in Table 1 [1]. This chapter deals with the first two categories of congenital cardiac lesions.

MINOR LESIONS

A good example of a minor lesion is the bicuspid aortic valve. Most bicuspid aortic valves of normal histology are competent or have only minor regurgitation; however, occasionally these valves can be severely incompetent. Of the two complications seen with these valves, the most important is infective endocarditis. Antibiotic prophylaxis for dental procedures or surgery through contaminated areas is required to decrease the possibility of endocarditis developing. Other complications include the development of aortic insufficiency or calcification and severe aortic stenosis at 40 to 50 years of age. A large proportion of people with bicuspid aortic valves never have any complications and can live a normal life span without problems.

Clues that the valve is bicuspid come from physical examination. Because the valve does not open properly, these patients can have an ejection click and a short systolic ejection murmur. The murmur is similar to an innocent ejection murmur, but if it is associated with an ejection click, a diagnosis of abnormal aortic valve is

TABLE 1 MOST COMMON PRESENTATIONS OF CONGENITAL HEART DISEASE IN ADULTS

Minor lesions without hemodynamic consequence

Major lesions that were not diagnosed previously

Major lesions that were previously diagnosed but at present are not amenable to surgery, including irreversible pulmonary vascular disease and cyanotic patients with extremely small pulmonary arteries that would not support a shunt

Lesions recognized, operated on, and anatomically and/or physiologically "corrected"

Lesions operated on and "cured" —an extremely small category consisting of some secundum atrial septal defects and patent ductus arteriosus that are closed

probable. Because there is difficulty with coaptation at the aortic leaflets, minimal aortic regurgitation may be present, the murmur of which can be increased in loudness by a handgrip or by squatting. The diagnosis can be made with Doppler echocardiography. When this lesion is recognized, the major appropriate treatment is prophylaxis at the time of dental procedure and at other times of bacteremia to prevent endocarditis.

Other lesions that may cause problems in differential diagnosis are 1) dextrocardia and situs inversus and 2) a pulmonary varix (or pulmonary varicose vein), which may appear as a solitary nodule on the chest roentgenogram. The varix presents as a rounded density in the lung, usually near the cardiac silhouette on the left or the right side and frequently in association with a disease that increases left atrial pressure, such as mitral stenosis. Under fluoroscopy, the lesion can be seen to collapse during a Valsalva maneuver.

Many other minor lesions are important to recognize, such as the right-sided aortic arch that can be mistaken for a paratracheal mass. The major challenge with most is recognizing the lesion, and thus, avoiding the mistake of diagnosing a more serious problem.

RECOGNITION OF COMMON CONGENITAL HEART DISEASE PROBLEMS

The unoperated, hemodynamically important congenital heart disease problems likely to be seen in the adult are relatively few. Adult patients with pulmonary atresia and tetralogy of Fallot can be seen previously undiagnosed. McNamara and Latson [2], looking at the number of children born with congenital heart disease, showed that atrial septal defect, interventricular septal defect, patent ductus arteriosus (PDA), tetralogy of Fallot, and coarctation of the aorta constituted approximately 60% of the cases of congenital heart disease in adults. If Ebstein's disease, aortic stenosis, pulmonic valve stenosis, and bicuspid aortic valve are added, the vast majority of the important congenital heart disease lesions seen in adulthood are accounted for.

Predominant Left-to-Right Shunts with Normal or Moderately Increased Pulmonary Vascular Resistance

Predominant left-to-right shunts with normal or moderately increased pulmonary vascular resistance can occur at the atrial level, the ventricular level, or the pulmonary artery level. All of these shunts result in the return of pulmonary venous blood to the right side of the heart. This increase in pulmonary blood flow increases pulmonary vascular markings on chest roentgenography (Fig. 1). If the shunt is large, ventricular enlargement along with pulmonary hypertension results, leading to right ventricular hypertrophy and finally right-sided heart failure.

Interatrial septal defect

Anatomy

Three types of atrial septal defects are 1) ostium secundum (the most common type), 2) ostium primum (results in a low-lying atrial septal defect where the atrial septum joins the confluence of the mitral and tricuspid rings), and 3) sinus venosus defects (the least common type, it is most often either superior near the entrance of the superior vena cava or inferior near the inferior vena cava and the ostium of the coronary sinus).

Pathophysiology

Because the right ventricle is more compliant than the left ventricle, it fills more readily. In diastole, blood just returning from the lung to the left atrium goes through the defect into the right side of the heart, resulting in a right ventricular end-diastolic volume and subsequent stroke volume that are larger than those on the left. The blood flow through the lung is markedly increased. The pathophysiology is similar in the three types of atrial septal defects.

Physical, electrocardiographic, and roentgenographic findings

The physical, electrocardiographic, and chest roentgenographic findings in atrial septal defect are listed in Table 2.

Echocardiography (ECG)

There is an increased right ventricular volume and a flattening of the interventricular septum at end-diastole, with systolic paradoxical motion of the septum. Doppler echocardiography shows a continuous flow across the atrial septum (Fig. 2). With the intravenous injection of agitated saline (intravenous contrast injection), microbubbles are seen filling the right atrium and right ventricle, and a negative-contrast jet may be seen flowing across the atrial septum from right to left.

Complications

Pulmonary hypertension. The most important complication of atrial septal defect is the development of severe pulmonary vascular disease, which occurs only with large atrial septal defects with large left-to-right shunts and produces a form of Eisenmenger's syndrome. It occurs in fewer than 10% of

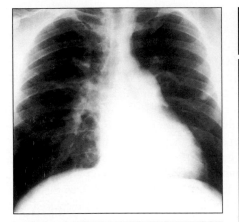

Figure 1 Chest x-ray, posterior-anterior projection of 40-year-old man with a secundum atrial septal defect with a pulmonary blood flow/systemic blood flow ratio of 2:1.

Table 2 Physical, Electrocardiographic, and Chest Roentgenographic Findings in Atrial Septal Defect

Finding	Comment
Systolic ejection murmur in the second left intercostal space	Produced by the increased right ventricular stroke volume
Increase in the pulmonary vascular markings on chest roentgenography	Caused by the increased pulmonary blood flow
Diastolic flow rumble at the left sternal border	Produced by an increase in flow across the tricuspid valve
Wide, fixed splitting of the second heart sound	Caused by the increased right ventricular filling in diastole, which is unaffected by respiration
rSR' in V_1 on the electrocardiogram	Caused by the increased right ventricular diastolic filling, which increases the size of the right atrium and the right ventricle

patients with large atrial septal defects. It almost always occurs after puberty, and if the patient reaches 30 to 40 years of age without developing pulmonary hypertension, the later development of pulmonary vascular disease is rare. There is an increase in right ventricular and pulmonary artery systolic pressure, with the subsequent development of right ventricular hypertrophy. Eventually, the shunt becomes a right-to-left one, and cyanosis occurs.

The pulmonary artery branches maintaining high, even systemic, pressures dilate, and they may become atherosclerotic and calcified. The patient now has the complications of systemic arterial desaturation, with polycythemia and the subsequent clotting and bleeding problems. In addition, the patient may develop syncopal episodes, probably from arrhythmias, dyspnea, hemoptysis, and anginal chest pain. Pregnancy is poorly tolerated, with fetal wastage high and the maternal mortality rate increased.

Congestive heart failure. With the increased volume load on the right ventricle, right ventricular dilatation and hypertrophy occur. Eventually, right ventricular systolic dysfunction supervenes, and the right ventricle dilates further, interfering with left ventricular filling in diastole. With failure, both the right and the left ventricle filling pressures rise together, as do the right and the left atrial pressures, which must remain equal because of the large connection between them.

Atrial arrhythmias. Atrial arrhythmias (*ie*, atrial fibrillation and atrial tachycardias) are not uncommon, especially in patients older than 40 years of age. Once they occur, surgical correction does not eliminate the possibility that they will recur.

Treatment

Young patients with an atrial septal defect of any type who have a pulmonary-to-systemic blood flow ratio of greater than or equal to 1.8:1 should have repair of their defect. If the right ventricle is dilated, even lesser-volume shunts should be repaired. The surgery is very low risk, and many of the complications mentioned will probably be avoided. In

sinus venosus defects, the anomalous pulmonary veins can be redirected to drain into the left atrium.

Age is not a contraindication to repair. There is good evidence that repair, even after age 40, improves the patient's functional capacity and decreases symptoms [3•].

Because there is no jet formation to disrupt the endocardium and create a site for the development of infective endocarditis and if no associated lesions such as mitral valve prolapse or clefting of the mitral valve with mitral regurgitation are present, antibiotic prophylaxis to prevent endocarditis is not needed in patients with atrial septal defect.

Alternatives to surgical closure of the secundum atrial septal defect are being developed. These approaches consist of patches, or "clam shells," which can be affixed by means

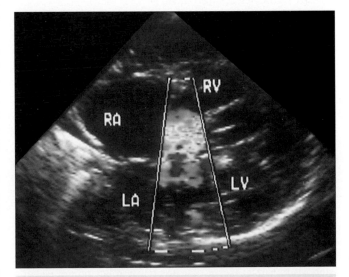

Figure 2 Echo-Doppler, subcostal view of a 40-year-old man with an ostium primum atrial septal defect. Doppler signal shows abnormal continuous jet from left atrium to right atrium across the low-lying atrial septal defect. RA—right atrium; RV—right ventricle; LA—left atrium; LV—left ventricle. (*See* Color Plate.)

of catheters. So far, this treatment is available at relatively few institutions and must still be considered to be under development.

Interventricular septal defect

Interventricular septal defect is the most commonly recognized congenital heart lesion in infants. A large percentage of these defects close in early infancy; therefore, only approximately 10% of adult patients with congenital heart disease have a large ventricular septal defect (VSD) [4].

Pathophysiology

The effect of the VSD depends on its size, its position, and the relative ratio of pulmonary vascular resistance to systemic vascular resistance. Ventricular septal defects can be 1) perimembranous, 2) supracristal, 3) a posterior or atrioventricular canal defect, or 4) muscular.

Small ventricular septal defect. With small VSDs, there is a connection between the high-pressure left ventricle and the low-pressure right ventricle. In systole, a high-velocity, small-volume jet of blood is directed from the left to the right ventricle. This left-to-right shunt adds little to the pulmonary blood flow. Therefore, the effect is to create a loud pansystolic murmur without any change in cardiac size or ventricular function. This type of defect, called *Roger's disease*, is commonly seen in the adult.

Moderate-sized ventricular septal defect. With the moderate-sized VSD, the left-to-right shunt is larger, but the defect is not large enough to create a common chamber with equal pressure between the right and the left ventricles. The right-to-left shunt is determined by the size of the VSD and the magnitude of the pulmonary vascular resistance relative to that of the systemic vascular resistance. The right ventricular pressure can be raised owing to the increased pulmonary blood flow, but it is not equal to the left ventricular pressure because the size of the defect is too small.

Large ventricular septal defect. With the large VSD, the area of the VSD is more than half of the area of the aortic ring, making the right ventricle and the left ventricle a common chamber. With the large VSD, the increased pulmonary blood flow and high pulmonary artery pressure result in irreversible pulmonary vascular disease and Eisenmenger's syndrome, usually by the end of the first or the second decade of life.

Physical findings

Small ventricular septal defect. Because the left-to-right shunt is small, there is no volume overload of the ventricles, no cardiac enlargement, and no increase in pulmonary vascular markings. The major finding is the presence of a loud pansystolic murmur along the left sternal border, usually in the third and fourth interspace and usually of grade IV to VI intensity.

The supracristal VSD murmur can simulate a pulmonic stenosis murmur, except that it is pansystolic and not ejection in type. If aortic regurgitation develops, a diastolic murmur comes directly off the second heart sound (S_2) and can be confused with the murmur of PDA and other lesions causing continuous murmurs.

Moderate-sized ventricular septal defect. In addition to the pansystolic murmur along the left sternal border, enlargement of the left atrium and dilatation and hypertrophy of the left ventricle may be noted on chest roentgenography and electro-cardiography (ECG). The S_2 may be increased in intensity, and in adolescents and thin adults, a diastolic flow rumble of increased blood flow across the mitral valve may be heard at the apex. A ventricular gallop (S_3) resulting from an increased rate of left ventricular filling is not unusual.

Large ventricular septal defect. By the time patients reach adolescence or adulthood, they most often have severe pulmonary hypertension. If they still have an appreciable left-to-right shunt, a pansystolic murmur is still present. The pulmonic heart sound (P_2) is always increased and now may be coincident with the aortic second sound (A_2), so that there is a single loud S_2. The left ventricle is laterally displaced and hypertrophied, as is the right ventricle.

As the pulmonary vascular resistance increases relative to the systemic vascular resistance, the left-to-right shunt decreases. The size of the left ventricle decreases; the systolic murmur decreases in intensity and is no longer present throughout systole, finally disappearing altogether. At this point, predominant right ventricular hypertrophy may be present. With pulmonary hypertension, pulmonic valvular regurgitation causes a high-frequency blowing diastolic murmur that is heard along the left sternal border, similar to the murmur of aortic regurgitation. With right ventricular failure and dilatation, the tricuspid ring dilates and tricuspid regurgitation occurs, causing a systolic murmur along the left sternal border that may increase with inspiration.

Diagnosis

With the left-to-right shunt, pansystolic murmur is the best clue to the diagnosis. The enlarged left ventricle and left atrium and increased pulmonary vascular markings are seen on chest roentgenography. Echocardiography identifies the chamber enlargement and the increased left ventricular stroke volume, and Doppler echocardiography demonstrates the position of the jet across the interventricular septum (Fig. 3). From the velocity of the jet, the gradient in systole can be estimated. With low pressure in the right ventricle, the jet is high velocity. As the systolic gradient between the right and the left ventricles decreases as the VSD becomes larger, the velocity of the jet also decreases.

Complications

The development of irreversible pulmonary vascular disease is the most common complication of the large VSD (Table 3). High pulmonary blood flow and pressure, and high shear forces damage the intima of the small pulmonary arteries, resulting in intimal hyperplasia, medial hypertrophy of the small pulmonary arteries, and fewer small pulmonary vessels. All of these changes, which are irreversible, result in pulmonary vascular disease and pulmonary hypertension with left-to-right shunting and cyanosis with its complications. Eventually, dilatation of the right ventricle occurs, as does severe left- and right-sided heart failure.

With large left-to-right shunts, left ventricular failure can occur. In my experience, the high-flow, low-pressure VSD, sufficient to cause heart failure, is extremely unusual in adults. With large VSDs, the most common presentation in the adult is that of Eisenmenger's syndrome.

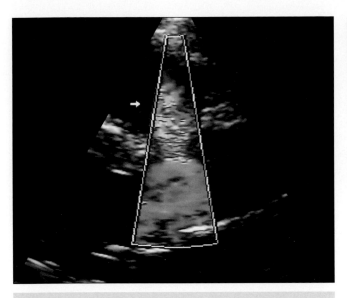

FIGURE 3 Echo-Doppler, parasternal long-axis view of a 32-year-old man with a moderate sized ventricular septal defect. Systolic jet is seen through the ventricular septal defect from left ventricular outflow tract to right ventricle. (*See* Color Plate.)

Ventricular septal defect	Complication
Small VSD	Infective endocarditis
Supracristal VSD	Progressive aortic regurgitation
Moderate and large VSD	Congestive heart failure
	Infective endocarditis
	Pulmonary vascular disease

TABLE 3 COMPLICATIONS OF VENTRICULAR SEPTAL DEFECT

VSD—ventricular septal defect.

In some patients, hypertrophy of the crista supraventricularis causes infundibular stenosis, converting the clinical picture to that of a "pink" tetralogy of Fallot. The severity of the obstruction caused by the infundibular stenosis is such that a right-to-left shunt may occur through the VSD, and the clinical picture becomes that of a tetralogy of Fallot.

Infective endocarditis. The high-velocity jet injures the endocardium. Vegetations occur on the right ventricular side of the VSD or on the tricuspid or pulmonic valve. Emboli therefore occur most often to the lungs.

Prolapse of the right coronary cusp of the aortic valve and aortic regurgitation with supracristal VSD.

Treatment

Small VSDs without hemodynamic significance need only antibiotic prophylaxis to prevent endocarditis. If infective endocarditis recurs in a patient with a small VSD despite adequate antibiotic prophylaxis, then consideration should be given to closing the VSD.

In patients with large VSDs with a large left-to-right shunt and with a pulmonary blood flow–to–systemic blood flow ratio of 2:1 or greater, surgical closure is indicated. This type of VSD is unusual in the adult. With pulmonary hypertension, if a left-to-right shunt is still present in the range of 1.8:1, the pulmonary vascular resistance is not greater than 7.5 Wood units, and the arterial saturation is greater than 90%, then closure can be considered.

With Eisenmenger's syndrome and cyanosis, operative closure is contraindicated because it would require all the systemic venous return to go through the lungs and would precipitate severe right-sided heart failure. Phlebotomy is indicated only for a very high hematocrit level (> 65) or if the "polycythemic syndrome" of headache, lethargy, and excessive fatigue occurs. The only hope that these patients have is lung transplantation with or without heart transplantation. This approach is still available in only a few centers.

Patent ductus arteriosus

Anatomy

Patent ductus arteriosus completes the "big three" of left-to-right shunts. It is by far the most common cause of a continuous murmur and results from persistent patency of the fetal ductus arteriosus, which connects the proximal descending aorta just beyond the takeoff of the left subclavian artery with the pulmonary artery just to the left of the bifurcation [5].

Pathophysiology

With a small PDA, the high-pressure aorta is connected with the pulmonary artery, which results in a high-velocity jet of low volume into the pulmonary artery. The larger the ductus, the more the shunt is determined by the ratio of pulmonary vascular resistance to systemic vascular resistance. If the patent ductus is large enough, there is equalization of pressure in the pulmonary artery and the aorta; then, the size of the shunt depends completely on the ratio of pulmonary vascular resistance to systemic vascular resistance. As with the VSD, the high pressure and high flow result in irreversible changes in the pulmonary vasculature, an irreversible increase in pulmonary vascular resistance, and Eisenmenger's syndrome.

Physical findings

Small patent ductus arteriosus. The continuous jet from the aorta to the pulmonary artery results in a high-pitched, continuous murmur, with peaking of the murmur at the time of the S_2. The murmur is best heard in the second interspace to the left of the sternum and under the left clavicle. If the shunt is small, there is no increase in heart size and no increase in pulmonary vascular markings.

Moderate-sized patent ductus arteriosus. The volume of the left-to-right shunt is increased; the murmur becomes louder and coarser, still peaking at the S_2; and the pulmonary artery pressure may be increased, causing an increased P_2. Because of the increased flow across the mitral valve, there may be a mitral diastolic flow rumble and an S_3 at the apex. Left ventricular hyperactivity and possibly a right ventricular lift are present because of the high right ventricular pressure.

Patent ductus arteriosus with pulmonary hypertension. As the pulmonary artery and aortic pressures equalize, the left-to-right shunt is totally dependent on the ratio of pulmonary vascular resistance to systemic vascular resistance. As the pulmonary vascular resistance approaches the systemic vascular resistance, the murmur may be heard only in late systole. Finally, with a further increase in pulmonary vascular resistance, there is little left-to-right shunt and

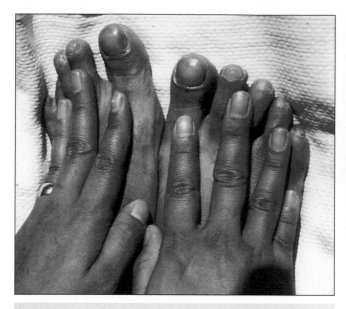

FIGURE 4 Hands and feet of a 20-year-old woman with patent ductus arteriosus and pulmonary vascular disease. Note cyanosis and clubbing of the toes, and pink nonclubbed fingers. (*See* Color Plate.)

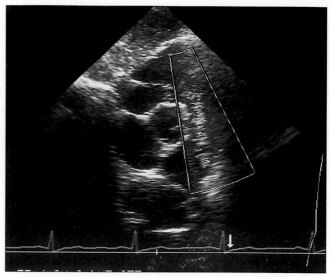

FIGURE 5 Echo-Doppler, short-axis view at level of aortic valve. The color of Doppler shows an abnormal jet in the main pulmonary artery which, on motion, showed that jet through the patent ductus entered at the bifurcation of the pulmonary artery and went down the main pulmonary artery. (*See* Color Plate.)

no murmur is heard. The P_2 is then loud and coincident with the A_2, creating a loud single S_2. The findings are those of pulmonary hypertension, frequently with a diastolic decrescendo murmur of pulmonic regurgitation. With right ventricular dilatation, right-sided heart failure and tricuspid regurgitation may result.

With pulmonary vascular disease, a right-to-left shunt occurs, with arterial desaturation occurring downstream from where the patent ductus enters. This event results in the finding of "differential cyanosis," pink fingers and cyanosis and clubbing of the toes (Fig. 4).

Diagnosis

The best clue to the presence of a PDA is the continuous murmur. With the larger shunts, the ascending aorta, the left atrium, and the left ventricle should be dilated and hypertrophied, which can be seen on both chest roentgenography and ECG. Echocardiography reveals the chamber enlargement, and Doppler echocardiography demonstrates the abnormal high-velocity jet entering the main pulmonary artery, swirling down one side of the pulmonary artery and up the other, that is characteristic of a PDA (Fig. 5).

As pulmonary vascular resistance increases, the jet may be less obvious or even absent, and the findings are those of pulmonary hypertension and right ventricular failure, with an increased S_2, pulmonic regurgitation, tricuspid regurgitation, right-sided S_3 and atrial gallop (S_4) sounds, and an elevated jugular venous pressure. Here, the presence of differential cyanosis can make the diagnosis.

The differential diagnosis of a continuous murmur is important and consists of problems that create a continuous murmur at the base of the heart to the left of the sternum (Table 4). Four conditions must be considered when a continuous murmur is heard: 1) aorta–pulmonary artery window, in which a connection exists between the ascending aorta and the main

pulmonary artery; 2) ruptured sinus of Valsalva aneurysm into the outflow tract of the right ventricle; 3) supracristal VSD with aortic regurgitation; and 4) coronary artery–pulmonary artery fistula. Of all of these conditions, PDA is by far the most common.

Another lesion that is important to exclude is a venous hum loud enough to be heard in the second interspace on the left. The murmur can be obliterated by pressing firmly over the internal jugular vein and occluding it. In addition, a mammary souffle in the pregnant or postpartum woman with lactating breasts can be confusing. Blood flow to the breasts is markedly increased, creating continuous bruits; here, finding the position of the loudest bruit and pressing firmly with the

TABLE 4 DIFFERENTIAL DIAGNOSIS OF A CONTINUOUS MURMUR
Confusion with PDA
Aortic-pulmonary window
Sinus of Valsalva aneurysm rupturing into the right atrium or right ventricle
Supracristal VSD with aortic regurgitation
Coronary artery to pulmonary artery fistula
Venous hum
Other causes of continuous murmurs
Mammary souffle in pregnant women with lactating breasts
Coronary arteriovenous fistula
Coronary cameral fistula
Pulmonary arteriovenous fistula
Systemic arteriovenous fistula
PDA—patent ductus arteriosus; VSD—ventricular septal defect.

stethoscope can obliterate the bruit. Other causes of continuous murmur, such as coronary arteriovenous fistulas, coronary-cameral fistulas, pulmonary arteriovenous fistulas, and systemic arteriovenous fistulas, are usually loudest in different areas of the chest and are usually not confused.

Complications

The complications of PDA are similar to those of VSD, although a large left-to-right shunt and a lower-pressure pulmonary artery are more often seen in adults with PDA than in those with VSD. The danger of a small PDA is the development of infective endarteritis, and its presence requires antibiotic prophylaxis at the time of dental or other procedures causing bacteremias.

Treatment

A small PDA should be closed in children and young adults because the perioperative mortality rate is low and the operation is curative. As the patient gets older, the ductus becomes atherosclerotic and is therefore more easily torn at surgery, increasing the danger of a surgical mishap. In patients older than 60 years of age, the danger of the surgery is similar to or greater than the danger of developing infective endarteritis, and I do not recommend surgery. With a large PDA and a large shunt, especially in a symptomatic patient, I recommend surgery at any age.

In a patient with pulmonary vascular disease and little or no left-to-right shunt, surgical closure is contraindicated, and lung transplantation is the patient's only hope.

Pure Valvular Lesions
Aortic stenosis
Anatomy

Congenital aortic stenosis can occur at any level of the left ventricular outflow tract and ascending aorta. The most common type is caused by valvular abnormalities. If its histology is normal, the bicuspid aortic valve does not create severe aortic stenosis, but it may be incompetent, resulting in aortic regurgitation. Severe aortic stenosis may occur with the bicuspid valve early in infancy if the valve is dysplastic. If the histology of the valve is normal, a minority of patients with bicuspid aortic valve will develop fibrosis and calcification and severe aortic stenosis between 40 and 50 years of age [6].

The aortic valves that are congenitally stenotic in childhood are those with only one commissure; the bicuspid valve with a fused commissure or a unicuspid valve; and those without any normally formed commissures, the so-called acommissural valves. Much less often, left ventricular outflow tract obstruction above (supravalvular) or below (subvalvular) the aortic valve occurs. Supravalvular aortic stenosis can be caused by a discrete membrane, an hourglass constriction, or a hypoplastic ascending aorta. These obstructions are usually above the takeoff of the coronary arteries. The subvalvular obstructions can be discrete and membranous, caused by abnormal hypertrophy (so-called hypertrophic cardiomyopathy), or caused by a fibromuscular tunnel involving both the interventricular septum and the anterior leaflet of the mitral valve. These problems are more difficult to treat surgically.

Pathophysiology

The obstruction to the left ventricular outflow tract results in a systolic afterload burden to the left ventricle, which causes left ventricular hypertrophy, and the pathophysiologic consequences are similar in all ways to those seen in the adult with acquired aortic stenosis.

The increase in left ventricular mass, the high left ventricular systolic pressure, the relatively low aortic diastolic pressure, and the high extramural pressure on the intramural coronary arteries all result in an increase in myocardial oxygen demand and a decrease in coronary blood supply. The pathophysiologic factors result in myocardial ischemia, which can lead to angina pectoris and myocardial infarction.

Ventricular arrhythmia and sudden death can result from myocardial ischemia. Exertional syncope can be caused by an inability to increase stroke volume with exercise and therefore a decrease in systolic blood pressure, but it may be caused by sudden self-limited ventricular arrhythmias or inappropriate reflexes that cause vasodilation and bradycardia at a time when the aortic systolic pressure is falling.

Physical findings

The systolic ejection murmur at the base, which radiates into the carotid arteries, is the most valuable diagnostic sign of aortic stenosis. With valvular aortic stenosis, because the valve is flexible in the young adult, there is frequently a systolic ejection click. In half of the patients, minimal aortic regurgitation is audible. If the chest wall has a normal configuration and the cardiac output is normal, the murmur is usually loud enough to create a systolic thrill. Therefore, in a young person, the absence of a thrill is powerful evidence against severe aortic stenosis. However, in an older person, who may have decreased cardiac output and an increased anteroposterior diameter of the chest, the absence of a systolic thrill is less valuable in predicting the absence of severe aortic stenosis.

Left ventricular hypertrophy is the natural compensation for severe aortic stenosis, so a sustained point of maximal impulse and an S_4 are also good evidence of the increased severity of aortic stenosis. With left ventricular failure, there is dilatation of the left ventricle and an S_3, but they are present very late in the natural history of the disease. The absence of a systolic ejection click should lead the clinician to suspect calcification of the aortic valve or an unusual type of aortic stenosis, either supravalvular or subvalvular.

Diagnosis

The systolic ejection murmur is the best clue to the diagnosis of aortic stenosis. Chest roentgenography usually shows post-stenotic dilatation of the ascending aorta, but the cardiac silhouette is usually normal. The ECG in severe aortic stenosis usually demonstrates left ventricular hypertrophy (Fig. 6), although approximately 15% to 20% may show only ST-T wave changes or be within normal limits. In these situations, echocardiography shows left ventricular hypertrophy if the aortic stenosis is severe, usually without dilatation of the left ventricle. In young adults, left ventricular contractility is usually preserved. Supravalvular aortic stenosis, subvalvular aortic stenosis, and hypertrophic cardiomyopathy can be diagnosed with echocardiography, which is the best way to visualize the discrete membranous type of subaortic stenosis. Doppler echocardiography can reliably identify minimal-velocity and high-velocity jets, and therefore minimal and large systolic gradients, and is a good way of detecting an increase in the severity of the lesion over the years.

Complications and treatment

The complications of congestive heart failure, angina pectoris including non–Q wave myocardial infarction, exertional syncope, arrhythmias, sudden death, and infective endocarditis are all similar to those seen with acquired aortic stenosis. In adolescents and young adults, the presence of severe aortic stenosis with a systolic gradient of 50 mm Hg, or an aortic valve area of less then 0.8 cm², is an indication for surgical correction. With commissurial fusion and an uncalcified valve, correction can be achieved by repair rather than by replacement. In children and some young adults, balloon valvotomy can be just as effective as surgical valve repair. If the valve is calcified, as it is in almost all patients older than 40 years of age, valvular replacement is necessary.

When valve repair is possible, it is highly likely that a second surgical procedure, and even replacement of the valve, will be necessary after 15 to 20 years.

Valvular pulmonary stenosis

Anatomy

Valvular pulmonary stenosis is a relatively uncommon problem in adults. Although stenosis of the right ventricular outflow tract can be at, below, or above the pulmonic valve, valvular pulmonary stenosis is by far the most common as an isolated lesion. Infundibular stenosis without a VSD and supravalvular pulmonary stenosis are extremely rare.

Pathophysiology

Valvular pulmonary stenosis is caused by an abnormally formed pulmonic valve. The obstruction to right ventricular outflow causes an afterload burden on the right ventricle, resulting in right ventricular hypertrophy. There is a large gradient across the pulmonic valve, and the jet causes post-stenotic dilatation of the main pulmonary artery and frequently of the left pulmonary artery but not of the right.

Physical findings

The obstruction across the pulmonic valve results in a high-velocity jet created by the entire stroke volume. This jet results in a loud ejection murmur, best heard in the second intercostal space to the left of the sternum. It radiates into the lung fields and less well into the neck. The flexible stenotic valve and poststenotic dilatation result in an ejection click.

Right ventricular hypertrophy results in a systolic precordial lift. A prominent "A" wave may also be present in the jugular venous pulse. If there is a right-to-left shunt through a patent foramen ovale, cyanosis may be present.

Diagnosis

The systolic ejection murmur in the second interspace to the left of the sternum is the first clue to the diagnosis. The ejection click, which decreases with inspiration, is an excellent clue to the valvular abnormality. With severe pulmonic valve stenosis, right ventricular hypertrophy is seen on the ECG. Doppler echocardiography demonstrates right ventricular hypertrophy and the high-velocity jet across the pulmonic valve, allowing for an estimation of the systolic gradient.

Complications

Valvular pulmonary stenosis is a rare disease in adults. If it occurs in adults severely enough to cause right ventricular hypertrophy, then repair of the pulmonic valve is indicated. If the patient has signs of right ventricular failure, the lesion should be repaired at any age. If pulmonic valvular stenosis is present, even if it is mild, antibiotic prophylaxis to prevent endocarditis is indicated.

Coarctation of the aorta

Anatomy

In adults, coarctation of the aorta constitutes approximately 5% of cases of congenital cardiovascular disease. The most common form consists of a relatively short constriction of the descending aorta just beyond the takeoff of the left subclavian

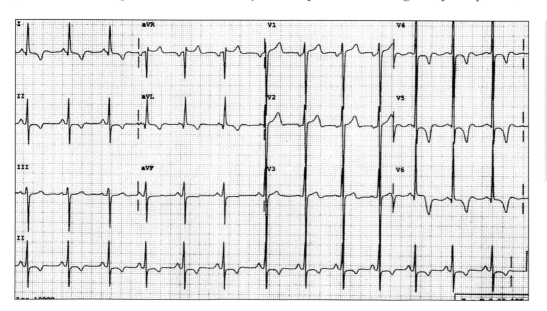

FIGURE 6 Electrocardiogram showing left ventricular hypertrophy and left atrial abnormality in a 45-year-old man with a calcified bicuspid aortic valve and a mean systolic gradient across the aortic valve of 80 mm Hg.

artery at the level of the ligamentus arteriosus. Occasionally, the aorta proximal to this point can be markedly hypoplastic, resulting in a longer length of constriction.

A bicuspid aortic valve is the most commonly associated abnormality and may be present in up to 80% of patients. In addition, associated congenital aneurysms may be present in the aorta either proximal or distal to the coarctation or in arteries of the circle of Willis (so-called berry aneurysms). Associated abnormalities such as PDA, aortic valve and subvalvular stenosis, and mitral valve abnormalities are not uncommon.

Pathophysiology

Coarctation of the aorta results in higher blood pressure in the aorta and arteries proximal to the obstruction and lower blood pressure distally. With severe coarctation of the aorta, collateral circulation develops that bypasses the obstruction. This collateral circulation involves the branches of the subclavian and cervical arterial system, the intercostal arteries, and the internal mammary and periscapular arteries, all of which have connections to arteries arising distal to the coarctation. These vessels dilate and elongate, becoming enlarged and tortuous.

The variables that determine the clinical picture depend on the severity of the obstruction. Minor obstructions cause almost no collateral formation and produce only a dampening of the distal aortic pressure, whereas severe to total occlusion of the aorta causes marked damping of the pulse beyond the coarctation and decreases in distal arterial blood pressure. The size and number of collaterals are also important. The collaterals can be so large and extensive that distal aortic flow is not impaired, and even distal pulse pressure and mean blood pressure may be only mildly decreased. However, the proximal aortic hypertension results in left ventricular hypertrophy and can eventually cause congestive heart failure.

Physical findings

The diagnosis of coarctation of the aorta is easily made by noting a decreased or an absent femoral arterial pulse compared with the brachial pulse. In some patients, the femoral pulses may be difficult to feel; in this case, the diagnosis can be made by comparing the systolic blood pressure in the right arm with the blood pressure in the leg, with both being taken with appropriately sized cuffs. It is important to take the blood pressure in both arms to pick up the unusual coarctation that begins proximal to the takeoff of the left subclavian artery. Normally, the indirect systolic blood pressure by cuff should be 10 mm Hg or higher in the leg than in the arm. If the systolic blood pressure is lower in the leg than in the arm, a diagnosis of aortic obstruction is made; in the proper setting, the etiology is coarctation of the aorta.

The murmur generated by flow past the obstruction is a late systolic bruit heard at the base of the heart anteriorly and as well or better in the interscapular area to the left of the spine. If the patient has a bicuspid aortic valve, an ejection click, a blowing diastolic murmur of aortic regurgitation, or both may also be heard. With the patient leaning forward with the arms crossed over the chest, intercostal and periscapular arterial pulsations can be felt with palpation over the posterior chest wall, and systolic bruits may be heard over the enlarged, tortuous collateral vessels.

Diagnosis

The ECG findings can be within normal limits or show left ventricular hypertrophy. On chest roentgenography, the ascending aorta is frequently dilated; there is a large aortic "knob" because of the lateral displacement of the left subclavian artery. At times, notching of the descending aorta can be seen at the point of the constriction, and poststenotic dilatation can be noted below the coarctation. Rib notching, especially of the third rib and lower, is seen because of the enlarged tortuous intercostal arteries. On barium swallow, a proximal and distal impingement on the barium-filled esophagus of the aorta above and below the coarctation can be seen. On two-dimensional echocardiography, only hypertrophy of the left ventricle and abnormalities of the aortic valve may be seen. With transesophageal echocardiography, the area of the coarctation can be visualized and Doppler echocardiography can reveal the high-velocity jet of blood across the coarctation.

Complications and treatment

Eventually, left-sided heart failure can occur, as can infective endarteritis distal to the coarctation and infective endocarditis on the bicuspid aortic valve. Berry aneurysm rupture can cause a cerebrovascular bleed, and dissection of the aorta proximal to the coarctation has been reported.

In coarctation of the aorta that is severe enough to cause an increase in proximal aortic blood pressure and the development of collateral circulation, resection of the coarctation should be done, especially in young people. If the coarctation is mild, without collateral formation and with minimal difference in blood pressure proximal and distal to the coarctation, there is little evidence that resection of the coarctation is better than treatment with antihypertensive agents.

Even after coarctation repair, antibiotic prophylaxis to prevent infective endocarditis is recommended.

Cyanotic Lesions
(Lesions with Right-to-Left Shunts)

Cyanotic lesions are characterized by a right-to-left shunt large enough to cause arterial desaturation. For a patient to be cyanotic, the reduced hemoglobin concentration must be at least 5 g/dL. Lesser concentrations, for instance in patients with anemia, will not result in cyanosis. The right-to-left shunting can occur at any cardiac level. Table 5 lists examples of lesions in this group and the cardiac level at which shunting occurs.

Although several congenital heart lesions are included in this group, relatively few are seen in the adult without previous surgery.

Eisenmenger's syndrome

Eisenmenger's syndrome lesions have already been discussed under the section dealing with atrial septal defects, VSDs, and PDA. When pulmonary hypertension occurs, it is clinically difficult to make a distinction between these lesions. All are characterized by the findings of pulmonary hypertension (ie, a loud P_2, right ventricular hypertrophy, possibly pulmonic valve regurgitation, right-sided heart failure, dilatation of the right ventricle with tricuspid regurgitation, and right-sided S_3 and S_4 sounds). The murmurs are no longer characteristic, the proximal pulmonary arteries are large, and the peripheral lung fields

TABLE 5 RIGHT-TO-LEFT SHUNTS CLASSIFIED BY CARDIAC LEVEL	
Level at which shunting occurs	**Examples of lesions**
Venous	Total anomalous pulmonary venous drainage; anomalous drainage of the superior vena cava into the left atrium
Atrial	Atrial septal defect with pulmonary hypertension; tricuspid atresia; Ebstein's disease; valvular pulmonary stenosis with blown-open foramen ovale
Ventricular	Ventricular septal defect with pulmonary hypertension; tetralogy of Fallot; pulmonary atresia; patent ductus with pulmonary hypertension
Arterial	Transposition of the great vessels; truncus arteriosus; double-outlet right ventricle; pulmonary arteriovenous fistula

are clear because of extreme narrowing of the more distal pulmonary vessels, or so-called pruning (Figs. 7 and 8). The definitive differential diagnosis can be made with two-dimensional Doppler echocardiography.

Tetralogy of Fallot

Anatomy

Beyond infancy, tetralogy of Fallot is the most common lesion causing cyanosis. It is characterized by obstruction in the right ventricular outflow tract and a VSD, usually proximal to the outflow obstruction. The right ventricular obstruction is usually infundibular, with or without valvular pulmonic stenosis. Least common is valvular pulmonic stenosis alone. The other two lesions inferred from the "tetralogy" are right ventricular hypertrophy and an aortic root that overrides the VSD.

Pathophysiology

The clinical picture depends on the severity of the right ventricular outflow tract obstruction, the size of the VSD, and the systemic vascular resistance. As mentioned in the section on VSD, in patients with large VSDs and pulmonary hypertension, right ventricular hypertrophy is at times accompanied by hypertrophy of the crista supraventricularis, which can form an acquired infundibular obstruction. In many of these patients, the obstruction is mild enough so that left-to-right shunting still occurs, and although a systolic gradient is present across the infundibular obstruction, there is still a predominant left-to-right shunt.

With the congenital malformation of the right ventricular outflow tract that defines the true tetralogy of Fallot, the right ventricular outflow tract is severely stenotic, and the shunt through the VSD is from right to left. The murmur is therefore that of infundibular pulmonary stenosis and not that of VSD.

Physical findings and diagnosis

In infundibular pulmonary stenosis with hypertrophy of the crista supraventricularis and VSD, the murmur may still be pansystolic, loudest at the left sternal border. With obstruction, the predominant systolic murmur is that of infundibular pulmonary stenosis: in other words, a loud ejection murmur without an ejection click. The pulmonary arteries may still be large on roentgenography and echocardiography. In this disease, the magnitude of a right-to-left shunt is usually small at rest.

With tetralogy of Fallot, the right ventricular outflow tract is severely obstructed, the pulmonary blood flow is never large, and the main pulmonary artery and its branches

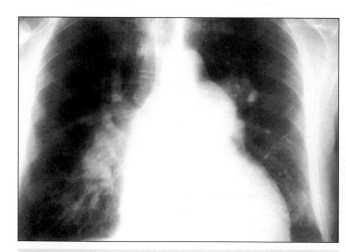

FIGURE 7 Chest x-ray, posteroanterior projection of a 50-year-old man with a large ventricular septal defect, pulmonary hypertension, and pulmonary vascular disease. Note huge main pulmonary artery, large right and left proximal pulmonary arteries, and absence of pulmonary vascular markings in the lateral one third of lung fields ("pruning"). The cardiac silhouette is enlarged, with dilated left ventricle.

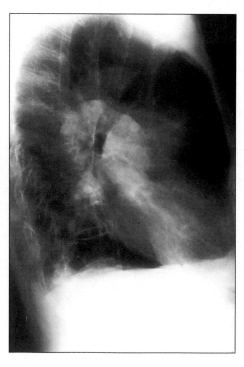

FIGURE 8 Chest x-ray, right lateral view. Same patient as in Figure 7.

are small. It is common for patients with these lesions in infancy to have cyanosis of the mucous membranes of the mouth, nail beds, and conjunctiva and to have clubbing of the fingers and toes. Right ventricular hypertrophy is invariably noted on ECG. Although a definitive diagnosis can be made with two-dimensional Doppler echocardiography, it is recommended that these patients have catheterization, mainly to look at the size of the pulmonary artery and its branches and at the origin and disposition of the coronary arteries. In 15% of cases, the left anterior descending coronary artery anomalously arises from the right coronary artery or the anterior sinus of Valsalva and crosses the right ventricular outflow tract.

Treatment

In most cases in which tetralogy of Fallot is found in the adult, complete correction is indicated. This is true even if the patient is doing well with a Blalock-Taussig or Potts shunt.

Pulmonary arteriovenous fistula

Anatomy

Pulmonary arteriovenous fistulas can be single, multiple, or even microscopic in number and size. They are often associated with hereditary hemorrhage telangiectasia (Rendu-Osler-Weber disease).

Pathophysiology

A right-to-left shunt exists because the arteriovenous fistula bypasses the pulmonary capillary bed. Because these arteriovenous fistulas are low-resistance shunts in the low-resistance pulmonary circuit, there is no afterload or preload burden on either the right or the left ventricle. The main problem is arterial desaturation and its consequences: polycythemia, clubbing, and the possibility of endarteritis. The heart itself is not abnormal from the pulmonary arteriovenous fistulas per se.

Physical findings

Telangiectasis on the mucous membranes and a personal or family history of gastrointestinal bleeding can be seen in patients with Rendu-Osler-Weber disease. The fistulas are subpleural, and if they are at the lung surface and have a large flow, they create a continuous murmur. At times, this murmur can be difficult or impossible to hear. The murmur may be mainly systolic. Because most of these fistulas are in the lower lobes, the murmur is usually in the anterior or lateral chest. Findings of cyanosis and clubbing are present.

Diagnosis

The lesions are commonly seen on plain chest films. With the roentgenographic findings and cyanosis, even without the diagnostic continuous murmur, a diagnosis can be made. Doppler echocardiography is of help in ruling out the other, more common causes of continuous murmurs and central cyanosis. With the injection of microbubbles, bubbles can be seen to fill the left side of the heart after filling the right side. It may not be possible to tell how the microbubbles get into the left side of the heart by transthoracic echocardiography.

Angiocardiography is essential in defining how many arteriovenous fistulas exist and where they are located (Fig. 9).

Complications

These fistulas create cyanosis and its complications. Hemoptysis is not uncommon. Gastrointestinal bleeding associated with Rendu-Osler-Weber syndrome can be seen. Finally, endarteritis caused by infection of arteriovenous fistulas has occurred. Systemic embolization through arteriovenous fistulas has been described, as have brain abscess and meningitis.

Treatment

A single fistula or a limited number of pulmonary arteriovenous fistulas that create a large right-to-left shunt can be surgically excised by partial lobectomy. Catheter embolization of pulmonary arteriovenous fistulas can be accomplished, with elimination of or marked diminution in the shunt. This approach may be preferable to surgical excision, even with a single fistula. It is the preferred technique for multiple arteriovenous fistulas.

Ebstein's disease

Anatomy

Ebstein's disease is a congenital lesion that is characterized by displacement of a portion of the tricuspid valve attachment

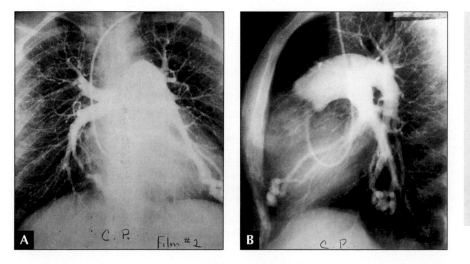

FIGURE 9 **A**, Angiocardiogram, pulmonary artery injection in the posteroanterior projection of a 30-year-old woman with pulmonary vascular disease who suddenly developed a continuous murmur lateral to the cardiac apex. Two pulmonary arteriovenous fistulae are visible, one in the right middle lobe and one on the left lower lobe. **B**, Angiocardiogram, pulmonary artery injection in the left lateral projection. Note the filling of the retrosternal space by the enlarged right ventricle as well as the two arteriovenous fistulae. Same patient as in *A*.

into the anatomic right ventricle. The posterior and septal leaflets are usually involved, and the displacement varies from mild to severe, resulting in enlargement of the chamber above the tricuspid valve (the "right atrium") and compromise of the chamber below (the "right ventricle"). There is frequently an atrial septal defect or an open foramen ovale.

Pathophysiology

The tricuspid valve is usually incompetent, resulting in a varying degree of tricuspid regurgitation. The "right atrium" is enlarged. If the tricuspid regurgitation is sufficient, the right atrial pressure is abnormally high, and if an atrial septal defect is present, a right-to-left shunt at the atrial level can cause arterial desaturation and even cyanosis.

There is frequently a muscle connection between the right atrium and the right ventricle, or a bundle of Kent; therefore, the anatomic substrate for Wolff-Parkinson-White syndrome exists in approximately 20% of patients.

Physical findings

The patient may have a precordial lift in the area of the outflow tract of the right ventricle. There may be signs of tricuspid regurgitation with an increased "V wave." The large anterior leaflet may move toward the atrium one or more times during ventricular systole, causing one or more nonejection clicks. The murmur of tricuspid regurgitation with its enhancement on inspiration is common as is a short diastolic inflow murmur. The S_1 and S_2 are frequently widely split, so that it often sounds as if there are several systolic clicks. The patient may be cyanotic with clubbing.

Approximately 20% of patients have supraventricular tachycardias.

Diagnosis

The chest roentgenogram shows a wide sweep of the right atrial border. The heart looks globular, but the pulmonary vascular markings are always normal or diminished, never plethoric. The ECG usually shows a right bundle branch block with a low-voltage rSR' or a qR in V_1 and occasionally demonstrates first-degree atrioventricular block or Wolff-Parkinson-White syndrome, usually with a posteriorly directed delta wave. Two-dimensional Doppler echocardiography can make the diagnosis because the attachment of the posterior or septal leaflet, which is displaced toward the apex, is clearly visualized on echocardiography (Fig. 10).

Complications

Most patients with Ebstein's disease who survive to adulthood do quite well. Cyanosis in childhood is a bad prognostic sign. Symptoms are related to the degree of tricuspid regurgitation and the presence and magnitude of a right-to-left shunt. The most troublesome problem that many people experience is with paroxysmal atrial tachycardia. Evidence indicates that the bundle of Kent can be interrupted by radiofrequency catheter ablation, which should be accomplished for those with recurrent paroxysmal atrial tachycardia.

For patients who are symptomatic and have easy fatigability, cyanosis, or shortness of breath, surgical correction should be considered. Various techniques of plication of the portion of the right ventricle above the tricuspid valve have been advocated, together with closing of the atrial septal defect, and tricuspid valve replacement has also been described. In patients who are minimally symptomatic or are asymptomatic, no surgery or ablation techniques are indicated.

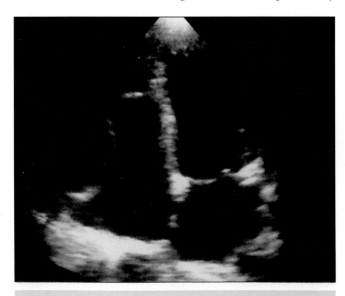

FIGURE 10 Two-dimensional echocardiogram, four-chamber view of a 50-year-old man with Ebstein's anomaly. Note displacement of the septal leaflet of the tricuspid valve down into the right ventricle almost to the apex.

REFERENCES AND RECOMMENDED READING

Recently published papers of particular interest have been highlighted as:
• Of interest
•• Of outstanding interest

1. Cheitlin MD: Congenital heart disease in the adult. *Mod Concepts Cardiovasc Dis* 1986, 55:20–24.
2. McNamara DG, Latson LA: Long-term follow-up of patients with malformations for which definitive surgical repair has been available for 25 years or more. *Am J Cardiol* 1982, 50:560–568.
3.• Konstantinides S, Geibel A, Olschewski M, *et al.*: A comparison of surgical and medical therapy for atrial septal defect in adults. *N Engl J Med* 1995; 333:469–473.
4. Ellis JH IV, Moodie DS, Sterba R, *et al.*: Ventricular septal defect in the adult: natural and unnatural history. *Am Heart J* 1987, 114:115–120.
5. Morgan JM, Gray HH, Miller GA, *et al.*: The clinical features, management and outcome of persistence of the arterial duct presenting in adult life. *Int J Cardiol* 1990, 27:193–199.
6. Fenoglio JJ Jr, McAllister HA Jr, DeCastro CM, *et al.*: Congenital bicuspid aortic valve after age 20. *AM J Cardiol* 1977, 39:164–169.

SELECT BIBLIOGRAPHY

Cheitlin MD, Sokolow M, McIlroy MB: Congenital heart disease (with special references to adult cardiology). In *Clinical Cardiology*, edn 6. Norwalk, CT: Appleton & Lange; 1993:358–406.

Liberthson RR: *Congenital Heart Disease: Diagnosis and Management in Children and Adults.* Boston: Little Brown; 1989.

Congenital Heart Disease in the Adult Postoperative Patient

32

John S. Child

Key Points

- Cardiac operations for congenital heart disease, now common in adults, have resulted in the survival of many previously operated infants and children to adulthood.

- Understanding of the basic malformation, the nature of the surgical operation, and any potential residua, sequelae, and complications is mandatory for proper care of adults with operated congenital heart disease.

- Residua and sequelae generally can be categorized as electrophysiologic or as anatomic with attendant hemodynamic consequences.

- Superimposed, adult acquired diseases such as hypertension, aortic stenosis, or coronary artery disease may result in deterioration of ventricular function despite a good operative outcome, and they require proper diagnosis and treatment.

- Knowledge of how to integrate sophisticated imaging and hemodynamic assessment, the mainstay being echocardiography, into the care of the patient is important.

Because of advances in cardiovascular surgical techniques during the past 25 years, there are many long-term survivors of cardiac operations during infancy and childhood, and physicians are faced with caring for an increasing number of patients with congenital heart disease [1••,2,3]. Caring for adults with congenital heart disease requires knowledge of the original defect, the hemodynamic and anatomic problems caused by that defect, and the progressive age-related changes in anatomy and physiology. Proper patient care after catheterization or surgical palliation or repair requires intimate knowledge of the nature and effects of the intervention and of the postoperative residua, sequelae, and complications (Table 1) [1••,2,3].

The success of these interventions is judged by the patient's quality of life, survival time, and need for reoperation. The general practitioner must be knowledgeable about currently applied techniques and materials as well as outmoded techniques previously applied during infancy and childhood. Adults who underwent surgery 20 or more years ago are alive because of their operations, but they may have had inadequate myocardial protection or have degenerating prosthetic materials.

GENERAL POSTOPERATIVE CONSIDERATIONS

Except for ligation of an uncomplicated patent ductus arteriosus and suture closure of a secundum atrial septal defect, all other surgery for cardiac anomalies leaves behind or causes some obligatory abnormality, ranging from trivial to serious (Tables 1 and 2). Postoperative residua and sequelae can be broadly categorized as electrophysiologic or anatomic (valvular, myocardial, vascular), or related to the durability of prosthetic materials and valves.

TABLE 1 REPRESENTATIVE RESIDUA AND SEQUELAE AFTER INTRACARDIAC REPAIR FOR CONGENITAL HEART DISEASE

Residua (defects only partially or not corrected)	Sequelae (defects caused by the form of operative intervention)
Bicuspid aortic valve (coarctation)	Mechanical—ventricular function (ventriculotomy), intraventricular or venous baffle obstruction (*eg*, Mustard or Rastelli repair).
Cleft mitral leaflet (ostium primum atrial septal defect)	Electrophysiologic—atrial arrhythmias and sinus node dysfunction (atrial septal, Mustard intraatrial baffle, Fontan) conduction defects (central right bundle-branch block or left anterior fascicular block after ventricular septal patch, *eg*, tetralogy of Fallot), ventriculotomy-induced ventricular arrhythmias or conduction defects
Residual ventricular outflow obstruction	
Atrioventricular valve regurgitation (after Fontan procedure for tricuspid atresia or single ventricle)	
Systemic hypertension (coarctation) or pulmonary hypertension (shunts)	Valvular—aortic or pulmonic regurgitation (valvotomy, tetralogy of Fallot), mitral regurgitation or stenosis after repair of cleft mitral leaflet (primum atrial septal defect)
Myocardial function—long-term ability of right ventricle (transposition) or single ventricle to function as systemic ventricle; effects of previous volume/pressure overload, prolonged cyanosis and erythrocytosis on coronary reserve and myocardial contractility	Prosthetic materials—patches (deterioration with time, ventricular septal patch leaks), conduits (kinking or progressive intraluminal obstruction), valves (bioprosthetic deterioration with stenosis/regurgitation) or disk valves with thrombosis, fracture, or stenosis; anticoagulant complications
Cyanosis—residual left superior vena cava to left atrium with or without coronary sinus atrial septal defect	Cyanosis—pulmonary arteriovenous fistulae (Glenn shunt)

Electrophysiologic Sequelae

Electrophysiologic sequelae include atrial and ventricular arrhythmias caused by scar or aneurysm formation after atrial or ventricular incisions or patch suturing. Insertion of intracardiac patches or conduits may cause disruption of the conduction system. For example, repair of tetralogy of Fallot includes a right ventricular outflow tract incision and ventricular septal defect patch. If the right ventricular outflow tract or pulmonary artery obstruction is inadequately relieved by the operation, the resultant right ventricular pressure overload superimposed on the right ventricular outflow tract scar or aneurysm may cause ventricular arrhythmias.

Anatomic Sequelae and Residua

Important anatomic sequelae and residua must be sought. Bicuspid aortic valves are often associated with aortic coarctation and continue to pose risks of progressive stenosis, regurgitation, and endocarditis after coarctation repair. Variations on a parachute mitral valve, often found in conjunction with coarctation and other stenoses in sequence on the left-sided circulation, may have gone undetected. Repair of an ostium primum atrial septal defect includes cleft mitral valve repair; residual mitral regurgitation may exist and is occasionally progressive. Subaortic, discrete stenosis may coexist and should be recognized.

Repaired tetralogy of Fallot may have pulmonary regurgitation because of a valvulotomy or a transannular incision and patch. Isolated mild to moderate low-pressure pulmonary regurgitation is common and well-tolerated. Severe pulmonary regurgitation may cause right ventricular failure and tricuspid regurgitation, particularly if there is any residual right ventricular outflow, pulmonary valvular or arterial (*eg*, branch stenosis) obstruction. Also, muscular ventricular septal defects may have been missed preoperatively. Postoperative aortic regurgitation is common in the adult whose malforma-

tion was associated with a dilated aortic root or trunk (*eg*, tetralogy of Fallot, transposition of the great arteries, single ventricle in association with pulmonic stenosis, truncus arteriosus). Atrioventricular valve regurgitation is common preoperatively in candidates for the Fontan procedure and may progress postoperatively. These valvular lesions pose a continuing risk for endocarditis and may affect long-term ventricular performance.

Prosthetic Materials

Use of prosthetic materials such as septal patches, mechanical or bioprosthetic valves, and intracardiac and extracardiac conduits may have long-term consequences. Prosthetic valves are associated with a risk for thrombus formation and infective endocarditis. Bioprosthetic valves may undergo premature degeneration and calcification. External conduits may kink or develop internal intimal thickening ("peel formation"), and valved conduits frequently undergo valvular degeneration that may result in severe obstruction. An internal conduit holds a risk for conduit leaks, internal obstruction, and kinking, or it may partially obstruct the chamber within which it sits. Examples of procedures using external and internal conduits include the Fontan repair with an external conduit from the right atrium to the pulmonary artery (for tricuspid atresia or single ventricle with pulmonic stenosis), and the Rastelli repair with an external conduit from the right ventricle to the pulmonary artery (for D-transposition or double-outlet right ventricle) and an intraventricular conduit to route the left ventricle to the aorta via the ventricular septal defect.

Transthoracic echocardiography with Doppler and color-flow imaging is the mainstay for detailed anatomic and hemodynamic postoperative evaluation of patients with congenital heart disease. These studies are best done in laboratories having extensive experience with these abnormalities [4]. Transesophageal echocardiography (TEE) is needed

TABLE 2 POTENTIAL RESIDUA AND SEQUELAE AFTER REPAIR OF SPECIFIC COMMONLY OPERATED CONGENITAL HEART DEFECTS

Original defect	Residua	Sequelae
Bicuspid aortic valve	Aortic regurgitation or stenosis (if valvotomy) Left ventricular enlargement or left ventricular hypertrophy	Prosthetic valve malfunction Anticoagulation
Coarctation	Bicuspid aortic valves Hypertension Residual coarctation Left ventricular hypertrophy Coronary disease Intracranial aneurysms	Recurrent coarctation
Atrial septal defect secundum	Atrial arrhythmias Mitral prolapse/mitral regurgitation Right atrial and right ventricular enlargement Right ventricular failure Tricuspid regurgitation Pulmonary hypertension	Atrial fibrillation/stroke
Atrial septal defect primum	Residual cleft mitral valve/mitral regurgitation Discrete subaortic stenosis (missed) Right ventricular, right atrial, left atrial enlargement Tricuspid regurgitation Pulmonary hypertension Atrial arrhythmias	Mitral stenosis Subaortic stenosis caused by chordal attachments to ventricular septum and suture of mitral valve cleft Patch leak Atrial arrhythmias
Tetralogy of Fallot	Right ventricular outflow tract obstruction Ventricular septal defect patch leak Branch pulmonary stenosis Right ventricular hypertrophy Aortic regurgitation (dilated aorta)	Ventricular septal defect patch right bundle-branch block (aortic regurgitation as a complication) Right ventricular outflow tract incision Pulmonary regurgitation Right bundle-branch block Ventricular arrhythmia Conduit obstruction
Transpositions	Decreased systemic right ventricular function Aortic regurgitation	Intracardiac conduit leak/obstruction Extracardiac conduit obstruction Intraatrial baffle leak or obstruction Caval or pulmonary venous obstruction Atrial and ventricular arrhythmias, sinus node dysfunction
Univentricular hearts (tricuspid atresia, single ventricle)	Atrioventricular valve regurgitation Myocardial dysfunction Aortic regurgitation	Fontan conduit obstruction/thrombus Atrial patch leak Atrial and ventricular arrythmias Pulmonary arteriovenous fistulae (Glenn shunt)

when transthoracic echocardiography is not technically adequate and structures are not readily accessible to surface echocardiography (*eg*, aortic coarctation) [5]. Magnetic resonance imaging (MRI) is complementary for imaging abnormalities of the great vessels. If the echocardiographic and MRI data are not definitive, they conflict with the clinical picture, or reoperation is indicated, goal-directed diagnostic cardiac catheterization may be necessary. Intraoperative TEE improves results by detecting unexpected anomalies, refining known anatomic details, or allowing detection and re-repair of unsatisfactory results while the patient is still in the operating room.

SPECIFIC POSTOPERATIVE LESIONS

Congenital aortic stenosis caused by a bicuspid aortic valve is one of the most common congenital cardiac malformations, although it may go unrecognized early in life. It may be directly repaired in younger patients (< 21 years old) by valvotomy or balloon dilation using percutaneous catheter techniques if the valve is pliant and noncalcified with obstruction caused by congenital fusion of the commissures. There is often some degree of aortic regurgitation after valvotomy or balloon valvuloplasty, and the inherent abnormal valve remains a site for recurrent stenosis or infective endocarditis.

Aortic regurgitation usually progresses gradually but can suddenly increase because of infective endocarditis. Generally, recurrent aortic stenosis slowly progresses, and reoperation is often necessary. Echocardiographic quantitation of aortic valve area, aortic regurgitation, and left ventricular size and ejection fraction should be done routinely on a yearly basis. For the older patient, direct valve replacement is often preferable. Surgically important aortic regurgitation requires directly proceeding with valve replacement to remove the left ventricular volume overload and to preserve ventricular function. Despite the best attempts at selecting patients, some may exhibit late myocardial dysfunction and ventricular arrhythmias. The type of aortic prosthesis used affects its long-term durability, and the need for anticoagulation therapy and possible reoperation. Anti-infective endocarditis prophylaxis is required for life.

Valvular pulmonic stenosis (isolated) usually can be readily repaired with excellent results. Minimal residua and sequelae are expected if the valve repair is performed when the patient is young (< 21 years old), even if mild degrees of pulmonic stenosis and regurgitation remain. If severe pulmonic stenosis is operated on after 21 years of age, the outlook is excellent; however, the longstanding right ventricular pressure overload and hypertrophy can result in right ventricular failure. Balloon dilation has largely replaced surgical valvotomy, except for dysplastic valves, and short-term results have been excellent.

Ebstein's anomaly is the most common cause of surgically important congenital tricuspid valvular regurgitation. If the anterior tricuspid leaflet is shown by echocardiography to be long and mobile, a surgeon experienced with this anomaly can achieve a good repair. Residual, mild to moderate, low-pressure tricuspid regurgitation is usually well tolerated. Valvular reconstruction reduces right ventricular volume overload and improves right ventricular function. An interatrial communication (a commonly associated defect) should be closed at the same time to eliminate cyanosis and avoid future risk of paradoxic embolization. Wolff-Parkinson-White syndrome is a common association. During the same operation, right-sided atrioventricular bypass tracts are surgically interrupted to prevent the accelerated ventricular response to supraventricular arrhythmias. Postoperative supraventricular arrhythmias may still recur but usually respond to pharmacologic treatment with standard, type-I antiarrhythmic agents. If amiodarone therapy or radiofrequency ablation becomes necessary, consultation with a specialist is needed. Valve replacement, occasionally required, has a long-term mortality rate of 10% to 15%. Tissue valves are preferred because of concerns about the risk of pulmonary embolization from mechanical prostheses despite anticoagulation. Improvement after surgical intervention notwithstanding, there are obligatory residual abnormalities of ventricular size and function.

Isolated, left-sided, atrioventricular valve incompetence may occur with congenital transposition of the great arteries. The left-sided tricuspid valve may have an Ebstein-like malformation, with severe left atrioventricular valve regurgitation initially mistaken for mitral regurgitation until echocardiographic study elucidates the inverted ventricles. Replacement is usually required when regurgitation is severe. The possibility of complete heart block (approximately 2% accrued incidence per year) and right ventricular failure (the systemic subaortic ventricle) warrants annual electrocardiograms and echocardiograms.

SURGICAL PROCEDURES

Intra-atrial Surgery

Atrial septal defects, particularly the secundum variety, are some of the most common congenital heart defects. Early closure of these defects prevents subsequent right ventricular dysfunction or pulmonary hypertension. Surgical closure achieves excellent long-term results, particularly if performed by the age of 40 years. Nonetheless, even patients older than 60 years benefit from repair symptomatically and prognostically, but they do experience more arrhythmias and pulmonary problems than patients operated on before age 40 [6••,7,8].

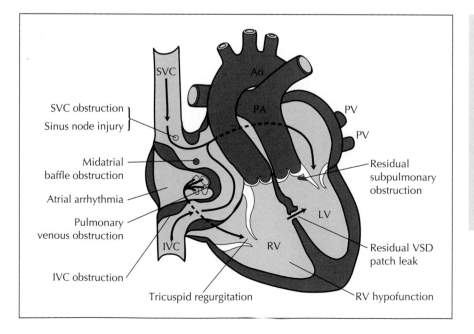

FIGURE 1 Postoperative Mustard repair procedure for D-transposition of the great arteries. The intraatrial baffle can be seen to connect the superior and inferior vena cavae (SVC, IVC) to the left ventricle (LV), which directs deoxygenated blood to the lungs via the pulmonary artery (PA). Pulmonary veins (PV) are routed to the right ventricle (RV), which directs oxygenated blood to the body via the aorta (Ao). As such, the circulation in series is reconstituted. This schematic displays the various potential sequelae or complications. VSD—ventricular septal defect.

Removal of the left-to-right shunt usually decreases the right ventricular size to normal if done during childhood, whereas adults who undergo repair usually have some residual right ventricular enlargement. Long-term right ventricular dysfunction is infrequent. Even if a patient has preoperative tricuspid regurgitation and right ventricular failure, right ventricular function usually improves postoperatively. Significantly increased pulmonary vascular resistance decreases long-term improvement and survival.

The incidence of atrial arrhythmias increases each decade in adults with an unrepaired atrial septal defect. The later the operation is performed, the less preventable these arrhythmias. With repair after age 40, as many as 50% of patients with preoperative sinus rhythm will have late postoperative atrial fibrillation.

Intra-atrial "switch" surgery has primarily been performed for complete transposition of the great arteries (Fig. 1). Such procedures redirect the systemic venous flow to the left ventricle (which supplies blood to the lungs via the pulmonary artery) and the pulmonary venous flow to the right ventricle (which ejects blood to the body via the aorta). Currently, the trend is to perform an arterial switch procedure during infancy, but a large number of today's young adults have previously had a Mustard or Senning atrial switch procedure. Although approximately 80% of these patients survive to adulthood, long-term complications are the rule (Tables 1 and 2) [9,10]. Routine follow-up electrocardiograms should be obtained. Atrial arrhythmias are common; injury to the sinus node may cause bradycardias and junctional escape rhythms, which may require inserting a permanent pacemaker. Because of the unusual intracardiac pathways, the pacemaker should be inserted by a physician experienced in dealing with these patients.

Long-term concerns about the functioning of the right ventricle in the systemic subaortic position persist, with some patients developing cardiomyopathy and ventricular failure. Echocardiography should be performed at least yearly to detect this complication. Afterload reduction with angiotensin-converting enzyme (ACE) inhibitors may be needed if the right ventricular ejection fraction is decreased or systemic arterial hypertension is detected.

Intraventricular Surgery

Intraventricular surgery includes repair of ventricular septal defects and tetralogy of Fallot as well as Rastelli procedures. Intraventricular surgery may be performed via a right atriotomy or ventriculotomy. Long-term outcome is affected by the adequacy of myocardial protection, degree of residual ventricular pressure or volume overload, subsequent electrophysiologic sequelae, and durability of prosthetic conduits, valves, and patches.

The most representative malformation is tetralogy of Fallot. Patients who received palliative aortopulmonary shunts (Blalock-Taussig, Pott's, or Waterston) and subsequent intracardiac repair at approximately 2 years of age have a nearly 90% survival rate 20 years after operation. Before complete repair, these shunts may gradually obstruct and result in increased cyanosis because of decreased pulmonary

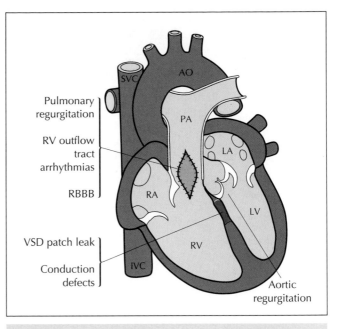

FIGURE 2 Representative corrective repair for tetralogy of Fallot. The misaligned ventricular septal defect (VSD) has been closed with a patch. Obstruction to flow from the right ventricle (RV) to the pulmonary artery (PA) may occur in the right ventricular outflow tract, pulmonary annulus or valve, or the PA. Here, a transannular patch is enlarging the right ventricular outflow tract and annulus after resection of obstructing right ventricular outflow tract muscle via the right ventricular incision. Potential sequelae or complications of the VSD patch and transannular incision and patch are shown. The aortic root, once overriding the VSD, may result in long-term aortic regurgitation. AO—aorta; LA—left atrium; LV—left ventricle; RA—right atrium; RBBB—right bundle branch block; SVC—superior vena cava.

blood flow, or they may be too large and either result in left ventricular volume overload or increased pulmonary vascular resistance and pulmonary hypertension. Adults who received palliative shunts as children benefit from complete repair. Although patients older than 40 years at the time of repair have a late mortality rate of approximately 15%, long-term survival is enhanced by intracardiac repair, and most of these patients lead essentially normal lives [11,12].

Approximately 15% of persons with tetralogy of Fallot require reoperation for residua and sequelae of the previous intracardiac repair, including residual right ventricular outflow tract obstruction and ventricular septal defect patch leaks (Figs. 2 and 3). Severe pulmonary regurgitation may occur if the pulmonary valve is excised and can result in right ventricular failure and tricuspid regurgitation requiring reoperation to insert a bioprosthetic valve. In patients with severe hypoplasia of the pulmonary valve or pulmonary atresia, a right ventricular–to–pulmonary artery conduit may be necessary. As previously noted, this can result in late obstruction because of intimal buildup or degeneration of a tissue valve within the conduit. Such hemodynamic abnormalities cause pressure and volume overload of a right ventricle with an incisional scar and, occasionally, a right ventricular aneurysm. This is the substrate for ventricular arrhythmias and sudden death. Bundle-branch blocks or high-grade

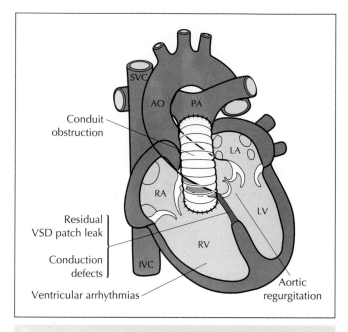

FIGURE 3 Rastelli repair of severe tetralogy of Fallot/pulmonary atresia. The ventricular septal defect (VSD) is patched, and the right ventricle (RV)–to–pulmonary artery (PA) connection is made by a conduit, usually containing a bioprosthetic valve. Potential sequelae, residua, and complications are noted.

ventricular dysfunction, even though volumes increase postoperatively. Because of concerns about long-term left ventricular function in adults with repaired tetralogy of Fallot, systemic arterial hypertension must be treated, preferably with afterload-reducing agents (ACE inhibitors). Aortic regurgitation (common in the adult with tetralogy of Fallot) may become severe and cause ventricular failure. It is also susceptible to infective endocarditis and requires lifelong prophylaxis. Two-dimensional echocardiography and Doppler evaluation are necessary to evaluate the right ventricular outflow tract and pulmonary artery anatomy for obstruction and to measure right ventricular systolic pressure and ventricular septal patch leaks.

Central Arterial Surgery

Central arterial surgery includes palliative aortopulmonary shunts and repair of patient ductus, coarction of the aorta, or sinus of Valsalva aneurysms. Surgical division of an isolated small patent ductus arteriosus in a child is an extracardiac operation and as close to a curative operation as can be performed. Currently, a potentially competing technique is transcatheter closure. If the ductus is moderate to large, surgical division in childhood usually allows regression of the left atrial and ventricular size. If a large ductus is not closed early, pulmonary hypertension and pulmonary vascular disease may occur.

Surgical repair of coarctation of the aorta relieves the obstructive gradient in most instances [13]. A bicuspid aortic valve often coexists and requires endocarditis prophylaxis. Even in the well-repaired aortic coarctation, yearly follow-up for late hypertension is needed. Patients should undergo treadmill stress testing with the specific goal of detecting an inordinate rise in arterial blood pressure that may occur despite normal resting blood pressure. Resting and immediate postexercise blood pressures should be taken in both the arms and legs to detect a residual coarctation gradient. Recurrent coarctation may require repeat surgery or balloon dilation if severe. Resid-

heart block may result from incision and resection of the right ventricular outflow tract and insertion of the ventricular septal defect patch.

Late postoperative left ventricular function relates to the adequacy of myocardial protection at operation, age at time of repair, and degree of left-side heart volume overload from prior palliative shunt procedures. There are also concerns that the duration of cyanosis before repair may relate to progressive myocardial fibrosis and late ventricular dysfunction. Patients with severe cyanotic tetralogy of Fallot may have reduced left ventricular volume and ejection fraction. Repair after 2 years of age leaves residual left

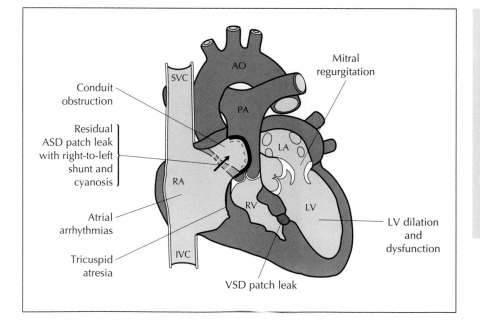

FIGURE 4 Right atrium (RA)–to–pulmonary artery (PA) connection for tricuspid atresia, functionally a univentricular heart, is a common variation on the Fontan connection seen on patients operated on within the last few years. (Now, a total cavopulmonary connection with a lateral tunnel is more commonly performed.) The obligatory atrial septal defect (ASD) is closed. Flow from the left ventricle (LV) to the PA is removed by closing a ventricular septal defect (VSD) as shown or by oversewing the pulmonary valve. Potential residua, sequelae, and complications also are depicted.

ual coarctation should be quantified by TEE or MRI of the descending thoracic aorta.

Caval to Pulmonary Arterial Connections

Fontan or Glenn shunts are performed to increase pulmonary blood flow in malformations with a basic underlying problem of a "univentricular heart" with pulmonic stenosis and intracardiac shunts (Fig. 4). Cyanosis is relieved, and symptoms are improved or alleviated [14]. Long-term problems relate mainly to arrhythmias and ventricular function; atrial fibrillation or flutter is poorly tolerated. Cardiac output and systemic venous congestion decrease. Ventricular function can deteriorate over time and may cause or be compounded by atrioventricular valve regurgitation. Routine echocardiographic evaluation of ventricular function and valvular regurgitation is necessary. The caval and right atrial connections to the right ventricle or pulmonary artery are better imaged by transesophageal echocardiography.

Infective endocarditis prophylaxis is necessary for patients with valvular regurgitation. Hypertension must be normalized with afterload reduction (by ACE inhibitors) to decrease the load on the ventricle. Ventricular dysfunction occasionally becomes sufficiently severe to require orthotopic cardiac transplantation.

KEY REFERENCES

Recently published papers of outstanding interest, as identified in *References and Recommended Reading*, have been annotated.

•• Perloff JK and Child JS: Congenital Heart Disease in Adults. Philadelphia, W.B. Saunders, 1997.
Most complete and current in-depth review of the spectrum of issues in these patients; excellent overall reference or for specific questions and detailed bibliography.

•• Konstantinides S, Geibel A., Olschewski M, *et al.*: A comparison of surgical and medical therapy for atrial septal defect in adults. *N Engl J Med* 1995, 333:469–473.
This retrospective study shows that closure of an atrial septal defect in adults over 40 years old improves survival and prevents functional deterioration and heart failure but does not prevent atrial arrhythmias. As such, these patients require continued followup for atrial arrhythmias so as to reduce the risk of thromboembolic complications.

REFERENCES AND RECOMMENDED READING

Recently published papers of particular interest have been highlighted as:
• Of interest
•• Of outstanding interest

1.•• Perloff JK and Child JS: *Congenital Heart Disease in Adults.* Philadelphia, W.B. Saunders, 1997.

2. Twenty-second Bethesda Conference: Congenital heart disease after childhood: an expanding patient population. *J Am Coll Cardiol* 1991, 18:311–342.

3. Morris CD, Menashe VD: Twenty-five year mortality after surgical repair of congenital heart defect in childhood. *JAMA* 1991, 266:3447–3542.

4. Child JS: Echo-Doppler and color-flow imaging in congenital heart disease. *Cardiology Clinics* 1990, 8:289–313.

5. Child JS: Congenital heart disease. In *Multiplane Transesophageal Echocardiography*. Edited by Roelandt JRTC, Pandian NG. New York: Churchill Livingstone; 1996:173–198.

6.•• Konstantinides S, Geibel A, Olschewski M, *et al.*: A comparison of surgical and medical therapy for atrial septal defect in adults. *N Engl J Med* 1995, 333:469–473.

7. St. John Sutton MG, Tajik AJ, McGoon DC: Atrial septal defect in patients 60 years and older: operative results and long-term postoperative followup. *Circulation 1981, 84:402–409.*

8. Steele PM, Fuster V, Cohen M, *et al.*: Isolated atrial septal defect with pulmonary vascular obstructive disease—long term followup and prediction of outcome after surgical correction. *Circulation* 1987, 76:1037–1042.

9. Gelatt M, Hamilton RM, McCrindle BW, *et al.*: Arrhythmia and mortality after the Mustard procedures: a 30-year single-center experience. *J Am Coll Cardiol* 1997, 29:194–201.

10. Warnes CA, Somerville J: Transposition of the great arteries: late results in adolescents and adults after the Mustard operation. *Br. Heart J* 1987, 58:148–155.

11. Hu DCK, Seward JB, Puga FJ, *et al.*: Total correction of tetralogy of Fallot at age 40 years or older: long-term follow-up. *J Am Coll Cardiol* 1985, 5:4-–44.

12. Waien SA, Liu PP, Ross BL , *et al.*: Serial follow-up of adults with repaired tetralogy of Fallot. *J Am Coll Cardiol* 1992, 295–300.

13. Cohen M, Fuster V, Steele PM, *et al.:* Coarctation of the aorta. Long-term follow-up and prediction of outcome after surgical correction. *Circulation* 1989, 80:840-845.

14. Driscoll DJ, Offord KP, Feldt RH, *et al.*: Five-to-fifteen year followup after the Fontan operation. *Circulation* 1992, 85:469-496.

Pulmonary Hypertension 33

Stuart Rich

Key Points

- Severe pulmonary hypertension can result from many common cardiopulmonary conditions.
- The accurate diagnosis of pulmonary hypertension requires multiple tests to evaluate all possible contributing factors.
- General treatment measures appear to be helpful for patients with pulmonary hypertension of many etiologies.
- The assessment of drug effects and drug initiation should be left to experienced specialists.
- The prognosis of patients with severe primary and secondary forms of pulmonary hypertension may markedly improve with appropriately focused, aggressive treatments.

Although not common, pulmonary hypertension usually overwhelms the clinical course of a patient whether its etiology is primary or secondary. For this reason, early diagnosis of pulmonary hypertension could have important implications for patients regarding their responsiveness to treatment and clinical course. There are many causes of pulmonary hypertension that can affect the pulmonary vascular bed in similar ways. Injury to the pulmonary vascular endothelium produces a cascade of effects including pulmonary vasoconstriction and thrombosis that is self-perpetuating and can lead to extreme pulmonary hypertension and right-side heart failure. Some patients have pulmonary hypertension from more than one cause, such as chronic obstructive pulmonary disease as well as pulmonary thromboembolism. For these patients, distinguishing the relative contribution of each underlying disease to the overall clinical state can be quite difficult.

Many physicians are confused when a patient has pulmonary hypertension that appears to be out of proportion to the underlying disease. The response of the pulmonary vascular bed to all types of stimuli is markedly variable, however. Some patients may have only minimal elevations in pulmonary hypertension when exposed to hypoxia; other patients may have a pronounced effect. Appreciating the variability of the pulmonary vascular response to injury explains why many patients have pulmonary hypertension that appears to be more severe than the extent of the underlying disease process.

ROLE OF THE GENERALIST

Patients suspected of having pulmonary hypertension should be referred to a specialist in the field because of the complexity of pulmonary hypertensive disease and the morbidity associated with both diagnostic testing and therapies. Early diagnosis of pulmonary hypertension is fundamental to successfully treating the patient, however, and in this regard, heightened suspicion by the primary-care physician is

TABLE 1 CAUSES OF PULMONARY HYPERTENSION AND CONFIRMING DIAGNOSTIC TESTS	
Cause	**Test**
Lung disease (*eg*, parenchymal, hypoxic)	Chest radiography or high-resolution computed tomography Pulmonary function tests
Heart disease (*eg*, congenital, abnormal left heart filling)	Echocardiography Catheterization
Pulmonary vascular obstruction (*eg*, thromboembolism, mediastinal fibrosis)	Lung scan Pulmonary angiography
Collagen vascular diseases	Serologic tests High-resolution chest computed tomography
Primary pulmonary hypertension (diagnosis of exclusion)	Catheterization

TABLE 2 CONDITIONS ASSOCIATED WITH UNEXPLAINED PULMONARY HYPERTENSION
Exogenous substance ingestion Anorexigens Toxic rapeseed oil L-Tryptophan Crack cocaine Human immunodeficiency virus infection (with or without AIDS) Portal hypertension

critical in making an early diagnosis. After patients with pulmonary hypertension have been evaluated and placed on long-term treatment, the generalist should be able to manage the patient, with periodic consultation from the cardiologist or pulmonologist. Because there are so few centers of excellence in this area, it is essential for the generalist to reassume day-to-day care.

DIAGNOSIS

An algorithm to diagnose the cause of pulmonary hypertension has been established through the National Institute of Health Registry on Primary Pulmonary Hypertension (Table 1) [1].

Because the underlying cause of pulmonary hypertension may not be readily apparent, a physician needs to assess all possible etiologies, even when there is no clinical history or overt signs of an underlying disease process. There also is an association between unexplained pulmonary hypertension and other conditions, particularly HIV infection and ingestion of anorexigens [2•] (Table 2).

Chest radiography is helpful in evaluating parenchymal lung disease. Pulmonary hypertension often manifests with cardiomegaly and enlarged central pulmonary arteries (Fig. 1). Tapering of the pulmonary vasculature and oligemia are nonspecific findings. The lung fields on the chest x-ray film may appear normal in spite of interstitial lung disease; hence, if interstitial lung disease is suspected, a high-resolution chest computed tomographic (CT) scan is the test of choice. Its sensitivity for detecting interstitial abnormalities may preclude the need for open-lung biopsy.

Patients with pulmonary hypertension generally have limited exercise tolerance and may have exercise-induced syncope. Exercise tolerance is an important prognostic indicator, however, and assessing it may help in the early detection of patients with mild pulmonary hypertension when

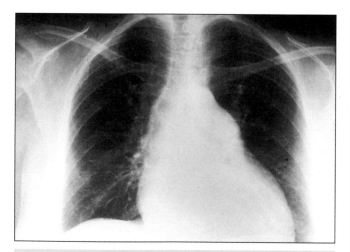

FIGURE 1 Chest radiographic (posteroanterior view) of a patient with unexplained pulmonary hypertension. Cardiomegaly with a large central pulmonary artery, prominent right descending pulmonary artery, and tapering of the vessels towards the periphery. The lung fields are clear. This could be a radiograph of a patient with pulmonary hypertension from almost any etiology.

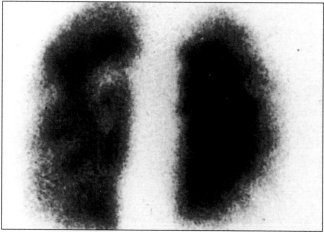

FIGURE 2 Perfusion lung scan (posterior upright view) of a patient with primary pulmonary hypertension. Patchy distribution of tagged albumin is marked but not in any anatomic segmental or subsegmental distribution suggesting pulmonary thromboembolism. This lung-scan pattern also may be seen in patients with pulmonary hypertension of other etiologies.

symptoms are manifest primarily with effort. The concomitant measurement of systemic oxygen saturation with pulse oximetry will confirm abnormal cardiopulmonary performance and help guide the physician toward the need for oxygen therapy. Patients whose history suggests limited effort tolerance should be studied using modified or low-level treadmill protocols.

Pulmonary Function Testing and Echocardiography

Pulmonary function tests are necessary to establish whether an obstructive airways disease or restrictive lung disease is present. Patients who develop pulmonary hypertension from obstructive airways disease should have associated clinical findings, but restrictive lung disease can be more difficult to ascertain. Increased pulmonary artery pressure produces restrictive changes in the lungs to a moderate degree. Thus, the diagnosis of restrictive lung disease requires a combination of restrictive changes on pulmonary function testing and evidence of parenchymal lung disease either by chest radiography, high-resolution CT scan, or lung biopsy. Although diffusion capacity from carbon monoxide may be reduced with pulmonary hypertension of any etiology, extremely low levels may reflect interstitial lung disease when it is not obvious from other tests.

The ventilation-perfusion lung scan will reveal patients with a high likelihood of having thromboembolism. Because thromboembolism that produces pulmonary hypertension is usually silent, this lung scan needs to be performed on every patient regardless of a history of deep-vein thrombosis or previous pulmonary embolism. Patients with primary pulmonary hypertension also may have abnormal, patchy distribution of radionuclide (Fig. 2). Abnormal distribution or retention of xenon in the ventilation scan may indicate underlying parenchymal lung disease.

Echocardiography is very helpful in revealing underlying congenital heart disease. Use of saline contrast and color Doppler will aid in detecting intracardiac shunts, which usually are bidirectional or reversed in patients with pulmonary hypertension. When in doubt, transesophageal echocardiography can be instrumental in differentiating an atrial septal defect from a patent foramen ovale.

Pulmonary Angiography and Cardiac Catheterization

Although pulmonary angiography carries increased risk in patients with pulmonary hypertension, it is mandatory for patients whose lung scan suggests the possibility of pulmonary thromboembolism. Hypotensive episodes after pulmonary angiography may be vagally mediated, and pretreating patients with 1 mg of atropine and using low-osmolar, nonionic agents may make the procedure safer in this regard.

Because the clinical management of the patient with pulmonary hypertension can be complex, cardiac catheterization is advised for every patient in whom the diagnosis of pulmonary hypertension is suspected. In addition to confirming the etiology, catheterization will help to establish the prognosis by directly measuring cardiac output and pulmonary

artery saturation, both of which predict survival. It is also essential to accurately determine pulmonary-capillary wedge pressure to assess left ventricular end-diastolic pressure. The pulmonary-capillary wedge pressure may be difficult to obtain in these patients, but a conclusion that the patient had a "falsely elevated wedge pressure" is unacceptable. Catheterization of patients with advanced disease can be quite difficult; these patients should be referred to physicians with considerable experience.

CAUSES OF PULMONARY HYPERTENSION AND TREATMENT

Chronic thromboembolic obstruction of the proximal pulmonary arteries is an established treatable cause of pulmonary hypertension.

Primary Pulmonary Hypertension

Primary pulmonary hypertension is a diagnosis of exclusion and can be made only when all secondary causes have been eliminated. The natural history of primary pulmonary hypertension is poor, with a mean survival of 2.8 years from the time of diagnosis [1]. As many as 30% of these patients however, can return to a normal lifestyle and have improved survival if they are diagnosed early and respond to high doses of calcium channel blockers (Fig. 3) [3]. The titration of calcium blockers at high doses can be extremely hazardous and should be done by physicians with established experience and expertise. Patients who fail to respond to calcium channel blockers

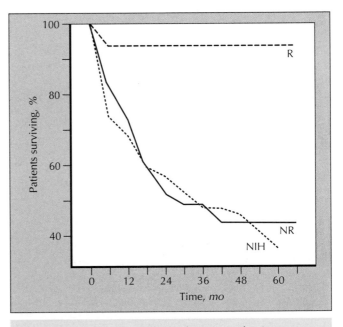

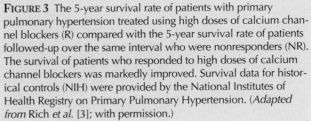

FIGURE 3 The 5-year survival rate of patients with primary pulmonary hypertension treated using high doses of calcium channel blockers (R) compared with the 5-year survival rate of patients followed-up over the same interval who were nonresponders (NR). The survival of patients who responded to high doses of calcium channel blockers was markedly improved. Survival data for historical controls (NIH) were provided by the National Institutes of Health Registry on Primary Pulmonary Hypertension. (*Adapted from* Rich *et al.* [3]; with permission.)

should be given intravenous prostacyclin therapy, although long-term experience suggests that most patients have improved quality of life and survival [4••]. Patients who continue to deteriorate in spite of medical management should be considered for lung transplantation [5]. The use of single- or bilateral lung transplantation is still controversial and may differ from center to center.

Obstructive Lung Disease

The development of pulmonary hypertension in patients with chronic obstructive pulmonary disease results in increased mortality. The only established, effective treatment of pulmonary hypertension in these patients has been chronic supplemental oxygen therapy [6]. Although it rarely reduces pulmonary artery pressure in the short term, oxygen retards progression of the pulmonary hypertension. Monitoring the response to oxygen therapy with arterial blood gases is important to check for carbon dioxide retention.

Vasodilators have been tested in patients with pulmonary hypertension from chronic obstructive pulmonary disease, but little documentation of their effectiveness exists. More importantly, however, vasodilators may worsen gas exchange, reduce arterial oxygen saturation, and cause pronounced systemic hypoxemia [7]. Vasodilators are not recommended, but if they are given to patients with lung disease, careful monitoring of the arterial blood gases before and after their administration is important.

Collagen Vascular Disease

Pulmonary hypertension complicating collagen vascular disease is becoming increasingly recognized since virtually all of the collagen vascular diseases have been reported to be associated with pulmonary hypertension [8]. The mechanism may be associated interstitial lung disease, direct effects on the pulmonary vasculature causing vasoconstriction or thrombosis, or both.

Experience with using vasodilators for these patients has been unsatisfactory, which probably reflects that the disease process had been ongoing for a long time before the pulmonary hypertension was recognized. Although use of immunosuppressive therapy may be justifiable in some patients for treating their pulmonary hypertension, more studies need to be conducted before recommendations can be made.

Mitral Valve Stenosis

Pulmonary hypertension is a common complication of mitral valve stenosis because of the increased left atrial pressure transmitted backward into the pulmonary vascular bed. The severity of pulmonary hypertension in mitral stenosis varies and it results from reactive vasoconstriction occurring in addition to the increased left atrial pressure. The definitive treatment for these patients has been mitral valve surgery. Although operative mortality increases among patients with severe pulmonary hypertension, no level of pulmonary artery pressure precludes mitral valve replacement or valvotomy, because pulmonary artery pressure should regress by at least 50% postoperatively [9].

More recent experience using balloon valvuloplasty for mitral stenosis has been quite similar—the level of pulmonary hypertension usually falls to a modest degree initially and continues to fall over time [10].

Congenital Heart Disease

Pulmonary hypertension secondary to congenital heart disease is well recognized in infants and children and is occasionally seen in adults. The fundamental principle in managing congenital heart disease with pulmonary hypertension is surgical correction before the pulmonary vascular disease becomes advanced. A patent intracardiac shunt associated with pulmonary hypertension usually results in right-to-left shunting with systemic hypoxemia. Patients with pulmonary hypertension and reversed shunting (Eisenmenger's syndrome) are considered inoperable. The use of vasodilators with these patients can be quite hazardous, because they may lower systemic vascular resistance and worsen the right-to-left shunting. At present, heart–lung or lung transplantation is considered to be the best therapeutic option for patients with congenital heart disease and Eisenmenger's syndrome.

Left Ventricular Diastolic Dysfunction

Physicians are familiar with the concept of pulmonary hypertension as a result of increased left atrial pressure from mitral stenosis. It is less well appreciated that similar levels of pulmonary hypertension can develop in patients with hypertensive or ischemic heart disease (or both) who have increased left ventricular end-diastolic pressure [11]. The correct diagnosis can be established by cardiac catheterization demonstrating high left ventricular end-diastolic filling pressures. The treatment of these patients (as for patients with other secondary forms of pulmonary hypertension) is focused on the underlying cause. Thus, patients with hypertensive heart disease should have their systemic blood pressures aggressively treated, because the pulmonary artery pressures would be expected to respond accordingly. Similarly patients with ischemic heart disease should have the left ventricular ischemia aggressively managed. Once these patients develop right ventricular failure, managing the left ventricular dysfunction becomes extraordinarily difficult.

General Treatment Measures

General treatment measures for patients with primary and secondary pulmonary hypertension are indicated in Table 3. Digitalis has recently been shown to have similar effects for the treatment of pulmonary hypertension as it does for left heart failure. Diuretics will help to relieve venous congestion and reduce dyspnea. Oxygen is of unproven benefit for treating pulmonary hypertension without chronic obstructive pulmonary disease, but it may be useful for patients with severe hypoxia. Warfarin anticoagulation therapy improves survival in patients with primary pulmonary hypertension, especially those unresponsive to oral vasodilators [3]. Low-dose anticoagulation therapy, to prolong the international normalized ratio to 2 to 3 times the control value, appears to be effective and is

TABLE 3 GENERAL TREATMENT MEASURES FOR PATIENTS WITH PULMONARY HYPERTENSION

Treatment	Comments
Daily activity	General activity advised, isometric and strenuous activity should be avoided
Supplemental oxygen	Continuous in hypoxic lung disease, supplemental in instances of profound hypoxemia (exercise/altitude)
Cardiac glycosides	Unproven, may be helpful in overt right ventricular failure
Diuretics	Relieve venous congestion and edema, may require large doses or multiple drugs
Anticoagulants	Improve survival in some patients, low doses effective

associated with a minimal risk of bleeding. Patients with liver dysfunction from venous congestion may be very sensitive to anticoagulants and need particularly close monitoring.

Because patients with pulmonary hypertension often have a limited cardiac output, they need to be advised regarding changes in their lifestyle. Isometric activities in particular should be avoided as they may induce syncope. On the other hand, patients with advanced pulmonary hypertension may lead productive lives as they learn to limit their stress, and these patients should be encouraged to be as active as possible.

WHEN TO REFER

Diagnosing and managing pulmonary hypertension is highly specialized and associated with increased risks. Specifically, commonly used tests such as lung scanning and echocardiography may show subtle abnormalities that are difficult to accurately interpret for patients with severe pulmonary hypertension. Other tests, such as exercise testing, pulmonary angiography, and right-side heart catheterization are associated with increased morbidity and mortality. Therefore, patients with the clinical features of pulmonary hypertension should be referred to specialists with expertise in this area for an accurate diagnosis.

Even more important, however, is the need for referring patients with a confirmed diagnosis of pulmonary hypertension to recognized experts for treatment. Although high doses of calcium channel blockers improve survival for some patients with primary pulmonary hypertension, many physicians are uncomfortable about initiating calcium blockers at high doses, and patients who may have been helped remain chronically, inappropriately treated. Similarly, surgical interventions requiring mitral valve replacement, repair of congenital heart disease, or thromboendarterectomy require particular expertise, because operative morbidity and mortality are clearly increased in patients with pulmonary hypertension. These patients must be referred to institutions with proven experience in these specialized areas.

As pulmonary hypertension is probably more common than we appreciate, the generalist retains a critical role in making the initial diagnosis, initiating the workup, and the ongoing management of patients on therapy. Many treatment measures are both new and complex, so frequent communica-

tion between the generalist and the specialist are important to maintain a high level of day-to-day care.

KEY REFERENCES

Recently published papers of outstanding interest, as identified in *References and Recommended Reading*, have been annotated.

•• Barst RJ, Rubun LJ, Long WA, *et al.*: A comparison of continuous intravenois etroprostenol (prostacyclin) with conventional therapy for primary pulmonary hypertension. *N Engl J Med* 1996, 334:296–301.
The first randomized prospective trial showing hemodymanic and survival benefit of prostacyclin for patients with primary pulmonary hypertension.

REFERENCES AND RECOMMENDED READING

Recently published papers of particular interest have been highlighted as:

• Of interest

•• Of outstanding interest

1. Rich S, Dantzker DR, Ayres SM, *et al.*: Primary pulmonary hypertension: a national prospective study. *Ann Intern Med* 1987, 107:216–223.

2.• Aberhaim L, Moride Y, Brenot F, *et al.*: Appetite suppressant drugs and the risk of primary pulmonary hypertension. *N Engl J Med* 1996, 335:609–616.

3. Rich S, Kaufmann E, Levy PS: The effect of high doses of calcium-channel blockers on survival in primary pulmonary hypertension. *N Engl J Med* 1992, 327:76–81.

4.•• Barst RJ, Rubun LJ, Long WA, *et al.*: A comparison of continuous intravenois etroprostenol (prostacyclin) with conventional therapy for primary pulmonary hypertension. *N Engl J Med* 1996, 334:296–301.

5. Pasque MK, Trulock EP, Kaiser LD, Cooper JD: Single lung transplantation for pulmonary hypertension: three month hemodynamic follow-up. *Circulation* 1991, 84:2275–2279.

6. Timms RM, Khaja FU, Williams GW, *et al.*: Hemodynamic response to oxygen therapy in chronic obstructive pulmonary disease. *Ann Intern Med* 1985, 103:29–36.

7. Melot C, Hallemans R, Naeije R, *et al.*: Deleterious effect of nifedipine on pulmonary gas exchange in chronic obstructive pulmonary disease. *Am Rev Respir Dis* 1984, 130:612–616.

8. Kasukawa R, Nishimaki T, Takagi T, *et al.*: Pulmonary hypertension in connective tissue disease. Clinical analysis of sixty patients in multi-institutional study. *Clin Rheumatol* 1990, 9:56–62.

9. Zener JC, Hancock EW, Shumway NE, *et al.*: Regression of extreme pulmonary hypertension and mitral valve surgery. *Am J Cardiol* 1972, 30:820–826.

10. Ribeiro PA, Al Zaibag M, Abdullah M: Pulmonary artery pressure and pulmonary vascular resistance before and after mitral balloon valvotomy in 100 patients with severe mitral valve stenosis. *Am Heart J* 1993, 125:1110–1113.

11. Kessler KM, Willens HJ, Mallon SM: Diastolic left ventricular dysfunction leading to severe reversible pulmonary hypertension. *Am Heart J* 1993, 126:234–235.

SELECT BIBLIOGRAPHY

Christman BW, McPherson CD, Newman JH, *et al.*: An imbalance between the excretion of thromboxane and prostacyclin metabolites in pulmonary hypertension. *N Engl J Med* 1992, 327:70–75.

D'Alonzo GG, Barst RJ, Ayres SM, *et al.*: Survival in patients with primary pulmonary hypertension: results from a national prospective registry. *Ann Intern Med* 1991, 115:343–349.

Kaiser LR, Cooper JD: The current status of lung transplantation. *Adv Surg* 1992, 25:259–307.

Mette SA, Palevsky HI, Pietra GG, *et al.*: Primary pulmonary hypertension in association with human immunodeficiency virus infection. *Am Rev Resp Dis* 1992, 145:1196–1200.

Rubin LJ: Primary pulmonary hypertension. *N Engl J Med* 1997, 336:111–117.

Voelkel NF, Tuder RM: Cellular and molecular mechanisms in the pathogenesis of severe pulmonary hypertension. *Eur Respir J* 1995, 8:2129–2138.

Pulmonary Embolism 34

Paul D. Stein
Russell D. Hull

> ### *Key Points*
>
> - It is critical to employ a method of prophylaxis against deep venous thrombosis that is effective for that particular condition in which deep venous thrombosis is likely to occur: low-dose heparin is effective in only some conditions.
>
> - Anticoagulant therapy is the primary treatment for deep venous thrombosis and pulmonary embolism; for treatment, intravenous or subcutaneous heparin should be administered in doses sufficient to prolong the activated partial thromboplastin time to a range that corresponds to a level of 0.2 to 0.4 U/mL. Heparin and warfarin therapy can be started together, and warfarin should be administered to achieve an international normalized ratio of 2.0 to 3.0 and continued for at least 3 months.
>
> - Low-molecular-weight heparin is at least as safe and effective as unfractionated heparin for the treatment of deep venous thrombosis.
>
> - The bedside evaluation of pulmonary embolism is meaningful and helps determine the extent to which diagnostic tests should be pursued; a sound bedside impression also contributes strongly to formulating a noninvasive diagnosis of pulmonary embolism.
>
> - The diagnostic validity of ventilation-perfusion lung scanning is enhanced when this technique is combined with prior clinical assessment.
>
> - Strategies of diagnosis developed based on diagnosing and treating deep venous thrombosis as an alternative to the diagnosis of pulmonary embolism spare many patients the necessity of pulmonary angiography.
>
> - Transvenous inferior vena cava occlusion is indicated if there is a contraindication to anticoagulant use, a continuing predisposition to pulmonary embolism, or a recurrence of pulmonary embolism on full-dose anticoagulants.
>
> - Thrombolytic therapy for pulmonary embolism is indicated if the patient is hypotensive or hypoxic on high levels of oxygen or has acutely induced right ventricular failure.

Pulmonary embolism (PE) is a complication of deep venous thrombosis (DVT). The most frequent predisposing factor for PE (and for DVT) is bed rest, usually following surgery (Table 1).

DEEP VENOUS THROMBOSIS

Diagnosis

Deep venous thrombosis of the thigh veins is more likely to cause PE than thrombosis of the veins of the calves. Techniques for diagnosing DVT include impedance plethysmography, B-mode ultrasonography, magnetic resonance imaging, venography, and radionuclide scanning. Radionuclide scanning is more sensitive for detecting venous thrombosis in the calves than venous thrombosis in the thighs. Therefore, in view of the greater danger of DVT of the thighs, the value of radionuclide scanning of the legs is limited. Impedance plethysmography is sensi-

	TABLE 1 PREDISPOSING FACTORS FOR ACUTE PULMONARY EMBOLISM	
Factor		**Patients with positive angiographic findings, %***
Immobilization (≤3 mo)		54
Surgery (≤3 mo)		42
Coronary artery disease (ever)		20
Thrombophlebitis (ever)		19
Malignancy		18
Myocardial infarction		13
Trauma (lower extremities)		12
Congestive heart failure (right or left)		12
Chronic obstructive pulmonary disease		10
Stroke (ever)		10
Asthma		7
Pneumonia (acute)		7
History of pulmonary embolism		6
Collagen vascular disease		4
Postpartum (≤3 mo)		2
Interstitial lung disease		2
Sickle cell disease		1
Vasculitis		1
Self-administered drug use		1

*Patients may have more than 1 predisposing factor; n=383.

Data from the National Collaborative Study of the Prospective Investigation of Pulmonary Embolism Diagnosis (PIOPED) [22].

tive for the detection of DVT of the thighs [1,2], and B-mode ultrasonography using compression has a sensitivity equal to or higher than that of impedance plethysmography for the detection of DVT [3,4,5]. Both methods are valid alternatives to contrast venography [5]. Most centers employ B-mode ultrasonography. Sparse data suggest that magnetic resonance imaging is sensitive and specific, but expensive; its role requires confirmation by further testing [6•]. Venography, which is an invasive procedure, generally does not need to be performed in view of the excellent results shown with noninvasive techniques.

Prevention and Treatment

Fatal PE resulting from untreated, clinically symptomatic DVT occurs more frequently (37%) than fatal PE in patients with asymptomatic, early DVT diagnosed by refined techniques (5%) [7,8]. Recommendations for the prevention of DVT, by the American College of Chest Physicians Consensus Conference on Antithrombotic Therapy, are outlined in Table 2 [9••]. Antithrombotic prevention of DVT differs from anticoagulant therapy in that the dose of heparin is lower. Intermittent pneumatic compression is beneficial in preventing DVT. Graded-pressure elastic stockings also may be beneficial, but aspirin is generally not [9••].

Anticoagulant therapy for DVT, based on recommendations by the American College of Chest Physicians Consensus Conference on Antithrombotic Therapy, is outlined in Table 3 [10••]. An attempt should be made to achieve a critical therapeutic level within the first 24 hours [11]. Heparin is administered to increase the activated partial thromboplastin time (APTT) to 1.5 times the mean of the control value or 1.5 times the upper limit of the normal APTT range. This value corresponds to a heparin blood level of 0.2 to 0.4 U/mL by the protamine sulfate titration assay and 0.35 to 0.70 by the factor Xa assay. However, there is wide variability in the APTT and heparin blood levels with different reagents and even with different batches of the same reagent [12]. It is therefore vital for each laboratory to establish the minimal therapeutic level of heparin, as measured by the APTT, that will provide a heparin blood level if at least 0.2 U/mL by the protamine titration assay for each batch of thromboplastin reagent used, particularly if the reagent is provided by a different manufacturer [12]. Therapeutic levels of heparin should be maintained for 5 or 6 days. Warfarin should be administered to maintain the international normalized ratio (INR) at 2.0 to 3.0 [10••,13]. Heparin should be continued until the INR is within this therapeutic range for two consecutive days. Low-molecular-weight heparins have several advantages over unfractionated heparin: 1) low-molecular-weight heparins have a greater bioavailability when given by subcutaneous injection, 2) the duration of the anticoagulant effect is greater, permitting once or twice daily administration, and 3) the anticoagulant response (anti Xa activity) is highly correlated with body weight, permitting administration of a fixed dose [14]. Laboratory monitoring is not necessary. When these agents become more available for treatment, they may replace unfractionated heparin in the initial management of patients with thromboembolism. Warfarin therapy should be continued for at least 3 months. Warfarin should be continued longer if a predisposition to DVT exists. It is helpful to obtain an impedance plethysmogram or B-mode ultrasound image of the legs at the time that anticoagulants are about to be discontinued: this is to be certain that no continuing DVT is present.

PULMONARY EMBOLISM

Clinical Diagnosis

It is useful to consider PE in terms of the syndrome of presentation: the syndrome of pulmonary hemorrhage or infarction, of uncomplicated PE (*ie*, PE not complicated by pulmonary hemorrhage or infarction and not complicated by circulatory collapse), and of circulatory collapse or shock [15]. The PE is least severe in patients with the pulmonary infarction syndrome, and most severe in patients with circulatory collapse [15]. One-third of patients with PE die within 1 or 2 hours and the diagnosis of PE in about 70% is unsuspected [16]. Most patients who survive long enough for a diagnosis to be made have the syndrome of pulmonary infarction (pleuritic pain or hemoptysis).

Among patients with no prior cardiopulmonary disease in whom a clinical diagnosis was made, the vast majority had either dyspnea or tachypnea, or pleuritic pain (Table 4) [17].

TABLE 2 RECOMMENDATIONS FOR THE PREVENTION OF DEEP VENOUS THROMBOSIS

Patients undergoing general surgery

General surgery patients who are undergoing minor operations, younger than 40 y of age, and have no clinical risk factors require no specific prophylaxis other than early ambulation

General surgery patients who are older than 40 y of age and undergoing major operations but who have no additional clinical risk factors for venous thromboembolism require low-dose heparin (5000 U SQ q 12 h) or intermittent pneumatic compression; combining graded-pressure elastic stockings with low-dose heparin may give better protection than either alone

General surgery patients who are older than 40 y of age, undergoing major operations, and have additional risk factors require heparin (5000 U SQ q 8 h) or low-molecular-weight heparin

General surgery patients (as profiled in the third recommendation) prone to bleeding or wound infection should be treated with intermittent pneumatic compression or dextran

General surgery patients with multiple risk factors should be treated with low-dose heparin or low-molecular-weight heparin or dextran combined with intermittent pneumatic compression

In selected high-risk general surgery patients, perioperative warfarin may be used at an INR of 2.0–3.0.

Aspirin is not recommended for prophylaxis in patients undergoing general surgery

Patients undergoing orthopedic surgery

In patients undergoing total hip replacement, warfarin (INR, 2.0–3.0), low-molecular-weight heparin, and subcutaneous heparin in doses adjusted to keep the activated partial thromboplastin time in the upper-normal range (31–36 s) 6 h after injection are the most effective prophylactic agents; in patients with a high risk for bleeding, intermittent pneumatic compression is recommended as an alternative

In patients with hip fractures, warfarin (INR, 2.0–3.0) or low-molecular-weight heparin is recommended

In patients undergoing knee surgery, either low-molecular-weight heparin or intermittent pneumatic compression is recommended

In selected high-risk orthopedic and multiple-trauma patients in whom other forms of prophylaxis would be contraindicated or ineffective, placement of a prophylactic inferior vena cava filter may be considered

In multiple-trauma patients, intermittent pneumatic compression, warfarin, and low-molecular-weight heparin are recommended when feasible

Patients who have neurologic disorders or have had neurosurgery

In patients undergoing intracranial neurosurgery, intermittent pneumatic compression with or without elastic stockings is recommended

In patients with acute spinal cord injury with paralysis, subcutaneous heparin in doses adjusted to keep the activated partial thromboplastin time in the upper-normal range (31–36 s) 6 h after injection or low-molecular-weight heparin is recommended for prophylaxis; warfarin also may be effective; low-dose heparin and intermittant pneumatic compression when used alone appear to be ineffective and are not recommended

In patients with ischemic stroke and lower extremity paralysis, low-dose heparin and low-molecular-weight heparin are effective; warfarin is probably effective. Intermittent pneumatic compression is an effective alternative in patients with hemorrhagic complications of stroke

Medical patients

In patients with clinical risk factors, particularly congestive heart failure and/or chest infections, low-dose heparin (5000 U q 8 h or q 12 h) or low-molecular-weight heparin are recommended

In patients with long-term indwelling central venous catheters, warfarin (1 mg/d) is recommended to prevent axillary-subclavian venous thrombosis

INR—international normalized ratio; q 8 h—every 8 hours; q 12 h—every 12 hours; SQ—subcutaneously.

Adapted from Clagett *et al.* [9••]; with permission.

Patients with deep venous thrombosis or pulmonary embolism should be treated with intravenous or subcutaneous heparin sufficient to prolong the activated partial thromboplastin time to a range that corresponds to a blood heparin level of 0.2 to 0.4 µg/mL

Heparin and warfarin therapy can be started together; heparin therapy should be discontinued on day 5 or 6 if the prothrombin time is therapeutic; for massive pulmonary embolism or ileofemoral thrombosis, a longer period of heparin therapy may be considered

Therapy should be continued for at least 3 mo using oral anticoagulants to prolong the prothrombin time to an international normalized ratio of 2.0–3.0; heparin to prolong the activated par-

tial thromboplastin time to a range that corresponds to a blood heparin level of 0.2 to 0.4 µg/mL may be used when oral anticoagulants are either contraindicated (*eg*, pregnancy) or inconvenient

Patients with multiple episodes of recurrent venous thrombosis or a continuing risk factor should be treated indefinitely

Symptomatic isolated calf vein thrombosis should be treated with anticoagulation for 3 mo; if for any reason anticoagulation cannot be given, serial noninvasive studies of the lower extremity should be performed to assess for proximal extension of thrombus

Adapted from Hyers *et al.* [10••]; with permission.

Pleuritic pain is more common than hemoptysis among patients with no prior cardiopulmonary disease, and almost all have dyspnea, tachypnea, pleuritic pain, unexplained evidence of atelectasis, or a parenchymal abnormality on the chest radiograph [18]. Conversely, clinically detectable PE is rare in patients without one of these findings. Signs of pulmonary hypertension or right ventricular failure (eg, an accentuated pulmonary component of the second sound or a right ventricular lift) are uncommon. Qualitative signs of DVT, including erythema, palpable cord, tenderness, Homans' sign, or edema, occur in less than one third of patients with PE, but the addition of calf asymmetry of 1 cm or more to these signs increased the prevalence of a detectable abnormality of the lower extremities from 27% to 56% [19]. Nevertheless, DVT is the cause of PE in most patients [20].

Sudden, unexplained shortness of breath in a patient who is a likely candidate for PE (a patient who has had recent surgery, is debilitated, or is immobilized) is a finding that leads to a diagnosis. The electrocardiogram is usually abnormal [17,21••]. The typical electrocardiographic abnormalities are nonspecific ST-segment or T-wave changes (> 40% of patients) (Table 5) [17,21••]. Right ventricular hypertrophy, right bundle-branch block, right-axis deviation, P pulmonale, and an $S_1Q_2T_3$ pattern are uncommon [17,21••]; in fact, new left-axis deviation occurs more often than right-axis deviation. Rhythm disturbances are uncommon [17,21••].

The chest radiograph frequently shows unexplained parenchymal abnormalities, small pleural effusions, or elevation of a hemidiaphragm (Table 6) [17]. Vascular signs on chest radiography (decreased pulmonary vascularity, a prominent central pulmonary artery, or both) are uncommon or difficult to recognize.

Ventilation-Perfusion Lung Scan

Pulmonary embolism is present in 87% of patients whose ventilation-perfusion lung scan shows a high probability of PE [22]

TABLE 4 SYMPTOMS AND SIGNS OF ACUTE PULMONARY EMBOLISM IN PATIENTS WITH NO PREEXISTING CARDIAC OR PULMONARY DISEASE

Symptoms or signs	Patients with symptom or sign, %*
Dyspnea	73
Pleuritic pain	66
Cough	37
Leg swelling	28
Leg pain	26
Hemoptysis	13
Palpitations	10
Wheezing	9
Anginalike pain	4
Tachypnea (≥20/min)	70
Rales (crackles)	51
Tachycardia (>100/min)	30
Fourth heart sound	24
Increased pulmonary component of second sound	23
Deep venous thrombosis	11
Diaphoresis	11
Temperature >38.5°C	7
Wheezes	5
Homans' sign	4
Right ventricular lift	4
Pleural friction rub	3
Third heart sound	3
Cyanosis	1

*n=117.
From Stein et al. [17].

TABLE 6 CHEST RADIOGRAPHIC FINDINGS IN PULMONARY EMBOLISM IN PATIENTS WITH NO PREVIOUS CARDIAC OR PULMONARY DISEASE

Chest radiographic finding	Patients with finding, %†
Atelectasis or pulmonary parenchymal abnormality	68
Pleural effusion	48
Pleural-based opacity	35
Elevated diaphragm	24
Decreased pulmonary vascularity	21
Prominent central pulmonary artery	15
Cardiomegaly	12
Westermark's sign*	7

*Prominent central pulmonary artery and decreased pulmonary vascularity.
†n=117.
From Stein et al. [17].

TABLE 5 ELECTROCARDIOGRAPHIC MANIFESTATIONS IN PATIENTS WITH PULMONARY EMBOLISM AND NO PRIOR CARDIAC OR PULMONARY DISEASE

Electrocardiographic finding	Patients with finding, %*
Normal electrocardiographic findings	30
Rhythm disturbances	
Atrial flutter	1
Atrial fibrillation	4
Atrial premature contractions	4
Ventricular premature contractions	4
P wave	
P pulmonale	2
QRS abnormalities	
Right-axis deviation	2
Left-axis deviation	13
Incomplete right bundle-branch block	4
Complete right bundle-branch block	6
Right ventricular hypertrophy	2
Pseudoinfarction	3
Low voltage (frontal plane)	3
ST segment and T wave	
Nonspecific ST-segment or T-wave abnormalities	49

*Some patients had more than one abnormality; n=89.
From Stein et al. [17].

(Fig. 1). If lung scan findings are normal, PE is excluded (Table 7). If the probability is intermediate, there is no information, with PE being present in approximately 30% of patients. If the probability is low, PE is present in 14%. Therefore, a low-probability ventilation-perfusion lung scan does not exclude PE [22]. Prior clinical assessment combined with interpretation of the ventilation-perfusion lung scan improves the diagnostic validity (Table 7) [22]. If the ventilation-perfusion scan is interpreted as high probability for PE, and if the clinical impression is concordantly high, then the prevalence of PE is 96%. If the ventilation-perfusion scan is low probability and the clinical suspicion is concordantly low, then pulmonary embolism is excluded in 96% of patients [22]. Similarly, if the ventilation-perfusion scan findings indicate a low probability of PE and the clinical suspicion is concordantly low, PE can be excluded in 96% of patients.

The probability of PE can be determined based on the number of mismatched perfusion defects [23,24]. A further refinement of probability can be made if the ventilation-perfusion lung scan is interpreted after patients are stratified according to prior cardiopulmonary disease (Fig. 2) [23]. Fewer mismatched perfusion defects are required to diagnose PE in patients with no prior cardiopulmonary disease. Adding clinical assessment to the stratification results in a more accurate evaluation (Fig. 3 and 4) [25].

Pulmonary Angiography

Pulmonary angiography (Fig. 5) is associated with serious complications in approximately 1% of patients [26]. When needed, pulmonary angiography is useful, and it remains the

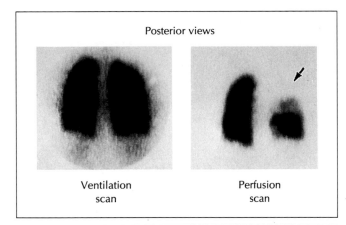

FIGURE 1 Posterior views of ventilation lung scan (*left*) and perfusion lung scan (*right*) showing normal ventilation with absent perfusion in the right upper lobe (*arrow*).

	TABLE 7 PROBABILITY OF PULMONARY EMBOLISM USING CLINICAL ASSESSMENT IN COMBINATION WITH VENTILATION-PERFUSION LUNG SCANS			
	Ratio of PE-positive patients to total patients, *n/n (%)*			
Scan category	**CP of 80%–100%**	**CP of 20%–79%**	**CP of 0%–19%**	**All probabilities**
High probability	28/29 (96)	70/80 (88)	5/9 (56)	103/118 (87)
Intermediate probability	27/41 (66)	66/236 (28)	11/68 (16)	104/345 (30)
Low probability	6/15 (40)	30/191 (16)	4/90 (4)	40/296 (14)
Near-normal to normal	0/5 (0)	4/62 (6)	1/61 (2)	5/128 (4)
Total	61/90 (68)	170/569 (30)	21/228 (9)	252/887 (28)

CP—clinical probability; PE—pulmonary embolism.

*PE positive indicates an angiographic reading that shows PE or the determination of PE by the outcome classification committee on review. PE status is based on angiographic interpretation for 713 patients, on angiographic interpretation and outcome classification committee reassignment for 4 patients, and on clinical information alone (without definitive angiography) for 170 patients.

From A Collaborative Study by the PIOPED Investigators [22]; with permission.

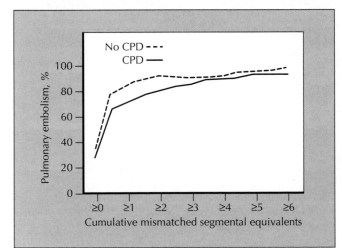

FIGURE 2 Predictive value of pulmonary embolism relative to the cumulative number of mismatched segmental equivalent perfusion defects among patients with no prior cardiopulmonary disease (CPD) and those with prior CPD. Significant differences occurred with 0.5 or more and 1.0 or more segmental equivalents (*P* < 0.01) and with 1.5 or more segmental equivalents (*P* < 0.05). (*From* Stein *et al.* [23].)

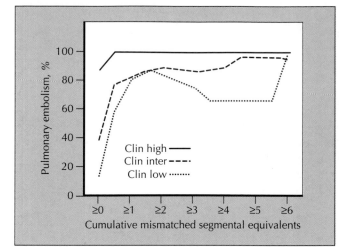

FIGURE 3 Predictive value of pulmonary embolism relative to the cumulative number of mismatched segmental equivalent perfusion defects among patients with no prior cardiopulmonary disease. Patients were categorized as having high-probability (Clin high), intermediate-probability (Clin inter), or low-probability clinical assessment (Clin low). The variability of the low-probability curve is because of the small numbers of patients in that group. (*From* Stein *et al.* [25].)

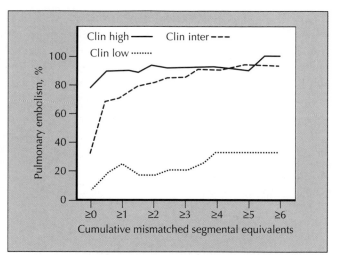

FIGURE 4 Predictive value of pulmonary embolism relative to the cumulative number of mismatched segmental equivalent perfusion defects among patients with prior cardiopulmonary disease. Patients were categorized as having high-probability (Clin high), intermediate-probability (Clin inter), or low-probability clinical assessment (Clin low). (*From* Stein *et al.* [25].)

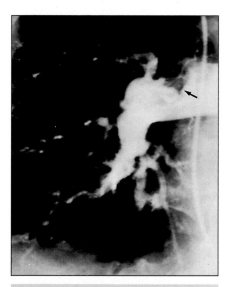

FIGURE 5 Pulmonary arteriogram of right pulmonary artery showing multiple intraluminal filling defects, one of which occludes the artery to the right upper lobe (*arrow*).

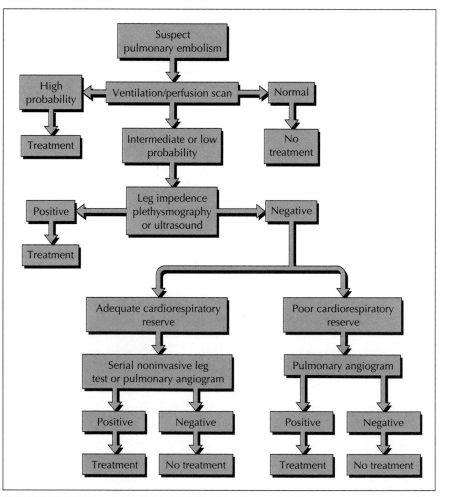

FIGURE 6 Strategy for the diagnosis and treatment of patients with suspected acute pulmonary embolism based on use of a ventilation-perfusion scan as the first diagnostic test. (*From* Stein *et al.* [30••]; with permission.)

Cardiology for the Primary Care Physician

diagnostic "gold standard" for PE. Patients in whom the risk of complications from PE are greatest are those referred for angiography from the medical intensive care unit. Frequently, such patients are receiving respiratory support and are in an unstable condition. The presence or absence of PE and the magnitude of pulmonary hypertension does not relate to the frequency of morbidity from angiography [26]. Elderly patients (ie, 70 years of age or older) are at greater risk for renal impairment from the injection of contrast material than younger patients [27].

Residual Impairment

A residual abnormality of perfusion 1 year after acute PE is more frequent in patients with prior cardiopulmonary disease than in those with no prior cardiopulmonary disease [28]. A posttherapy baseline ventilation-perfusion lung scan is useful in the event of suspected recurrent PE. This baseline lung scan will assist in determining if abnormalities on a later ventilation-perfusion lung scan are new or residuals of prior PE.

Strategy for Diagnosis

Strategies have been developed to reduce the number of pulmonary angiograms that may be required [20,29,30••]. If the patient has a high-probability ventilation-perfusion scan, particularly in association with a high clinical suspicion, treatment with anticoagulants generally is indicated (Fig. 6). In patients with a high-probability ventilation-perfusion scan and an uncertain or low clinical suspicion, studies of the leg veins may assist the clinician in reaching a decision about therapy. If ventilation-perfusion lung scan findings are normal, treatment is not indicated. If lung scan findings show an intermediate or low probability of PE, a noninvasive evaluation of the proximal veins of the legs for DVT is useful. Spiral contrast enhanced computed tomography also may be useful, particularly for the detection of central PE [6•,31]. If such tests are positive, then treatment is indicated. If the findings are negative, the clinician should obtain either a pulmonary angiogram to clarify the diagnosis, or if cardiorespiratory reserve is adequate, follow the patient with serial studies of the legs (using impedance plethysmographic or B-mode Doppler studies) [30••]. The latter strategy is safe, and the risk of PE is low among patients in whom serial investigations of the legs show no DVT [32–34]. It may be more economical or convenient to obtain studies of the legs before ventilation-perfusion scanning. Lung scans are recommended, however, if there is a suspicion of PE, regardless of the results of leg studies.

Preliminary data suggest that a D-dimer level of less than 500 μg/L would tend to exclude PE [35]. An elevation of the D-dimer level to 500 μg/L or higher, however, provides no diagnostic information and may occur under various conditions other than PE.

Treatment

Antithrombotic therapy for PE is the same as antithrombotic therapy for DVT (Table 3). Inferior vena cava occlusion is indicated if there is a contraindication to anticoagulant use, a continuing predisposition to PE, or a recurrence of PE on full-dose anticoagulants.

Thrombolytic therapy is indicated if the patient is hypotensive or hypoxic on 100% oxygen. Thrombolytic therapy is not indicated for the routine treatment of PE. It is generally recommended that pulmonary angiograms be obtained in patients with suspected PE who may be candidates for thrombolytic therapy. Pulmonary angiography, however, markedly increases the risk of major bleeding with thrombolytic therapy. Therefore, thrombolytic therapy perhaps may be administered to unstable patients on the basis of a strong clinical impression and a high-probability ventilation-perfusion lung scan [36].

Key References

Recently published papers of outstanding interest, as identified in *References and Recommended Reading*, have been annotated.

•• Clagett GP, Anderson FA Jr, Heit J, *et al.*: Prevention of venous thromboembolism. *Chest* 1995, 108(suppl):312S–334S.
Fully referenced authoritative review and guideline of great value and importance.

•• Hyers TM, Hull RD, Weg JG: Antithrombotic therapy for venous thromboembolic disease. *Chest* 1995, 108(suppl):335S–351S.
Fundamentally important authoritative guideline for therapy.

•• Stein PD: Acute pulmonary embolism. *Dis Month* 1994, 40:465–524.
Extensive and detailed review article.

•• Stein PD, Hull RD, Pineo G: Strategy that includes serial noninvasive leg tests for diagnosis of thromboembolic disease in patients with suspected acute pulmonary embolism based on data from PIOPED. *Arch Intern Med* 1995, 155:2101–2104.
Strategy of diagnosis that combines the traditional angiographic approach with the Canadian approach of diagnosing "thromboembolic disease." The strategy incorporates serial noninvasive leg tests.

References and Recommended Reading

Recently published papers of particular interest have been highlighted as:
• Of interest
•• Of outstanding interest

1. Moser KM, LeMoine JR: Is embolic risk conditioned by location of deep venous thrombosis? *Ann Intern Med* 1981, 94:439–444.

2. Hull RD, Hirsh J, Carter CJ, *et al.*: Pulmonary angiography, ventilation lung scanning, and venography for clinically suspected pulmonary embolism with abnormal perfusion lung scan. *Ann Intern Med* 1983, 98:891–899.

3. White RH, McGahan JP, Daschbach MM: Diagnosis of deep-vein thrombosis using duplex ultrasound. *Ann Intern Med* 1989, 111:297–304.

4. Becker DM, Philbrick JT, Abbitt PL: Real time ultrasonography for the diagnosis of lower extremity deep venous thrombosis. *Arch Intern Med* 1989, 149:1731–1734.

5. Heijboer H, Cogo A, Buller HR, *et al.*: Detection of deep vein thrombosis with impedance plethysmography and real-time compression ultrasonography in hospitalized patients. *Arch Intern Med* 1992, 152:1901–1903.

6.• ACCP Consensus Committee on Pulmonary Embolism: Second report opinions regarding the diagnosis and management of venous thromboembolic disease. *Chest*, in press.

7. Byrne JJ: Phlebitis: a study of 748 cases at the Boston City Hospital. *N Engl J Med* 1955, 253:579–586.

8. Collins R, Scrimgeour A, Yusuf S, Peto R: Reduction in fatal pulmonary embolism and venous thrombosis by perioperative administration of subcutaneous heparin. *N Engl J Med* 1988, 318:1162–1173.

9.•• Clagett GP, Anderson FA Jr, Heit J, *et al.*: Prevention of venous thromboembolism. *Chest* 1995, 108(suppl):312S–334S.

10.•• Hyers TM, Hull RD, Weg JG: Antithrombotic therapy for venous thromboembolic disease. *Chest* 1995, 108(suppl):335S–351S.

11. Hull RD, Raskob GE, Hirsch J, *et al.*: Continuous heparin compared with intermittent subcutaneous heparin in the initial treatment of proximal-vein thrombosis. *N Engl J Med* 1986, 315:1109–1114.

12. Brill-Edwards P, Ginsberg S, Johnston M, *et al.*: Establishing a therapeutic range for heparin therapy. *Ann Intern Med* 1993, 119:104–109.

13. Hirsh J, Dalen JE, Deykin D, Poller L: Oral anticoagulants: mechanism of action, clinical effectiveness, and optimal therapeutic range. *Chest* 1992, 102(suppl):312S–326S.

14. Hirsh J, Levine MN: Low molecular weight heparin. *Blood* 1992, 79:1–17.

15. Stein PD, Willis PW III, DeMets DL: History and physical examination in acute pulmonary embolism in patients without preexisting cardiac or pulmonary disease. *Am J Cardiol* 1981, 47:218–223.

16. Stein PD, Henry JW: Prevalence of acute pulmonary embolism among patients in a general hospital and at autopsy. *Chest* 1995, 108:978–981.

17. Stein PD, Terrin ML, Hales CA, *et al.*: Clinical, laboratory, roentgenographic and electrocardiographic findings in patients with acute pulmonary embolism and no pre-existing cardiac or pulmonary disease. *Chest* 1991, 100:598–603.

18. Stein PD, Saltzman HA, Weg JG: Clinical characteristics of patients with acute pulmonary embolism. *Am J Cardiol* 1991, 68:1723–1724.

19. Stein PD, Henry JW, Godalakrishman D, Relyea B: Asymmetry of the calves in the assessment of patients with suspected acute pulmonary embolism. *Chest* 1995, 107:936–939.

20. Stein PD, Hull RD, Saltzman HA, Pineo G: Strategy for diagnosis of patients with suspected acute pulmonary embolism. *Chest* 1993, 103:1553–1559.

21.•• Stein PD: Acute pulmonary embolism. *Dis Month* 1994, 40:465–524.

22. A Collaborative Study by the PIOPED Investigators: Value of the ventilation/perfusion scan in acute pulmonary embolism: results of the prospective investigation of pulmonary embolism diagnosis (PIOPED). *JAMA* 1990, 263:2753–2759.

23. Stein PD, Gottschalk A, Henry JW, Shivkumar K: Stratification of patients according to prior cardiopulmonary disease and probability assessment based upon the number of mismatched segmented equivalent perfusion defects: approaches to strengthen the diagnostic value of ventilation/perfusion lung scans in acute pulmonary embolism. *Chest* 1993, 104:1461–1467.

24. Stein PD, Henry JW, Gottschalk A: Mismatched vascular defects: an easy alternative to mismatched segmental equivalent defects for the interpretation of ventilation/perfusion lung scans in pulmonary embolism. *Chest* 1993, 104:1468–1472.

25. Stein PD, Henry JW, Gottschalk A: The addition of clinical assessment to stratification according to prior cardiopulmonary disease further optimizes the interpretation of ventilation/perfusion lung scans in pulmonary embolism. *Chest* 1993, 104:1472–1476.

26. Stein PD, Athanasoulis C, Alavi A, *et al.*: Complications and validity of pulmonary angiography in acute pulmonary embolism. *Circulation* 1992, 85:462–469.

27. Stein PD, Gottschalk A, Saltzman HA, Terrin ML: Diagnosis of acute pulmonary embolism in the elderly. *J Am Coll Cardiol* 1991, 18:1452–1457.

28. Urokinase Pulmonary Embolism Trial: Chapter VIII. Perfusion lung scanning. *Circulation* 1973, 47(suppl):II-46–II-50.

29. Dalen JE: When can treatment be withheld in patients with suspected pulmonary embolism? *Arch Intern Med* 1993, 153:1415–1418.

30.•• Stein PD, Hull RD, Pineo G: Strategy that includes serial noninvasive leg tests for diagnosis of thromboembolic disease in patients with suspected acute pulmonary embolism based on data from PIOPED. *Arch Intern Med* 1995, 155:2101–2104.

31. Remy-Jardin M, Remy J, Dechildre F, *et al.*: Diagnosis of pulmonary embolism with spiral CT: comparison with pulmonary angiography and scintigraphy. *Radiology* 1996, 200:699–706.

32. Hull RD, Raskob GE, Carter CJ: Serial impedance plethysmography in pregnant patients with clinically suspected deep-vein thrombosis. *Ann Intern Med* 1990, 112:663–667.

33. Huisman MV, Buller HR, Ten Cate JW, Vreeken J: Serial impedance plethysmography for suspected deep venous thrombosis in outpatients. *N Engl J Med* 1986, 314:823–828.

34. Hull RD, Raskob GE, Ginsberg JS, *et al.*: A noninvasive strategy for the treatment of patients with suspected pulmonary embolism. *Arch Intern Med* 1994, 154:289—297.

35. Bounameaux H, Cirafici P, DeMoerloose P, *et al.*: Measurement of D-dimer in plasma as a diagnostic aid in suspected pulmonary embolism. *Lancet* 1991, 337:196–200.

36. Stein PD, Hull RD, Raskob G: Risks for major bleeding from thrombolytic therapy: consideration of noninvasive management. *Ann Intern Med* 1994, 12:313–317.

SELECT BIBLIOGRAPHY

Hull RD, Pineo GF, eds: *Disorders of Thrombosis.* Philadelphia: WB Saunders; 1996.

Hull RD, Raskob GE, Pineo GF, eds: *Venous Thromboembolism: An Evidence-Based Atlas.* Armonk, NY: Futura Publishing; 1996.

Stein PD: *Pulmonary Embolism.* Media, PA: Williams & Wilkins; 1996.

Cardiac Tumors 35

Navin C. Nanda
Elizabeth O. Ofili

Key Points

- Although most primary cardiac tumors are histologically "benign," clinical manifestations can be devastating and include cerebrovascular and peripheral emboli, cardiac arrhythmias, valvular obstruction, pericardial constriction or tamponade, and death.
- A high index of suspicion is necessary for early diagnosis. Echocardiography usually provides rapid and accurate diagnosis; chest radiography tends to be nonspecific.
- Surgical excision is curative in most cases, although some myxomas may recur. Periodic postoperative clinical and echocardiographic surveillance is important.
- Metastatic tumors are uniformly fatal; surgery is largely palliative.

Cardiac tumors can be primary or metastatic and can involve the heart or pericardium. Advances in diagnostic imaging now allow accurate diagnosis in most patients. Clinical manifestations and hemodynamic features of cardiac tumors can mimic virtually all other forms of heart disease. Thus, a high index of suspicion is necessary for making an accurate diagnosis.

PRIMARY CARDIAC TUMORS

Primary tumors of the heart and pericardium are rare, with an incidence of 0.002% to 0.250% in autopsy series [1,2]. Figure 1 shows the relative incidence of primary tumors of the heart. Although 75% of primary cardiac tumors are histologically benign, clinical manifestations can be quite devastating, with complications such as death caused by arrhythmia, pericardial constriction or tamponade, valvular obstruction, and cerebral arterial embolism [2].

Benign Tumors

Myxomas are the most common cardiac tumors, accounting for 30% to 50% of benign cardiac tumors in most series [3]. Over 90% of myxomas occur sporadically. Women are more commonly affected, with a typical age range of 30 to 60 years; however, patients as young as 3 years and as old as 80 years have also been reported [3]. Most myxomas are solitary tumors and are often pedunculated and attached to the limbus of the fossa ovalis of the left atrium by a short stalk. Myxomas are noted for their protean clinical manifestations. Constitutional signs and symptoms, obstructive manifestations, and embolic phenomena are the classic triad of myxoma presentation [4,5]. Presenting symptoms may include syncope, episodic dizziness, episodic dyspnea, and weight loss (Table 1). Symptoms may vary with positional change. Syncope is particularly ominous and not infrequently associated with sudden death. Multiple systemic emboli may mimic systemic vasculitis or infective endocarditis, particularly when associated with fever, weight loss, and arthralgias. The neurologic consequences of embolization include transient ischemic attacks, seizures, syncope, and cerebral infarction.

Atrial myxomas may mimic mitral or tricuspid valve disease on physical examination (Table 2). The sudden movement of tumor from atrium to the ventricle has been associated with an early diastolic sound or "tumor plop." This high-frequency diastolic sound, in addition to a diastolic murmur and (in some cases) a systolic murmur of a valvular regurgitation, has been described. Left atrial myxomas frequently mimic mitral stenosis. Right atrial myxomas may present with recurrent pulmonary emboli and right heart failure. Right atrial myxomas have been reported to mimic the carcinoid syndrome, constrictive pericarditis, tricuspid stenosis, or Ebstein's anomaly.

Familial myxomas make up 7% of all myxomas and are transmitted by an autosomal dominant trait. Compared with patients with sporadic myxomas, patients presenting with familial myxomas are usually younger (mean age in the twenties), more likely to have multiple myxomas involving chambers other than the left atrium, and more likely to have a recurrence of myxoma postoperatively [6,7]. Because cardiac myxomas may be familial, routine echocardiographic screening of first-degree relatives is appropriate, particularly in young patients who have multiple or right-sided tumors [8]. Clinical manifestations of other benign cardiac tumors are listed in Table 3.

Malignant Tumors

Malignant cardiac tumors account for 25% of all primary heart tumors. They include mesotheliomas, which typically involve the pericardium. Sarcomas involve the myocardium, and malignant vascular tumors can affect both the pericardium and the myocardium (Table 4).

METASTATIC OR SECONDARY CARDIAC TUMORS

Metastatic tumors of the heart are 25 times more common than primary cardiac tumors. All major types of tumors can metastasize to the heart, with an average frequency of 10% in autopsy series. The highest percentages of metastases to the heart occur with melanoma (64%), leukemia (43%), and malignant lymphoma (35%) [9]. Lung and breast cancers predominate as the major sites of origin for cardiac metastases because of their high prevalence and contiguous anatomic location. Pericardial metastases are most frequent, and endocardial metastases occur rarely. Discrete nodules or diffuse infiltration may occur as a result of pericardial metastases. Fibrinous pericarditis and pericardial effusion usually are present. The effusion may not be bloody. Pericardial metastases may be diffuse or present as discrete nodules.

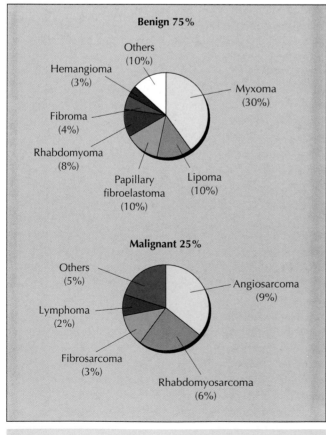

FIGURE 1 Relative incidence of primary cardiac tumors.

TABLE 1 CARDIAC MYXOMAS

Clinical manifestations

Symptoms	Incidence, %
Dyspnea on exertion	>75
Fever	50
Weight loss	50
Dizziness or syncope	20
Sudden death	15
Hemoptysis	15

Clinical presentation of cardiac myxoma in 130 patients	Patients, *n*
Signs and symptoms of mitral valve disease	57
Embolic phenomena	36
Incidental finding	16
Signs and symptoms of tricuspid valve disease	6
Sudden death	5
Pericarditis	4
Myocardial infarction	3
Signs and symptoms of pulmonary valve disease	2
Fever of unknown origin	2

Location of cardiac myxomas

Site	Incidence, %
Left atrium	75.0
Right atrium	20.0
Left ventricle	2.5
Right ventricle	2.5
Multiple myxomas	<5.0

From McAllister and Fenoglio [27], Meller *et al.* [28], and Vidaillet *et al.* [29]; with permission.

Leukemic involvement typically causes effusion because of infiltration of the interstitium by leukemic cells. Mural thrombi and embolization secondary to metastatic cardiac tumors are quite rare. Metastatic cardiac tumors do not interfere with cardiac function until myocardial involvement is extensive. Cardiac metastases are almost always associated with widespread metastatic involvement in other organs.

The vast majority of patients with cardiac involvement because of metastatic tumor have few or no cardiac symptoms (Table 5) [1]. Despite autopsy evidence of cardiac metastases

TABLE 2 CONDITIONS MIMICKED BY ATRIAL MYXOMAS

Left atrium

Rheumatic mitral valve disease (stenosis, insufficiency)

Pulmonary hypertension

Cerebral emboli

Endocarditis

Myocarditis

Vasculitis

Right atrium

Rheumatic tricuspid valve disease (stenosis, insufficiency)

Pulmonary hypertension

Pulmonary emboli

Constrictive pericarditis

Ebstein's anomaly

Carcinoid heart disease

TABLE 3 COMMON MANIFESTATIONS OF OTHER BENIGN CARDIAC TUMORS

Tumor	Manifestations
Rhabdomyoma	Most common childhood benign primary tumor; associated with systemic tuberous sclerosis; ventricular tachyarrhythmia
Fibroma	Second most common childhood tumor; may cause left ventricular outflow obstruction
Lipomas	Left ventricle, right atrium, and atrial septum affected in that order; rarely cause problems (valvular obstruction and conduction abnormalities)
Lipomatous hypertrophy	Adipose tissue accumulation in atrial septum; not true neoplasm; most common in the obese, elderly, and women; usually not pathologic
Papillary fibroelastoma	Affects heart valves; may embolize rarely or cause valvular dysfunction
Hemangioma and lymphangioma	Rare vascular tumors; may cause heart block and sudden death
Bronchogenic cysts, pericardial cysts, teratomas, and dermoid cysts	Most common benign pericardial tumor; usually in young children; can compress great vessels and rupture into pericardium

TABLE 4 COMMON MANIFESTATIONS OF MALIGNANT PRIMARY CARDIAC TUMORS

Tumor	Manifestations
Sarcomas	Affect young adults; right side of heart common; rapid downhill course; death within 2 years of symptoms; local infiltration and metastases to lungs, lymph nodes, sternum and vertebral column; cardiac tamponade, right heart failure, and vena caval obstruction may occur
Angiosarcomas	Including Kaposi's sarcoma and malignant hemangioendotheliomas; 2:1 male:female ratio; usually from right atrium, attached to septum; course and clinical manifestations as for other sarcomas, including rapid downhill course
Pericardial mesothelioma	Usually affects in third to fifth decade; more in men; no association with asbestos exposure; symptomatic late in course; survival less than 1 year after diagnosis

TABLE 5 CLINICAL MANIFESTATIONS OF CARDIAC METASTATIC TUMORS

Manifestation	Description
Pericardial effusion and tamponade	Most common manifestations of metastatic disease (less common but may occur with benign tumors); cytologic examination of fluid or pericardial biopsy may be diagnostic; effusive constrictive pericarditis can occur if prior irradiation
Heart failure	May be dilated or restrictive right, left, or biventricular failure; leukemic infiltration and irradiation can cause restrictive cardiomyopathy; doxorubicin cardiomyopathy is dose related (> 400–500 mg/m^2); sudden onset; resistant to conventional treatment
Myocardial ischemia and infarction	May be from large transmural tumor nodules or, rarely, tumor embolization; usually widespread metastases and poor prognosis; death within several weeks
Embolization	Most common with benign atrial myxomas but can be seen with metastatic tumors
Conduction defects and arrhythmias	Heart block is common in mesothelioma of the atrioventricular node; arrhythmias are common with metastatic myocardial disease

TABLE 6 RADIOLOGIC FINDINGS IN CARDIAC TUMORS
Cardiac enlargement (chamber enlargement; pericardial effusion)
Mediastinal widening (hilar-mediastinal adenopathy)
Calcification (rhabdomyoma, fibroma, teratoma, myxoma)

TABLE 7 DIAGNOSTIC WORK-UP OF CARDIAC TUMORS
History and physical examination (may be nonspecific)
Chest radiography
Transthoracic two-dimensional or Doppler echocardiography (left ventricular tumors, left atrial, and right atrial myxomas)
Transesophageal echocardiography (if suboptimal, inconclusive, or nondiagnostic transthoracic echocardiogram)
Computed tomography and magnetic resonance imaging (extent of myocardial invasion; pericardial or extracardiac extension)
Coronary angiography (for coronary anatomy)
Surgical exclusion or biopsy
Periodic two-dimensional echocardiogram for follow-up after surgery

in 10% to 20% of patients with widespread metastatic disease, antemortem symptoms or physical findings of cardiac involvement occur only in approximately 8% of the cases [10]. This may be because cardiac abnormalities are often overlooked by clinicians in the presence of widespread neoplastic disease.

DIAGNOSTIC TECHNIQUES

Noninvasive diagnostic cardiac evaluation is increasingly used to confirm a suspected intracardiac tumor. As a result, it is not unusual for cardiac tumors to be diagnosed and cured in patients who are totally asymptomatic or without signs of cardiovascular disease. Chest radiography tends to be nonspecific but may provide important diagnostic clues (Table 6). Careful use of noninvasive modalities such as two-dimensional echocardiography, transesophageal echocardiography, and in some instances, magnetic resonance imaging help in the preoperative localization and assessment of tumor extent; invasive procedures such as cardiac catheterization are therefore unnecessary. Table 7 summarizes a diagnostic and surveillance algorithm for evaluation of cardiac tumors. Patients presenting with clinical manifestations of cardiogenic emboli should be referred for echocardiography. A high index of suspicion is necessary for early diagnosis, particularly in patients with nonspecific symptoms such as dyspnea, atypical chest pain, or palpitations.

Echocardiography

Two-dimensional echocardiography, when carefully performed, provides adequate information regarding the pres-

ence or absence of an intracardiac tumor as well as its size, attachment, and mobility to allow for operative resection without preoperative angiography (Figs. 2 and 3). This technique is sensitive for detecting small tumors and is especially useful in the diagnosis of atrial and ventricular tumors. Furthermore, color Doppler flow studies allow for the assessment of the hemodynamic consequences of valvular obstruction or insufficiency caused by cardiac tumors [11].

Transesophageal Echocardiography

Transesophageal echocardiography provides an unimpeded view of both atria and interatrial septum. It allows a more accurate evaluation of the attachment of atrial myxomas and differentiation of atrial thrombi from cardiac tumors [12]. Transesophageal echocardiography is complementary to the

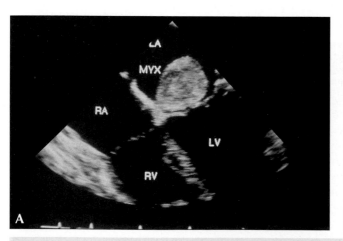

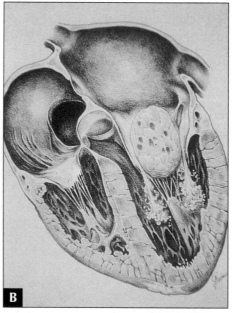

FIGURE 2 Transesophageal echocardiogram in a patient with left atrial myxoma. **A,** A large left atrial myxoma (MYX) attached to the base of interatrial septum is viewed in four-chamber view. **B,** Schematic of *panel A*. LA—left atrium; LV—left ventricle; RA—right atrium; RV—right ventricle. *From* Nanda and Mahan [30]; with permission.

transthoracic approach in providing additional visualization and superior resolution. It should be requested when the transthoracic echocardiogram is suboptimal or additional information regarding the tumor attachment and extent of involvement is needed. Transesophageal echocardiography is superior for the evaluation of right heart tumors and involvement of the vena cava [13,14••].

Computed Tomography

Computed tomography (particularly ultrafast computed tomography and electron beam computed tomography) may allow tissue discrimination with definition of the degree of intramural tumor extension. It is useful for assessing the degree of myocardial invasion and involvement of pericardial and extracardiac structures [15,16•].

Magnetic Resonance Imaging

This technique may be of considerable value in the detection and delineation of cardiac tumors, and in some cases, it may show the size, shape, and surface characteristics of the tumor

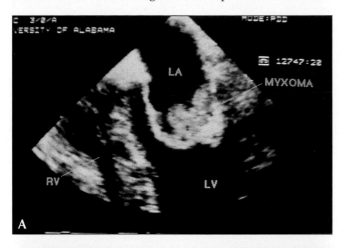

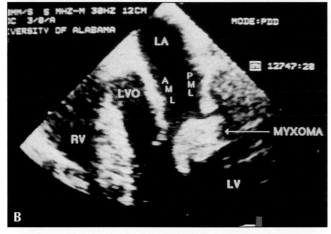

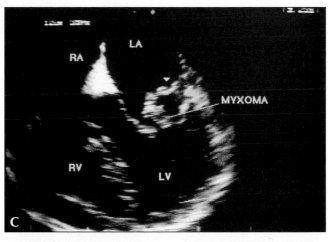

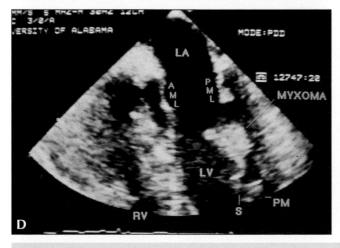

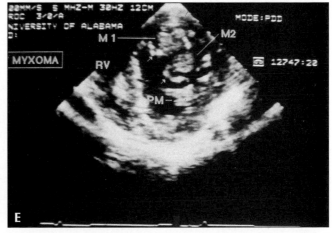

FIGURE 3 Transesophageal echocardiogram in a patient with multicentric left ventricular myxomas mimicking a left atrial tumor. In systole (**A**), a large tumor mass is seen within the left atrium (LA) behind the closed position of the mitral leaflets imaged in the four-chamber plane. In diastole (**B**), the mass has moved from LA into the left ventricle (LV), mimicking the motion pattern of a left atrial tumor. Intermittently, especially during the transesophageal study in the awake state, the mass was also visualized in LA in diastole, suggesting intermittent trapping of the tumor in the left atrium. The *arrowhead* points to the thinner portion of the mass in contact with the LA free wall (**C**). There is no evidence in **A**, **B**, or **C** to suggest (LV) attachment of the tumor. In (**D**), the attachment of the tumor to a papillary muscle (PM) head in LV by a long stalk (S) is clearly delineated. The long stalk makes it possible for the tumor to prolapse into LA in systole and move back into LV in diastole as well as for trapping in LA to occur. In the transgastric LV short-axis view (**E**), two separate tumors (M_1, M_2) with their stalks (*arrows*) are seen in the vicinity of the papillary muscles. AML—anterior mitral leaflet; PML—posterior mitral leaflet; RA—right atrium; RV—right ventricle. (*From* Samdarshi *et al.* [31]; with permission.)

more clearly than two-dimensional echocardiography [17]. The larger field-of-view with magnetic resonance imaging also may provide a better definition of tumor prolapse, secondary valve obstruction, and cardiac tumor size than two-dimensional echocardiography [15]. Spin echo and cine magnetic resonance images may allow morphologic and histologic characterization of cardiac myxomas [18].

Angiography

Cardiac catheterization and selective angiocardiography are not necessary in all cases of cardiac tumors, especially with the use of transesophageal echocardiography, ultrafast and electron beam tomography, and magnetic resonance imaging. Cardiac tumors that are amenable to surgery frequently can be diagnosed by these noninvasive techniques. In some cases, however, cardiac catheterization may allow visualization of the vascular supply of the tumor and identify the source of its blood supply and its relationship to the coronary arteries. The major risk of angiography is embolization resulting from dislodgement of tumor fragment or associated thrombus [19]. Therefore, its use before surgery is becoming increasingly less common, except perhaps for the sole purpose of assessing the coronary anatomy.

TREATMENT AND PROGNOSIS

Benign Tumors

Operative excision is the treatment of choice for most benign tumors (Table 8) and in many cases results in complete cure [20••]. Despite the histologically benign nature of these cardiac tumors, they are potentially lethal because of clinical manifestations of valvular obstruction, embolization, cardiac-rhythm disturbances, conduction defects, or sudden death. It is not uncommon for patients to die or experience a major complication while awaiting surgery. It is therefore mandatory to carry out the operation promptly after the diagnosis has been established [21]. Open heart surgery with cardiopulmonary bypass is required in most cases. This procedure allows for adequate inspection and removal of all tumor fragments. The dislodgement of tumor fragments represents a major risk during surgery and may result in embolization. Because early surgery is curative, patients with recurrent unexplained, albeit nonspecific cardiac symptoms should undergo

echocardiographic evaluation. The high sensitivity of this technique permits adequate screening in most patients provided that the technical quality is adequate for diagnosis.

Numerous reports have documented complete cure of left and right atrial myxomas during a follow-up of up to 22 years [21,22]. Causes of recurrent atrial myxomas include incomplete resection of the original tumor with regrowth or intracardiac implantation from the original tumor. Castells and coworkers [23] reported a low recurrence rate of 4.7%. Patients with a familial history of cardiac myxoma or features of a complex myxoma syndrome may have tumor recurrence in 12% to 22% of cases as opposed to 1% of cases with sporadic atrial myxoma. Echocardiographic follow-up is important for detecting recurrent tumors in such patients. Following resection of myxoma, it is generally recommended that all patients have periodic follow-up by two-dimensional echocardiography for detection of recurrence. Although no criteria have been established, echocardiographic follow-up every 2 to 5 years is reasonable depending on patient symptomatology; suspected complex myxoma requires closer follow-up.

Other benign tumors also have been excised with a high degree of success. These include rhabdomyoma, hamartoma, fibroma hemangioma, and papillary fibroelastomas (Table 8). Spontaneous resolution occurs in some childhood rhabdomyomas [24••].

Malignant Tumors

Surgery is not an effective treatment for the great majority of primary malignant tumors of the heart, either because of the large mass of cardiac tissue involved or the presence of metastases [20]. A major role for surgery in such cases may be to establish the diagnosis and to explore the possibility of a curable benign tumor. Percutaneous transesophageal echocardiography guided transvenous biopsy may preclude surgery in some cases [25•]. Survival times from 1 to 3 years have been reported following partial resection with additional chemotherapy or radiation therapy. Lymphosarcoma of the heart frequently responds to chemotherapy, radiation therapy, or both [26]. Most reports indicate a failure to alter the course of cardiac sarcomas even with various combinations of surgery, chemotherapy, and radiation therapy. Surgery for metastatic cardiac tumors is largely palliative; surgically placed pericardial windows are commonly used to treat large pericardial effusions and cardiac tamponade.

KEY REFERENCES

Recently published papers of outstanding interest, as identified in *References and Recommended Reading*, have been annotated.

•• Lynch M, Clements SD, Shenewise JS: Right-sided cardiac tumors detected by transesophageal echocardiography and its usefulness in differentiating the benign from the malignant ones. *Am J Cardiol* 1997, 79(6):781–784.

In right sided tumors identified by transesophageal echocardiography, tumors arising within the right atrium are usually benign. Tumors extending into the right atrium are typically malignant. Right ventricular tumors are rare, and likely to be malignant.

•• Perchinsky MJ, Lichtenstein SV, Tyers GF: Primary cardiac tumors: forty years' experience with 71 patients. *Cancer* 1997, 79(9):1809–1815.

This study of 71 patients confirms the rarity of primary cardiac tumors. Left atrial tumors are benign in 70% of cases with 96% successful complete resection. Up to 50% of right atrial tumors are malignant and less amenable to surgical cure.

•• DiMario FJ Jr, Diana D, Leopold H, Chameides L: Evolution of cardiac rhabdomyoma in tuberous sclerosis complex. *Clin Pediatr* 1996, 35(12):615–619.

Gradual but complete spontaneous tumor resolution was documented in this longitudinal cohort study of cardiac rhabdomyomas in patients with tuberous sclerosis. Regression was usually complete by the age of 6 years.

REFERENCES AND RECOMMENDED READING

Recently published papers of particular interest have been highlighted as:
• Of interest
•• Of outstanding interest

1. Fine G: Primary tumors of the pericardium and heart. *Cardiovasc Clin* 1973, 5:207–238.

2. Prichard RW: Tumors of the heart: review of the subject and report of 150 cases. *Arch Pathol* 1951, 51:98–128.

3. Bulkley BH, Hutchins GM: Atrial myxomas: a fifty year review. *Am Heart J* 1979, 97:639–643.

4. Peters MN, Hall RJ, Cooley DA, *et al.*: The clinical syndrome of atrial myxoma. *JAMA* 1974, 230:695–701.

5. McDevitt HO, Bodomer WF: Protean clinical manifestations of primary tumors of the heart. *Am J Med* 1972, 52:1–8.

6. Farah MG: Familial cardiac myxoma. A study of relatives of patients with myxoma. *Chest* 1994, 105:65–68.

7. McCarthy PM, Piehler JM, Schaff HV, *et al.*: The significance of multiple recurrences and "complex" cardiac myxomas. *Thorac Cardiovasc Surg* 1986, 91:389–396.

8. Carney JA: Difference between nonfamilial and familial cardiac myxomas. *Am J Surg Pathol* 1983, 9:53–55.

9. Harvey WP: Clinical aspects of cardiac tumors. *Am J Cardiol* 1968, 21:328–343.

10. Roberts WC, Glancy DL, DeVita VT Jr: Heart in malignant lymphoma (Hodgkin's disease, lymphosarcoma, reticulum cell sarcoma and mycosis fungoides). A study of 196 autopsy cases. *Am J Cardiol* 1968, 22:149–153.

11. Panidis IP, Mintz GS, McAllister MO: Hemodynamic consequence of left atrial myxoma assessed by Doppler ultrasound. *Am Heart J* 1986, 111:927–931.

12. Ofili EO, Labovitz AJ: Transesophageal echocardiography in the evaluation of cardiac source of embolus and intracardiac masses. *J Invasive Cardiol* 1992, 4:349–358.

13. Leibowitz G, Keller NM, Daniel WG, *et al.*: Transesophageal versus transthoracic echocardiography in the evaluation of right atrial tumors. *Am Heart J* 1995, 130:1224–1227.

14.•• Lynch M, Clements SD, Shenewise JS: Right-sided cardiac tumors detected by transesophageal echocardiography and its usefulness in differentiating the benign from the malignant ones. *Am J Cardiol* 1997, 79(6):781–784.

15. Jack CM, Cleland J, Geddes JS: Left atrial rhabdomyosarcoma and the use of digital gated computed tomography in its diagnosis. *Br Heart J* 1986, 55:305–307.

16.• Mousseaux E, Hernigou A, Azencot M, *et al.*: Evaluation by electron beam computed tomography of intracardiac masses suspected by transesophageal echocardiography. *Heart* 1996, 76(3):256–263.

17. Freedberg RS, Kronzon I, Rumancik WM, Liebeskind D: The contribution of magnetic resonance imaging to the evaluation of intracardiac tumors diagnosed by echocardiography. *Circulation* 1988, 77:96–103.

18. Matsuoka H, Hamada M, Honda T, *et al.*: Morphologic and histologic characterization of cardiac myxomas by magnetic resonance imaging. *Angiology* 1996, 47:693–698.

19. Pindyck F, Pierce EC, Baron MG, Lukban SB: Embolization of left atrial myxoma after transeptal cardiac catheterization. *Am J Cardiol* 1972, 30:569–571.

20.•• Perchinsky MJ, Lichtenstein SV, Tyers GF: Primary cardiac tumors: forty years' experience with 71 patients. *Cancer* 1997, 79(9):1809–1815.

21. Semb BK: Surgical considerations in the treatment of cardiac myxoma. *J Thorac Cardiovasc Surg* 1984, 87:251–259.

22. Bortolotti V, Maraglino G, Rubino M, *et al.*: Surgical excision of intracardiac myxomas: a 20 year follow up. *Ann Thorac Surg* 1990, 49:449–453.

23. Castells E, Ferran V, Octavio de Toledo MC, *et al.*: Cardiac myxomas: surgical treatment, long term results and recurrence. *J Cardiovasc Surg* 1993, 34:49–53.

24.•• DiMario FJ Jr, Diana D, Leopold H, Chameides L: Evolution of cardiac rhabdomyoma in tuberous sclerosis complex. *Clin Pediatr* 1996, 35(12):615–619.

25.• Malouf JF, Thompson RC, Maples WJ, Wolfe JT: Diagnosis of right atrial metastatic melanoma by transesophageal echocardiographic-guided transvenous biopsy. *Mayo Clin Proc* 1996, 71(12):1167–1170.

26. Vergnon JM, Vincent M, Perinett M, *et al*: Chemotherapy of metastatic primary cardiac sarcomas. *Am Heart J* 1985, 110:682–684.

27. McAllister HA, Fenoglio JJ: Tumors of the cardiovascular system. In *Atlas of Tumor Pathology*. Washington, DC: Armed Forces Institute of Pathology; 1978.

28. Meller J, Teichholz LE, Pichard AD, *et al.*: Left ventricular myxoma: echocardiographic diagnosis and review of the literature. *Am J Med* 1977, 66:816–823.

29. Vidaillet HJ Jr, Seward JB, Fyke FE III, *et al.*: Syndrome myxoma: a subset of patients with cardiac myxoma associated with pigmented skin lesions and peripheral and endocrine neoplasms. *Br Heart J* 1987, 57:247–255.

30. Nanda NC, Mahan EF III: Transesophageal echocardiography. American Heart Association Council Clinical Cardiology Newsletter; Summer, 1990:3–22.

31. Samdarshi TE, Mahan EF III, Nanda NC, *et al.*: Transesophageal echocardiography diagnosis of multicentric left ventricular myxomas mimicking a left atrial tumor. *J Thorac Cardiovasc Surg* 1992, 103:471–474.

Nonpenetrating Cardiac Trauma 36
A. James Liedtke

> ### *Key Points*
> - Rapid deceleration impact injuries are a major cause of myocardial contusion.
> - A 12-lead electrocardiogram is the time-tested *sine qua non* of diagnosing myocardial contusion.
> - Current assessment of outcome statistics of cardiac complications secondary to myocardial contusion provides prospective clues to identifying high- and low-risk patients.
> - It is now possible to develop a triage algorithm for managing patients with myocardial contusion.
> - Direct injury to coronary arteries threatens myocardial perfusion and viability.
> - Therapeutic strategies for coronary artery disease may be applicable to lesions resulting from coronary trauma.

Cardiac injury secondary to severe, nonpenetrating, blunt chest-wall injury is a perilous, unpredictable consequence of deceleration impact injuries. It commonly occurs in motor vehicle accidents, is sometimes fatal, and is difficult to diagnose, particularly if accompanied by more obvious injuries of other organ systems. Parmley and coworkers [1], in one of the initial reviews on this topic, noted that cardiovascular involvement (most commonly contusion and rupture) in nonpenetrating trauma was not infrequent but was routinely unrecognized. Hospitals and trauma centers throughout the United States have dedicated increasingly greater staff and resources to the triage and management of trauma victims with suspected cardiac lesions.

This dedication has resulted in impressive results—in patients with even the most morbid of injuries, such as cardiac chamber rupture, survival following surgical repair is now possible [2]. Nevertheless, debate is still ongoing as how best to diagnose and manage this patient group. Some trauma experts have argued that current strategies for evaluation of the majority of these patients may be excessive and have argued that diagnostic and management systems be reevaluated to justify their cost. They further propose critically reviewing and possibly revamping utilization criteria for those triage algorithms, which necessitate intensive care facilities and expensive diagnostic and therapeutic procedures. This chapter focuses on two cardiac lesions: myocardial contusion and direct coronary artery trauma.

MYOCARDIAL CONTUSION

Diagnostic Criteria

Myocardial contusion has nonspecific diagnostic criteria and an uncertain clinical outcome, including major cardiac complications and, occasionally, cardiac death. One early view of this disorder (*ie*, that myocardial contusion is analogous to myocardial infarction) is probably flawed or incomplete and is not substantiated by

TABLE 1 MECHANISM OF INJURY IN PATIENTS WITH SUSPECTED MYOCARDIAL CONTUSION FOLLOWING BLUNT CHEST TRAUMA

Mechanism	Patients, *n*
Car or truck accident	214
Pedestrian accident	30
Motorcycle accident	16
Fall	26
Other	26
Total (227 men; 85 women)	312

From McLean *et al.* [10]; with permission.

recent literature. Evidence in 1973 [3] was biased by the more dramatic expressions of myocardial trauma and contusion. With a more complete database developed from recent observations, the spectrum of injury expression is more complete. The perspectives of morbidity and mortality are being adjusted; however, myocardial contusion lacks definitive diagnostic criteria.

Myocardial infarction and myocardial contusion differ markedly with respect to the specificity of their diagnostic clues. Symptom presentation of chest-wall pain and thoracic tenderness in patients with trauma is nonspecific. Physical examination is only helpful in defining certain complications of major cardiac injury, such as pericardial tamponade, cardiac arrhythmias, primary or secondary valvular insufficiency, and heart failure. Historically, acquisition of serum enzymes (*ie*, serum glutamic-oxaloacetic transaminase and lactate dehydrogenase) leukocyte count, and sedimentation rate lacked specificity. Their modern replacements (creatine kinase [CK] isoenzymes) still do. The most reliable means of establishing the diagnosis is a 12-lead electrocardiogram, which remains the keystone of diagnosing myocardial contusion and is further enhanced as a predictive marker by the observed abnormalities in rhythm that occur early after injury.

Current literature encompasses a large population of patients studied with detailed workups [4–11]. It can be reviewed to determine which diagnostic maneuvers stand the test of time, what has been learned in terms of population outcome data to triage, and how to stratify patients as low-risk or more likely to suffer cardiac complications.

Myocardial contusion is an injury of the twentieth century. Most cases occur because of rapid deceleration events (before the era of air bags) secondary to motor-vehicle accidents or auto–pedestrian accidents [4,10] (Table 1, Fig. 1). Representative diagnostic clinical criteria for patients with suspected myocardial contusion are listed in Table 2. These criteria reflect the lack of specific diagnostic signs, symptoms, and laboratory parameters while heightening awareness of the possible presence of cardiac injuries. This list includes mechanisms of injury at the scene of the accident, any symptoms and physical evidence if present, electrocardiographic findings suggestive of ischemia and infarction, conduction delays and dysrhythmias, and any other biochemical evidence suggestive for tissue injury of the heart muscle.

Updated outcome statistics of cardiac complications secondary to myocardial contusion confirm its reputation as a potentially life-threatening condition, both as a primary consequence of blunt chest-wall injury and as a disorder associated with other complications. For example, in traumatic thoracic aortic rupture, myocardial contusion worsens perioperative morbidity and mortality by promoting cardiac instability and cardiac arrest [12]. Deaths have also been reported [4,10,13] (Table 3). This complication is infrequent, however, and typically occurs with severe injury to other organ systems. Other complications are more frequent and include pericardial tears and effusions, nonlethal and lethal cardiac ruptures, acute myocardial infarction, transient myocardial ischemia, congestive heart failure, pulmonary edema and atrial thrombus, and cardiac dysrhythmias [4–8,10,11,13] (Table 3). Cardiac dysrhythmias include atrial ectopy, atrial fibrillation, sinoatrial nodal arrest, ventricular ectopy, ventricular tachycar-

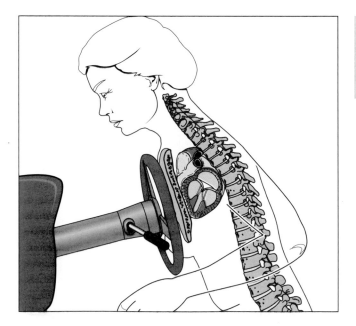

FIGURE 1 Typical impact injury to the anterior chest wall when the driver is thrust against the fixed steering column. Myocardial contusion results from high-speed deceleration accidents, most typically experienced by motor-vehicle and motorcycle crashes and auto–pedestrian accidents.

TABLE 2 REPRESENTATIVE DIAGNOSTIC CLINICAL CRITERIA OF PRESUMPTIVE MYOCARDIAL CONTUSION*

Study	Criteria
Foil and coworkers [7]	Presence of chest pain, chest-wall contusion or tenderness, or sternal tenderness; a likely mechanism of injury such as rapid deceleration injury, bent or broken steering wheel, or a blow to the chest, dysrhythmias or ECG abnormalities (exclusive of sinus tachycardia)
Norton and coworkers [8]	ECG pattern consistent with evolving or resolving pattern of acute injury; CK-MB isoenzyme fraction ≥5 % of the total CK concentration, or an elevated CK concentration with a "positive" MB fraction; an abnormal ECHO (hypokinesis, pericardial effusion, acute valvular injury; apical thrombus; wall thickening with edema or hemorrhage)
Miller and coworkers [4]	History of direct blows to the chest, broken steering-wheel accidents; likely mechanism of injury; physical evidence of anterior chest-wall injury, precordial bruising, fractured sternum, or anterior rib fractures
Ross and coworkers [5]	ECG and CK-MB isoenzyme assay monitored over the first 72 hours
	ECG criteria: arrhythmias, atrial or ventricular ectopy, conduction defects, any ischemic changes; CK-MB percentage >2.5%

*Exclusive of autopsy results.
CK—creatine kinase; ECG—electrocardiogram; ECHO—echocardiogram.

dia, ventricular fibrillation, nodal rhythm, atrioventricular conduction block, and intraventricular conduction delay. These rhythm disturbances sometimes require medical treatment or pacemaker insertion.

Blunt chest wall injury can also precipitate sudden cardiac death. Maron and coworkers [14••] reviewed a registry of 25 children and young adults who dies in sporting activities due to chest impact trauma. Cardiopulmonary resuscitation performed in 19 of these victims was unsuccessful to long-term survival. Autopsies were obtained in 22 of the 25 patients. Twelve victims had small chest contusions; most were located directly over the left ventricle. Also described were bruises, lacerations, and puncture wounds involving the chest wall, heart, pericardium, and lungs. The authors speculated that the sudden chest blow "presumably delivered at an electrically vulnerable phase of ventricular excitability," affected cardiac arrest due to ventricular dysrhythmias.

Updated statistics confirm that myocardial contusion is hazardous and requires careful diagnostic and electrical monitoring, dedicated professional staff, and the availability of sophisticated resources to conduct complex diagnostic and rapid therapeutic intervention; however, is this labor-intensive and costly triage algorithm mandatory for all patients with presumed myocardial contusion? Several reports agree on the markers defining a high-risk population of patients with myocardial contusion [4,8,10,11]. Cardiac complications strongly correlate with the presence and severity of multiorgan injuries as defined by the Injury Severity Score (ISS) [15]. This score derives from the Abbreviated Injury Scale, which was created by the Committee on Medical Aspects of Automotive Injury of the American Medical Association [16], revised in 1985 [17], and subsequently rendered "user-easy" [18] (Tables 4A–C).

Using multivariant analysis, Norton and colleagues [8] proposed that an abnormal electrocardiogram on admission and an ISS of 10 or higher were highly predictive of a myocardial contusion, and that in their absence the probability of contusion (1%) was virtually excluded. Probability estimates from their analysis are shown in Table 5. They further noted

that because these two predictive markers are easily acquired in the emergency department, a patient population at high risk for myocardial contusion could be rapidly identified and triaged to the appropriate intensive care unit.

Cachecho and coworkers [11] also observed a relationship between ISS and cardiac complications in a stable group of young patients with asymptomatic myocardial contusion. Increasing the ISS from 6.6 ± 6.1 to 23.5 ± 16.2 led to an increase in the occurrence of cardiac complications and dysrhythmias from 0% to 29%. Other important prognosticators were electrocardiogram abnormalities, which were either present on arrival at the emergency department or developed within the first 4 to 24 hours [4,7]; an adverse clinical course including hemodynamic shock [4]; and the occurrence or presence of atrial fibrillation, which in one study [10] was shown to be an increased risk factor for predicting cardiac deaths. Also important was the identity of patients at low risk for either the diagnosis of contusion or its complications. Foil and coworkers [7] noted that a normal electrocardiogram on admission and the lack of development of cardiac dysrhythmias in the first 4 hours of observation virtually excluded significant cardiac sequelae, even in patients with physical findings of chest-wall contusion. They further proposed that these patients did not warrant hospitalization. These findings were again confirmed by Cachecho and coworkers [11], who observed in their patients that a normal or only minimally abnormal electrocardiogram did not require sophisticated cardiac monitoring during hospitalization and that the hospital stay strongly correlate with ISS.

Dubrow and coworkers [6] defined their entrance criteria based on radionuclide angiography. This technique is insensitive to smaller lesions and is only diagnostic for those injuries with observably decreased global left ventricular ejection fraction or induced abnormalities in segmental wall motion. The ISS range was correspondingly higher (12.7 to 30.7) in three patient subgroups. Despite the higher absolute ISS values, mortality rates were lower than those predicted by their ISS ranking. This disparity was so wide (10% to 20% predicted vs. 0.58% observed) that the authors concluded that in stable

Study	Patients reviewed, n	Patients with presumed or suspected MC, n	Deaths secondary to MC, n	Other cardiac complications
Wisner and coworkers [13]	3010	110	27*	19 Dysrhythmias (4 required treatment) 2 Cardiac rupture
Foil and coworkers [7]	1936	524	0	23 Dysrhythmias (19 required treatment) 3 Myocardial infarctions 2 Pericardial effusions 4 Hemodynamic instability
Cachecho and coworkers [11]	336	336	0	13 Atrial fibrillation (4 required treatment) 12 Supraventricular tachycardia/sinoatrial node dysfunction (7 required treatment) 24 Ventricular irritability (4 required treatment for ventricular tachycardia or ventricular bigeminy/trigeminy) 19 BBB or atrioventricular block 18 Ischemia 4 Congestive heart failure (all required treatment)
McLean and coworkers [10]	312	312	35 (at least 4 had MC)	27 With ventricular ectopic score > 3, Including 17 ventricular tachycardia (2 required treatment) 14 Atrial fibrillation or sinus arrest or both (at least 5 treated) 11 New Q waves (4 died)
Dubrow and coworkers [6]	243	172	1 (MC not causal)	1 Ventricular ectopy 4 Ventricular tachycardia (2 required treatment) 3 Atrial ectopy 1 Atrial fibrillation 1 right BBB 1 Ischemia 1 Myocardial infarction
Miller and coworkers [4]	172	28	At least 3 (MC not necessarily causal in 2)	12 Dysrhythmia (4 required treatment) 4 Pericardial effusions
Norton and coworkers [8]	88	27	0	2 Atrial dysrhythmia 6 Ventricular dysrhythmias (5 required treatment) 8 Conduction delays 3 Myocardial infarction (all required treatment) 3 Cardiogenic shock (all required treatment) 1 Apical thrombus (required treatment)
Ross and coworkers [5]	64	58	0	25 ECG changes with ST-T wave abnormalities 10 Ventricular ectopy 9 right BBB 3 Atrioventricular block 2 Atrial ectopy 3 Atrial fibrillation 4 Operative complications: ventricular ectopy, ventricular fibrillation, nodal rhythm, pulmonary edema

*Includes cardiac rupture, pericardial tear, coronary arterial injury.
BBB—bundle-branch block; ECG—electrocardiogram; MC—myocardial contusion.

AIS Score	Head/neck	Face	Thorax
1 (Minor)	Headache/dizziness 2° to head trauma C spine strain with no fracture or dislocation	Corneal abrasion Superficial tongue laceration Nasal or mandibular ramus† fracture Tooth fracture/avulsion or dislocation	Rib fracture* Thoracic spine strain Rib-cage contusion Sternal contusion
2 (Moderate)	Amnesia from accident Lethargic/stuporous/obtunded; can be roused by verbal stimuli Unconsciousness < 1 h Simple vault fracture Thyroid contusion Brachial plexus injury Dislocation or fracture spinous or transverse process of C spine Minor compression fracture (≤ 20%) C spine	Zygoma, orbit,† body,† or subcondylar mandible† fracture LeFort I fracture Scleral/corneal laceration	2–3 rib fractures* Sternum fracture Dislocation or fracture spinous or transverse process T spine Minor compression fracture (≤ 20%) T spine
3 (Severe, not life-threatening)	Unconsciousness 1–6 h Unconsciousness < 1 h with neurologic deficit Fracture base of skull Comminuted compound or depressed vault fracture Cerebral contusion/subarachnoid hemorrhage Intimal tear/thrombosis carotid A Contusion larynx, pharynx Cervical cord contusion Dislocation or fracture of lamina body, pedicle or facet of C spine Compression fracture > 1 vertebra or > 20% anterior height	Optic nerve laceration LeFort II fracture	Lung contusion/laceration ≤ 1 lobe Unilateral hemo- or pneumothorax Diaphragm rupture ≥ 4 rib fractures* Intimal tear/minor laceration/thrombosis subclavian or innominate artery Inhalation burn, minor Dislocation or fracture of lamina body, pedicle or facet of T spine Compression fracture ≥ 1 vertebra or > 20% height Cord contusion with transient neurologic signs
4 (Severe, life-threatening)	Unconsciousness 1–6 h with neurologic deficit Unconsciousness 6–24 h Appropriate response only to painful stimuli Fractured skull with depression > 2 cm, torn dura or tissue loss Intracranial hematoma ≤100 cc Incomplete cervical cord lesion Laryngeal crush Intimal tear/thrombosis carotid A with neurologic deficit	LeFort III fracture	Multilobar lung contusion or laceration Hemopneumomediastinum Bilateral hemopneumothorax Flail chest Myocardial contusion Tension pneumothorax Hemothorax > 1000 cc Tracheal fracture Intimal aortic tear Major laceration subclavian or innominate A Incomplete cord syndrome
5 (Critica, survival uncertain)	Unconsciousness with inappropriate movement Unconscious > 24 h Brain stem injury Intracranial hematoma > 100 cc Complete cervical cord lesion C4 or below	—	Major aortic laceration Cardiac laceration Ruptured bronchus/trachea Flail chest/inhalational burn requiring mechanical support Laryngotracheal separation Multilobar lung laceration with tension pneumothorax hemopneumomediastinum, or > 1000 cc hemothorax Cord laceration or complete cord lesion
6 (Maximum injury)	Crush fracture, crush/laceration brain stem Decapitation Cord crush/laceration or total transection with or without fracture C3 or above	—	Total severence aorta Chest massively crushed

*Add AIS 1 if associated with hemothorax, pneumothorax, or hemopneumomediastinum. †Add AIS 1 to these fractures if open, displaced, or comminuted.
AIS—Abbreviated Injury Scale; C—cervical; T—thoracic.
From Civil and Schwab [18]; with permission.

AIS score	Abdomen	Extremities	External
1 (Minor)	Abrasion/contusion superficial laceration scrotum, vagina, vulva, perineum Lumbar spine strain Hematuria	Contusion elbow, shoulder, wrist, ankle Fracture/dislocation finger, toe Sprain A-C joint, shoulder, elbow, finger, wrist, hip, ankle, toe	Abrasions/contusions ≤ 25 cm on face/hand ≤ 50 cm on body Superficial lacerations ≤ 5 cm on face/hand ≤ 10 cm on body 1° burn up to 100% 2° or 3° burn/degloving injury < 10% total body
2 (Moderate)	Contusion/superficial laceration stomach, mesentery, SB, bladder, ureter, urethra Minor contusion/laceration kidney, liver, spleen, pancreas Contusion duodenum/colon Dislocation or fracture spinous or transverse process L-spine Minor compression fracture (≤ 20%) L spine Nerve root injury	Fracture humerus,* radius,* ulna,* fibula, tibia,* clavicle, scapula, carpals, meta-carpals, calcaneus tarsals, metatarsals, pubic rami or simple pelvic fracture Dislocation elbow, hand, shoulder, A-C joint Major muscle/tendon laceration Intimal tear/minor laceration axillary, brachial, popliteal A; axillary, femoral, popliteal vein	Abrasions/contusions > 25 cm on face or hand > 50 cm on body Laceration > 5 cm on face or hand > 10 cm on body 2° or 3° burn or degloving injury 10%–19% of total body
3 (Severe, not life-threatening)	Superficial laceration duodenum/colon/rectum Perforation SB/mesentery/bladder ureter/urethra Major contusion/or minor laceration with major vessel involvement, or hemoperitoneum > 1000 cc of kidney/liver/spleen/pancreas Minor iliac artery or vein laceration Retroperitoneal hematoma Dislocation or fracture of lamina body, facet or pedicle of L spine Compression fracture > 1 vertebra or > 20% anterior height Cord contusion with transneurologic signs	Comminuted pelvic fracture Fractured femur Dislocation wrist/ankle/knee/hip Below knee or upper extremity amputation Rupture knee ligaments Sciatic nerve laceration Intimal tear/minor laceration femoral artery Major laceration ± thrombosis axillary or popliteal artery; axillary, popliteal, or femoral vein	2° or 3° burn or degloving injury 20%–29% of total body
4 (Severe, life-threatening)	Perforation stomach duodenum/colon/rectum Perforation with tissue loss stomach/bladder SB/ureter/urethra Major liver laceration Major iliac artery or vein laceration Incomplete cord syndrome Placental abruption	Pelvic crush fracture Traumatic above knee amputation/crush injury Major laceration femoral or brachial artery	2° or 3° burn or degloving injury 30%–39% total body
5 (Critical)	Major laceration with tissue loss or gross contamination of duodenum/colon/rectum Complex rupture liver, spleen/kidney/pancreas Complete cord lesion	Open pelvic crush fracture	2° or 3° burn or degloving injury 40%–89% total body
6 (Maximum injury)	Torso transection	—	2° or 3° burn or degloving injury ≥ 90% total body

*Add AIS 1 to these fractures if open, displaced, or comminuted. AIS—Abbreviated Injury Scale; L—lumbar; SB—small bowel; T—thoracic.
From Civil and Schwab [18]; with permission.

TABLE 4C CALCULATION OF INJURY SEVERITY SCORE		
ISS body region	**AIS score**	**Square of AIS score**
Head/neck	_____	_____
Face	_____	_____
Thorax	_____	_____
Abdomen	_____	_____
Extremities	_____	_____
External	_____	_____

ISS = sum of squares of 3 most severe only.

ISS–Injury Severity Score; AIS–Abbreviated Injury Scale.
From Civil and Schwab [18]; with permission.

their patients with myocardial contusion would not have been so diagnosed. Other data, however, have not been confirmatory. In one study of 138 patients with severe injury, including possible myocardial contusion [11], only 1.4% had positive isoenzymes compared with 32% who had diagnostic electrocardiographic changes. Another study [7] found no significant association between CK isoenzyme changes and the occurrence of cardiac-related complications, and a third [4] observed that combined findings of electrocardiogram abnormalities and elevated CK isoenzymes were of no higher predictive value in defining patients at higher risk than using the electrocardiogram alone. In a final report of 182 patients with significant blunt chest wall trauma [22], the authors concluded that "CK-MB determinations in patients with suspected blunt myocardial injury were unjustifiably expensive and added confusion to an already vague clinical area." The problem of enzyme analysis is compounded in trauma cases by the presence of skeletal muscle injury, which almost always occurs in severe blunt chest-wall injury and lowers the CK-MB fraction (< 3%) relative to the total CK concentration in blood [23]. Adams and coworkers [24] have proposed the use of cardiac troponin I as a less ambiguous way of detecting cardiac injury since it is not elevated by skeletal muscle injury.

patients, "myocardial contusion does not by itself increase the risk of complication, does not necessitate intensive care unit monitoring, should be devalued when computing ISS scores, may account for lengthy and often unnecessary hospitalization, and in patients at risk for complications may be (more easily) identified by ECG abnormalities on arrival to the Emergency Department." [6]

Similar results were reached by Paone and coworkers [19]. They evaluated 159 cases of major blunt chest injury using several forms of diagnostic testing, including ECG monitoring, cardiac isoenzyme patterns and lactate dehydrogenase, and two-dimensional echocardiograms. They concluded that laboratory testings had "poor predictive value," and that clinical "observations with ECG monitoring" plus treatment of any symptomatic dysrhythmias were "an adequate and cost-conscious" approach. A meta-analysis survey by Maenza [20] also concluded that the ECG and the CPK-MB isoenzyme were the diagnostic parameters of most merit in evaluating patients with clinically significant myocardial contusion.

However, the value of CK-MB isoenzyme analysis is contested. Fabian and coworkers [21] reported that in 140 of 1110 patients suffering nonpenetrating trauma and at increased risk for blunt cardiac injury, 56 had likely evidence for myocardial contusion as estimated either by increased CK-MB concentrations in blood or by abnormalities on the admission electrocardiogram. The authors cautioned, however, that elevated isoenzymes were transient and required careful sampling (at admission and every 6 hours for the first 24 hours). If these sampling times were missed, up to 75% of

Imaging Modalities

It is probably too early to cast final judgment on the newer imaging modalities being employed to diagnose myocardial contusion, but the available data are not encouraging for either radionuclide angiography or two-dimensional transthoracic echocardiography. This may relate to the size and severity of the contusion injury, which *a priori* must be at least moderate to large or severe to affect a motion abnormality visible by noninvasive testing. An association has been described among patients with positive radionuclear imaging and mortality [10], but when a more complete population of trauma patients is surveyed, the sensitivity and specificity of this testing mode is reduced.

Radionuclide angiography

McLean and colleagues [9] performed radionuclear angiography in 163 patients who suffered thoracic trauma. Only seven patients had abnormal studies; five of them died. Postmortem findings in four patients showed evidence of prior infarction in three and one new anterior infarction in the fourth. Another report [10] noted that a radionuclear study performed 1 week

TABLE 5 CALCULATION OF THE PROBABILITY OF MYOCARDIAL CONTUSION USING ISS AND ECG IN 88 PATIENTS			
Predictors of myocardial contusion		**Probability of myocardial contusion**	**Patients with myocardial contusion, *n***
ISS>10	**Abnormal ED ECG**		
Yes	Yes	0.8656	9
No	Yes	0.3538	12
Yes	No	0.0396	4
No	No	0.0396	0

ECG—electrocardiogram; ED—emergency department; ISS—Injury Severity Score.
From Norton *et al.* [8]; with permission.

after injury showed normal wall motion and ejection fractions in a patient with biventricular contusions who died late. A third study reported a positive relationship between the extent of blunt trauma estimated by ISS and cardiac-gated, blood-pool scintigraphy using labeled technetium-99m, but with much less accuracy than with using electrocardiographic abnormalities [11].

The results of a small series of patients studied by coronary perfusion imaging using thallium-201 are more encouraging [25]. Approximately 70% of these patients with blunt chest trauma had scintigraphic defects related to areas of myocardial contusion, and all patients with these defects had either paroxysmal dysrhythmias or electrocardiogram abnormalities. Godbe and coworkers [26] reported that thallium-201 imaging with single-photon emission computed tomography is useful in predicting those patients suffering severe chest-wall trauma at increased risk for developing cardiac dysrhythmias. Another approach has used indium-111 antimyosin scintigraphy as the imaging probe. However, in one report [27], focal antimyosin uptake was uncommon in a series of 17 patients with severe multisystem trauma and suspected myocardial contusion.

Transthoracic echocardiography

Mixed results have confounded the use of two-dimensional transthoracic echocardiography. In animal studies, the diagnosis of contused myocardium seemed well-suited to two-dimensional echocardiography using the criteria of (1) increased end-diastolic wall thickness, (2) increased echo brightness, and (3) impaired regional systolic function" [28]. The precision and merits of this tool, however, have not been generally confirmed in clinical trials. In 172 patients with either blunt chest trauma or suspected or proven myocardial contusion evidenced by other clinical or laboratory criteria, myocardial contusion by echocardiography criteria was not obvious in 49% [29], 74% [4], 81% [13], and 86% [21] of cases. Another 7% to 15% of cases were either technically inadequate or nondiagnostic in quality. In those echocardiographic studies that were positive, myocardial contusion, wall-motion disorders, and small pericardial effusions were noted. It is presumed that as with radionuclear imaging, two-dimensional transthoracic echocardiography is only helpful in confirming large-sized contusions sufficient either to affect regional contractility or to produce other complications such as pericardial effusion. Conversely, it is inferred that the specificity and sensitivity of this procedure for smaller-sized injury is sufficiently reduced to jeopardize the accuracy of diagnosis.

Transesophageal echocardiography

Transesophageal echocardiography is a new imaging strategy in patients with blunt chest-wall trauma. The modality has a better signal-to-noise ratio and imaging capability than transthoracic echocardiography. Nineteen prospective patients with severe chest-wall injury were evaluated by transesophageal echocardiography [30]. Patients were studied within 12 hours of trauma. No procedural complications were reported. Investigations were undertaken for widened mediastinum (> 8 cm on chest film), and a variety of lesions were noted, including tricuspid, mitral, and aortic insufficiency; pericardial effusions; myocardial contusions; and aortic hematoma. In 5 of 19 patients with hypokinetic motion abnormalities compatible with myocardial contusion, isoenzyme analysis was negative.

Transesophageal echocardiography was also successful in characterizing traumatic aortic transection in one patient suffering blunt chest-wall trauma [31]. In addition, it was deemed critical in another patient for selecting medical over surgical treatment for trauma-induced mitral regurgitation with leaflet prolapse [32].

CORONARY ARTERY TRAUMA

In 1973, the question of coronary artery trauma in blunt chest-wall injury was speculative because of a deficiency in essential information and too few unequivocal cases with direct documentation of the diagnosis using coronary cineangiography [3]. This literature is still not available in large series comparable to those described for myocardial contusion. In 1979, Allen and Liedtke [33] listed five categories to characterize the case material:

1. Cardiac contusion (or myocardial infarction) in the absence of sustained injury to a major coronary artery,
2. Cardiac contusion (or myocardial infarction) associated with perfusion abnormalities of a major coronary artery,
3. Coronary artery fistula formation,
4. Coronary artery rupture, and
5. Animal experiments evaluating the effect of blunt trauma on the coronary vasculature.

It is difficult to separate myocardial infarction from myocardial contusion without mechanisms that specifically relate tissue injury with flow abnormalities in the major coronary vessels, particularly for contusions or infarctions in the presence of normal coronary arteries. In this instance, tissue damage may reflect primary myocardial injury, including trauma to the microcirculation; transient epicardial arterial spasm; or clot formation with secondary lysis, which cannot be adequately described by subsequent arteriography. Literature is limited to several case reports that detail the relationship between arterial damage and tissue necrosis. Chest injury has resulted from sporting accidents, accidents of childhood, and workplace events, as well as from traffic accidents [34–39]. In almost every circumstance in which coronary trauma was established or suspected, there were electrocardiographic findings of acute myocardial infarction.

In contrast to recommendations developed for the early triage of patients with myocardial contusion, myocardial infarct occurred 3 and 15 days after the initial traumatic event in two patients in these reports [37,39]. Either delayed vasomotor spasm or a hypercoagulopathy may contribute to the late clinical development of infarction. Accompanying these coronary injuries were examples of hypotension or shock, intraarterial clot formation, posttraumatic angina with an abnormal exercise tolerance evaluation, severe myocardial injury with depressed left ventricular ejection fraction and left ventricular aneurysm formation, tachyarrhythmias (nonsustained ventricular tachycardia), and complete heart block requiring temporary pacemaker insertion [35–39]. This latter finding confirms previous observations of complete heart block noted in the setting of blunt chest-wall trauma [40].

Therapy

These coronary injuries are well-suited to the therapeutic strategies developed for managing acute myocardial infarction. For example, intracoronary urokinase was infused for 2 hours in a patient with left anterior descending coronary arterial thrombus that had occluded both the anterior descending artery and first diagonal branch of that perfusion system [35]. Also, Lijoi and coworkers [39] attempted percutaneous transluminal coronary angioplasty of a totally obstructed left anterior descending coronary artery and were initially successful. The vessel reoccluded at 24 hours, and the patient was subsequently managed with surgical revascularization. In a 6-year-old boy with complicated cardiac trauma from a crush injury, cardiac surgery was employed to excise a left ventricular aneurysm that extended from the coronary sulcus to the apex of the heart and was filled with thrombus [36]. The operation was successful, and symptoms of heart failure that had developed before surgery resolved.

Coronary artery rupture secondary to blunt chest-wall injury is life-threatening. Heyndricks and associates [41] reported a 62-year-old patient involved in a car accident who presented with acute inferior myocardial infarction and hypotension. The patient received several supportive maneuvers, including assisted ventilation, pacemaker insertion, resuscitation, and pericardiocentesis. Treatment was unsuccessful, and the patient died 9 hours after injury. Autopsy revealed 13 rib fractures and the presence of blood bilaterally in both pleural spaces. One bone splinter had perforated the left pleura, lacerated the pericardium, and torn the right coronary artery from its origin on the aorta. There was also a smaller, transverse tear of the intima of the left coronary artery as well as a nonperforating tear of the aorta distal to the left subclavian artery. Histologic and histochemical examination confirmed the presence of an extensive, inferior myocardial infarction.

Consequences of Coronary Injury

In animal studies with controlled injuries to the coronary arteries, Sabbah and coworkers [42,43] described multiple coronary lesions by either microscopic examination or selective coronary arteriograms. They noted complete and partial obstructions to major coronary vessels, extravasation of blood from traumatic vascular wounds, accompanying extravascular hemorrhages, and a small arteriovenous fistula. Despite the angiographic severity of these lesions, which were evident by the third day after trauma, almost all findings resolved to near-normal or normal by 2 to 5 weeks of follow-up.

Even in the absence of demonstrable anatomic lesions, (ie, no spasm, thrombosis, hemorrhage, or laceration), functional consequences of direct coronary injury occur [44]. In our report, the epicardial-to-endocardial flow ratios measured by radioactive microspheres increase in absolute magnitude after injury and were accompanied by decreased coronary vascular resistance in the vascular bed distal to the

impact site. Other coronary abnormalities included a reduction in reactive hyperemia reflective of decreased coronary flow reserve and concomitant declines in regional systolic shortening, left ventricular pressure development, and left ventricular maximum rate of pressure development during isovolumic contraction. Metabolically, myocardial oxygen consumption and lactate extraction were decreased.

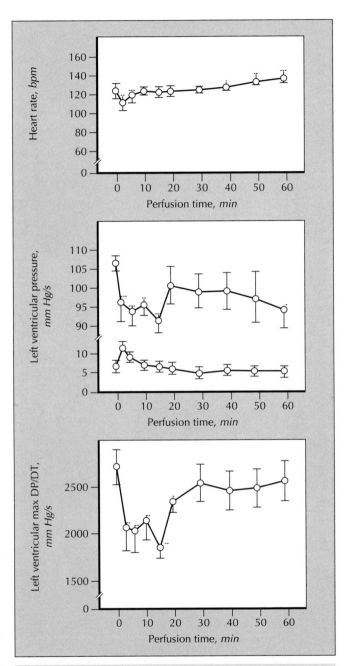

FIGURE 2 Changes in various parameters in global hemodynamic function in traumatized hearts. The major interval of mechanical dysfunction occurs early after the impact injury. **Middle panel**, *bottom open circles* represent left ventricular end-diastolic pressure; *top circles* represent left ventricular peak systolic pressure. *Dots* represent statistical significance by paired Student's *t*-test comparisons with pretrauma values: .—$P < 0.05$; ..—$P < 0.01$; ...—$P < 0.005$. *Bars* represent ± 1 SEM. Max DP/DT—maximum rate of pressure development during isovolumic contraction.

One unifying interpretation of these data is that there is an adverse reflex pattern of coronary perfusion with distribution of flow away from the subendocardial zone. This flow is sufficient to decrease coronary oxygen delivery and mechanical performance and to alter glucose metabolism, suggestive of early myocardial ischemia (Figs. 2 and 3, Table 6). These data *in toto* suggest that the coronary vasculature is not immune from direct injury after blunt chest-wall trauma; that consequences of this trauma may be expressed in a variety of clinical conditions, including life-threatening myocardial infarction or contusion; and that even without anatomic obstruction, derangements in coronary flow, which are functionally adverse

(particularly to the subendocardium) may occur with subsequent mechanical and metabolic sequelae.

KEY REFERENCES

Recently published papers of outstanding interest, as identified in *References and Recommended Reading*, have been annotated.

•• Maron BJ, Poliac LC, Kaplan JA, Mueller FO: Blunt impact to the chest leading to sudden death from cardiac arrest during sports activities. *New Engl J Med* 1995, 333:337–342.
The authors speculate that ventricular dysrhythmias induced by a blow to the precordium and delivered during an electrically vulnerable period of ventricular excitability is the cause of sudden deaths in chest impacts not associated with traumatic injury.

REFERENCES AND RECOMMENDED READING

Recently published papers of particular interest have been highlighted as:
• Of interest
•• Of outstanding interest

1. Parmley FF, Manion WC, Mattingly TW: Nonpenetrating traumatic injury of the heart. *Circulation* 1958, 18:371–396.
2. Fenton J, Myers ML, Lane P, Casson AG: Blunt cardiac trauma: survival after bichamber rupture. *Ann Thorac Surg* 1993, 55:1256–1257.
3. Liedtke AJ, DeMuth WE: Nonpenetrating cardiac injuries: a collective review. *Am Heart J* 1973, 86:687–697.
4. Miller FB, Shumate CR, Richardson JD: Myocardial contusion: when can the diagnosis be eliminated? *Arch Surg* 1989, 124:805–808.
5. Ross P, Degutis L, Baker CC: Cardiac contusion: the effect on operative management of the patient with trauma injuries. *Arch Surg* 1989, 124:506–507.

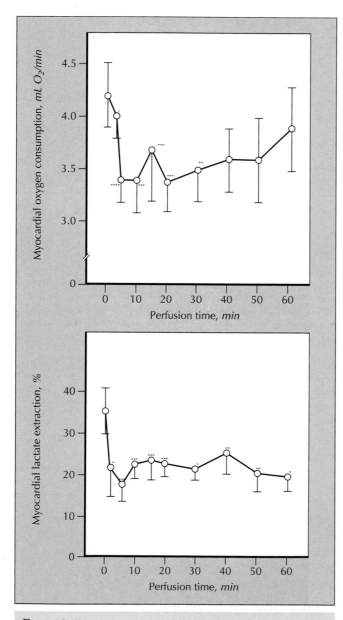

FIGURE 3 Changes in regional metabolism for oxygen consumption and lactate extraction in the perfusion distribution of the traumatized artery. The metabolic consequences of coronary injury, particularly for depressed lactate extraction, appear to last longer than for mechanical dysfunction. *Dots* represent statistical significance by paired Student's *t*-test comparisons with pretrauma values: .—*P* < 0.05; ..—*P* < 0.01; ...—*P* < 0.005. *Bars* represent ± 1 SEM.

TABLE 6 PERFUSION DATA IN FOUR TRAUMATIZED ANIMALS INJECTED WITH MICROSPHERE

	Epicardial/endocardial flow ratio		
	Impact	**LAD**	**LCF**
Pretrauma			
Mean	0.94	0.97	1.36
SEM	0.15	0.09	0.24
5 Min after trauma			
Mean	1.60	1.30	1.42
SEM	0.36	0.07	0.36
P	< 0.025	< 0.005	NS
55 Min after trauma			
Mean	1.54	1.25	1.17
SEM	0.26	0.06	0.16
P	< 0.005	< 0.001	NS

Impact—LAD perfusion system directly beneath and around the impact site; LAD—left anterior perfusion system; LCF—left circumflex perfusion system; NS—not significant; *P*—statistical comparisons with pretrauma data; SEM—standard error of the mean.
From Liedtke [43]; with permission.

6. Dubrow TJ, Mihalka J, Eisenhauer DM, *et al.*: Myocardial contusion in the stable patient: what level of care is appropriate? *Surgery* 1989, 106:267–274.

7. Foil MB, Mackersie RC, Furst SR, *et al.*: The asymptomatic patient with suspected myocardial contusion. *Am J Surg* 1990, 160:638–643.

8. Norton MJ, Stanford GG, Weigelt JA: Early detection of myocardial contusion and its complications in patients with blunt trauma. *Am J Surg* 1990, 160:577–582.

9. McLean RF, Devitt JH, Dubbin J, McLellan BA: Incidence of abnormal RNA studies and dysrhythmias in patients with blunt chest trauma. *J Trauma* 1991, 31:968–970.

10. McLean RF, Devitt JH, McLellan BA, *et al.*: Significance of myocardial contusion following blunt chest trauma. *J Trauma* 1992, 33:240–243.

11. Cachecho R, Grindlinger GA, Lee VW: The clinical significance of myocardial contusion. *J Trauma* 1992, 33:68–73.

12. Kram HB, Appel PL, Shoemaker WC: Increased incidence of cardiac contusion in patients with traumatic thoracic aortic rupture. *Ann Surg* 1988, 208:615–618.

13. Wisner DH, Reed WH, Riddick RS: Suspected myocardial contusion: triage and indications for monitoring. *Ann Surg* 1990, 212:82–86.

14.•• Maron BJ, Poliac LC, Kaplan JA, Mueller FO: Blunt impact to the chest leading to sudden death from cardiac arrest during sports activities. *N Engl J Med* 1995, 333:337–342.

15. Copes WS, Champion HR, Sacco WJ, *et al.*: The Injury Severity Score revisited. *J Trauma* 1988, 28:69–77.

16. Committee on Medical Aspects of Automotive Safety: Rating the severity of tissue damage. 1. The Abbreviated Injury Scale. *JAMA* 1971, 215:277–280.

17. *The Abbreviated Injury Scale (AIS)—1985 revision.* Des Plaines, IL: American Association for Automotive Medicine; 1985.

18. Civil ID, Schwab CW: The Abbreviated Injury Scale, 1985 revision: a condensed chart for clinical use. *J Trauma* 1988, 28:87–90.

19. Paone RF, Peacock JB, Smith DLT: Diagnosis of myocardial contusion. *South Med J* 1993, 86:867–870.

20. Maenza RL, Seaberg D, D'Amico F: A meta-analysis of blunt cardiac trauma: ending myocardial contusion. *Am J Emerg Med* 1996, 14:237–241.

21. Fabian TC, Mangiante EC, Patterson CR, *et al.*: Myocardial contusion in blunt trauma: clinical characteristics, means of diagnosis, and implications for patient management. *J Trauma* 1988, 28:50–57.

22. Keller KD, Shatney CH: Creatine phosphokinase-MB assays in patients with suspected myocardial contusion: diagnostic test or test of diagnosis? *J Trauma* 1988, 28:58–63.

23. Sobel BE, Jaffe AS: The value and limitations of cardiac enzymes in the recognition of acute myocardial infarction. *Heart Dis Stroke* 1993, 2:26–32.

24. Adams JE III, Dávila-Román VG, Bessey PQ, *et al.*: Improved detection of cardiac contusion with cardiac tropinin I. *Am Heart J* 1996, 131:308–312.

25. Bodin L, Rouby J-J, Viars P: Myocardial contusion in patients with blunt chest trauma as evaluated by thallium-201 myocardial scintigraphy. *Chest* 1988, 94:72–76.

26. Godbe D, Waxman K, Wang FW, *et al.*: Diagnosis of myocardial contusion: quantitative analysis of single photon emission computed tomography scans. *Arch Surg* 1992, 127:888–892.

27. Hendel RG, Cohn S, Aurigemma G, *et al.*: Focal myocardial injury following blunt chest trauma: a comparison of indium-111 antimyosin scintigraphy with other noninvasive methods. *Am Heart J* 1992, 123:1208–1215.

28. Pandian NG, Skorton DJ, Doty DB, Kerber RE: Immediate diagnosis of acute myocardial contusion by two-dimensional echocardiography: studies in a canine model of blunt chest trauma. *J Am Coll Cardiol* 1983, 2:488–496.

29. Reid CL, Kawanishi DT, Rahimtoola SH, Chandraratna PAN: Chest trauma: evaluation by two-dimensional echocardiography. *Am Heart J* 1987, 113:971–976.

30. Shapiro MJ, Yanofsky SD, Trapp J, *et al.*: Cardiovascular evaluation in blunt thoracic trauma using transesophageal echocardiography (TEE). *J Trauma* 1991, 31:835–840.

31. Brooks SW, Cmolik BL, Yong JC, *et al.*: Transesophageal echocardiographic examination of a patient with traumatic aortic transection from blunt chest trauma: a case report. *J Trauma* 1991, 31:841–845.

32. Turabian M, Chan K-L: Rupture of mitral chordae tendineae resulting from blunt chest trauma: diagnosis by transesophageal echocardiography. *Can J Cardiol* 1990, 6:180–182.

33. Allen RP, Liedtke AJ: The role of coronary artery injury and perfusion in the development of cardiac contusion secondary to nonpenetrating chest trauma. *J Trauma* 1979, 19:153–156.

34. de Feyter PJ, Roos JP: Traumatic myocardial infarction with subsequent normal coronary arteriogram. *Eur J Cardiol* 1977, 6:25–31.

35. Ledley GS, Yazdanfar S, Friedman O, Kotler MN: Acute thrombotic coronary occlusion secondary to chest trauma treated with intracoronary thrombolysis. *Am Heart J* 1992, 132:518–521.

36. Cizmarova E, Simkovic I, Zelenay J, Masura J: Post-traumatic coronary occlusion and its consequences in a young child. *Pediatr Cardiol* 1988, 9:117–120.

37. Foussas SG, Athanasopoulos GD, Cokkinos DV: Myocardial infarction caused by blunt chest injury: possible mechanisms involved—case reports. *Angiology* 1989, 40:313–318.

38. Pringle SD, Davidson KG: Myocardial infarction caused by coronary artery damage from blunt chest injury. *Br Heart J* 1987, 57:375–376.

39. Lijoi A, Tallone M, Parodi E, *et al.*: Coronary occlusion secondary to blunt chest trauma: a first attempt at balloon angioplasty. *Tex Heart Inst J* 1992, 19:291–293.

40. Brennan JA, Field JM, Liedtke AJ: Reversible heart block following nonpenetrating chest trauma. *J Trauma* 1979, 19:784–788.

41. Heyndricks G, Vermeire P, Goffin Y, Van den Bogaert P: Rupture of the right coronary artery due to nonpenetrating chest trauma. *Chest* 1974, 65:577–579.

42. Sabbah HN, Stein PD, Hawkins ET, *et al.*: Extrinsic compression of the coronary arteries following cardiac trauma in dogs. *J Trauma* 1982, 22:937–943.

43. Sabbah HN, Mohyi J, Stein PD: Coronary arteriography in dogs following blunt cardiac trauma: a longitudinal assessment. *Cathet Cardiovasc Diagn* 1988, 15:155–163.

44. Liedtke AJ, Allen RP, Nellis SH: Effects of blunt cardiac trauma on coronary vasomotion, perfusion, myocardial mechanics, and metabolism. *J Trauma* 1980, 20:777–785.

Diseases of the Aorta 37

Gregg M. Yamada
Joseph S. Alpert

Key Points

- Seventy-five percent of arteriosclerotic aortic aneurysms involve the infrarenal abdominal aorta.
- Thoracic aneurysms most commonly result from atherosclerosis; most involve the descending thoracic aorta.
- Abdominal aortic aneurysms 4 cm or more in diameter and thoracic aortic aneurysms more than 6 to 7 cm in diameter require surgical repair.
- Magnetic resonance imaging, computed tomography, and transesophageal echocardiography are highly sensitive and specific for the diagnosis of aortic dissection.
- Untreated aortic dissections are associated with a high mortality.
- Arteritis syndromes including Takayasu's arteritis, giant cell arteritis, and the seronegative spondyloarthropathies are associated with varying degrees of aortic involvement.
- Most aortoiliac emboli are cardiac in origin.
- Embolization of small cholesterol crystals may follow surgical or catheter manipulation, leading to the cholesterol emboli syndrome.

A complex array of diseases, either congenital or acquired, may affect the aorta (Table 1). This chapter reviews the pathogenesis, clinical manifestations, and therapy of the most common aortic processes, including arteriosclerotic aneurysms, dissection, arteritis, and thromboembolic disease.

ARTERIOSCLEROTIC AORTIC ANEURYSMS

Arteriosclerotic aortic aneurysms include both abdominal and thoracic aortic aneurysms.

Abdominal Aortic Aneurysms

Pathophysiology

Seventy-five percent of aortic aneurysms involve the abdominal aorta distal to the origin of the renal arteries. Approximately 25% occur within the thoracic aorta. Most of these aneurysms are fusiform and result from arteriosclerotic weakening of the elastic media; other causes of aortic aneurysms are listed in Table 2. Aneurysmal dilatation leads to increased aortic wall tension, which results in further enlargement of the aneurysm.

Presentation

Most patients who present with abdominal aortic aneurysms are asymptomatic. The diagnosis is suspected when routine physical examination reveals a pulsatile midepigastric mass or when aortic calcification is seen on abdominal radiographs (Fig. 1).

TABLE 1 DISEASES OF THE AORTA

Arteriosclerotic aortic aneurysms
Aortic dissection
Aortic arteritis
   Takayasu's arteritis
   Giant cell arteritis
   Ankylosing spondylitis
   Psoriatic arthritis
   Reiter's syndrome
Aortic thromboembolic disease
Aortic bacterial infection (syphilis, tuberculosis)
Traumatic injuries of the aorta
Aortic tumors
Coarctation and pseudocoarctation of the aorta
Hypoplastic aortic syndromes

TABLE 2 CAUSES OF AORTIC ANEURYSMS

Acquired
Atherosclerosis
Cystic medial degeneration
Infection (syphilis, tuberculosis)
Aortitis (infectious)
Trauma

Congenital
Aortitis (noninfectious)
Aneurysms associated with coarctation and patent ductus
   arteriosus

Diagnosis

The diagnosis may be confirmed with computed tomography (CT), magnetic resonance imaging (MRI), angiography, or ultrasonography. Abdominal ultrasonography is the most practical and cost-effective method for determining and monitoring aneurysm size [1,2], although CT provides additional preoperative information, delineating possible suprarenal extension or other abdominal abnormalities [3,4].

Treatment and prognosis

Prognosis is related to the size of the aneurysm, with larger aneurysms (> 5 cm in diameter) expanding more rapidly and being more likely to rupture than smaller aneurysms [5,6,7]. Aneurysm expansion rate is approximately 0.5 cm/y. Asymp-

tomatic aneurysms 4 cm or more in diameter (or twice the diameter of the infrarenal aorta) should be surgically repaired [8], and symptomatic or rapidly expanding aneurysms require immediate repair. The operative mortality rate for elective repair is approximately 3% to 5% [9].

Thoracic Aortic Aneurysms
Pathophysiology

Atherosclerosis is the most common cause of thoracic aortic aneurysms. Less common causes include annuloaortic ectasia, syphilis or other infections, and aortic valve disease. Arteriosclerotic thoracic aneurysms occur most frequently in the descending aorta and are typically fusiform, with the ascending aorta and the aortic arch less commonly involved. Patients with descending thoracic aortic aneurysms also may have associated abdominal aortic aneurysms [10]. Syphilitic aneurysms, which have a predilection for the ascending aorta, are often saccular.

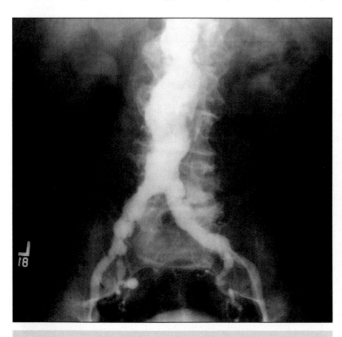

FIGURE 1 Abdominal aortogram demonstrating a fusiform infrarenal abdominal aortic aneurysm. (*From* Cipriano *et al.* [21]; with permission.)

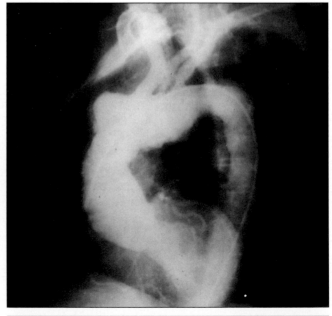

FIGURE 2 Thoracic aortogram demonstrating a saccular thoracic aortic aneurysm. (*From* Cipriano *et al.* [21]; with permission.)

TABLE 3 FACTORS PREDISPOSING TO AORTIC DISSECTION	

Primary or secondary cystic medial degeneration
  combined with:
Atherosclerosis
Hypertension
Advanced age
Aortic valve disease
Coarctation of the aorta
Aortic trauma, including iatrogenic trauma
Pregnancy

Aneurysms caused by cystic medial degeneration may involve the aortic sinuses and aortic valve, resulting in myocardial ischemia and valvular insufficiency.

Presentation

Descending aortic aneurysms are usually asymptomatic. In contrast, ascending aortic aneurysms are more likely to be symptomatic because of their impingement on adjacent thoracic structures. Patients may complain of a deep, aching anterior chest discomfort. Less common symptoms include dyspnea, cough, and hoarseness.

Palpable pulsations may be present along the anterior chest wall at either sternal border, the sternoclavicular borders, or the suprasternal notch. Aortic insufficiency and signs of Marfan's syndrome may be noted. Tracheal deviation, hoarseness, superior vena cava syndrome, and discrepant pulses and blood pressure also may be found.

Diagnosis

Thoracic aortic aneurysm may be suspected from routine posteroanterior and lateral radiographs, and it may be confirmed by angiography in patients requiring surgical resection (Fig. 2). Computed tomography, MRI, and transesophageal echocardiography (TEE) are sufficient to make the diagnosis, however, if surgery is not being considered.

Treatment and prognosis

Less information is available on the natural history of thoracic aortic aneurysms than for abdominal aneurysms. Symptomatic thoracic aneurysms are associated with a 5-year survival rate of 27%, compared with 58% in asymptomatic patients. Symptomatic thoracic aneurysms, or those over 6 to 7 cm in diameter in either the ascending or descending thoracic aorta, require prompt surgical attention [11]. Because of the high prevalence of associated cardiovascular disease (eg, coronary artery disease), patients must be carefully selected for surgery. Early surgical mortality is approximately 5% to 10% and most often results from myocardial infarction, congestive heart failure, stroke, renal failure, or sepsis [12].

AORTIC DISSECTION

Pathophysiology

Aortic dissection results from a sudden intimal rupture followed by the formation of a dissecting hematoma along or within the aortic media separating the intima from the adventitia. Two thirds of all aortic dissections occur in the ascending aorta 2 to 5 cm above the aortic valve. The descending aorta, just distal to the origin of the left subclavian artery, is the second most common site of aortic dissection.

Cystic degenerative changes of the elastic and smooth muscle elements of the aortic media predispose the patient to the development of aortic dissection [13]; other factors associated with aortic dissection are listed in Table 3. Aortic dissection is more common in men, and hypertension is present in most patients with descending aortic dissection. Aortic dissection occurs in various connective tissue disorders associated with prominent, congenital cystic medial degeneration (eg, Marfan's syndrome, Ehlers-Danlos syndrome). An increased frequency of aortic dissection is also seen in patients with aortic coarctation, congenital bicuspid aortic valve, aortic stenosis, and pregnancy. Iatrogenic causes include cardiac catheterization, cardiac surgery, intra-aortic balloon counterpulsation, cardiopulmonary bypass, and prosthetic valve surgery.

The most widely cited classification for aortic dissection is that of DeBakey [14], which uses the location of the intimal tear and the extent of the aortic dissection as points of classification (Table 4) [14]. Type I dissections arise just above the aortic valve and extend into the descending aorta. Type II dissections are localized within the ascending aorta. Type III dissections originate in the descending aorta just distal to the origin of the left subclavian artery and extend into the abdominal aorta (Fig. 3).

A simpler classification (ie, the DeBakey classification) identifies the DeBakey types I and II dissections as proximal or ascending (type A) dissections and DeBakey type III dissections as distal or descending (type B) dissections (Fig. 4) [15]. Acute aortic dissections are those present for less than 2 weeks.

TABLE 4 DEBAKEY CLASSIFICATION OF AORTIC DISSECTION	

Classification	Description
I	Originates in the ascending aorta and propagates distal to the brachiocephalic artery
II	Originates in and is confined to the ascending aorta
III	Originates in the descending aorta near the ligamentum arteriosum
IIIA	Dissection does not extend below the diaphragm
IIIB	Dissection extends below the diaphragm

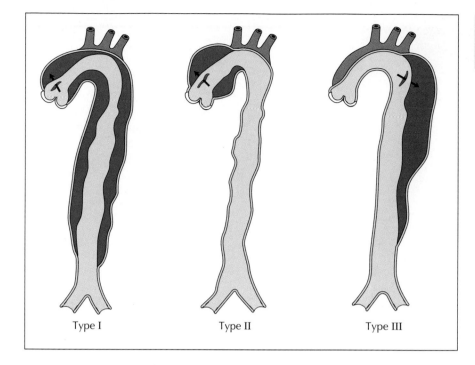

FIGURE 3 The DeBakey classification of aortic dissection. (*From* Eagle and DeSanctis [17]; with permission.)

Type I   Type II   Type III

Presentation

Severe chest pain described as "stabbing," "ripping," or "tearing" in character is present in most patients. Unlike the presentation of myocardial ischemia, which often develops over several minutes, the intensity of the pain is extreme at onset. The site of dissection may be suggested by the location of the pain, but the pain commonly migrates into the neck, back, and extremities as the dissection extends along the aorta.

Aortic insufficiency, pulse abnormalities, neurologic deficits, and evidence of cardiac tamponade may be present in patients with ascending aortic dissection. Pulse deficits are less common in distal aortic dissections but if present may involve the femoral and left subclavian arteries. Although most patients present with hypertension, hypotension may signify aortic rupture, cardiac tamponade, or subclavian artery dissection.

Diagnosis

The diagnosis of aortic dissection may be suspected from the history and physical examination, and it can be confirmed with echocardiography, CT, MRI, or angiography. Routine posteroanterior radiographs may reveal progressive mediastinal widening (Fig. 5). Separation of intimal calcification from the adventitial border by more than 1 cm is highly suggestive of dissection. Magnetic resonance imaging, CT and TEE are highly sensitive diagnostic methods. Because of the limitations of monoplane imaging probes, TEE was initally considered to be less sensitive [16]. However, the introduction of biplane and omniplane imaging probes has increased the specificity to 98% for type A and B dissections [17]. Due to the availability

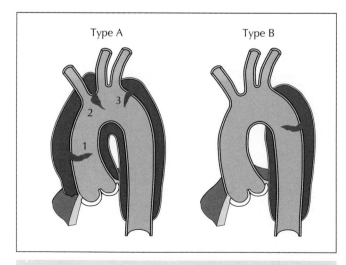

Type A   Type B

FIGURE 4 The DeBakey classification of aortic dissection. (*From* Miller *et al.* [22]; with permission.)

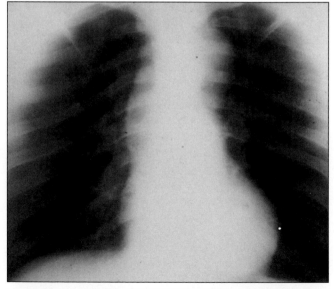

FIGURE 5 Posteroanterior chest radiograph demonstrating mediastinal widening caused by aortic dissection of the ascending aorta. (*From* Kidd *et al.* [23]; with permission.)

and rapidity of obtaining both omniplane TEE and CT scanning, either of these methods should be considered as the initial mode of evaluation in patients with high clinical suspicion for aortic dissection. In addition, TEE may be more suitable in unstable patients. MRI is the superior method for following chronic or repaired dissections. Transthoracic echocardiography allows the clinician to visualize proximal dissections, whereas TEE, CT, and MRI allow better visualization of distal dissections. Aortography is still recommended on the rare occasion when the diagnosis remains in question despite TEE, CT or MRI (Fig. 5) [17].

Treatment and Prognosis

Acute type A (ascending) aortic dissections (Fig. 6) almost invariably require immediate surgical therapy. Acute type B (descending) aortic dissections and chronic dissections of any location are first managed medically; surgery is reserved for complications such as rupture, expansion, continued pain, or distal ischemia. Untreated aortic dissections are associated with a 21% mortality at 24 hours, a 37% mortality at 48 hours, a 74% mortality at 2 weeks, and a 90% mortality at 3 months [17].

All patients with suspected aortic dissection require intensive monitoring for cardiac arrhythmias, hypotension, declining renal function, and other signs of systemic hypoperfusion before definitive diagnostic procedures are performed. The aim of medical therapy is to decrease both systemic arterial pressure and the rate of rise in aortic pressure. Analgesics and sedatives should be administered as needed. Intravenous β-blockers (eg, metoprolol) in combination with vasodilators (eg, sodium nitroprusside) should be administered to all patients with hypertension. Patients with hypotension require transfusion and emergent surgical correction [17]. The surgical technique used depends on the location of the dissection.

AORTIC ARTERITIS

Aortitis results from a variety of vasculitic syndromes and is characterized by obstruction of the aorta and its branches with dilatation and aneurysm formation. Aortic arteritis includes Takayasu's arteritis, giant cell arteritis, and other arteritis syndromes with rare origins.

Takayasu's Arteritis
Pathophysiology

Takayasu's arteritis is a chronic vasculitis involving the aorta and its primary branches, and it affects adolescent and young women. Asian, African, Native American, and Hispanic women are affected more often than white women. The cause of Takayasu's arteritis is unknown, but an immunopathogenic mechanism is suspected. Prominent intimal proliferation and fibrosis are characteristic, with involvement of the media, adventitia, and vasa vasorum resulting in luminal narrowing and aneurysm formation. The subclavian, carotid, vertebral, and renal arteries are the most frequently affected.

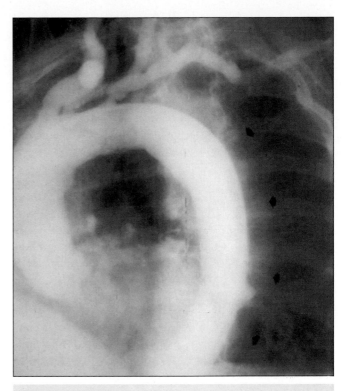

FIGURE 6 Ascending aortogram demonstrating type A aortic dissection. (*From* Cigarroa *et al.* [24]; with permission.)

Presentation

Fatigue, fever, malaise, weight loss, night sweats, and arthralgias predate ischemic manifestations. Pain and tenderness develop over the involved arteries, with diminished pulses, bruits, hypertension, heart failure, and retinopathy present on examination. Less common manifestations include coronary ischemia caused by ostial involvement of the coronary arteries, myocarditis, aortic regurgitation, and pulmonary hypertension.

Diagnosis

The diagnosis of Takayasu's arteritis is suspected in any woman younger than 40 years of age who develops bruits with diminished or discrepant peripheral pulses and blood pressures. The characteristic vascular abnormalities on angiography (ie, luminal irregularity, narrowing, dilatation, and aneurysm) are confirmatory. More comprehensive diagnostic criteria have been proposed [18]. Laboratory abnormalities are nonspecific and include an elevated erythrocyte sedimentation rate (ESR), anemia of chronic inflammation, and thrombocytosis.

Treatment and prognosis

The clinical course of Takayasu's arteritis varies, but slow progression is typical. Steroids are effective in alleviating symptoms and arresting disease progression; and cyclophosphamide is helpful in patients unresponsive to steroids. Renovascular hypertension is responsive to angiotensin-converting enzyme inhibitors and should be treated aggressively. The role of ASA or chronic anticoagulation in decreasing ischemic symptoms is not established [18].

Giant Cell Arteritis

Giant cell (or temporal) arteritis is a vasculitis affecting medium-sized arteries, typically those of the head and neck. The aorta and its primary branches are involved less commonly. White women over 50 years of age are most often affected.

Patchy or segmental granulomatous arterial inflammation is present. The etiology of giant cell arteritis is unknown, but an autoimmune mechanism is possibly responsible. Symptoms may develop gradually and include fatigue, headache, polymyalgia rheumatics, jaw claudication, and visual loss. Aortic arch involvement similar to that of Takayasu's arteritis may be seen, and patients are usually febrile on examination, with tenderness over the temporal arteries. Laboratory studies reveal a markedly elevated ESR, decreased serum albumin level, and moderate anemia of chronic inflammation. The diagnosis is confirmed by temporal artery biopsy. Corticosteroids are the treatment of choice and are continued for 1 to 2 years.

Other Arteritis Syndromes

Ankylosing spondylitis, psoriatic arthritis, Reiter's syndrome, and Behçet's syndrome are rare causes of aortitis. Typical findings include aortic root dilatation with thickened and retracted aortic valve leaflets and aortic valvular insufficiency. Histopathologic changes reveal destruction of elastic medial elements with an obliterative endarteritis of the vasa vasorum. The clinical course varies, and treatment is directed at the underlying disease process. Aortic valve replacement may be required.

AORTIC THROMBOEMBOLIC DISEASE

Aortic thromboembolic disease includes aortic and atheromatous emboli.

Aortic Embolism

Pathophysiology

Acute aortoiliac occlusion may result from thromboembolic disease or, less commonly, acute thrombosis. Most aortoiliac emboli originate from the left heart, with only a minority arising from a thrombus overlying an arteriosclerotic aortic plaque. Predisposing factors for aortic thromboembolism are listed in Table 5.

TABLE 5 FACTORS PREDISPOSING TO AORTIC THROMBOEMBOLISM
Myocardial infarction with mural thrombus
Ventricular aneurysm
Prosthetic valves
Atrial fibrillation
Cardiomyopathy
Endocarditis (bacteria, marantic)
Paradoxic embolism (patent foramen ovale or atrial septal defect)
Atrial myxoma
Idiopathic origin

Presentation

Acute, severe lower extremity pain with numbness, paresthesias, and weakness in the ischemic distribution is typical. The lower extremities are cold, pale, and cyanotic, with diminished or absent pulses.

Diagnosis

Clinical presentation is suggestive of the diagnosis, and angiography is confirmatory. Transesophageal echocardiography is useful in identifying cardiac sources of emboli [19].

Treatment and prognosis

Transfemoral artery catheter embolectomy is the procedure of choice and is performed by cardiovascular specialists. All patients are initially heparinized, and chronic anticoagulation is usually required.

Atheromatous Emboli (Cholesterol Emboli Syndrome)

Pathogenesis

Embolization of small cholesterol crystals into distal arterial beds may follow manipulation of an atherosclerotic segment of the aorta during surgery or catheterization. Spontaneous embolization is less common.

Presentation

Clinical presentation may include livedo reticularis, ecchymotic and gangrenous extremities, renal failure, hypertension, pancreatitis, abdominal pain, and neurologic deficits [20].

Diagnosis

Diagnosis is suspected clinically and is confirmed by demonstrating intra-arterial cholesterol crystals in muscle or skin.

Treatment and prognosis

Treatment for cholesterol microembolism is supportive, with prevention of necrosis and infection being the mainstays of therapy. Anticoagulation may exacerbate further embolization, and its use is controversial.

REFERENCES

1. Littooy FN, Steffan G, Greisler HP, *et al.*: Use of sequential B-mode ultrasonography to manage abdominal aortic aneurysms. *Arch Surg* 1989, 124:419–421.

2. Shapira OM, Pasik S, Wassermann JP, *et al.*: Ultrasound screening for abdominal aortic aneurysms in patients with peripheral vascular disease. *J Cardiovasc Surg* 1990, 31:170–172.

3. Gomes MN, Choyke PL: Pre-operative evaluation of abdominal aortic aneurysms: ultrasound or computed tomography. *J Cardiovasc Surg* 1987, 28:159–166.

4. Pillari G, Chang JB, Zito J, *et al.*: Computed tomography of abdominal aortic aneurysm. *Arch Surg* 1988, 123:727–732.

5. Sterpetti AV, Schultz RD, Feldhaus RJ, *et al.*: Abdominal aortic aneurysm in elderly patients: selective management based on clinical status and aneurysmal expansion rate. *Am J Surg* 1985, 150:772–776.

6. Naevoid MP, Ballad DJ, Hailed J: Prognosis of abdominal aortic aneurysms: a population-based study. *N Engl J Med* 1989, 321:1009–1014.

7. Ernest CB: Abdominal aortic aneurysm. *N Engl J Med* 1993, 328:1167–1172.

8. Hollier LH, Taylor LM, Ochsner J: Recommended indications for operative treatment of abdominal aortic aneurysms: report of a subcommittee of the joint council of the Society for Vascular Surgery and the North American Chapter of the International Society for Cardiovascular Surgery. *J Vasc Surg* 1992, 15:1046–1056.

9. Sullivan CA, Rohrer MJ, Cutler BS: Clinical management of the symptomatic but unruptured abdominal aortic aneurysm. *J Vasc Surg* 1990, 11:799–803.

10. Crawford ES, Cohen ES: Aortic aneurysm. A multifocal disease. *Arch Surg* 1982, 117:1393–1400.

11. Crawford ES, Crawford JL, Hazim SJ, *et al.*: Thoracoabdominal aortic aneurysms: preoperative and intraoperative factors determining immediate and long-term results of operations in 605 patients. *J Vasc Surg* 1986, 3:389–404.

12. Moreno-Cabral CE, Miller C, Mitchell S, *et al.*: Degenerative and atherosclerotic aneurysms of the thoracic aorta. *J Thorac Cardiovasc Surg* 1984, 88:1020–1032.

13. Dale JR, Pape LA, Cohn LH, *et al.*: Dissection of the aorta: pathogenesis, diagnosis, and treatment. *Prog Cardiovasc Dis* 1980, 23:237–242.

14. DeBakey ME, McCollum CH, Crawford ES, *et al.*: Dissection and dissecting aneurysms of the aorta: twenty year follow-up of five hundred twenty seven patients treated surgically. *Surgery* 1982, 92:1118–1134.

15. Erbel R, Delert H, Meyer J, *et al.*: Effect of medical and surgical therapy on aortic dissection evaluated by transesophageal echocardiography: implications for prognosis and therapy. *Circulation* 1993, 87:1604–1615.

16. Nienaber CA, von Kodolitsch Y, Nicolas V, *et al.*: The diagnosis of thoracic aortic dissection by noninvasive imaging procedures. *N Engl J Med* 1993, 328:1–9.

17. Keren A, Kim CB, Hu BS, *et al.*: Accuracy of biplane and multiplane transesophageal echocardiography in diagnosis of typical acute aortic dissection intramural hematoma. *J Am Coll Cardiol* 1996, 28:627–636.

18. Ishikawa K: Diagnostic approach and proposed criteria for the clinical diagnosis of Takayasu's arteriopathy. *J Am Coll Cardiol* 1988, 12:964–972.

19. Karalis DG, Krishnaswamy D, Victor MF, *et al.*: Recognition and embolic potential of intraaortic atherosclerotic debris. *J Am Coll Cardiol* 1991, 17:73–78.

20. Hendel RC, Cuenoud HF, Giansiracusa DF, Alpert JS: Multiple cholesterol emboli syndrome: bowel infarction after retrograde angiography. *Arch Intern Med* 1989, 2371–2374.

21. Ciprano PR, Alonso DR, Baltaxe HA, Gay WA: Multiple Aortic aneurysms in relapsing polychondritis. *Am J Cardiol* 1976, 37:1097–1102.

22. Miller DC, Stinson EB, Oyer PE, *et al.*: Operative treatment of aortic dissections: experience with 125 patients over a sixteen-year period. *J Thorac Cardiovasc Surg* 1979, 78:365–369.

23. Kidd JN, Reul GJ, Cooley DA, *et al.*: Surgical treatment of aneurysms of the ascending aorta. *Circulation* 1976, 54(suppl 3):111–119.

24. Cigarroa JE, Isselbacher EM, DeSanctis RW, Eagle KA: Diagnostic imaging in the evaluation of suspected aortic dissection: old standards and new directions. *N Engl J Med* 1993, 328:35–43.

SELECT BIBLIOGRAPHY

Baron JF: Dipyridamole-thallium scintigraphy and gated radionuclide angiography to assess cardiac risk before abdominal aortic surgery. *N Engl J Med* 1994, 330:663–339.

Debeider A, Thomas M, Marrinan M: Traumatic rupture of the thoracic aorta diagnosed by transesophageal echocardiography. *Br Heart J* 1993, 70:393–394.

Geva T, Hornberger LK, Sanders SP, *et al.*: Echocardiographic predictors of left ventricular outflow tract obstruction after repair of interrupted aortic arch. *J Am Coll Cardiol* 1993, 22:1953–1960.

Roman MJ, Rosen SE, Kramerfox R, Devereux RB: Prognostic significance of the pattern of aortic root dilatation in the Marfan syndrome. *J Am Coll Cardiol* 1993, 22:1470–1476.

Thromboembolism to the Kidney and Atheroembolic Disease

38

Jack W. Coburn
João M. Frazão

Key Points

- Thromboembolism to the kidney causes acute renal failure, usually anuria or oliguria.

- Abdominal or flank pain, fever, leukocytosis, and enzyme elevations support the diagnosis of thromboembolism.

- A positive diagnosis of thromboembolism is important because anticoagulation may prevent emboli to other vital organs; local therapy (angioplasty or thrombolysis) may help restore renal function.

- A specific diagnosis of thromboembolism by renal flow scintiscan or angiography is useful for specific therapy (heparin, thrombolytic agents, angioplasty, or surgical revascularization).

- One or more of three underlying events commonly exist in atheroembolism to the kidney: recent surgery involving the major arteries or heart, arterial catheterization of the heart or a major artery, and anticoagulant or thrombolytic therapy. Less commonly, it develops spontaneously. It is most common in white men over 60 years of age, less common in women, and rare in black patients.

- Renal failure from atheroembolism is accompanied by multisystem features caused by emboli elsewhere (pancreas, skin, brain, gastrointestinal tract, muscle, and eyes).

- A specific diagnosis of atheroembolism is made from a biopsy of skin, muscle, or kidney. Eosinophilia and elevated erythrocyte sedimentation rate are common; hypocomplementemia can occur.

- Therapy for atheroembolism is unsatisfactory; anticoagulants should be avoided if possible; cholesterol-lowering agents may be useful.

Renal artery thromboembolism and atheroembolism to the kidney are two relatively common but clinically distinct disorders that produce renal failure. Thromboembolism generally leads to sudden acute renal failure, whereas atheroembolism most often leads to insidious, slowly progressive renal failure, although sudden renal failure can occur. Both are prone to develop in older patients with heart disease, particularly arteriosclerotic heart disease and generalized arteriosclerosis. These disorders are commonly overlooked, and an early and proper diagnosis can lead to proper therapy with greater chance of recovery and the avoidance of unnecessary and invasive diagnostic procedures.

THROMBOEMBOLISM TO THE RENAL ARTERY OR ARTERIES

Thromboembolism to the renal artery or arteries commonly presents as oliguric or anuric renal failure; less commonly, nonoliguric renal failure occurs. In fully established cases, the pathology is that of renal infarction, the extent of which is determined by the size of the thrombus and the vessel or vessels occluded. The heart is usually the source of the thrombus, with mural thrombi from a myocardial infarct or left atrial thrombi resulting from rheumatic valvular disease being the most common causes [1••]. Other causes of renal artery embolism are untreated bacterial endocarditis, tumor embolism, and fat embolism; the last two causes are rare. Atrial

TABLE 1 CLINICAL FEATURES OF THROMBOEMBOLIC DISEASE OF THE KIDNEY

Clinical finding	Prevalence, %
Pain and tenderness (in the flank, abdomen, back, or chest)	70–80
Nausea and vomiting	50
Gross hematuria	20–25
Worsened hypertension	10–20
Cardiac history (of myocardial infarction, atrial fibrillation, or rheumatic heart disease)	90–95

TABLE 2 LABORATORY FINDINGS IN RENAL ARTERY EMBOLISM

Laboratory finding	Prevalence, %
Leukocytosis (11,000–32,000 cells/mm^3)	95
Microscopic hematuria (> 15 red blood cells per high-power field)	90
Pyuria (> 10 white blood cells per high-power field)	80
Proteinuria (1+ to 4+)	95
Increased serum enzyme levels	
Lactate dehydrogenase	98–100
Aspartate aminotransferase	60–70
Alanine aminotransferase	50–60
Alkaline phosphatase*	30–40

*This increase occurs later than the other enzyme changes.

fibrillation or another arrhythmia is often present. With better control of arrhythmias and the use of anticoagulants for atrial fibrillation, the incidence of this condition is probably lower. Less common conditions that cause occlusion or thrombosis of the renal artery and lead to renal infarction are trauma, arteriosclerotic renal artery stenosis, a hypercoagulable state (*eg*, nephrotic syndrome), dissecting aneurysm of the renal artery, and renal aneurysm rupture or thrombosis (often during pregnancy) [1••].

In animal experiments, total occlusion of the renal artery for 2 hours or more causes irreversible renal infarction; however, the clinical observations that renal function can recover after anticoagulant therapy, fibrinolytic therapy, angioplasty, or surgical revascularization after a thromboembolic renal artery occlusion has existed for many hours or even days [2,3•] suggests that the occlusion occurring in nature is rarely total or that significant collateral circulation exists. Oliguria and significant azotemia commonly occur after embolism to one kidney, even though the contralateral renal artery remains totally patent [1••]. The explanation for impaired contralateral renal function is unknown.

Clinical and Laboratory Features

The clinical features of renal artery occlusion are quite variable (Table 1). Abdominal or flank pain can be severe, and the findings of abdominal distention, ileus, and even rebound tenderness can lead to a mistaken diagnosis of acute cholecystitis or intestinal obstruction. Flank pain can resemble that of nephrolithiasis or acute pyelonephritis. Fever is common, with a temperature of 101° to 102° F. Clinical features of embolism to the brain or extremities may coexist, or there may be a history of a remote event. Acute or worsened hypertension sometimes occurs, but the blood pressure is unchanged in many patients [1••]. Oliguria or anuria (urine output of < 50 mL/24h) is common. With small segmental infarctions, the clinical manifestations can be minimal.

The nonspecific laboratory features of renal artery embolism are listed in Table 2. The enzyme increments may help in the diagnosis; moreover, the enzyme levels are elevated longer after renal infarction than after myocardial infarction (Fig. 1). In addition, creatine phosphokinase levels are not increased with renal infarction, distinguishing this condition from myocardial infarction.

Diagnosis and Treatment

Isotopic renal flow scanning is the best noninvasive screening test. With a segmental embolism, dimercaptosuccinic acid scanning can identify a smaller infarct. Arteriography and/or renal angiography will identify the nature of the occlusion, and either is more sensitive and specific than renal scanning. However, such an invasive procedure is not indicated unless surgery, local thrombolytic therapy, and/or angioplasty is being contemplated (*see* later discussion). Contrast-enhanced computed tomography shows an area of decreased accentuation and a thin rim of cortical accentuation, but the use of intravenous contrast material is required. Intravenous urography and renal ultrasonography serve only to exclude nephrolithiasis and other causes of ureteral obstruction.

The optimal treatment for renal artery thromboembolism has not been established. Vascular patency can be established by surgery, through the use of thrombolytic agents, and with balloon angioplasty. However, there has been good success following long-term anticoagulation [1••], with morbidity and mortality substantially less than with surgery [4]. The thrombolytic agents, streptokinase and urokinase, and recombinant tissue plasminogen activator have been successful in restoring blood flow and renal function according to case reports [5,6]; these agents can be combined with balloon angioplasty [7]. With prolonged anuria or oliguria that does not respond to anticoagulation, or with bilateral embolism and oliguria, aggressive intervention should be strongly considered, even after a period of days to weeks [2,3•]. Anticoagulation should be lifelong after thromboembolism, unless a contraindication exists.

ATHEROEMBOLISM TO THE KIDNEY

Atheroembolic renal disease arises from the occlusion of multiple small arteries and arterioles by cholesterol plaques that are displaced from ulcerative atheromata of the aorta. Because the extent of occlusion of arterioles is scattered and variable, the degree of renal failure varies from mild to severe.

A progressive but variable course in some patients suggests that embolization may occur continuously or intermittently in "showers." The pathology involves cholesterol plaques present as crystals within the lumina of arterioles; there are various degrees of inflammation with foreign body reaction and multinucleated giant cells. Patchy areas of ischemia and small infarctions occur, with tubular and glomerular atrophy and ultimate hyalinization [1••,8••].

This disorder occurs in patients with severe ulcerative atheromatous disease. There are increasing reports of its occurrence [9,10,11•]. One or more of three precipitating factors is commonly present: 1) any surgical procedure involving the major vessels or heart, 2) angiography, arteriography, or arterial catheterization of the heart or great vessels, and 3) therapy with anticoagulants or thrombolytic agents [8••,12]. It is presumed that the last therapy prevents the deposition of fibrin or hastens its removal, thereby allowing cholesterol plaques to break free and enter the circulation. Not uncommonly, there is no precipitating event [8••]. With the advancing age of hospital patients, the increasing use of cardiac catheterization and performance of cardiovascular surgery, and the widespread use of anticoagu-

lants and therapy with thrombolytic agents, atheroembolic disease is found with increasing frequency [13].

Clinical and Laboratory Features

Renal failure may occur abruptly after cardiac catheterization or a similar procedure; alternatively, renal failure may appear insidiously up to 4 weeks after such a procedure. Males predominate over females 3:1, while white patients predominate over black patients 30:1 [8••]. Oliguria may be transient or even absent, and a progressive increase in the serum creatinine and urea nitrogen levels may be the only renal abnormality. Evidence of generalized arteriosclerosis is usually present [8••,14]. Features suggesting multisystem disease are common and arise because of embolization to other organs, such as the skin (livedo reticularis or other rashes), brain (transient ischemic attacks or strokes), pancreas (pancreatitis), gastrointestinal tract (abdominal pain or gastrointestinal bleeding), liver (hepatitis), spleen, and muscle. Another feature is the "blue toe syndrome." Hypertension can appear, worsen, or become refractory to treatment [8••,14]. Fever and leukocytosis may be prominent. Disseminated intravascular coagulation

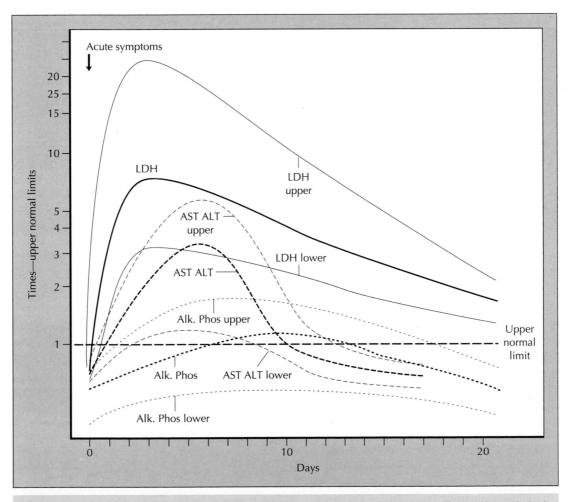

FIGURE 1 The time course of approximate changes in serum enzymes, LDH (*solid line*), AST and ALT (*dashed lines*), and alkaline phosphatase (*dotted lines*) after a renal thromboembolism with renal infarction. For the various enzyme levels, the data are shown in relation to the upper range of normal; the "average" is shown by the *heavy central line* and the upper and lower ranges for each, by *lighter lines*. ALT—alanine aminotransferase; Alk Phos—alkaline phosphatase; AST—aspartate aminotransferase; LDH—lactate dehydrogenase.

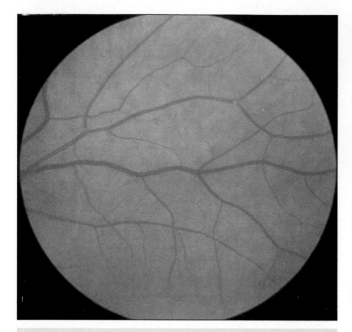

FIGURE 2 Optic fundus of a patient with atheroembolism showing the bright yellow refractile emboli, which characteristically lodge at the bifurcations of the arterioles. This finding is specific for the diagnosis of atheroemboli; however, only a fraction of afflicted patients exhibit this problem and a negative examination is not helpful. (*See* Color Plate.)

TABLE 3 DISORDERS THAT ATHEROEMBOLISM CAN MASQUERADE AS
Acute renal failure due to intravenous contrast material
Polyarteritis nodosa
Allergic vasculitis
Other collagen diseases
Acute hepatitis
Renal thromboembolism
Bacterial endocarditis
Septicemia
Disseminated intravascular coagulation

TABLE 4 SPECIFIC DIAGNOSIS OF ATHEROEMBOLISM AS A CLINICAL ENTITY
Renal biopsy
Skin biopsy
Muscle biopsy
Ophthalmoscopic examination (plaques)
Incidental finding on gastric biopsy, prostatic curettings, and so forth
Strong clinical suspicion

has been reported [15]. The finding on ophthalmoscopic examination of a cholesterol plaque in a retinal artery can confirm the diagnosis; unfortunately, this finding is not very common. Figure 2 shows the appearance of the optic fundus in a patient with atheroembolism, and Table 3 lists disorders atheroembolism can masquerade as.

The laboratory features of atheroembolic renal disease are not specific, and are only useful to exclude other disorders. Mild leukocytosis may occur, and eosinophilia is often present. The erythrocyte sedimentation rate is commonly elevated, serum complement levels can be reduced, and rarely, antineutrophil cytoplasmic antibodies (ANCA) may be present [16]. Urinalysis often shows mild proteinuria; less commonly, "nephrotic range" proteinuria may occur [17]. Microscopic hematuria can occur, with hyaline and granular casts. Eosinophiluria may occur, and a higher than expected serum urea nitrogen to creatinine ratio may arise as a result of decreased glomerular perfusion [18]. Biochemical features of renal infarction (as with thromboembolism) are uncommon, except in very severe cases with rapidly progressive renal failure.

Diagnosis and Treatment

Proof of this diagnosis requires histologic demonstration of the cholesterol emboli in various tissues. A biopsy of skin, muscle, or kidney often permits a definitive diagnosis (Table 4). However, the clinical features and a strong suspicion of this diagnosis are frequently adequate for clinical purposes.

The management is usually supportive, with the mortality rate reaching 60% or higher [8,11]. Anticoagulants should be withheld unless absolutely necessary. A very aggressive approach consisting of a cholesterol-lowering diet and drug

therapy may be helpful [19,20]. One major reason for establishing a specific diagnosis is to avoid unnecessary therapy for other suspected diagnoses (*eg*, prednisone or immunosuppressive therapy for suspected polyarteritis or other collagen vascular diseases). Transesophageal echocardiography can be used to identify large "dangling" aortic atheromata in high-risk patients [21•], and surgical "debridement" has been successfully carried out to prevent continued embolization [22].

KEY REFERENCES

Recently published papers of outstanding interest, as identified in *References and Recommended Reading*, have been annotated.

•• Llach F, Nikakhtar B: Renal thromboembolism, atheroembolism, and renal vein thrombosis. In *Diseases of the Kidney*, edn. 6. Edited by Schrier RW, Gottschalk CW. Boston: Little, Brown; 1997: 1893.
This chapter is an extensive and detailed review of a variety of vascular disorders affecting the renal arteries and veins. The entities described include acute thrombosis of the renal artery, thromboembolism to the renal artery, acute dissection of the renal artery, rupture of renal arterial aneurysms, and atheroembolic disease of the kidneys. There is an extensive bibliography of 256 references.

•• Saleem S, Lakkis FG, Martinex-Maldonado M: Atheroembolic renal disease. *Semin Nephrol* 1996, 16:309–318.
This review is an easy to read, complete, up-to-date description of atheroembolic renal disease. There are photos of kidney biopsies and tables summarizing the predisposing factors, clinical features, and laboratory findings. An extensive bibliography with 70 references is included.

References and Recommended Reading

Recently published papers of particular interest have been highlighted as:
• Of interest
•• Of outstanding interest

1.•• Llach F, Nikakhtar B: Renal thromboembolism, atheroembolism, and renal vein thrombosis. In *Diseases of the Kidney*, edn. 6. Edited by Schrier RW, Gottschalk CW. Boston: Little, Brown; 1997:1893.

2. Ramsay AG, D'Agati V, Dietz PA, *et al.*: Renal functional recovery 47 days after renal artery occlusion. *Am J Nephrol* 1983, 3:325–328.

3.• Fort J, Camps J, Ruiz P, *et al.*: Renal artery embolism successfully revascularized by surgery after 5 days anuria. Is it never too late? *Nephrol Dial Transplant* 1996, 11:1843–1845.

4. Nicholas GG, Demuth WE, Jr.: Treatment of renal artery embolism. *Arch Surg* 1984, 119:278–281.

5. Salam TA, Lumsden AB, Martin LG: Local infusion of fibrinolytic agents for acute renal artery thromboembolism: report of ten cases. *Ann Vasc Surg* 1993, 7:21–26.

6. Takeda M, Katayama Y, Takahashi H, *et al.*: Successful fibrinolytic therapy using tissue plasminogen activator in acute renal failure due to acute thrombosis of bilateral renal arteries. *Urol Int* 1993, 51:177–180.

7. Beraud J-J, Calvet B, Durand A, Mimran A: Reversal of acute renal failure following percutaneous transluminal recanalization of an atherosclerotic renal artery occlusion. *J Hypertens* 1989, 7:909–911.

8.•• Saleem S, Lakkis FG, Martinex-Maldonado M: Atheroembolic renal disease. *Semin Nephrol* 1996, 16:309–318.

9. Rhodes JM: Cholesterol crystal embolism: an important "new" diagnosis for the general physician. *Lancet* 1996, 347:1641.

10. Scoble JE, O'Donnell PJ: Renal atheroembolic disease: the Cinderella of nephrology? *Nephrol Dial Transplant* 1996, 11:1516–1517.

11.• Scolari F, Bracchi M, Valzorio B, *et al.*: Cholesterol atheromatous embolism: an increasingly recognized cause of acute renal failure. *Nephrol Dial Transplant* 1996, 11:1607–1612.

12. Blankenship JC: Cholesterol embolisation after thrombolytic therapy. *Drug Saf* 1996, 14:78–84.

13. Mayo RR, Swartz RD: Redefining the incidence of clinically detectable atheroembolism. *Am J Med* 1996, 100:524–529.

14. Dahlberg PJ, Frecentese DF, Cogbill TH: Cholesterol embolization: experience with 22 histologically proven cases. *Surgery* 1989, 105:737–746.

15. Thibault GE: One more hypothesis. *N Engl J Med* 1993, 329:38–42.

16. Peat DS, Mathieson PW: Cholesterol emboli may mimic systematic vasculitis. *BMJ* 1996, 313:546–547.

17. Haggie SS, Urizar RE, Singh J: Nephrotic-range proteinuria in renal atheroembolic disease: report of four cases. *Am J Kidney Dis* 1996, 28:493–501.

18. Clinicopathologic conference: Progressive renal failure with hematuria in a 62 year old man. *Am J Med* 1981, 71:468–474.

19. Cabili S, Hochman I, Goor Y: Reversal of gangrenous lesions in the blue toe syndrome with lovastatin: A case report. *Angiology* 1993, 44:821–825.

20. Kawakami Y, Hirose K, Watanabe Y, *et al.*: Management of multiple cholesterol embolization syndrome—a case report. *Angiology* 1990, 41:249–252.

21.• Kronzon I, Tunick PA: Atheramatous disease of the thoracic aorta: pathologic and clinical implications. *Ann Intern Med* 1997, 126:629—637.

22. Bojar RM, Payne DD, Murphy RE, *et al.*: Surgical treatment of systematic atheroembolism from the thoracic aorta. *Ann Thorac Surg* 1997, 61:1389–1393.

Diseases of Peripheral Arteries and Veins 39

John A. Spittell, Jr.
Peter C. Spittell

Key Points

- In addition to the evaluation of peripheral arterial pulsations, elevation-dependency tests provide confirmation of occlusive arterial disease in an extremity and a rough estimation of the degree of any ischemia.

- The most sensitive indicator of occlusive arterial disease in a lower extremity is an abnormal ankle:brachial index 1 minute after standard exercise.

- Arteriography is not necessary for the diagnosis of atherosclerotic occlusive peripheral arterial disease; it is indicated when restoration of pulsatile flow is planned.

- In the nondiabetic person with only intermittent claudication, restoration of pulsatile flow is elective.

- Features that suggest an uncommon type of occlusive peripheral arterial disease include a young person, involvement of the upper extremity and/or digits, and presentation as acute ischemia without prior symptoms of occlusive peripheral arterial disease.

- Atheroembolism (blue toes and livedo reticularis) may occur spontaneously from an atherosclerotic aorta or aneurysm, with the initiation of anticoagulant therapy, or follow arterial interventions or surgery.

- When venous thromboembolism recurs in the face of adequate anticoagulant effect, a secondary cause should be strongly suspected.

- Chronic indurated cellulitis (*ie*, lipodermatosclerosis), a complication of inadequately controlled chronic venous insufficiency, may mimic infection but can be relieved by good elastic support to the affected limb.

When symptomatic, diseases of peripheral arteries and veins cause pain, swelling, changes in skin color, or ulceration of the extremities or digits. The ease with which arterial and venous circulation of the extremities can be evaluated by physical examination and noninvasive methodology makes clinical diagnosis an office or bedside exercise in many cases.

DISEASES OF PERIPHERAL ARTERIES

Peripheral arterial disease is common and can present as either an acute or a chronic disorder, the latter being more common. Because occlusive and aneurysmal diseases are principally atherosclerotic in origin, they are the most frequently encountered disorders, but the less common types present the generalist with interesting diagnostic problems. Although the abnormalities presented by peripheral arterial disorders usually can be identified by a careful patient history and physical examination, noninvasive diagnostic studies are readily available to provide objective confirmation of clinical findings.

Occlusive Peripheral Arterial Disease

Occlusive peripheral arterial disease can be chronic or acute. The lower extremities are much more frequently involved than the upper extremities. Acute arterial occlusion can be thrombotic or embolic. Chronic occlusive arterial disease is most often caused by atherosclerosis, but thromboangiitis obliterans (Buerger's disease), giant cell arteritis, trauma, and external arterial compression (entrapment), although less common, are important for the clinician to keep in mind [1•,2].

Diagnosis

A useful way to think of occlusive peripheral arterial disease is the Fontaine classification (Table 1). The classic feature of symptomatic occlusive arterial disease in the lower extremities is intermittent claudication, which is characterized by aching, cramping, or tiredness that occurs with walking and is relieved by standing still. It may be mimicked by musculoskeletal disorders, chiefly pseudoclaudication from lumbar spinal stenosis (Table 2). When more severe ischemia develops, the patient experiences pain at rest (ischemic rest pain) and, with even minor trauma, ischemic ulceration (Fig. 1, Table 3) occurs.

Reduced or absent pulsation of the extremity arteries is the classic physical finding in occlusive arterial disease. Arterial narrowing upstream may cause audible systolic bruits over large arteries, and when the lumen becomes more narrowed (usually > 80%) creating a gradient in diastole, the bruit may extend into diastole. A useful clinical estimate of the degree of ischemia can be obtained by observing development of pallor on elevation of the extremity and then the time required for return of color to the skin and the superficial veins to fill on dependency of the extremity or extremities after elevation (Table 4). In the upper extremity, the

TABLE 1 FONTAINE CLASSIFICATION	
Stage	**Clinical feature**
1	Silent
2	Intermittent claudication
3	Rest ischemia
4	Ulceration or gangrene

From Fontaine *et al.* [13].

TABLE 2 CONDITIONS CONFUSED WITH INTERMITTENT CLAUDICATION	
Site of claudication	**Confused conditions**
Foot	Foot strain
	Tight shoes
	Plantar neuroma
Calf	Muscle strain
	Flat feet
	Osteoarthritis of knee
Thigh	Sciatica
	Pseudoclaudication caused by spinal stenosis
Hip	Osteoarthritis of hip
	Pseudoclaudication caused by spinal stenosis

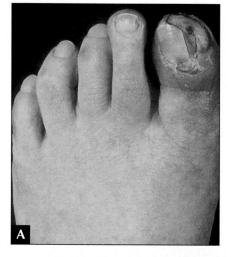

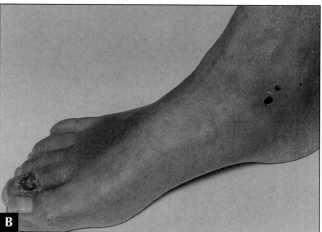

FIGURE 1 A, Ischemic ulceration, first toe. **B,** Ischemic ulceration, second toe and medial aspect of ankle.

TABLE 3 CHARACTERISTICS OF ISCHEMIC AND VENOUS STASIS ULCERATION		
	Ischemic	**Venous stasis**
Location	Toe, heel, foot	Medial distal leg
Pain	Severe	Only when infected
Surrounding skin	± inflamed	Stasis pigmentation
Ulcer edge	Discrete	Shaggy
Ulcer base	Pale, eschar	Healthy

TABLE 4 OFFICE ESTIMATION OF THE DEGREE OF ISCHEMIA

Degree	Elevation pallor, *sec**	CR, *sec†*	VFT, *sec‡*
None	None in 60	10	15
Moderate	Pallor in 30–60	15–20	20–30
Severe	Pallor in < 30	40+	40+

*Elevation of extremity at an angle of 60° above level.
†Color return (CR) to skin of foot on dependency after elevation.
‡Superficial venous filling time (VFT) on dependency after elevation.

Allen test (Fig. 2) to evaluate circulation in the hand and the thoracic outlet maneuvers (Fig. 3) are useful when occlusive arterial disease is present.

When taken with the patient supine using a standard blood pressure cuff and a handheld continuous-wave Doppler, the systolic brachial and ankle blood pressures provide an objective measure of lower extremity arterial circulation. Normally, the systolic blood pressure at the ankle exceeds that at the brachial level. When these pressures are determined before and after standard exercise (Table 5), functional as well as semiquantitative assessment of the occlusive arterial disease can be made. Arteriography is usually not needed unless restoration of pulsatile flow is being considered or some unusual type of occlusive arterial disease is suspected.

Differential diagnosis

As noted, arteriosclerosis is by far the most common cause of occlusive peripheral arterial disease. Uncommon types of occlusive arterial disease are suggested by their occurrence in young persons, acute (often digital) ischemia, or associated systemic symptoms.

Arteriosclerosis is more common in men over 40 years of age, particularly those with the risk factors of tobacco use, hyperlipidemia, or diabetes mellitus. It affects large- and medium-sized extremity arteries as well as the coronary and cerebral arteries.

Less common types of occlusive peripheral arterial disease include thromboangiitis obliterans (Buerger's disease), traumatic (repetitive, blunt-type) occlusive arterial disease in the hand, occlusive disease caused by compression of a peripheral artery (popliteal artery entrapment [Table 6] and thoracic outlet compression of the subclavian artery), and the arteritides (giant cell arteritis and connective tissue disorders). In connective tissue disorders, the occlusive disease is usually digital. Giant cell (temporal, cranial) arteritis affects persons over 60 years of age whose dominant symptoms are headache and those of a systemic illness, whereas Takayasu's arteritis typically affects the branches of the aortic arch in young women.

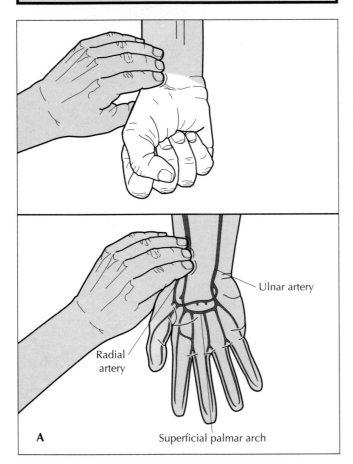

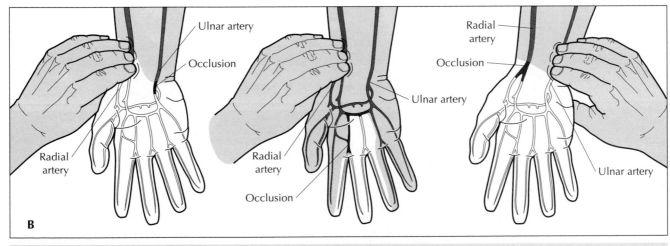

FIGURE 2 Allen test. **A,** Normal (negative) result, indicating patency of ulnar artery and superficial palmar arch. **B,** Abnormal (positive) results caused by occlusion of ulnar artery (*left*), superficial palmar arch (*bottom center*), and radial artery (*right*). (*From* Spittell [15]; with permission.)

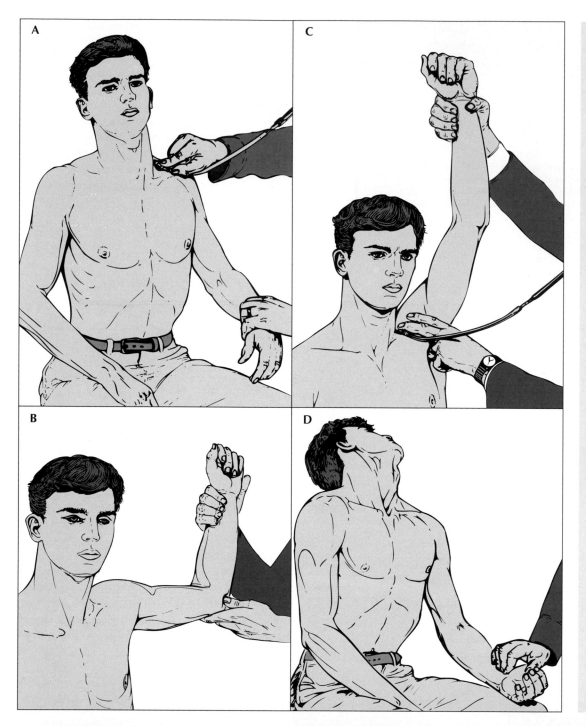

FIGURE 3 **A,** Costoclavicular maneuver, active. Auscultation over subclavian artery, above or below midportion of clavicle, may reveal systolic bruit as artery is compressed. Radial pulse and bruit over subclavian artery disappear when complete compression of subclavian artery occurs. **B,** Costoclavicular maneuver, passive. **C,** Hyperabduction maneuver. Axillary artery may be completely or incompletely compressed. In the latter case, bruit may be heard above or below the clavicle or, on occasion, deep in the axilla. **D,** Scalene or Adson maneuver. This test is used in both cervical rib or anomalous first thoracic rib syndrome and scalenus anticus syndrome. Auscultation over subclavian artery being tested may reveal bruit when the artery is partially compressed. (*From* Fairbairn *et al.* [16]; with permission.)

TABLE 5 NONINVASIVE LABORATORY ASSESSMENT OF ARTERIAL INSUFFICIENCY OF LEGS

	Standard exercise		Systolic blood pressure index*	
Degree of insufficiency	Claudication	Duration, *min*	Before exercise	After exercise
Minimal	0	5	Normal to mildly abnormal	Abnormal
Mild	Present	5	> 0.8	> 0.5
Moderate	Present	< 5	< 0.8	< 0.5
Severe†	Present	< 3	< 0.5	< 0.15

*Systolic pressure index is obtained by dividing the systolic ankle blood pressure by the systolic brachial blood pressure, both measured with the patient supine (normal, 0.95 or greater).

†Often, the systolic ankle blood pressure is less than 50 mm Hg.

From Spittell [14].

TABLE 6 CLINICAL FEATURES OF LESS COMMON TYPES OF OCCLUSIVE PERIPHERAL ARTERIAL DISEASE

Thromboangiitis obliterans (Buerger's disease)

Men affected more than women

Tobacco use

Age < 30 y

Small arteries upper and lower extremities involved

Claudication of arch or calf

Migratory superficial phlebitis common

Occlusive arterial disease of hands from repetitive blunt trauma

Often occupational—tools, "hammerhand"

Dominant hand

Tobacco use (predisposing factor)

Popliteal artery entrapment

Young men affected more than women

Symptoms unilateral

Calf pain with walking not running

Decreased or absent pedal pulses

Diagnosis by magnetic resonance angiography

Thoracic outlet compression

Clinical presentations

  Mass, supraclavicular area

  Unilateral Raynaud's

  Unilateral digital ischemia

  Axillary-subclavian vein thrombosis

Prognosis

Survival of persons with arteriosclerosis is shortened because of associated coronary and cerebral artery disease. The risk of limb loss for the person without diabetes whose only symptom is intermittent claudication is approximately 5% in 5 years; when the ischemia is more severe (ischemic pain at rest or ischemic ulcer), the risk is approximately 12% in 5 years [3].

When arteriosclerosis obliterans (ASO) is symptomatic in the person with diabetes, the prognosis for limb loss is approximately fourfold that of the person without diabetes [4].

In thromboangiitis obliterans, the risk of limb loss is greater than in ASO. It depends mainly on the severity of the ischemia at the time of diagnosis and whether the patient stops using tobacco permanently.

In chronic occlusive arterial disease caused by repetitive, blunt trauma to the hand, loss of digits can occur if the cause is not recognized and corrected (Fig. 4). Limb or digital loss can occur with arterial compression syndromes as a result of embolization from mural thrombus that develops in the post-stenotic aneurysm because of chronic arterial compression. In occlusive arterial disease caused by arteritis, frequency of limb loss depends on the severity of ischemia at the time of diagnosis and how much control over the arteritis is achieved.

Management

Definitive management of chronic occlusive arterial disease should be individualized according to its etiology, severity, disability, and prognosis, but the physician should have all patients take general measures to protect the ischemic limb from trauma and avoid vasoconstrictive influences. These general measures include the following:

1. Stop tobacco use,
2. Avoid trauma,
3. Wear proper footwear,
4. Attend to regular foot care and hygiene,
5. Walk on a regular basis,
6. Avoid vasoconstriction, and
7. Control atherosclerosis risk factors.

For all persons, conservative measures are indicated; control of risk factors (hyperlipidemia, hypertension, and diabetes) is indicated to delay progression of the atherosclerosis. The importance of discontinuing tobacco use should be emphasized. Continued smoking increases the risk of limb loss tenfold [3]. A regular walking program may increase the walking distance, and a trial of pentoxifylline [5] may provide additional symptomatic relief of intermittent claudication. Careful attention to foot care and hygiene as well as selection

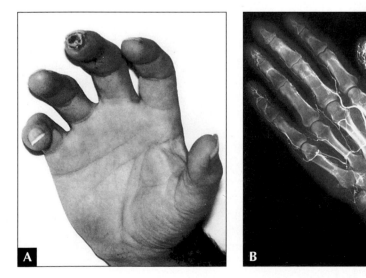

A

B

FIGURE 4 Right hand of a 42-year-old, right-handed millwright. **A,** Ischemic ulceration of the finger. **B,** Arteriogram showing a narrowed ulnar artery and occlusion of the ulnar portion of the superficial palmar arch.

of proper footwear is important. In the management of associated coronary and hypertension disease, drugs that may cause vasoconstriction (β-blockers and clonidine) are best avoided when alternative agents can be safely used.

In persons with traumatic occlusive disease, measures to protect the hand (regular use of gloves and avoiding blunt trauma) in addition to general measures are important to prevent progression. If ischemic ulceration has already occurred, an α-blocking agent or sympathectomy can be used to hasten healing and provide longer-term protection of the ischemic digit [6]. When occlusive arterial disease is caused by arteritis, management should include therapy of the systemic process and general measures to protect the ischemic limb.

When to refer

In symptomatic arteriosclerosis obliterans, restoration of pulsatile flow by either arterial surgery or percutaneous angioplasty can be used to relieve disabling claudication in the nondiabetic person. It is also indicated (when feasible) for the management of ischemic rest pain, ischemic ulceration, and symptomatic occlusive arterial disease in persons with diabetes. The frequency of coronary artery disease as a comorbid condition must always be kept in mind during preoperative evaluation and risk stratification if restoration of pulsatile flow is planned for persons with atherosclerotic occlusive peripheral arterial disease [7,8]. The appropriate management of arterial compression syndromes is surgical relief.

Acute Peripheral Arterial Occlusion

Acute occlusion of a peripheral artery can be thrombotic or embolic. Symptoms can be dramatic with one or all of the five *P*'s (pain, pallor, paresthesia, paralysis, and pulseless) or may be more subtle (*eg*, abrupt onset of intermittent claudication or shortening of walking distance in a person with existing claudication). The distinction between embolic and thrombotic arterial occlusion is frequently inferential (Table 7) but may be important, as either type can be a clue to an otherwise occult systemic or cardiovascular disorder.

Differential diagnosis

The differential diagnosis of acute peripheral arterial occlusion includes arterial spasm from drugs (*eg*, ergotism) or associated with extensive, acute, deep venous thrombosis.

Management

Initial management of acute arterial occlusion should include protection of the ischemic limb (do not heat, cool, or elevate) and heparin therapy to protect the collateral circulation while the etiology is being determined. Definitive management options include thrombolytic therapy, surgical thromboembolectomy, or antithrombotic therapy. Factors influencing the choice of therapy include size of the artery occluded, condition of the limb, etiology of the occlusion, and the general and cardiac status of the patient.

Atheroembolism from proximal aortic or arterial atherosclerotic plaques or aneurysms is now being recognized with increasing frequency as a result of improving noninvasive imaging techniques, particularly transesophageal echocardiography [9]. Features suggestive of atheroembolism include livedo reticularis, cyanotic digits, hypertension, renal insufficiency, transient eosinophilia, and an elevated sedimentation rate.

When to refer

Management is difficult unless the origin of the atheroembolic material can be surgically removed.

Peripheral Arterial Aneurysm

Like occlusive peripheral arterial disease, arterial aneurysms are most often atherosclerotic, more frequent in lower than in upper extremity arteries, and much more common in men than in women.

Diagnosis

Until an aneurysm becomes symptomatic as a result of complications (Table 8), the diagnosis depends on a careful physical examination or incidental recognition on radiography or ultrasonography performed for some other reason. Iliac artery aneurysms are usually associated with abdominal aortic aneurysms. Symptomatic iliac artery aneurysms may cause groin or perineal pain, iliac vein obstruction, or obstructive urologic symptoms [10].

Aneurysms of the femoral and popliteal arteries rarely occur in women. Popliteal aneurysms are bilateral approximately 50% of the time, and in over 40% of cases, they are associated with aneurysms elsewhere in the body, most often the abdominal area.

TABLE 7 ACUTE ARTERIAL OCCLUSION

Conditions suggesting embolic arterial occlusion
Heart failure
Atrial fibrillation
Recent myocardial infarction
Proximal atherosclerosis
Proximal arterial aneurysm

Conditions suggesting thrombotic arterial occlusion
Symptomatic peripheral arterial disease
Acute arterial trauma
Myeloproliferative disease
Active arteritis
Acute aortic dissection

TABLE 8 COMPLICATIONS OF ANEURYSMS

Pressure on surrounding structures
Thrombosis
Distal embolization
Rupture
Infection

Differential diagnosis

Peripheral artery aneurysm may be confused with other types of mass, but differentiation is readily made with ultrasonography.

When to refer

Untreated peripheral artery aneurysms frequently produce complications, most often thromboembolic, that may threaten the limb, so elective surgical treatment before complications occur gives the best results. Arteriography before surgery is needed to evaluate the arterial circulation proximal and distal to the aneurysm.

DISEASES OF VEINS

Clinicians are appropriately most interested in acute deep venous thrombosis because of its embolic potential, but other disorders of veins (varicose veins and chronic venous insufficiency) are frequent causes of complications and morbidity, much of which can be prevented by proper management.

Venous Thrombosis

Both superficial and deep venous thrombosis are important clinical events from the diagnostic and therapeutic aspects.

Diagnosis

Superficial thrombophlebitis, presenting as a reddened, tender nodule or cord in the course of a superficial vein, is readily diagnosed on physical examination. Deep venous thrombosis, however, is notorious for its variable clinical manifestations depending on the location and extent of the venous occlusion. Symptoms may include pain or swelling in the limb, and findings on physical examination may include tenderness over the involved vein and, when proximal to the calf, pitting edema distally and increased superficial (collateral) venous pattern.

The variability of clinical findings have made duplex ultrasonography the diagnostic procedure of choice in proximal deep vein thrombosis [11], but when only calf veins are involved, contrast venography remains the diagnostic gold standard. Impedance plethysmography is a useful noninvasive diagnostic test for deep vein obstruction, particularly in cases of recurrent proximal deep venous thrombosis.

Differential diagnosis

Superficial thrombophlebitis is easily differentiated from acute lymphangitis, because the latter is accompanied by chills and high fever. Occasionally, nodular conditions (erythema nodosum or vasculitis) require biopsy to confidently differentiate them.

Deep venous thrombosis involves a much more complicated differential diagnosis that includes nonthrombotic (chronic) venous obstruction, sciatica, muscle strain or tear, and acute lymphangitis and cellulitis. Unless physical findings, noninvasive diagnostic studies or duplex ultrasonsgraphy permit confident differential diagnosis, contrast venography is necessary.

Management

Therapy of superficial thrombophlebitis is basically symptomatic: local warm moist packs, analgesics, and elevation of the extremity. If the process extends despite such treatment, a short course of oral anticoagulant therapy may be used to effect resolution.

Therapy for acute deep venous thrombosis continues to be heparin initially, followed by oral anticoagulant therapy for 3 or preferably 6 months. Treatment of selected patients with proximal deep vein thrombosis with low-molecular-weight heparin on an outpatient basis is being evaluated [12]. Thrombolytic therapy is usually reserved for acute, extensive, deep venous thrombosis (*eg*, axillary subclavian vein thrombosis or phlegmasia cerulea dolens [Fig. 5] in young persons to obtain rapid resolution and lessen the chances of venous valvular damage). Anticoagulant therapy must be instituted as soon as thrombolytic therapy ends so as to prevent rethrombosis. An algorithm for management of the patient with suspected deep venous thrombosis is shown in Figure 6.

Recurring superficial or deep venous thrombosis is an important clinical problem, both diagnostically and therapeutically. Causes that need to be considered are shown in Table 9. Oral anticoagulant therapy provides effective management of the primary types and coagulation disorders, but particularly in secondary types, recurrences may occur despite adequate oral anticoagulant therapy.

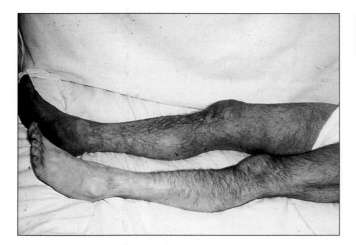

> **FIGURE 5** Phlegmasia cerulea dolens (extensive venous thrombosis of the whole right lower extremity).

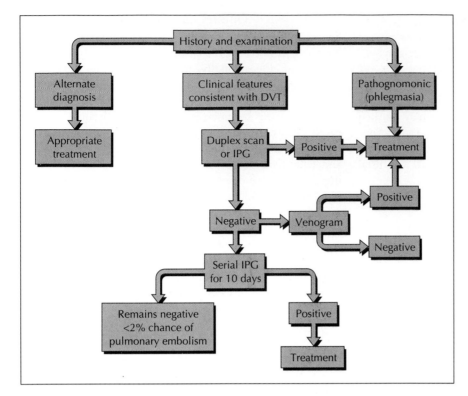

FIGURE 6 Algorithm for clinically suspected deep venous thrombosis (DVT). IPG—impedance plethysmography.

Flowchart content:

History and examination
→ Alternate diagnosis → Appropriate treatment
→ Clinical features consistent with DVT → Duplex scan or IPG → Positive → Treatment
→ Pathognomonic (phlegmasia) → Treatment

Duplex scan or IPG → Negative → Venogram → Positive → Treatment
Venogram → Negative
Negative → Serial IPG for 10 days → Remains negative <2% chance of pulmonary embolism
Serial IPG for 10 days → Positive → Treatment

TABLE 9 RECURRENT VENOUS THROMBOSIS

Primary (idiopathic)	**Coagulation disorders**
Familial	Hereditary
Nonfamilial	Activated protein C resistance
Secondary	Antithrombin III deficiency
Thromboangiitis obliterans	Protein C deficiency
Ulcerative bowel disease	Protein S deficiency
Myeloproliferative disease	Dysfibrinoginemia
Connective tissue disease	Acquired antiphospholipid antibody syndromes
Oral contraceptives	Circulating anticoagulant with systemic lupus
Neoplasms	Nonlupus types

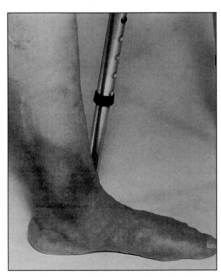

FIGURE 7 Chronic indurated cellulitis.

When to refer

Superficial phlebitis of a varicose vein is generally an indication for surgical removal.

Chronic Venous Insufficiency

An important and often neglected sequel of deep venous thrombosis is chronic deep venous insufficiency resulting from postphlebitic venous stasis. Regular use of properly fitted, adequate (30 to 40 mm Hg compression at the ankle) elastic stockings can prevent complications of chronic venous insufficiency.

The generalist is likely to be consulted by the patient who develops chronic tender induration of the medial distal leg because of uncontrolled chronic deep venous insufficiency (Fig. 7). The reddened, tender, indurated features of this complication (termed *lipodermatosclerosis* or *chronic indurated cellulitis*) suggest infection, but the problem is chronic venous stasis and its management the use of adequate support (Fig. 8) when the patient is ambulatory. The process gradually recedes with use of good elastic support over a foam pad for a period of several weeks. When resolved, recurrence can be prevented by the regular, daily use of adequate elastic support when ambulatory.

Venous stasis ulceration (Fig. 9), when early and small (< 1.0 cm), often can be managed on an ambulatory basis with the same type of elastic support described for chronic indurated cellulitis applied over a sterile dressing. Larger stasis ulcers are best managed by rest and elevation with moist dressings (sterile normal saline or 0.25% aluminum subacetate) until clean and, if needed, skin grafting. After healing, adequate elastic support (described earlier), often with the addition of a foam pad over the previously ulcerated area, should be used when ambulatory.

Varicose Veins

Varicose veins are the most common venous disorder seen by the generalist. They may be primary or secondary to postphlebitic chronic deep venous insufficiency. Obesity, pregnancy, and right heart failure are aggravating factors.

Frequently, the only complaint of the patient with varicose veins is cosmetic. Others may complain of "heaviness" in the affected leg or dependent edema.

Distinction between primary and secondary varicose veins is important if surgical treatment is being considered. Associated chronic deep venous insufficiency can be identified by Doppler ultrasonography of deep veins if surgical treatment of the varicose veins is an option.

Management

Use of adequate elastic support is indicated for asymptomatic primary varicose veins and for those associated with chronic deep venous insufficiency. Sclerotherapy may be used for minor primary varicose veins and for cutaneous venous stars.

When to refer

Surgical treatment (stripping) is indicated for primary varicose veins causing symptoms or venous stasis that is not controlled with elastic support and when there is acute superficial varicose vein thrombophlebitis. Surgery is also indicated to remove large varicosities for cosmetic reasons.

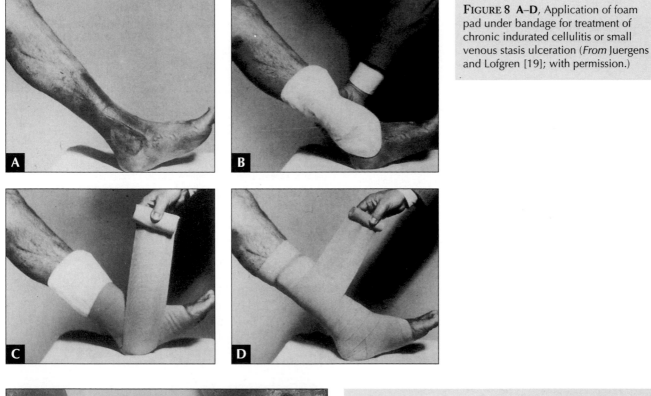

FIGURE 8 A–D, Application of foam pad under bandage for treatment of chronic indurated cellulitis or small venous stasis ulceration (*From* Juergens and Lofgren [19]; with permission.)

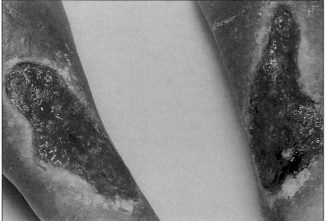

FIGURE 9 Large venous stasis ulcerations of both lower extremities.

REFERENCES AND RECOMMENDED READING

Recently published papers of particular interest have been highlighted as:
- • Of interest
- •• Of outstanding interest

1.• Spittell JA Jr: Peripheral arterial disease. *Dis Mon* 1994, 40:641–704.

2. Spittell JA Jr: Some uncommon types of occlusive peripheral arterial disease. *Curr Probl Cardiol* 1983, 8:3–35.

3. McDaniel MD, Cronenwett JL: Basic data related to natural history of intermittent claudication. *Ann Vasc Surg* 1989, 3:273–277.

4. Reiber GE, Pecoraro RE, Koepsell TD: Risk factors for amputation in patients with diabetes. *Ann Intern Med* 1992, 117:97–105.

5. Lindgarde F, Jehres R, Bjorkman H, *et al.*: Conservative drug treatments in patients with moderately severe chronic occlusive peripheral arterial disease. *Circulation* 1989, 80:1549–1556.

6. Spittell PC, Spittell JA Jr: Occlusive arterial disease of the hand due to repetitive blunt trauma. *Int J Cardiol* 1993, 38:281–292.

7. Gersh BJ, Rihal CS, Rooke TW, Ballard DJ: Evaluation and management of patients with both peripheral vascular and coronary artery disease. *J Am Coll Cardiol* 1991, 18:203–214.

8. ACC/AHA Task Force Report: Guidelines for perioperative cardiovascular evaluation for noncardiac surgery. *Circulation* 1996, 93:1278–1317.

9. Kronzon I, Tuvick PA: Atheromatous disease of the thoracic aorta: Pathologic and clinical implication. *Ann Intern Med* 1997, 126:629–637.

10. Lipoff O, Hoover EL, Diaz C, *et al.*: Initial report of a mycotic aneurysm of the common iliac artery with compression of the ipsilateral ureter and femoral vein. *Texas Heart Inst J* 1986, 13:321–324.

11. Heliboer H, Bueller HR, Lansing AWA, *et al.*: A comparison of real-time compression ultrasonography with impedance plethysmography for the diagnosis of deep-vein thrombosis in symptomatic outpatients. *N Engl J Med* 1993, 329:1365–1369.

12. Levine M, Gent M, Hirsh J, *et al.*: A comparison of low molecular weight heparin administered primarily at home with unfractionated heparin administered in the hospital for proximal deep vein thrombosis. *N Engl J Med* 1996, 334:677–681.

13. Fontaine R, Kreay R, Gaugloff JM, *et al.*: Long-term results of restorative arterial surgery in obstructive diseases of the arteries. *J Cardiovasc Surg* 1964, 5:463–472.

14. Spittell JA Jr: Recognition and management of chronic atherosclerotic occlusive peripheral arterial disease. *Mod Concepts Cardiovasc Dis* 1981, 50:19–23.

15. Spittell JA Jr: Occlusive peripheral arterial disease: guidelines for office management. *Postgrad Med* 1982, 71:137–151.

16. Fairbairn JF II: Clinical manifestations of peripheral vascular disease. In *Peripheral Vascular Diseases*, edn 5. Edited by Juergens JL, Spittell JA Jr, Fairbairn JF II. Philadelphia: WB Saunders; 1972:4–25.

17. Verstraete M: The diagnosis and treatment of deep-vein thrombosis. *N Engl J Med* 1993; 329:1418–1419.

18. Nichols WL, Heit JA: Activated protein C resistance and thrombosis. *Mayo Clin Proc* 1996, 71:897–898.

19. Juergens JL, Lofgren KA: Chronic venous insufficiency. In *Peripheral Vascular Disease*, edn 5. Edited by Juergens JL, Spittel JA Jr, Fairbairn JF II. Philadelphia: WB Saunders; 1980:820.

SELECT BIBLIOGRAPHY

Bergan JJ, Yao JST: *Venous Disorders*. Philadelphia: WB Saunders; 1991.

Spittell JA Jr: *Contemporary Issues in Peripheral Vascular Disease. Cardiovascular Clinics*. Philadelphia: FA Davis; 1992.

Thomas DP, Roberts HR: Hypercoagulability in venous and arterial thrombosis. *Ann Intern Med* 1997, 126:638–644.

Young JR, Olin JO, Bartholemew JR: *Peripheral Vascular Diseases*, edn 2. St. Louis: Mosby–Year Book; 1996.

Anticoagulation, Acute and Chronic: Indications and Methods

40

Jack E. Ansell

> **Key Points**
> - Salient aspects of anticoagulation therapy highlighted in this chapter include the following:
> - Failure to rapidly achieve a therapeutic level of heparin therapy is remedied by the use of heparing-dosing nomograms.
> - The activated partial thromboplastin time is highly inaccurate unless *ex vivo* heparin titration curves are used to establish a reagent-specific therapeutic range.
> - The advantages of low molecular weight heparin (LMWH) over unfractionated heparin relate to its subcutaneous use, the ability to perform daily dosing once or twice, and the absence of the need for monitoring.
> - Studies now document the equivalency or even superiority of LMWH over unfractionated heparin for the treatment of acute deep venous thrombosis. Home therapy is also a promising mode of treatment.
> - Warfarin therapy is associated with the fewest complications when managemenet is performed by a coordinated system of oversight referred to as *anticoagulation management service*.
> - Future models of warfarin management include patient self-testing and patient self-management.

Three major classes of antithrombotic drugs are currently in use: anticoagulants, antiplatelet agents, and thrombolytic or fibrinolytic agents. Thrombolytic agents have a direct effect on thrombi by hastening their dissolution, whereas anticoagulants and antiplatelet agents are always prophylactic in that they prevent *de novo* initiation of thrombosis (primary prophylaxis) or that they prevent extension of established thrombi (secondary prophylaxis). This chapter focuses on those anticoagulant agents of greatest current value: unfractionated heparin, low molecular weight heparin (LMWH), and warfarin.

Anticoagulation entered the therapeutic arena in the mid-1930s with the first clinical use of unfractionated heparin, a drug discovered more than 15 years earlier [1]. Shortly thereafter, the first coumarin-derived oral anticoagulant, dicoumarol, was isolated, and in 1941, it was first put to clinical use [2]. Some 35 years later, further refinements of unfractionated heparin resulted in the identification of LMWH as a suitable anticoagulant with properties more favorable than standard heparin [3]. In the 1990s, patients are beginning to reap the benefits of this newer antithrombotic agent. Unfractionated heparin and LMWH have an immediate onset of action and are indicated for the treatment of acute thromboembolic disorders. The coumarins have a delayed onset of action of several days and are indicated primarily for the long-term treatment of chronic thromboembolic disorders. All three agents are used for primary prophylaxis in patients at risk.

HEPARIN

Unfractionated heparin, also referred to simply as heparin, is a glycosaminoglycan made up of repeating disaccharide units of D-glucosamine and uronic acid with a

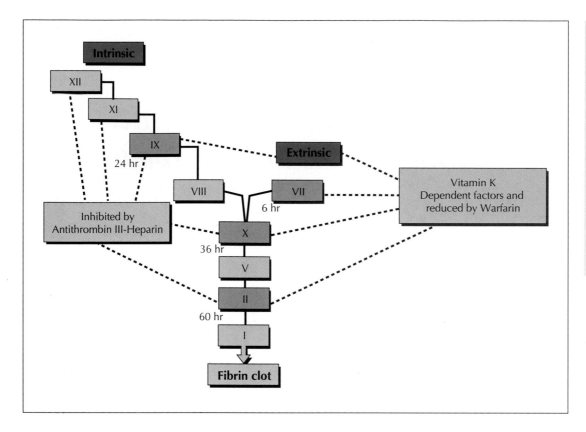

FIGURE 1 A simplified scheme of the coagulation cascade indicating the factors sensitive to heparin-antithrombin III neutralization and the vitamin K–dependent factors reduced by warfarin therapy and their respective half-lives (shaded factors).

wide range in molecular weights from 5,000 to 30,000 daltons [4]. It is commercially derived primarily from bovine lung or porcine intestinal mucosa. Heparin mediates its effect by binding to a plasma protein, antithrombin III (AT III), altering its conformation and thus enabling AT III to bind more rapidly and neutralize the serine protease coagulation factors (II_a, IX_a, X_a, XI_a, and XII_a) (Fig. 1). Its predominant activity is directed toward factors X_a and II_a. Heparin also binds to another inhibitor, heparin cofactor II, whose principal substrate is thrombin. Heparin contains a unique pentasaccharide essential for binding to AT III. To neutralize thrombin, the serine protease must bind to both AT III and heparin, forming a ternary complex (Fig. 2). This dual binding requires a minimal chain length of 18 monosaccharides. Factor X_a does not require simultaneous binding to heparin when bound to AT III, and thus smaller heparin chain lengths (containing the critical pentasaccharide) can serve to neutralize X_a.

Indications

Heparin is generally indicated as secondary prophylaxis in the treatment of acute thromboembolic disorders (*eg*, deep venous thrombosis or pulmonary embolism), or as primary prophylaxis when an increased risk of thromboembolism exists (*eg*, in surgical patients at risk for postoperative thromboembolism) [5]. The dose and method of administration are determined by the underlying condition and whether it is for primary or secondary prophylaxis. The principal indications for heparin therapy are outlined in Table 1.

Dosing

Although heparin has been an important anticoagulant for over 60 years, it has significant drawbacks as identified in

Table 2. Many of these drawbacks are eliminated or reduced by LMWH as discussed later in this chapter. A major problem with the administration of heparin is the failure to achieve a therapeutic level of anticoagulation early in the course of treatment [8–11]. This is principally the result of

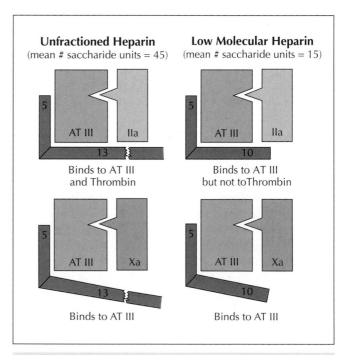

FIGURE 2 Schematic representation of the differential mechanism of heparin-antithrombin III's neutralizing effect on thrombin (II_a) and factor X_a compared with the action of low molecular weight heparin. (*Adapted from* Hirsh and Levine [3].)

TABLE 1 RECOMMENDED ANTITHROMBOTIC TREATMENT FOR VARIOUS INDICATIONS

Venous thromboembolic disease

Prevention of venous thromboembolism

Low-risk surgery patients	Early ambulation
Moderate-risk general surgery patients	Elastic stockings or intermittent pneumatic compression or low dose UFH (5000 U SC q 12 h)
High-risk general surgery patients	Low dose UFH (q8h) or LMWH
Very high-risk general surgery patients	Low dose UFH or LMWH combined with intermittent pneumatic compression
Hip and knee joint replacement	LMWH or warfarin (INR 2.0–3.0) or adjusted dose SQ UFH

Treatment of venous thromboembolism

Deep venous thrombosis or pulmonary embolism	Acute: UFH IV or adjusted dose SQ sufficient to prolong the activated partial prothrombin time to a plasma heparin level of 0.2–0.4 U/mL
	LMWH may be used in place of UFH (dosage varies with product)
	Long-term: Warfarin to maintain an INR 2.0–3.0 for at least 3 months

Arterial thromboembolic disease

Atrial fibrillation	Warfarin to maintain an INR 2.0–3.0 in high-risk patients (age > 65, previous TIA or stroke, hypertension, heart failure, clinical coronary artery disease, mitral stenosis or prosthetic heart valve, diabetes, or thyrotoxicosis)

Valvular heart disease

Rheumatic mitral valve disease	Aspirin can be used in low-risk patients
	History or systemic embolism or AF: warfarin (INR 2.0–3.0)
	Left atrial diameter > 5.5 cm: Consider warfarin
	Recurrent embolism despite warfarin: Add ASA (80–100 mg/d)
Aortic valve disease	History of systemic embolism, AF, or concomitant mitral valve disease: Oral anticoagulation (INR 2.0–3.0)
Mitral valve prolapse	History of TIA: ASA (160–325 mg/d)
	History of TIA on ASA, systemic embolism, or AF: Oral anticoagulation (INR 2.0–3.0)
	Ticlopidine (250 mg bid) if warfarin contraindicated
Mitral annular calcification	History of systemic embolism or AF: Oral anticoagulation (INR 2.0–3.0)

Prosthetic heart valves

Mechanical	Oral anticoagulation (INR 2.5–3.5); consider addition of ASA (80 mg/d) in high-risk patients; consider higher INR in patients with caged ball or disc valve prostheses
	History of systemic embolism: Oral anticoagulation and ASA

Bioprosthetic heart valves

Mitral position	Oral anticoagulation (INR 2.0–3.0) for 3 months
Aortic position	Oral anticoagulation optional for first 3 months; if not used, consider ASA (325 mg/d)
With AF, systemic embolism or atrial thrombus	Oral anticoagulation (INR 2.0–3.0)

Coronary artery disease

Myocardial infarction (acute)	See [7]
Post-MI (long-term)	ASA (160–325 mg/d) indefinitely unless oral anticoagulation used (warfarin with INR 2.5–3.5)
	Oral anticoagulation (INR 2.5–3.5) in high-risk patients (anterior Q wave MI, severe left ventricular dysfunction, CHF, mural thrombosis/systemic embolism) for up to 3 months
Coronary bypass grafts, angioplasty, stents, unstable and stable angina	See the study of Dalen and Hirsh [7]

Peripheral vascular disease/surgery

Treatment for acute events/surgery	See the study of Dalen and Hirsh [7]
Long-term treatment	ASA (80–325 mg/d) ± dipyridamole indefinitely
Post-carotid endarterectomy	ASA (80–650 mg bid) indefinitely

Continued on next page

TABLE 1   RECOMMENDED ANTITHROMBOTIC TREATMENT FOR VARIOUS INDICATIONS (CONTINUED)

Cerebrovascular disease	
Asymptomatic carotid stenosis/bruit	ASA (325 mg/d)
TIA/minor ischemic stroke	ASA (75–1300 mg/d)
Progressing ischemic stroke	Heparin 3–5 days (CT scan of brain to exclude hemorrhage)
Completed thrombotic stroke	ASA (325–1300 mg/d) or ticlopidine (250 mg bid)
Acute cardioembolic stroke	Small to moderate sized, no evidence of hemorrhage on CT/magnetic resonance image performed > 48 hrs later, nonhypertensive: UFH followed by oral anticoagulation (INR 2.0–3.0)
Large embolic stroke	Delay anticoagulation for 5–14 days

AF—atrial fibrillation; ASA—aspirin; CHF—congestive heart failure; CT—computed tomography; INR—international normalized ratio; IV—intravenously; LMWH—low molecular weight heparin; MI—myocardial infarction; SQ—subcutaneously; TIA—transient ischemic attack; UFH—unfractionated heparin.

(*Adapted from* Spencer and Becker [6], based on material in Dalen and Hirsh [7].)

TABLE 2   DRAWBACKS OF THERAPY WITH UNFRACTIONATED HEPARIN

Short half-life when given IV; longer when given SQ, but absorption is variable. Therefore usually given by continuous IV infusion.

Binds to plasma proteins, endothelial cells, leukocytes, and platelets leading to poor recovery and variable aPTT response.

Requires monitoring to maintain a therapeutic range.

Effects on platelets leading to thrombocytopenia and thrombosis.

Antithrombotic and hemorrhagic potential may reside in different structural components of heparin molecule.

aPTT—activated partial thromboplastin time; IV—intraveneously; SQ—subcutaneously.

inadequate dosing. To remedy this situation, a number of investigators have developed heparin dosing nomograms to standardize therapy across patients and dose adjustments within individual patients [9–11]. These nomograms, some of which are weight based whereas others call for fixed dosing, achieve more rapid therapeutic levels of heparin by requiring higher loading and maintenance doses of the drug. Table 3 outlines a popular dosing nomogram developed by Raschke and colleagues [10], but others are also available.

Monitoring

Another important aspect of therapy is an understanding of the limitations of the activated partial thromboplastin time (aPTT) as a measure of heparin effect. The aPTT's response to heparin is highly dependent on the reagent used in the test (similar to the variability of the prothrombin time in response to warfarin anticoagulation with different thromboplastins)[5]. There is no conversion or normalizing formula as exists for prothrombin time. Thus, every laboratory is obligated to perform an *in vitro* or *ex vivo* heparin titration curve with the reagent currently in use (even with new lots of reagent from the same manufacturer) and establish the reagent-specific therapeutic range (equivalent to 0.2–0.6 U/ml of heparin depending on the type of titration curve used)[12].

Heparin-Induced Thrombocytopenia

Besides the complication of bleeding, the major adverse effect of heparin is heparin-induced thrombocytopenia and thrombosis (HITT)[13]. This phenomenon is due to heparin binding to an endogenous platelet protein, platelet factor 4 (PF4), at the surface of platelets and eliciting an immune response to a newly created epitope. Binding of immunoglobulin leads not only to platelet destruction and thrombocytopenia, which by itself is rarely a problem, but it can lead to platelet clumping, thrombosis, and vascular occlusion in either the venous or arterial circulation, with the potential for catastrophic ischemic events. Once this problem is recognized, heparin therapy must be stopped immediately and, if necessary, an alternative anticoagulant substituted. The low molecular weight heparinoid, lomoparin, is currently the agent of choice in this situation, since cross reactivity of the antibody to lomoparin is minimal [14]. HIT occurs with a frequency of approximately 3% to 5% in patients treated with intravenous heparin for 5 or more days. It can, however, occur at shorter intervals in patients with previous heparin exposure and can also occur in patients receiving subcutaneous therapy or even heparin flushes used to maintain catheter patency. It appears more frequently with bovine lung-derived heparin. Platelet counts should be monitored at baseline in all patients who

TABLE 3 WEIGHT-BASED HEPARIN DOSING NOMOGRAM

Initial dose	80 U/kg bolus, then 18 U/kg/h
Maintenance dose	
aPTT < 1.2 x control	80 U/kg bolus, then 4 U/kg/h
aPTT 1.2–1.5 x control	40 U/kg bolus, then 2 U/kg/h
aPTT 1.5–2.3 x control	No change
aPTT 2.3–3 x control	Decrease infusion rate by 2 U/kg/h
aPTT > 3 x control	Hold infusion 1 hour, then decrease rate by 3 U/kg/h

aPTT—activated partial thromboplastin time. (*Adapted from* Raschke *et al.* [10].)

receive heparin and repeated approximately every 2 or 3 days thereafter in patients receiving intravenous therapy. The ideal frequency of assessing platelet counts in patients receiving low dose subcutaneous heparin is unknown, but periodic checks are recommended.

LOW MOLECULAR WEIGHT HEPARIN

Low molecular weight heparin is a fragment of unfractionated heparin and is produced by chemical or enzymatic depolymerization of unfractionated heparin [3]. Various preparations are available, most with an average molecular weight of between 4,000 and 6,500 daltons (Table 4). They are enriched with the essential pentasaccharide for AT III binding, enabling the AT III–LMWH complex to neutralize factor X_a, but they lack a substantial number of the larger monosaccharide chains (18 or more) required for binding to thrombin (see Fig. 2). Thus, the ratio of the relative neutralizing potency for X_a:II_a, which for unfractionated heparin is 1:1, is approximately 3:1 for LMWH. Low molecular weight heparins have qualities that make them a better anticoagulant than unfractionated heparin as

set out in Table 5. Most important, they have a significantly reduced ability to bind to plasma proteins, endothelial cells, and blood cells, making them more available for binding to AT III producing an anticoagulant effect. Consequently, they have a much greater bioavailability and predictability of response and do not require monitoring. They are also more uniformly absorbed from subcutaneous depots and have a longer plasma half-life, in the range of 2 to 4 hours. Although LMWHs are excreted predominantly from the kidney, alteration of dosing does not seem to be required in renal failure.

Indications

Initial clinical studies of LMWHs focused on primary prophylaxis in high-risk patients (*eg*, those undergoing hip and knee joint replacement)[15]. Other clinical situations have also been evaluated, but these were more limited studies, concerned with abdominal or thoracic surgery, spinal cord injury, trauma, cardiovascular conditions, medical patients, and pregnancy [15–18]. In the United States, a limited number of products are available with only a limited number of indications for each product. Because dosing recommendations and indications are product-specific, it is important to prescribe LMWH by name (generic or brand). Numerous clinical trials are ongoing to document to the satisfaction of the Food and Drug Administration, the efficacy and safety of LMWHs in other clinical situations including the acute treatment of venous thromboembolism. Such studies have been done elsewhere; LMWHs are used to varying degrees for primary and secondary prophylaxis (for acute venous thromboembolism) in many countries throughout the world. Indications for LMWH are listed in Table 1.

Although many of the early studies focused on primary prophylaxis in high-risk patients, a substantial body of evidence now supports the use of LMWH in the treatment of acute venous thromboembolic disease. Siragusa and coworkers [19••] recently published a meta-analysis of high quality studies identifying the benefits of LMWH. Figure 3, taken from this study,

TABLE 4 LISTING OF VARIOUS PREPARATIONS OF LOW MOLECULAR WEIGHT HEPARINS

Generic name	Trade name	Manufacturer
Enoxaparin	Lovenox	Rhone-Poulenc
Ardeparin	Normoflo	Wyeth Ayerst
Dalteparin	Fragmin	Kabi, Pharmacia
Tinzaparin	Logiparin	Novo-Nordisk
	Innohep	Leo Pharmaceuticals
Nadroparin	Fraxiparin	Sanofi-Winthrop
Certiparin	Sandoparin	Sandoz
Reviparin	Clivarin	Knoll AG
Parnaparum	Fluxum	Opocrin
Lomoparin*	Organan	Organon

*Heparinoid

TABLE 5 ADVANTAGES OF LOW MOLECULAR WEIGHT HEPARIN

Observation	Potential advantage
Lack of protein binding	Good bioavailability, predictable dose response, heparin-resistance less often encountered
Predictabel dose response	Fixed or weight-based dosing possible, monitoring not required
Longer half-life	Once or twice daily dosing possible
Smaller molecule	Better subcutaneous absorption
Less effect on platelets and endothelium	Less thrombocytopenia and bleeding

summarizes these benefits in terms of hard outcomes (thrombosis and bleeding). The full potential of LMWH has also recently been recognized in two studies assessing the safety and efficacy of home therapy with LMWH for deep venous thrombosis [20••,21••]. Table 6 summarizes these results.

Based on the results of clinical studies and on trends in other countries where LMWH is more fully available, LMWH is likely to replace unfractionated heparin as the anticoagulant of choice for acute thromboembolic disorders. What remains to be seen is what impact it may have in the long-term outpatient treatment of thrombotic disorders in which the oral anticoagulants have reigned supreme.

ORAL ANTICOAGULANTS

Although dicoumarol was the first coumarin anticoagulant identified and isolated from spoiled sweet clover by Link [22] in 1941, crystalline sodium warfarin has been the major formulation used in the United States for over 30 years. In 1994, it was the thirteenth most commonly prescribed medication in the United States and the fifth most prescribed cardiovascular medication [23]. In recent years, intense focus has been directed to identifying the appropriate indications for warfarin based on well-designed prospective randomized clinical trials and to qualifying the appropriate intensity of therapy based on an international normalized ratio (INR). Lately, attention has focused on improving the management of oral anticoagulation through coordinated clinical programs known as *anticoagulation management services* or *anticoagulation clinics*. The latest paradigm of oral anticoagulation management, however, is the model of patient self-management of therapy. This is a direct result of the development of portable, hand-held capillary–whole blood prothrombin time monitors that can yield results from a fingerstick sample of blood.

Mechanism of action

Warfarin exerts its effect by interfering with the reduction and recycling of vitamin K that is oxidized in the process of carboxylating glutamic acid moieties in the precursors of vitamin K-dependent coagulation factors (see Fig. 1)[24]. As a result, poorly functional coagulation precursors are secreted leading to a defective coagulation cascade. Factor VII has the shortest half-life (~6 hours) and its concentration falls most rapidly. Factor II has a half-life of ~60 hours; thus, several days of therapy are required for its concentration to fall,

accounting for the reason heparin and warfarin therapy must overlap for a minimum of 3 to 5 days so that all vitamin K–dependent factors are reduced.

Indications

The recent consensus conference of the American College of Chest Physicians [7] outlines in detail the many indications for oral anticoagulation therapy. Table 1 summarizes these indications. In the last 10 years, the scientific community has thoroughly documented the benefit of warfarin therapy for atrial fibrillation in patients 65 years or older [25]. The question of aspirin therapy in such individuals is no longer debated, since the high incidence of warfarin-associated intracranial hemorrhage found in the Stroke Prevention in Atrial Fibrillation (SPAF) II study [26] has not been confirmed by others.

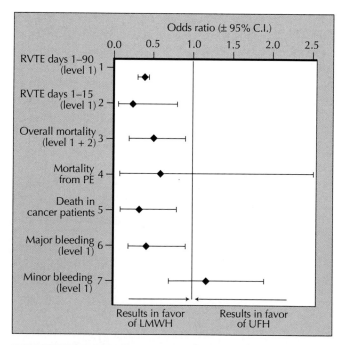

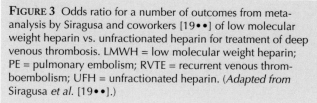

FIGURE 3 Odds ratio for a number of outcomes from meta-analysis by Siragusa and coworkers [19••] of low molecular weight heparin vs. unfractionated heparin for treatment of deep venous thrombosis. LMWH = low molecular weight heparin; PE = pulmonary embolism; RVTE = recurrent venous thromboembolism; UFH = unfractionated heparin. (*Adapted from* Siragusa *et al.* [19••].)

TABLE 6 OUTPATIENT THERAPY FOR TREATMENT OF DEEP VENOUS THROMBOSIS: LOW MOLECULAR WEIGHT HEPARIN VS. UNFRACTIONATED HEPARIN

	Levine [20••]		Koopman [21••]	
Drug	UFH	LMWH	UFH	LMWH
Patients	253	247	198	202
Recurrent thrombosis	17 (6.7%)	13 (5.3%)	17 (8.6%)	14 (6.9%)
Bleeding	3 (1%)	5 (2%)	4 (2%)	1 (0.5%)
Hospital stay (mean days)	6.5	1.1*	8.1	2.7†

*48% never hospitalized.
† 36% never hospitalized.
LMWH = low molecular weight heparin. UFH = unfractionated heparin.
(*Data from* Levine *et al.* [20••] and Koopman *et al.* [21••].)

Although the combination of aspirin (at low dosage) and warfarin (INR 2.5–3.5) has been shown to reduce the incidence of thromboembolism in patients with prosthetic cardiac valves [27] over warfarin alone, such combined therapy is not routinely used because of the higher risk of hemorrhage. Aspirin, however, is still the preferred choice of therapy to reduce the frequency of recurrent myocardial infarction even though studies have shown that warfarin (INR 2.5–3.5) can similarly reduce the incidence [28,29]. Aspirin is easier to use and may be associated with a reduced rate of hemorrhage in this setting. Recent trials [30], some still ongoing, to assess whether both low dose aspirin and warfarin (INR < 2.0) can further reduce the incidence of recurrent myocardial infarction with less bleeding have not been successful, suggesting at least in part, the need for therapeutic levels of warfarin (INR 2.0–3.0) for greatest effectiveness.

Management

Because warfarin has a narrow therapeutic index and patient responsiveness fluctuates, it requires careful monitoring of therapeutic intensity and management of dosing. Numerous studies have identified the risk of hemorrhage with excessive anticoagulation or thrombosis with inadequate anticoagulation [31,32]. Based on the recent study by Cannegeiter and colleagues [33•] of patients with prosthetic valves, a wide range of safety and efficacy exists between an INR of 2.0 and 4.5, although most investigators seek to identify a more narrow range of ideal effectiveness. Besides intensity, patient-specific characteristics also influence the risk of adverse events. Landefeld and Goldman [31] identified heart, liver and kidney disorders, cancer and anemia as risk factors as well as a history of stroke, myocardial infarction, or gastrointestinal bleeding. Hypertension, age, and other comorbid factors have also been associated as risk factors. Finally, because oral anticoagulation management is labor intensive and requires frequent patient contact and communication, a coordinated system of care has been suggested as the ideal system to produce good clinical and more cost effective outcomes[34••]. In a routine setting in which

patients are managed by their personal physician along with all other patients, several studies have indicated a high incidence of major hemorrhage in the range of 10% per treatment year. In a coordinated program, also known as an *anticoagulation clinic* or *anticoagulation management service*, the rate of major bleeding is closer to 2% to 4%, as is the rate of recurrent thromboembolism. Even these rates are higher than many of those shown in the large randomized studies reported for atrial fibrillation, but the latter involve selected patients monitored in a highly regulated fashion and with a uniform diagnosis. Based on individual studies comparing routine medical care with coordinated care, it is not surprising that a strong impetus exists for the creation of anticoagulation clinics throughout the country.

Patient Self-Testing and Self-Management

In 1987, a prothrombin [PT] time instrument was introduced that was able to measure prothrombin time from a fingerstick sample of capillary whole blood [35]. This instrument and subsequent models have been shown to be accurate and precise and are suitable for patient self-testing [36]. A number of small-scale studies demonstrated the ability of patients to perform their own PT [37,38]. Large scale studies showing benefit of patient self-testing (with management of dosing by the physician) have not been done, although White and coworkers [38] did demonstrate greater therapeutic effectiveness as measured by the PT in a small pilot study of 23 patients.

Of greater importance, however, is the potential impact of a self-management model of therapy in which patients adjust their own warfarin dose in response to their own INR testing. Ansell and colleagues [39•] recently completed a pilot trial with 20 patients who managed their own therapy, some for more than seven years. Table 7 summarizes the results of the study group compared with matched controls showing a better rate of therapeutic effectiveness as measured by the PT. Larger studies are needed to assess the rate of adverse events (hemorrhage or thrombosis) and whether a difference exists. Similar results have been generated by Bernardo [40]; this model of therapy is growing rapidly in Europe, especially in

TABLE 7 RESULTS OF PATIENT SELF-MANAGEMENT WITH STANDARD ANTICOAGULATION CLINIC MANAGEMENT.

Clinical outcomes	Self-managed patients	Control patients	P
Weekly warfarin dose (mean, mg)	37.5	34.8	>.10
Duration in study (median, range, months)	47 (3–87)	44 (3–86)	>.10
#Prothrombin times (mean)	2153 (107.7)	1608 (80.4)	>.05
Interval between PTs (mean days)	13.8	16.0	>.10
PTs above range (mean/patient)(%)	5.6 (5.2)	8.3 (10.3)	<.001
PTs below range (mean/patient) (%)	6.8 (6.3)	17.5 (21.8)	<.001
PTs in range (total number)(%)	1907 (88.6)	1093 (68.0)	<.001
Dose change (mean/patient)(%)	11.5 (10.7)	22.7 (28.2)	<.001

(*Data from* Ansell *et al.* [39•].)

Germany. In 1997, over 20,000 patients in Germany are managing their own anticoagulant dosing based on fingerstick PT times. These instruments are available for patient self-testing in the United States and studies are currently assessing the value of this model of therapy.

Interest in improving the management of oral anticoagulation is timely given the rapid expansion in use of oral anticoagulants. If the benefits of instituting therapy, such as in atrial fibrillation, are outweighed by the occurrence of fatal or serious complications, little has been gained in the effort to combat and prevent thromboembolic disease.

KEY REFERENCES

Recently published papers of outstanding interest, as indentified in *References and Recommended Reading*, have been annotated.

•• Sirgusa S, Cosmi B, Piovella F, *et al.*: Low molecular weight heparins and unfractionated heparin in the treatment of patients with acute venous thromboembolism: results of a meta-analysis. *Am J Med* 1996, 100:269–277.

A comprehensive meta-analysis of randomized studies comparing the safety and efficacy of low molecular weight heparin to a variety of antithrombotic agents in the treatment of acute deep venous thrombosis.

•• Levine M, Gent M, Hirsh J, *et al.*: A comparison of low molecular weight heparin administered primarily at home with unfractionated heparin administered in the hospital for proximal deep-vein thrombosis. *N Engl J Med* 1996, 334:677–681.

•• Koopman MMW, Prandoni P, Piovella F, *et al.*: Treamtent of venous thrombosis with intravenous unfractionated heparin administered in the hospital as compared with subcutaneous low molecular weight heparin administered at home. *N Engl J Med* 1996, 334:682–687.

Two key studies by Levine and coworkers and Koopman and coworkers establishing the possibility and potential of LMWH for outpatient (home) therapy of acute deep venous thrombosis. Both studies show LMWH to be safe and effective.

•• Ansell JE, Hughes R: Evolving models of warfarin management: anticoagulation clinics, patient self-monitoring, and patient self-management. *Am Heart J* 1996, 132:1095–1100.

Provides the basis for the value of coordinated anticoagulation care (anticoagulation clinics) and their ability to yield better clinical outcomes at reduced costs. Also reviews the literature pertaining to patient self-testing and patient self-management of anticoagulation therapy.

REFERENCES AND RECOMENDED READING

Recently published papers of particular interest have been highlighted as:

• Of interest

•• Of outstanding interest

1. Jacques LB: The new understanding of the drug heparin. *Chest* 1985, 88:751–754.

2. Butt HR, Allen EV, Bollman JL: A preparation from spoiled sweet clover which prolongs coagulation and prothrombin time of the blood: preliminary reports of experimental and clinical studies. *Mayo Clin Proc* 1941, 16:388–395.

3. Hirsh J, Levine MN: Low molecular weight heparin. *Blood* 1992, 79:1–17.

4. Hirsh J: Heparin. *N Engl J Med* 1991, 324:1565–1574.

5. Hirsh J, Raschke R, Warkentin TE, *et al.*: Heparin: Mechanism of action, pharmacokinetics, dosing considerations, monitoring, efficacy, and safety. *Chest* 1995, 108(Suppl):258S–275S.

6. Spencer F, Becker RC: Current approach to antithrombotic therapy: an abbreviated reference for practicing clinicians. *J Thromb Thrombolysis* 1996, 3:307–325, 317–318 (Table 3).

7. Dalen JE, Hirsh J: Fourth ACCP Consensus Conference on Antithrombotic Therapy. *Chest* 1995, 108(Suppl):225S–522S.

8. Fennerty A, Thomas P, Blackhouse G, *et al.*: Audit of control of heparin treatment. *BMJ* 1985, 290:27–28.

9. Cruickshank MK, Levine MN, Hirsh J, *et al.*: A standard heparin nomogram for the management of heparin therapy. *Arch Intern Med* 1991, 151:333–337.

10. Raschke RA, Reilly BM, Guidry JR, *et al.*: The weight-based heparin dosing nomogram compared with a standard care nomogram. *Ann Intern Med* 1993, 119:874–881.

11. Flaker GC, Bartolozzi J, Davis V, *et al.* and the Timi 4 Investigators: Use of a standardized heparin nomogram to achieve therapeutic anticoagulation after thrombolytic therapy in myocardial infarction. *Arch Intern Med* 1994, 154:1492–1496.

12. Brill-Edwards P, Ginsberg JS, Johnston M, Hirsh J: Establishing a therapeutic range for heparin therapy. *Ann Intern Med* 1993, 119:104–109.

13. Warkentin TE, Kelton JG: Heparin-induced thrombocytopenia. *Progr Hemost Thromb* 1991, 10:1–34.

14. Magnani HN: Heparin-induced thrombocytopenia (HIT): an overview of 230 patients treated with Orgaran (Org 10172). *Thromb Haemost* 1993, 70:554–561.

15. Green D, Hirsh J, Heit J, *et al.*: Low molecular weight heparin: A critical analysis of clinical trials. *Pharmacol Rev* 1994, 46:89–109.

16. Geerts WH, Jay RM, Code KI, *et al.*: A comparison of low dose heparin with low molecular weight heparin as prophylaxis against

venous thromboembolism after major trauma. *N Engl J Med* 1996, l335:701–707.

17. Becker RC, Spencer F: Adjunctive pharmacologic treatment: focus on the development of low molecular weight heparins. *J Thromb Thrombolysis* 1997, 4:197–205.

18. Melissari E, Parker CJ, Wilson NV, *et al.*: Use of low molecular weight heparin in pregnancy. *Thromb Haemost* 1992, 68:652–656.

19.•• Siragusa S, Cosmi B, Piovella F, *et al.*: Low molecular weight heparins and unfractionated heparin in the treatment of patients with acute venous thromboembolism: results of a meta-analysis. *Am J Med* 1996, 100:269–277.

20.•• Levine M, Gent M, Hirsh J, *et al.*: A comparison of low molecular weight heparin administered primarily at home with unfractionated heparin administered in the hospital for proximal deep-vein thrombosis. *N Engl J Med* 1996, 334:677–681.

21.•• Koopman MMW, Prandoni P, Piovella F, *et al.*: Treatment of venous thrombosis with intravenous unfractionated heparin administered in the hospital as compared with subcutaneous low molecular weight heparin administered at home. *N Engl J Med* 1996, 334:682–687.

22. Link KP: The discovery of dicumarol and its sequels. *Circulation* 1959, 19:97–107.

23. La Piana-Simonsen L: Top 200 drugs. *Pharm Times* 1995, 61:17–23.

24. Hirsh J, Dalen JE, Deykin D, *et al.*: Oral anticoagulants: mechanism of action, clinical effectiveness, and optimal therapeutic range. *Chest* 1995, 108(Suppl):231S–246S.

25.• Atrial Fibrillation Investigators: Risk factors for stroke and efficacy of antithrombotic therapy in atrial fibrillation. *Arch Intern Med* 1994, 154:1449–1457.

26. Stroke Prevention in Atrial Fibrillation Investigators: Warfarin versus aspirin for prevention of thromboembolism in atrial fibrillation: Stroke prevention in atrial fibrillation II study. *Lancet* 1994, 343:687–691.

27. Turpie AGG, Gent M, Laupacis A, *et al.*: A comparison of aspirin with placebo in patients treated with warfarin after heart-valve replacement. *N Engl J Med* 1993, 329:524–529.

28. Smith P, Arnesen H, Holme I: The effect of warfarin on mortality and reinfarction after myocardial infarction. *N Engl J Med* 1990, 323:147–152.

29. ASPECT Research Group: Effect of long-term oral anticoagulant treatment on mortality and cardiovascular morbidity after myocardial infarction. *Lancet* 1994, 343:499–503.

30. O'Gara P, Harrington R, Langer A, *et al.* and CARS Investigators: Coumadin Aspirin Reinfarction Study (CARS): relationship between event rates and INR. *Circulation* 1996, 94 (Suppl):I–80.

31. Landefeld GS, Goldman L: Major bleeding in outpatients treated with warfarin: incidence and prediction by factors known at the start of outpatient therapy. *Am J Med* 1989, 87:144–152.

32. Fihn SD, McDonell M, Martin D, *et al.*: Risk factors for complications of chronic anticoagulation. *Ann Intern Med* 1993, 118:511–520.

33.• Cannegeiter SC, Rosendaal FR, Wintzen AR, *et al.*: The optimal intensity of oral anticoagulant therapy in patients with mechanical heart valve prostheses: the Leiden artificial valve and anticoagulation study. *N Engl J Med* 1995, 333:11–17.

34.•• Ansell JE, Hughes R: Evolving models of warfarin management: anticoagulation clinics, patient self-monitoring, and patient self-management. *Am Heart J* 1996, 132:1095–1100.

35. Lucas FV, Duncan A, Jay R, *et al.*: A novel whole blood capillary technic for measuring the prothrombin time. *Am J Clin Pathol* 1987, 88:442–446.

36. Leaning KE, Ansell JE: Advanced in the monitoring of oral anticoagulation: point-of-care testing, patient self-monitoring, and patient self-management. *J Thromb Thrombolysis* 1996, 3:377–383.

37. White RH, McCurdy SA, von Marensdorff H, *et al.*: Home prothrombin time monitoring after initiation of warfarin therapy. *Ann Intern Med* 1989, 111:730–737.

38. Anderson D, Harrison L, Hirsh J: Evaluation of a portable prothrombin time monitor for home use by patients who require long-term oral anticoagulant therapy. *Arch Intern Med* 1993, 153:1441–1447.

39.• Ansell J, Patel N, Ostrovsky D, *et al.*: Long-term patient self-management of oral anticoagulation. *Arch Intern Med* 1995, 155:2185–2189.

40. Bernardo A: Experience with patient self-management of oral anticoagulation. *J Thromb Thrombolysis* 1966, 2:321–325.

Cerebrovascular Complications of Cardiac Disorders

41

Seemant Chaturvedi
Marc Fisher

Key Points
- Many cardiac conditions are associated with cerebral embolism.
- Patent foramen ovale and aortic arch plaques are receiving increased attention as embolic sources.
- Transesophageal echocardiography can increase the yield of embolism source detection, especially aortic atherosclerosis.
- Warfarin is effective in primary and secondary prevention in nonvalvular atrial fibrillation.

The relationship between cardiac disorders and stroke has become increasingly evident. A wide variety of cardiac abnormalities are associated with an enhanced potential for stroke occurrence. In addition, diagnostic and therapeutic modalities used in cardiology can contribute to cerebral ischemia or hemorrhage. Further adding to the cardiac-cerebrovascular link is the possibility that many of the therapeutic approaches employed for the treatment of acute myocardial ischemia may be relevant for acute ischemic stroke.

CARDIAC SOURCES OF STROKE

Cardioembolic stroke has assumed increasing importance as diagnostic advances for detecting cardiac sources for emboli have progressed [1•]. Currently, a cardioembolic source for stroke is recognized in 20% to 25% of the approximately 400,000 new strokes per year that occur in the United States. This percentage is even higher in younger stroke patients (*ie*, those younger than 50 years of age). Potential cardiac sources of emboli are shown in Figure 1, and the frequency of emboli attributed to various sources is shown in Figure 2.

Formation of intracardiac thrombi related to stasis, endothelial disruption, valvular abnormalities, and right-to-left shunts are common mechanisms for embolization in these disparate conditions. These cardiac emboli typically lodge in an intracranial vessel equal to their diameter at right angles to a larger parent artery, causing a clinical stroke syndrome related to the region of ischemic injury (Fig. 3). Cardioembolic stroke is the most likely diagnosis in a stroke patient who has a recognized cardiac disorder, associated embolization, and the abrupt onset of neurologic deficits. Supportive evidence includes the presence of prior or concurrent emboli in other organs or cerebral vascular territories and angiographic demonstration of vascular branch occlusion. The presence of a potential cardiac source for emboli does not conclusively establish the diagnosis of cardioembolic stroke because other potential stroke sources, such as large artery atherosclerosis or small intracranial vessel disease, are also present in approximately 33% of such patients. Therefore, the clinical diagnosis of cardioembolic source remains an educated guess. In reviewing the various

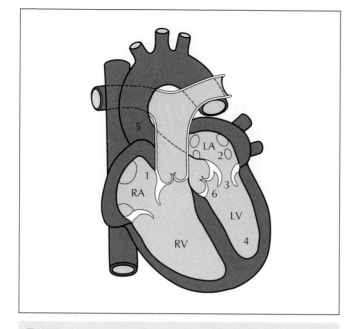

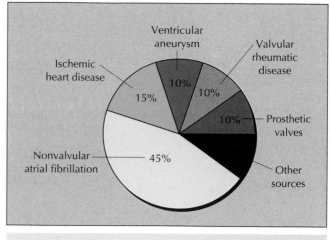

FIGURE 2 Sources of cardioembolism.

FIGURE 1 Sources of cardiogenic emboli: 1, paradoxical emboli (patent foramen ovale); 2, left atrium (LA) (atrial fibrillation, myxoma); 3, mitral valve (endocarditis, mitral valve prolapse, annulus calcification, prosthetic valve, other vegetations); 4, left ventricle (LV) (dyskinesia or akinesia, cardiomyopathy); 5, aorta (plaques); 6, aortic valve (endocarditis, prosthetic valve). RA—right atrium; RV—right ventricle.

etiologies for cardioembolic stroke, it is helpful to consider high-risk and medium-risk sources (Table 1).

High-Risk Sources

Nonvalvular atrial fibrillation (NVAF) is the most common cardiac disorder that predisposes to stroke occurrence. It is common in the elderly, and the annual stroke risk in untreated patients is approximately 5% (range 3% to 8%). Stroke risk increases with advancing age, history of hypertension, prior transient ischemic attack, stroke, and diabetes [2•]. Echocardiographically, left ventricular dysfunction and a dilated left atrium constituted the main predictive factors. Younger patients (< 60 years) without clinical risk factors have a low

risk for stroke. Acute myocardial infarction (MI) is associated with stroke development in approximately 1% of cases. Patients with transmural anterior wall MI have the greatest risk for thrombus formation and stroke occurrence. Most emboli occur within 4 weeks after the MI. The risk lessens 4 weeks to 6 months after MI, although at later dates akinetic ventricular segments and left ventricular aneurysms assume greater importance.

Rheumatic valvular disease has decreased in developed countries but remains an important source for stroke in developing countries. Rheumatic mitral valve disease has the highest incidence of systemic embolism among common forms of heart disease, and it is generally accepted that long-term anticoagulation is effective in lowering the frequency of systemic emboli.

Prosthetic cardiac valves remain an important source of cardiac stroke development, despite advances in valve design.

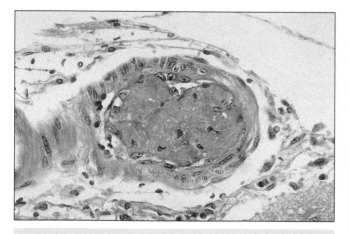

FIGURE 3 Embolus obstructing a cortical vessel.

TABLE 1 SOURCES OF CARDIOEMBOLIC STROKE

High-risk sources
Mechanical prosthetic valves
Mitral stenosis with atrial fibrillation
Atrial fibrillation
Left atrial thrombus
Sick sinus syndrome
Recent myocardial infarction (< 4 wk)
Left ventricular thrombus
Dilated cardiomyopathy
Akinetic segment
Myxoma
Infective endocarditis

Medium-risk sources
Mitral valve prolapse
Mitral annulus calcification
Mitral stenosis without atrial fibrillation
Patent foramen ovale
Nonbacterial thrombotic endocarditis
Hypokinetic segment
Myocardial infarction (> 4 wk, < 6 mo)

Cardiology for the Primary Care Physician

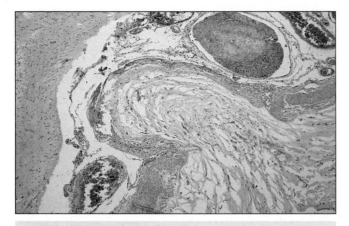

FIGURE 4 Myxomatous tissue within a cerebral vessel.

Mechanical valves pose a greater embolic threat than do biologic valves.

Infective endocarditis is a significant source of cardioembolic stroke in both young patients and the elderly. In one series of 203 patients, brain ischemia occurred in 19% of patients [3]. Echocardiographically documented vegetations did not always correlate with stroke risk. Most strokes occurred at the time of presentation, and recurrent strokes were uncommon if the primary infection was controlled.

Patients with sick sinus syndrome also have a substantial risk for stroke, and it is unclear if cardiac pacing reduces this risk. Predictors of stroke risk in patients with sick sinus syndrome are a history of cerebrovascular disease, ventricular pacing, and paroxysmal atrial fibrillation [4].

Two less-common entities that can still have a high rate of embolization are dilated cardiomyopathy and left atrial myxoma. In dilated cardiomyopathy, globally impaired ventricular performance promotes stasis and thrombus formation. The annual rate of embolization has been estimated at 3.5% [5].

Atrial myxomas are the most common primary cardiac tumors, and they are often quite friable (Fig. 4). Myxoma-related stroke occurs most often in persons ranging from 30 to 60 years of age, and recurrent emboli before surgery are common (Fig. 5) [6]. Anticoagulation is not always successful in preventing reembolization.

Medium-Risk Sources

Mitral valve prolapse (MVP) is a common, although heterogeneous, condition. It is estimated to have a prevalence of 5% in the general population [7]. Studies of stroke in young adults have had widely differing figures, ranging from 2% to more than 30% of strokes attributable to MVP. Certain subgroups of patients are believed to be at increased risk for developing infective endocarditis or peripheral embolization, or both (*eg*, men older than 45 years of age with systolic murmurs and patients with myxomatous degeneration of the valve leaflets and chordae). It is unclear if patients with MVP are at an increased risk for stroke [8].

Nonbacterial thrombotic endocarditis, or marantic endocarditis, is believed to be the most common cause of stroke in the cancer patient, at least based on autopsy studies [9]. This condition is characterized by the deposition of small, sterile thrombi on valves and may be responsible for multiple focal deficits in patients with neoplasms.

Recently, two new sources for embolic stroke—one in the heart and the other in the thoracic aorta—have been recognized. Paradoxical emboli were thought to be a rare cause of stroke; however, several studies in younger stroke patients employing contrast echocardiography have demonstrated that a patent foramen ovale (PFO) is four to five times more common in stroke patients than in age-matched controls. The prevalence of PFO is highest in those stroke patients who have no other obvious source for their stroke. One study compared the echocardiograms of patients with stroke of determined origin with those of patients with cryptogenic stroke [10]. In both the younger (< 55 years) and older age groups, a PFO was significantly more common in patients with cryptogenic stroke (48% vs 4% and 38% vs 8%, respectively). The presence of a PFO in a patient with an otherwise unexplained stroke certainly suggests a relationship, but conclusively establishing that paradoxical embolization has occurred remains difficult. The presence of venous or cardiac thrombus would be supportive.

Elevation of the right heart pressure is another related factor to paradoxical embolization with PFO, and the patient should be carefully questioned for any Valsalva-like episode before stroke onset. The natural history of recurrent stroke in patients with PFO is uncertain. The most appropriate intervention is also uncertain because only anecdotal information is currently available, but we currently recommend antiplatelet agents as initial therapy unless there is documented venous thrombosis. The risk of recurrent stroke with PFO appears to be low (22% per

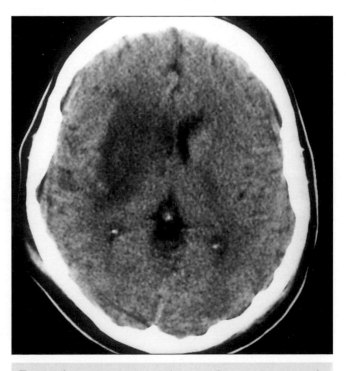

FIGURE 5 Computed tomography scan of a young woman with myxoma-related stroke.

year), but the patients are typically young, complicating decisions about management [11•].

Ulcerated plaques in the aortic arch (AA) are the other recently recognized source of cerebral emboli that can be classified as a pericardiac disorder. Previously, isolated case reports suggested the potential relationship between ulcerated plaques in the AA and embolic stroke. A more comprehensive, recent study evaluated the autopsies of 500 patients with neurologic disease [12]. It was found that 26% of cerebrovascular disease patients had AA plaques, whereas it was present only in 5% of controls with other neurologic disorders. In stroke patients with no other recognized cause, 61% had an ulcerated AA, as compared with 22% of stroke patients with another potential source.

Transesophageal echocardiography can evaluate the AA and detect ulcerated plaques, providing a relatively simple method to detect this potential source for embolic stroke. Information concerning the natural history and best therapeutic approach for stroke related to ulcerated AA plaques is not currently available. Plaques larger than 4 mm predict a higher stroke risk [13•].

The capability to noninvasively detect cardiac sources for embolic stroke has been the main reason for enhanced recognition of the relationship between the two disorders. Transthoracic echocardiography (TTE) is widely employed as an initial screening procedure to detect valvular heart disease, dyskinetic segments, intracardiac thrombi and masses, and cardiomyopathies. The addition of contrast agents, such as agitated saline, is helpful for detecting right-to-left shunts. However, TTE is relatively insensitive, especially for detecting thrombi and left atrial appendage abnormalities and for evaluating the atrial septum. Several studies have compared the diagnostic acumen of TTE with transesophageal echocardiography (TEE), which provides visualization of those abnormalities. Transesophageal echocardiography detects potential cardiac sources for emboli significantly better than TTE [14•]. TEE findings, such as spontaneous left atrial contrast and mitral valve strands, are associated with increased stroke risk. The best way to employ TEE in the evaluation of patients with ischemic stroke is continuing to evolve, but it should be considered in younger patients without an obvious stroke source, who have a nondiagnostic TTE.

STROKE PREVENTION

The substantial stroke risk associated with untreated NVAF prompted five large treatment trials, and the results are now available [15•]. In both the SPAF study and the Danish Atrial Fibrillation, Aspirin, Anticoagulation (AFASAK) study, patients were randomly assigned to receive warfarin, aspirin, or placebo; however, because the trial designs were different, a direct comparison of warfarin with aspirin is not possible. Both studies did demonstrate a significant reduction of ischemic stroke and systemic emboli by warfarin as compared with placebo (Table 2). In SPAF, 325 mg/d of aspirin also significantly reduced end-point occurrence, but in AFASAK, 75 mg/d of aspirin had no effect. A third open-label study, the Boston Area Anticoagulation Trial for Atrial Fibrillation (BAATAF), compared warfarin with placebo. The incidence of ischemic stroke was very low in the warfarin group, 0.4% per year, significantly less than the 3.0% per year rate in the placebo group.

Taken together, these studies and two others strongly support the beneficial effects of warfarin in low doses (international normalized ratio [INR] of 2.0 to 3.0, prothrombin time ratio of 1.2 to 1.5) to reduce primary stroke risk in NVAF patients. A lower INR is associated with less effective stroke prevention, whereas an INR higher than 4.0 has an increased risk for hemorrhage [16•]. The role of aspirin in primary stroke prevention in NVAF has not been established. In the Stroke Prevention in Atrial Fibrillation (SPAF) II trial a direct comparison of aspirin and warfarin demonstrated no overall difference. Although ischemic stroke incidence was lower in the warfarin group, the risk of hemorrhage was greater [17•]. In SPAF III a combination of very low-intensity warfarin (INR<1.5) and aspirin (325 mg/day) was less effective than standard intensity warfarin (INR 2–4) [18•]. Secondary stroke prevention in NVAF patients who have already suffered an initial stroke is another important consideration. The European Atrial Fibrillation Trial demonstrated the efficacy of warfarin in this setting as well, with a decrease in the annual stroke incidence from 12% in the placebo group to 4% in the warfarin group [19].

Therapy with a low-to-moderate dose of warfarin is indicated in patients with AF who can tolerate this therapy. Patients who are not good candidates for anticoagulation or

				Outcome events per year		
Study	Patients, *n*	Men, %	Mean age, *y*	Warfarin vs control, %/%	Aspirin vs control, %/%	Major bleeds per year, %
AFASAK	1007	64	74	2.2/5.5	4.7/5.5	0.8
SPAF	1330	71	67	2.3/7.4	3.6/6.3	1.5
BAATAF	420	72	68	0.4/3.0	—	0.8
CAFA	378	75	68	3.0/4.6	—	2.5
VA	525	100	67	0.9/4.3	—	1.3

TABLE 2 COMPARISON OF STUDIES OF WARFARIN FOR ISCHEMIC STROKE AND SYSTEMIC EMBOLI

AFASAK—The Danish Atrial Fibrillation, Aspirin, Anticoagulation Study; BAATAF—The Boston Area Anticoagulation Trial for Atrial Fibrillation Study; CAFA—The Canadian Atrial Fibrillation Study; SPAF—The Stroke Prevention in Atrial Fibrillation Study.

Cardiology for the Primary Care Physician

who do not wish to be placed on warfarin should consider aspirin (325 mg/d). Patients younger than 60 years of age with lone or paroxysmal AF should also consider aspirin use at this dosage [20]. It is unclear if aspirin or warfarin is better in patients older than 75 years.

The role of warfarin and aspirin for primary stroke prevention in other cardiac disorders has not been as well studied. Warfarin is widely used in patients with rheumatic valvular disease and prosthetic cardiac valves.

Patients with acute anterior MI and documented ventricular thrombi are also at high risk, and anticoagulants are frequently employed. There have been reports of up to a 55% reduction in the cerebral infarction rate in MI patients treated with long-term warfarin after the acute phase, but this area remains somewhat controversial [20].

Anticoagulants are frequently employed in dilated cardiomyopathy (especially when the ejection fraction is less than 15%), although the need for a clinical trial to study this issue has been raised. The role of anticoagulation in paradoxical embolization, marantic endocarditis, ventricular aneurysms, and other less-common disorders remains uncertain.

CONCLUSION

We believe that every patient with cerebral ischemia (either transient or with a completed stroke) should be evaluated by a neurologist, because many neurologic conditions can produce the same symptom complex. In addition, diagnostic and therapeutic advances are occurring at a rapid rate in cerebrovascular disease, and a stroke neurologist would be best apprised of the most recent developments.

In terms of cardiogenic embolism, technologic advances have contributed to the increasing recognition of the interconnection between cardiac disorders and stroke. Perhaps many of the currently cryptogenic stroke cases will eventually be assigned to the category of cardioembolic stroke. The similarity between ischemic injury in the heart and the brain implies that therapeutic advances in one area may be helpful and relevant to the other. The exchange of information between cardiologists and neurologists should remain of vital importance to both disciplines.

REFERENCES AND RECOMMENDED READING

Recently published papers of particular interest have been highlighted as:
• Of interest
•• Of outstanding interest

1.• Brickner ME: Cardioembolic stroke. *Am J Med* 1995, 100:465–474.

2.• Atrial Fibrillation Investigators: Risk factors for and efficacay of antithrombotic therapy in atrial fibrillation. *Arch Intern Med* 1994, 154:1449–1457.

3. Hart R, Foster J, Luther M, Kanter M: Stroke in infective endocarditis. *Stroke* 1990, 21:695–700.

4. Sgarbossa EB, Pinski SL, Maloney JD, *et al.*: Chronic atrial fibrillation and stroke in paced patients with sick sinus syndrome. *Circulation* 1993, 88:1045–1053.

5. Falk R: A plea for a clinical trial of anticoagulation in dilated cardiomyopathy. *Am J Cardiol* 1990, 65:914–915.

6. Knepper L, Biller J, Adams H, Bruno A: Neurologic manifestations of atrial myxoma. *Stroke* 1988, 19:1435–1440.

7. Cerebral Embolism Task Force: Cardiogenic brain embolism. *Arch Neurol* 1989, 46:727–743.

8. Orencia AJ, Petty GW, Khandheria BK, *et al.*: Risk of stroke with mitral valve prolapse in population-based cohort study. *Stroke* 1995, 26:7–13.

9. Rogers L, Cho E, Kempin S, Posner J: Cerebral infarction from non-bacterial thrombotic endocarditis. *Am J Med* 1987, 83:746–756.

10. DiTullio M, Sacco R, Gopal A, *et al.*: Patent foramen ovale as a risk factor of cryptogenic stroke. *Ann Intern Med* 1992, 117:461–465.

11.• Devuyst G, Bogousslavsky J, Ruchat P, *et al.*: Prognosis after stroke followed by surgical closure of patent foramen ovale: a prospective follow-up study with brain MRI and simultaneous transesophageal and transcranial Doppler ultrasound. *Neurology* 1996, 47:1162–1166.

12. Amarenco P, Duyckaerts C, Tzourio C, *et al.*: The prevalence of ulcerated plaques in the aortic arch in patients with stroke. *N Engl J Med* 1992, 326:221–225.

13.• Amerenco P, Cohen A, Tzourio C, *et al.*: Atherosclerotic disease of the aortic arch and the risk of ischemic stroke. *N Engl J Med* 1994, 331:1474–1479.

14.• Daniel WG, Mugge A: Transesophageal echocardiography. *N Engl J Med* 1995, 332:1268–1279.

15.• Albers GW: Atrial fibrillation and stroke. *Arch Intern Med* 1994, 154:1443–1448.

16.• Hylek EM, Skates SJ, Sheehan MA, Singer DE: An analysis of the lowest effective intensity of prophylactic anticoagulation for patients with nonrheumatic atrial fibrillation. *N Engl J Med* 1996, 335:540–546.

17.• Stroke Prevention in Atrial Fibrillation Investigators: Warfarin versus aspirin for the prevention of thromboembolism in atrial fibrillation. *Lancet* 1994, 343:687–691.

18.• Stroke Prevention in Atrial Fibrillation Investigators: Adjusted-dose warfarin versus low intensity, fixed dose warfarin plus aspirin for high-risk patients with atrial fibrillation. *Lancet* 1996, 348:633–638.

19. European Atrial Fibrillation Trial Study Group: Secondary prevention in non-rheumatic atrial fibrillation after transient ischemic attack or minor stroke. *Lancet* 1993, 342:1255–1262.

20. Albers G, Sherman D, Gress D, *et al.*: Stroke prevention in nonvalvular atrial fibrillation: a review of prospective randomized trials. *Ann Neurol* 1991, 30:511–518.

SELECT BIBLIOGRAPHY

Kanter M, Sherman D: Embolic stroke of cardiac origin. In *Current Therapy in Neurologic Disease*, edn 3. Edited by Johnson R. Philadelphia: BC Decker; 1990:181–186.

Koudstaal P: Cardioembolic stroke. In *Current Review of Cerebrovascular Disease*. Edited by Fisher M, Bogousslavsky J. Philadelphia: Current Medicine; 1993:41–47.

Sherman D: Prevention of cardioembolic stroke. In *Prevention of Stroke*. Edited by Norris J, Hachinski V. New York: Springer-Verlag; 1991:149–160.

Streifler J, Furlan A, Barnett H: Cardiogenic brain embolism: incidence, varieties, and treatment. In *Stroke*, edn 2. Edited by Barnett H, Mohr J, Stein B, Yatsu F. New York: Churchill Livingstone; 1992:967–994.

The Heart and Endocrine Diseases

42

Clifford J. Rosen

Key Points

- Diabetes mellitus profoundly accelerates atherosclerotic disease by micro- and macroangiopathic changes in coronary vessels.

- Coexistent hypertension and small vessel disease contribute to diabetic cardiomyopathy and congestive heart faliure.

- Cardiac function can be altered by chronic thyrotoxicosis through direct hormonal stimulation or indirectly via sympathetic overactivity.

- Reduction in cardiac output and asymptomatic pericardial effusions are classic signs of hypothyroidism.

- Atherosclerotic coronary disease is one of the major manifestations of Cushing's disease.

- Carcinoid heart disease is caused by endothelial fibrosis as a result of metastatic deposition on surfaces of the right heart and overproduction of vasoactive products such as serotonin.

Hormones are circulating peptides and sterols that regulate tissue activity at sites remote from their points of synthesis. The biologic activity of these endocrine effectors is dependent to a major degree on transport through the circulation. At the same time, the high metabolic requirements of the myocardium demand a fixed proportion of total cardiac output. Thus, as a circulatory pump and as a metabolic factory, the heart plays a central role in targeting hormonal action. A challenge for clinicians is to recognize that organic heart disease can be related to perturbations in hormonal factors or metabolic substrates. This chapter examines how hormonal excess or deficiency states can affect cardiac structure and function.

DIABETES MELLITUS AND THE HEART

The most common endocrine disorder associated with cardiac dysfunction is diabetes mellitus. Coronary heart disease (CAD) is the principle cause of premature death in both insulin-dependent diabetes mellitus (IDDM) and noninsulin-dependent diabetes mellitus (NIDDM) [1]. By the age of 55, one third of diabetics die of CAD compared with a mortality rate of 4% to 8% in the Framingham cohort of men and women without diabetes mellitus [2]. In particular, the incidence of CAD in females with diabetes is five times higher than in nondiabetics, and affected women have a much greater likelihood of dying from the disease than do women without diabetes [3]. Several studies have now confirmed that chronic hyperglycemia in men and women, whether symptomatic or asymptomatic, is a major risk factor for mortality from CAD, independent of all other factors [1–3].

Although diabetes mellitus ravages the heart by affecting large and small coronary vessels and autonomic nerves, the mechanisms that produce such injury are poorly understood. Several metabolic and structural perturbations seem likely to

TABLE 1 POSSIBLE PATHOGENETIC FACTORS CONTRIBUTING TO ACCELERATED ATHEROSCLEROTIC CORONARY ARTERY DISEASE IN DIABETES MELLITUS

Hyperglycemia
Direct toxic effects
Indirect via other risk factors (*e.g.*, insulin, IGF, LDL)

Hyperinsulinemia

Increased production of endothelial and smooth muscle growth factors
PDGF
IGF-I
EGF
FGF
TGF

Lipoprotein abnormalities including:
Increased LDL and VLDL
Decreased HDL

Altered hormonal milieu
Enhanced growth hormone secretion

Qualitative and quantitative changes in clotting factors

EGF—epidermal growth factor; FGF—fibroblast growth factor; HDL—high-density lipoprotein; IGF-I—insulin-like growth factor-I; LDL—low-density lipoprotein; PDGF—platelet-derived growth factor; TGF—transforming growth factor; VLDL—very low density lipoprotein.1

contribute to the high incidence of CAD in this disease (Table 1). Clearly the most consistent pathologic finding in diabetic heart disease is diffuse atherosclerosis. This *macroangiopathic* process is grossly, radiologically, and microscopically identical to atherosclerosis in coronary vessels of non-diabetic individuals. However, the development of atherosclerosis in diabetics is markedly accelerated [4]. Indeed, diabetic coronary macroangiopathy, irrespective of phenotype (IDDM vs NIDDM), is more severe and more diffuse than angiopathic disease in non-diabetic patients [5]. Although classical anginal symptoms are frequently reported by diabetics with underlying disease, there is often a mismatch between classic symptomatology and the extent of CAD. Unrecognized myocardial infarction (MI) is more common in persons with diabetes and accounts for 39% of diabetic infarctions compared with 22% in patients without diabetes [6]. Therefore, a high index of suspicion is necessary when evaluating diabetic patients for atypical chest pain, nausea, vomiting, or diaphoresis.

Objective tests (angiography, radionucleide studies, exercise examinations) to assess the severity of ischemia are indicated in patients suspected of having occult heart disease, even though exercise-induced angina during treadmill testing is considerably less common in diabetics than in non-diabetics [7]. The risk of coronary angiography in diabetic patients

(compared with non-diabetics of similar age and severity) is *not* increased unless there is superimposed renal disease, in which case pretreatment with intravenous fluids and mannitol can avert serious renal damage [8].

Treatment of myocardial ischemia and silent CAD in diabetics does not differ greatly from therapy for non-diabetics. Therapeutic options include coronary artery angioplasty, arterial stenting or coronary artery bypass graft (CABG) surgery. A recent multicenter study suggested that diabetics had a higher 5-year survival rate after CABG than after coronary angioplasty [9••]. This is in sharp contrast with non-diabetic patients, whose survival rates are similar for CABG and angioplasty.

If untreated, the macroangiopathic atherosclerotic process in diabetics can progress rapidly. Both early and later studies confirm significantly higher initial and one-year mortality rates in diabetics who suffer from myocardial damage compared with patients with heart disease but without glucose intolerance [10,11]. At particularly high risk are younger diabetics (who have a mortality rate three times that of non-diabetics) and diabetic women (who have twice the in-hospital mortality of non-diabetics) [11]. Despite this, the reason for the difference in death rates between diabetics and non-diabetics is not readily apparent. The extent of cardiac damage, the incidence of post-infarction arrhythmias, and the degree of left ventricular dysfunction are not significantly greater in patients with diabetes than in age-and sex-matched euglycemic patients. However, the coexistence of microvascular disease and altered diastolic compliance could be contributing factors. In addition, a higher incidence of coronary vasoconstriction related to autonomic neuropathy may jeopardize potentially viable myocardial tissue and enhance the risk of fatal arrythmias.

Although the management of acute myocardial infarctions (AMIs) for diabetics does not differ from that for non-diabetics, control of hyperglycemia and awareness of other diabetic complications are essential. In the end, increased awareness of the risk of CAD in diabetes should prompt early and aggressive intervention prior to a major myocardial event.

Microangiopathy, a process characteristic of diabetic retinopathy and nephropathy, also affects myocardial function and can result in congestive cardiomyopathy. In fact, diabetic cardiomyopathy without CAD is not rare and may account for nearly 25% of all cases of idiopathic cardiomyopathy [12]. In the cardiac microvessels and capillaries of both Type I IDDM and Type II NIDDM patients, basement membrane thickening and microaneurysm have been described [13]. However, macroangiopathic abnormalities often coexist, making it extremely difficult to interpret the full implication of these changes.

In addition to both micro-and macroangiopathic disease, there are also profound metabolic alterations in carbohydrates and lipids that can alter myocardial function at a cellular level. Reduced glucose uptake, increased fatty acid and triglyceride accumulation, and alterations in calcium transport in the myocardium can contribute to acute and diffuse myocardial dysfunction. The hemodynamic abnormalities described in diabetic cardiomyopathy include reduced cardiac output, impaired left ventricular compliance, increased ventricular wall stiffness, and end-diastolic pressure [14]. Whether these changes are reversible with control of the blood glucose remains controversial, although in vitro studies suggest there is a return to a normal contractile status when extracellular glucose is normalized [15].

Patients with diabetic cardiomyopathy exhibit classical signs of congestive heart failure (CHF) with reduced left ventricular compliance and recurrent pulmonary edema. Because of the high prevalence of atherosclerotic coronary disease in these patients, the premortem diagnosis of primary cardiomyopathy can be difficult. Further complicating the differential diagnosis are other disorders associated with diabetes that can accelerate the disease process, including hypertension and renal failure. Hemochromatosis can also present as a cardiomyopathy or as diabetes mellitus. The management of diabetic cardiomyopathy includes strict control of blood sugars, aggressive therapy for CHF, and control of hypertension.

The clinical course of diabetic heart disease can be dramatically altered by development of autonomic neuropathy. Sudden death, presumably cardiac, is responsible for the marked increase in mortality noted after development of autonomic neuropathy. Several events, in part related to chronic hyperglycemia, lead to autonomic dysfunction (Table 2). Parasympathetic nerve fibers are affected first. This results in a relative increase in sympathetic tone and a resting tachycardia [16]. Alterations in parasympathetic function can also exaggerate coronary vasoconstriction. Sympathetic dysfunction follows soon after parasympathetic involvement and produces orthostatic hypotension, which further reduces coronary artery perfusion [17]. Impaired neurogenic responsiveness to stressors, such as surgery or trauma, diminish cardiac performance and enhance the risk of major postoperative complications. Eventually, autonomic neuropathy can cause sudden death in diabetics. In part, this can be related to malignant arrhythmias from silent ischemia, although there is also evidence that

diabetic autonomic neuropathy and a prolonged QT interval shown on electrocardiogram (ECG) may increase the risk of life-threatening ventricular arrhythmias [18]. Other complications seen frequently in diabetics, such as transient hypokalemia, hypomagnesemia, and digitalis toxicity, may also multiply the relative risk of sudden death due to arrhythmia. Primary goals of therapy are correction of any underlying metabolic disorders and treatment of orthostatic hypotension.

THYROID DISEASES AND THE HEART

Hyperthyroidism

The cardiac manifestations of hyperthyroidism are usually the earliest and most prominent parts of the clinical presentation in this disease. Palpitations, tachycardia, and cardiomegaly were first described in hyperthyroid patients more than 200 years ago. Since then, numerous studies have documented the cardiovascular effects of thyrotoxicosis. In general, cardiac manifestations of thyroid overactivity can be divided into direct and indirect effects.

Excess circulating thyroxine *indirectly* affects the heart via the sympathetic nervous system. Anxiety, tremors, tachycardia, increased pulse pressure, and palpitations all can be attributed to the actions of thyroid hormone on the sympathoadrenal system. With active hyperthyroidism, catecholamine synthesis is enhanced and catecholamine uptake and breakdown are reduced. This results in enhanced pressor and chronotropic responses [19]. There also is increased sensitivity of myocardial tissue to catecholamines, possibly due to upregulation of adrenergic receptors [20]. Irrespective of the mechanism, enhanced sympathetic tone contributes greatly to the cardiovascular symptoms in patients with thyrotoxicosis.

Direct actions of thyroxine on the heart, independent of the sympathetic nervous system, have also been described [20]. Excess thyroid hormone can stimulate myocardial contractility, even during experimental states of catecholamine depletion. Furthermore, the marked increase in ionotropy during thyrotoxicosis is not ameliorated by coexistent administration of β blockers. This implies that myocardial activity is directly modulated by thyroxine. Stimulation of myocardial adenylate cyclase, changes in intracellular calcium transport, increases in Na/K pump activity, or induction of several contractile proteins contribute to augmented myocardial contractility [21].

The clinical stigmata and hemodynamic alterations that result from thyrotoxicosis often are very apparent. Increased heart rate, pulse pressure, cardiac output, stroke volume, and mean systolic ejection rate are coupled with diminished peripheral vascular resistance and increased circulating blood volume [22]. These findings correlate closely with oxygen utilization and the metabolic needs of the affected individual. Cardiac symptoms of hyperthyroidism also include dyspnea, palpitations, and angina. Patients can appear hypermetabolic, warm, and tachypneic, especially at rest. Frequently there is a third heart sound, and mitral valve prolapse and atrial fibrillation also are associated with thyrotoxicosis.

The diagnosis of hyperthyroidism in elderly individuals can be very elusive, although presenting symptoms are often

---

TABLE 2 DIABETIC AUTONOMIC NEUROPATHY AND ITS DELETERIOUS EFFECTS ON THE HEART

Parasympathetic dysfunction leading to:
Enhanced sympathetic tone
  Increased heart rate
  Coronary vasoconstriction

Sympathetic dysfunction leading to:
Orthostatic hypotension
  Reduced coronary perfusion
Impaired chronotropic response to stress and exercise

Conduction abnormalities leading to:
Sudden death
  Prolonged QT interval + sympathetic dysfunction
  Sympathetic dysfunction + hypokalemia or hypomagnesemia
Syncope

cardiac. For example, although "apathetic" thyrotoxicosis is associated with profound weight loss and lethargy, it is atrial fibrillation that often points clinicians toward the diagnosis of occult hyperthyroidism [23]. Atrial fibrillation alone occurs in 15% of all patients with hyperthyroidism and is frequently related to underlying CAD, especially in patients older than the age of 40 years. In most cases, atrial fibrillation due to hyperthyroidism is related to the severity of the thyrotoxicosis. It usually resolves following induction of the euthyroid state unless coexistent heart disease is present. Wolff-Parkinson-White syndrome, mitral valve prolapse with arrhythmias, and other supraventricular tachycardias have also been reported in patients with thyrotoxicosis. Echocardiography is generally not useful, although long-standing hyperthyroidism can lead to cardiac hypertrophy.

Treatment of hyperthyroid heart disease centers on controlling thyrotoxic symptoms through the use of beta blockers (primarily to slow the heart rate) and antithyroid medications (propylthiouracil or methimazole) to reduce intrathyroidal synthesis of thyroxine. As noted previously, induction of the euthyroid state can lead to spontaneous cardioversion. For acute episodes of supraventricular tachycardia, beta blockers or calcium channel blockers are frequently successful in slowing the heart rate [24••]. On the other hand, failure to control the ventricular response to atrial tachycardia with conventional doses of digitalis suggests that thyrotoxicosis may be an etiologic factor in the arrhythmia.

Thyroid storm is a clinical syndrome characterized by exaggerated organ responsiveness to high circulating levels of thyroxine. Cardiac tissue is particularly susceptible to acute rises in thyroid hormone, which results in very rapid heart rates (with or without atrial fibrillation), impending ischemia or infarction, and CHF. Besides beta blockers and antithyroid medications, high doses of glucocorticoids(which block T4 to T3 peripheral conversion), and iodides (which suppress hormone release from the thyroid gland) are usually employed. Subtle cardiac manifestations are also noted in long-standing, unrecognized hyperthyroidism or in patients treated with radioactive iodine but not adequately prepared with antithyroid medications prior to ablation.

Hypothyroidism

Not surprisingly, the cardiac manifestations of hypothyroidism are the opposite of those seen with thyrotoxic heart disease. However, in contrast to the overt cardiovascular symptoms that characterize hyperthyroidism (Table 3), signs of hypothyroid heart disease are often subtle. Cardiac signs and symptoms, which result from long-standing hypothyroidism, reflect a profound decrease in left ventricular performance [24]. This is manifested by a low cardiac output and prolongation of both pre-ejection time and isovolumic contraction. Reduced ionotropy from hypothyroidism can be attributed to altered calcium uptake and release in the myocyte [25]. However, there are also changes in expression of several myocardial contractile proteins. In addition, the slow heart rate can reduce cardiac output during stressful states. In the periphery, hypothyroidism increases systemic vascular resistance; hence, diastolic blood pressure may be very high.

TABLE 3 CARDIAC MANIFESTATIONS OF THYROID DYSFUNCTION
Hyperthyroidism
Cardiovascular effects
Increased sympathetic tone
Increased heart rate
Widened pulse pressure
Tachyarrythmias
Decreased peripheral vascular resistance
Increased ejection fraction
Increased blood volume
Direct effects from excess thyroxine
Increased ionotropy
Increased chronotropy
Shortened ejection and filling times
? Cardiac failure
Increased oxygen demand and utilization
Symptoms and signs
Dyspnea
Angina (electrocardiogram changes of ischemia)
Palpitations, tachycardia
Anxiety
Acute myocardial infarction
Apathy
Hypothyroidism
Cardiovascular effects
Bradycardia
Decreased ejection fraction
Reduced cardiac output
Narrow pulse pressure
Diastolic hypertension
Decreased blood volume
Symptoms and signs
Low body temperature
Decreased heart sounds
Apathy
Low voltage on electrocardiogram
Non-pitting edema

Surprisingly, blood volume is reduced even though hypothyroid patients often have non-pitting edema. The pathogenetic factors responsible for edema in hypothyroidism have not been fully elucidated.

As noted previously, few symptoms of hypothyroidism can be directly attributed to cardiac involvement. However, exertional dyspnea and exercise intolerance can be related to altered skeletal and cardiac muscle function. Angina pectoris may be more common in hypothyroidism, but it is unclear if myxedema alone can lead to CHF. Classically, patients with hypothyroidism have a slow heart rate, narrowed pulse pressure, and diminished heart sounds. In addition, diastolic hypertension is common. Laboratory studies generally show an increase in both cholesterol and triglycerides, which contributes to a greater risk of CAD in these patients. Serum creatine phosphokinase (CPK) activity is increased in approximately 30% of patients with hypothyroidism, although the isoenzyme pattern is skeletal rather than myocardial. This increase in enzyme activity is also related to impaired clearance from the circulation.

Electrocardiograms of patients with hypothyroidism show low voltage and sinus bradycardia. However, in contrast to hyperthyroidism, atrial and ventricular arrhythmias are not common. The low voltage noted on ECGs may be related to asymptomatic pericardial effusions, which occur in 30% to 50% of patients with overt hypothyroidism. The severity of pericardial effusion is directly related to the duration and extent of the hypothyroid state [26]. Pericardial aspirates reveal an exudative fluid with high concentrations of cholesterol and protein. However, the risk of pericardial tamponade is very low, with only a handful of cases reported.

Treatment of hypothyroidism reverses most cardiac manifestations. However, it may take a year or more for pericardial effusions to clear. In part this may be related to clinical practice patterns in which concern for arrhythmias in elderly patients has made practitioners more cautious in their approach to the rate of thyroid replacement. Generally, replacement therapy is initiated with very low doses of L-thyroxine (eg, 0.0125 or 0.025 mg/day) and increased gradually. Still, there is considerable controversy surrounding the rapidity of thyroxine replacement in the elderly. Despite anecdotal reports suggesting that thyroxine replacement in full doses to older individuals can increase the risk of arrhythmia, sudden death, or MI, there is little evidence to support that contention. In one prospective study of 55 patients with known symptomatic coronary disease, 38% improved with treatment of their thyroid disease, 46% had no change, and only 16% had more symptoms of ischemic heart disease [27]. Currently the issue of whether thyroid replacement can exacerbate CAD in patients with hypothyroidism remains unresolved. On the other hand, CABG can be safely performed without urgent thyroid replacement in patients with moderate or severe hypothyroidism [24]. Furthermore, therapeutic introduction of thyroxine immediately following CABG has not been associated with an increase in morbidity or mortality [24].

CALCIUM DISORDERS AND THE HEART

Hypercalcemia

Changes in serum calcium levels do not directly affect myocardial function but can influence electrical activity in the heart. High serum calcium is associated with a reversible shortening of the QT interval and prolongation of the PR interval [28]. First-degree atrioventricular block has been reported in hyperparathyroidism, but ventricular arrhythmias with acute or chronic hypercalcemia are rare. Ventricular arrhythmias are detected only when hypercalcemia is related to an infiltrative granulomatous disorder (eg, sarcoidosis). In contrast, hypertension is reported in nearly 50% of hyperparathyroid patients [29], which is at least two times higher than the incidence in other adult populations [29]. However,

the pathogenesis of hypertension in primary hyperparathyroidism is not well defined, especially after secondary causes of hypertension are excluded. For example, pheochromocytoma can coexist with primary hyperparathyroidism (multiple endocrine neoplasia Type II), and should always be considered in patients who present with hypercalcemia and hypertension. Similarly, chronic hypercalcemia can impair renal function because of nephrolithiasis or nephrocalcinosis. In turn this can lead to sustained hypertension. Still, when secondary causes of hypertension are excluded, the incidence of hypertension in hyperparathyroidism remains higher than in the normal population. Unfortunately, like other endocrine disorders associated with hypertension (aldosteronomas, pheochromocytomas), surgical removal of parathyroid adenomas does not always reverse systolic or diastolic hypertension.

Hypocalcemia

In contrast to hypercalcemia, low serum calcium can be extremely dangerous to the heart. Besides non-specific ECG changes including ST-T abnormalities, the corrected QT interval (QTc) can be prolonged, enhancing the likelihood of malignant ventricular arrhythmias [28]. Although this is not specific for hypocalcemia, its presence on ECG should alert the clinician to the possibility of hypocalcemia, especially in the setting of the critical care unit. In addition, reversible CHF has been reported in patients with severe hypocalcemia [30].

Hypocalcemia often coincides with another common electrolyte disorder, severe hypomagnesemia [31]. At least 10% of hospitalized patients are hypomagnesemic, and many of those are also mildly hypocalcemic. This occurs because low serum magnesium impairs parathyroid hormone (PTH) action and secretion. In addition, magnesium depletion blocks potassium conservation in the kidney, thereby setting up an ominous triad of hypocalcemia, hypokalemia, and hypomagnesemia. These three electrolyte disorders are a major cause of malignant ventricular arrhythmias and sustained atrial tachycardias. In particular, arrhythmias, which result from low serum magnesium, are notoriously resistant to anti-arrhythmic treatment unless the magnesium deficit is completely corrected. Principle causes of low calcium and low magnesium include primary hypoparathyroidism (surgery, radiation, or autoimmune), malabsorption due to gastrointestinal disorders (eg, Crohn's disease), vitamin D deficiency syndromes, alcohol, starvation, renal diseases, and diuretic use.

Therapy for hypocalcemia is often urgent in the intensive care setting and generally requires a rapid infusion of 10 cc of a 10% calcium gluconate solution (4.65 mEq (95 mg)/10 cc) over 10 minutes. This should be followed by a slower continuous infusion of 15 mg/kg over 12 to 24 hours. More importantly, theserum magnesium level must also be measured, and if it is low, it must be followed by immediate magnesium replacement (8 to 16 mEq over the first 2 hours followed by continuous infusion of 48 to 64 mEq of magnesium sulfate in 48 hours). Serum magnesium levels provide only a fair gauge of replacement since most magnesium is not found in the extracellular space. However, levels of serum magnesium greater than 1.8 mEq/L usually are indicative of adequate replacement.

ADRENAL DISORDERS AND THE HEART
Hyperfunction of the Adrenal Gland

Neoplasms of the adrenal gland secrete vasoactive substances (cortisol, aldosterone, epinephrine) that can alter myocardial function. Adrenocortical production of cortisol (Cushing's syndrome) can affect the cardiovascular system in several ways and is the major cause of death if the disease is not successfully treated [32]. More than 75% of patients with Cushing's disease (ie, adrenal hyperfunction caused by pituitary adenomas) have some degree of hypertension, itself a major risk factor for CAD [33]. Hypertension is caused by an increase in plasma volume and stimulation of the renin-angiotensin system, which can sensitize arterioles to the pressor effects of catecholamines [34]. Besides hypertension, lipid abnormalities and coexistent diabetes mellitus (related to insulin resistance) further increase the risk of atherosclerotic cardiovascular disease. Hypokalemia, which also can result from glucocorticoid excess, contributes to a much higher incidence of cardiac arrhythmias.

Aldosterone-producing adenomas (APAs) are characterized by marked diastolic hypertension and profound hypokalemia [35]. Hypertension is due to expansion of plasma volume and can contribute to concentric left ventricular hypertrophy. Malignant arrhythmias due to hypokalemia (and often hypomagnesemia) can strongly influence preoperative morbidity. Surgical removal of these relatively small APAs can reverse long-standing hypertension in the majority of cases and permanently correct the metabolic alkalosis and hypokalemia so characteristic of this syndrome.

Pheochromocytoma is often considered in the differential diagnosis of secondary hypertension, although establishing that diagnosis can be exceedingly difficult. The secretory products from a pheochromocytoma impact the heart and vasculature in several ways. Tachycardia and palpitations result from high circulating levels of norepinephrine or epinephrine [36]. Sustained or episodic hypertension can lead to a hypertensive crisis with heart failure, arrhythmia, or stroke as potential outcomes. Orthostatic hypotension from profound volume depletion following episodes of intense vasoconstriction is not uncommon.

Chronic catecholamine excess can lead to a congestive cardiomyopathy, in part due to sustained hypertension and in part due to a direct toxic effect from catecholamines on the myocardium [36]. Many of these manifestations are cured following surgical removal of solitary tumors, although hypertension persists in approximately 25% of patients after complete surgical resection. Medical treatment of hypertension from a pheochromocytoma is generally unsatisfactory and usually involves alpha blockade as well as competitive inhibition of tyrosine hydroxylation, a critical step in catecholamine synthesis [37]. Beta blockers can be used to treat tachyarrythmias, but only after complete alpha blockade has been accomplished. Phentolamine or nitroprusside can be used in the management of acute hypertensive crises.

Adrenal Insufficiency

The principle cardiovascular manifestation of primary adrenal insufficiency is orthostatic hypotension. It is a benchmark of this disorder and can be severe enough to cause syncope [38]. Although hyperkalemia and hyponatremia are frequently present in primary adrenal insufficiency, life-threatening arrhythmias are exceedingly rare. Peaked T waves and nonspecific ST-T changes have been reported in hyperkalemic patients with acute adrenal insufficiency. Secondary adrenal disorders rarely produce orthostasis or hyperkalemia, in part because aldosterone secretion is principally regulated by the renin-angiotensin system.

GROWTH HORMONE AND THE HEART

Cardiac disease is present in approximately one third of patients with growth hormone excess syndrome (ie, acromegaly) [39]. Cardiovascular complications are the most frequent cause of death in acromegalic patients and are a result of hypertension(which occurs in about 30% of all cases) and excess growth hormone (which can have a direct and deleterious effect on cardiac function). Concentric left ventricular hypertrophy, asymmetric septal hypertrophy, and a reduced ejection fraction are the most frequent signs of cardiac involvement. Cardiac hypertrophy can be very pronounced compared with enlargement of other organs [40]. ECGs are abnormal in more than 50% of patients with acromegaly and reveal nonspecific ST-T changes as well as left ventricular hypertrophy, conduction defects, and ventricular irritability. CAD is relatively frequent in acromegaly and, combined with myocardial dysfunction due to excess growth hormone, contributes to the high incidence of cardiovascular deaths in this disorder. In addition, the high frequency of the sleep apnea syndrome due to macroglossia enhances the likelihood of nocturnal oxygen desaturation, further aggravating latent ischemic disease. The severity of atherosclerotic disease in this syndrome has led some investigators to speculate that high circulating levels of insulin-like growth factor-I (IGF-I), a characteristic feature of acromegaly, enhance the propensity for atherogenesis by stimulating vascular smooth muscle hypertrophy. However, the pathogenesis of accelerated atherosclerosis in acromegaly remains unclear.

Since CAD and left ventricular hypertrophy frequently accompany this disease and may be advanced at the time of diagnosis, it is not surprising that CHF is relatively common in acromegaly. Whether chronic long-standing growth hormone excess results in an "acromegalic" cardiomyopathy remains debatable. In one longitudinal study of patients treated with surgical adenectomy, a sizable proportion of "cured" patients with acromegaly demonstrated improvement in left ventricular size and cardiac function [41]. However, as noted previously, heart disease in this syndrome is multifactorial and exceedingly difficult to define in a single clinical setting.

Recombinant human growth hormone (rhGH) recently was approved by the United States Food and Drug Administration for the treatment of adult patients with acquired growth hormone deficiency syndromes. Coincidental with the introduction of this peptide for replacement therapy, rhGH has also been tried experimentally in patients with end-stage cardiomyopathy. Such studies are still in their early stages but suggest there may be a limited role for this peptide in some people with end-stage heart disease [42••].

VASOACTIVE PEPTIDES AND THE HEART

The Carcinoid Syndrome

The carcinoid syndrome is characterized by flushing, diarrhea, and heart disease [43] Tumors that produce this syndrome are almost always metastatic at the time of clinical presentation and arise from enterochromaffin cells scattered throughout the body. Nonfunctioning carcinoids are frequent findings at autopsy, but true secretion of vasoactive material leading to clinical symptoms is relatively rare. Usually these tumors occur in the ileum, bronchus, stomach, ovary, or duodenum. Their secretory products are 5-hydroxytryptamine (serotonin), histamine, and 5-hydroxyindoleacetic acid (5-HIAA). The dramatic manifestations of the carcinoid syndrome occur after hepatic metastases, and heart disease is evident only when metastatic disease is clinically apparent. Cardiac symptoms are detected in approximately one third of patients with the carcinoid syndrome and are characterized by right heart failure, tricuspid regurgitation, and pulmonic stenosis [44]. In patients with metastatic bronchial carcinoid (not to the liver) left ventricular dysfunction can be found.

Carcinoid heart disease is caused by fibrosis of the endocardium, especially along the surfaces of the pulmonic and tricuspid valves. Metastatic tumor deposits, which travel directly from the liver to the right heart, are a major pathogenctic factor. However, high levels of serotonin also stimulate endocardial fibrosis and clearly contribute to the clinical manifestations of the carcinoid syndrome. The presentation of cardiac involvement in the carcinoid syndrome includes classic signs of right heart failure such as pitting edema, jugular venous distension, dyspnea, and ascites. Constrictive pericarditis has also been reported in this syndrome [44]. Occasionally the cardiac symptoms occur well after resection of the primary tumor.

Therapy for cardiac-related carcinoid disease centers on controlling metastases with chemotherapy or octreotide acetate while treating symptomatic heart disease with diuretics and afterload reduction. If possible, surgical removal of the primary disease can halt further cardiac fibrosis. In rare situations, tricuspid valve replacement has been performed [45]. However, cardiac involvement with the carcinoid syndrome usually implies a poor prognosis with a median survival time after diagnosis of 14 months [46].

Secretion of other vasoactive substances can cause orthostatic hypotension. However, they rarely have direct effects on the heart. Vasoactive intestinal peptide (VIP) is secreted from certain gastrointestinal tumors and can lead to diarrhea, hypokalemia, and hypercalcemia. Hypotension is common with vipomas, and increased cardiac contractility has also been reported [47]. The kinins and kallikreins are also produced by gastrointestinal tumors and have strong vasodilatory properties. These substances, however, do not directly affect cardiac function.

KEY REFERENCES

Recently published papers of outstanding interest, as identified in *References and Recommended Reading*, have been annotated.

•• Bypass Angioplasty Revascularization Investigation (BARI). Comparison of coronary artery bypass surgery with angioplasty in patients with multivesel disease. *N Engl J Med* 1996, 335:217–225.

This very large study (BARI) demonstrates for the first time that in diabetic patients CABG may be superior to angioplasty in terms of 5-year survival. This is not surprising considering the inherent potential for restenosis in diabetics due to the overproduction of local growth factors that accelerate atherosclerosis.

•• Klein I, Ojama K: Thyroid hormone and the cardiovascular system. *J Clin Endocrinol Metab* 1994, 78:1026–1030.

This is an outstanding review of the many and varied manifestations of cardiac disease in thyroidal conditions. In part, this article argues that thyroid hormone replacement in the elderly is not associated with adverse clinical outcomes despite the may anecdotes of numerous clinicians.

•• Fazio S, Salvatini D, Capaldo B, *et al.*: A preliminary study of growth hormone in the treatment of dilated cardiomyopathy. *N Engl J Med* 1996, 334:809–814.

Longstanding acromegaly is associated with cardiac hypertrophy. Short-term growth hormone treatment can increase cardiac function in part due to stimulation of local IGF-I production. Hence it is not surprising that recombinant human growth hormone has been considered as a potential therapeutic modality in end-stage heart disease. This trial is similar to other studies that have suggested that growth hormone can improve muslce performance in elders or in patients with growth hormone deficiency.

REFERENCES AND RECOMMENDED READING

Recently published papers of particular interest have been highlighted as:

• Of interest
•• Of outstanding interest

1. Dunn JP, Ipsen J, Elson KO, Ohtani M: Risk factors in coronary artery disease, hypertension and diabetes mellitus. *Am J Med Sci* 1970, 259:309–315.

2. Garcia MJ, McNamara PM, Gordon T: Morbidity and mortality in diabetics in the Framingham population. *Diabetes* 1974, 23:105–110.

4. Crall FV, Roberts WC: The extramural and intramural coronary arteries in juvenile diabetes mellitus: analysis of nine necropsy patients aged 19–38 years with onset of diabetes before age 15 years. *Am J Med* 1978, 64:221–230.

5. Martin BC, Warram JH, Manson J, Krolewski AS: The excess risk of coronary artery disease increases with duration of diabetes mellitus. *Diabetologia* 1988, 31:518A.

6. Marolis JR, Kannel WB, Feinlieb M, *et al*: Clinical features of unrecognized myocardial infarction-silent and symptomatic; 18 year follow up: the Framingham Study. *Am J Cardiol* 1977, 32:1–7.

7. Murray DP, O'Brien J, Mulrooney R, O'Sullivan DJ: Autonomic dysfunction and silent myocardial ischemia on exercise testing in diabetes mellitus. *Diabet Med* 1990, 7:580–584.

8. Viberti GC, Walker JD: Diabetic nephropathy: etiology and prevention. *Diabetes Metab Rev* 1988, 4:147–167.

9.•• Bypass Angioplasty Revascularization Investigation (BARI). Comparison of coronary artery bypass surgery with angioplasty in patients with multivesel disease. *N Engl J Med* 1996, 335:217–225.

10. Kessler II: Mortality experience of diabetic patients: a twenty six year follow-up study. *Am J Med* 1971, 51:715–720.

11. Kannel WB, McGee DL: Diabetes and cardiovascular disease: the Framingham study. *JAMA* 1979, 241:2035–2039.

12. Fein FS, Sonneblick EH: Diabetic cardiomyopathy. *Prog Cardiovasc Dis* 1985, 27:255–265.

13. Factor SM, Okun EM, Minase T: Capillary microaneurysms in the human diabetic heart. *N Engl J Med* 1980, 302:384–390.

14. Schaffer SW, Artman MF, Wilson GI: Properties of insulin idependent and noninsulin dependent diabetic cardiomyopathies. In: *Pathogenesis of Myocarditis and Cardiomyopathy.* Edited by Kawai C, Abelmann WH. Tokyo: University of Tokyo Press; 1987:149.

15. Schaffer SW, Tan FH, Wilson GL: Development of a cardiomyopathy in a model of noninsulin dependent diabetic. *Am J Physiol* 1985, 248:179–186.

16. Mackay JD, Page MM, Cambridge J, Watkins PJ: Diabetic autonomic neuropathy. *Diabetologia* 1980, 18:471–475.

17. Zander E, Schulz B, Heinke P: Importance of autonomic dysfunction in IDDM subjects with diabetic nephropathy. *Diabetes Care* 1989, 12:259–263.

18. Clark BF, Ewing DJ: Cardiovascular denervation in diabetic neuropathy. *Ann Intern Med* 1980, 92:304–310.

19. Levey GS, Klein I: Catecholamine-thyroid hormone interactions and the cardiovascular manifestations of hyperthyroidism. *Ann Intern Med* 1990, 88:642–650.

20. Klein I: Thyroid hormone and the cardiovascular system. *Am J Med* 1990, 88:651–656.

21. Balkman C, Ojamaa K, Klein I: Time course of the effects of thyroid hormone on cardiac gene expression. *Endocrinology* 1992, 130:2001–2004.

22. Morkin E, Flink IL, Goldman S: Biochemical and physiologic effects of thyroid hormone on cardiac performance. *Prog Cardiovasc Dis* 1983, 25:455–460.

23. Thomas FB, Massaferri EL, Killman TG: Apathetic thyrotoxicosis: a distinctive clinical and laboratory entity. *Ann Intern Med* 1970, 72:679–689.

24.•• Klein I, Ojama K: Thyroid hormone and the cardiovascular system. *J Clin Endocrinol Metab* 1994, 78:1026–1030.

25. Dillman WH: Biochemical basis of thyroid hormone action in the heart. *Am J Med* 1990, 88;626–635.

26. Kabadi UM, Kumar SP: Pericardial effusion in primary hypothyroidism. *Am Heart J* 1990, 120:1392–1397.

27. Klein I, Ojamaa K: The cardiovascular system in hypothyroidism. In *The Thyroid.* Edited by Bravrman LE, Utiger RD. Philadelphia: Lippincott-Raven Publishers: 1996:799–814.

28. Fitzpatrick L, Bilezikian JP: Primary hyperparathyroidism. In *Principles and Practice of Endocrinology and Metabolism.* Edited by Becker KL. Philadelphia: JB Lippincott Co.; 1991:430–438.

29. Scholz DA. Hypertension and hyperparathyroidism. *Arch Intern Med* 1977, 131:1123–1127.

30. Levine SN, Rheams CN: Hypocalcemic heart failure. *Am J Med* 1975, 78:1022–1032.

31. Rude RK, Singer FR: Magnesium deficiency and excess. *Ann Rev Med* 1981, 32:245–260.

32. Saruta T, Suzuki H, Handa M, *et al.*: Multiple factors contribute to the pathogenesis of hypertension in Cushing's Syndrome. *J Clin Endocrinol Metab* 1986, 62:275–279.

33. Krakoff LR, Nicolis G, Ansel B: Pathogenesis of hypertension in Cushing's syndrome. *Am J Med* 1975, 58:216–220.

34. Krakoff LR, Eisenfel AJ: Hormonal control of plasma renin substrate (angiotensionogen). *Circ Res* 1977, 41(suppl II):43–46.

35. Bravo EL, Tarazi RC, Dunston HP *et al.*: The changing clinical spectrum of primary aldosteronism. *Am J Med* 1983 ,74:641–651.

36. Hull CJ: Phaechromocytoma: Diagnosis, preoperative preparation and anaethestic management. *Br J Anaesthesiol* 1986, 58:1453–1459.

37. Engleman K: Pheochromocytoma. *Clin Endocrinol Metab* 1977, 6:769–789.

38. Loriaux DL: The polyendocrine deficiency syndromes. *N Engl J Med* 1983, 312:1568–1572.

39. Molitch ME: Clinical manifestations of acromegaly. *J Clin Endocrinol Metab* 1992, 21:597–613.

40. Martin JB, Kerber RE, Sherman BM, *et al.*: Cardiac size and function in acromegaly. *Circulation* 1977, 56:863–870.

41. McGuffin WL, Sherman BM, Roth J, *et al.*: Acromegaly and cardiovascular disorders. A prospective study. *Ann Intern Med* 1974, 81:11–15.

42.•• Fazio S, Salvatini D, Capaldo B, *et al.*: A preliminary study of growth hormone in the treatment of dilated cardiomyopathy. *N Engl J Med* 1996, 334:809–814.

43. Feldman JM: Carcinoid tumors and syndrome. *Semin Oncol* 1987, 14:237–257.

44. Maton PN: The Carcinoid tumor and the carcinoid syndrome. In *Principles and Practices of Endocrinology and Metabolism.* Edited by Becker KL. Philadelphia: JB Lippincott Co.; 1991:1641–1643.

45. Codd JE, Proxda J, Merjavy J: Palliation of carcinoid heart disease. *Arch Surg* 1987, 122:1076–1080.

46. Moertel CG: An odyssey in the land of small tumors. *J Clin Oncol* 1987, 5:1503–1507.

47. Said SI: Vasoactive intestinal peptide. *J Endocrinol Invest* 1986, 9:191–201.

SELECT BIBLIOGRAPHY

American Diabetes Association: Consensus statement on the detection and management of lipid disorders in diabetes. *Diabetes Care* 1993, 16:106–112.

Aron DC, Tyrrel JB: Cushing's syndrome. *Endocrinol Metab North Am* 1994 , 23:487–509.

Bonow R, Bohoman N, Hazzard W: Stratification in CAD and special populations. *Am J Med* 1996, 101(suppl)17–25.

Krahn AD, Klein GJ, Kerr CR, *et al.*: How useful is thyroid function testing with recent onset atrial fibrillation? *Arch Intern Med* 1996, 2221–2226.

Rheumatic Diseases and the Heart

43

Deborah M. DeMarco
David F. Giansiracusa

Key Points

- Physicians must have an awareness of the resurgence of rheumatic fever and the importance of antibiotic prophylaxis.
- Recognition of Lyme disease and spondyloarthropathies as a cause of bradycardia and conduction disturbances is important.
- There is potential involvement of all components of the heart in patients with systemic lupus erythematosus, rheumatoid arthritis, and scleroderma.
- Coronary artery thrombosis can be secondary to either phospholipid antibodies or vasculitis.
- The high frequency of asymptomatic cardiac involvement in scleroderma indicates the need for cardiac evaluation in all newly diagnosed patients.

The heart can suffer involvement in a spectrum of rheumatic diseases (Table 1). Cardiac disease is usually the result of the primary inflammatory, metabolic, or infiltrative process or is secondary to other organ system disease. Although the pathophysiologic mechanisms of these rheumatic diseases are quite diverse, some or all of the components of the heart may be affected by each of these conditions.

ACUTE RHEUMATIC FEVER

Acute rheumatic fever (ARF) is a rare sequela of group A streptococcal infection of the upper respiratory tract. Its manifestations, as outlined in the Jones criteria (Table 2) [1], remain the means of diagnosis for the initial attack. Carditis is its principal cardiac manifestation and has decreased in incidence in adults from 65% to 30% since the 1940s, but it remains at 70% to 90% in children. In chronic rheumatic heart disease, carditis may result in scarring of the heart valves and subsequent valvular heart disease. In a few patients, severe carditis occurs with rapid onset of complications, possibly leading to death.

Often, carditis in ARF is asymptomatic and is diagnosed by detection of a new murmur during the physical examination. Other major criteria for diagnosis include the presence of cardiomegaly, congestive heart failure, and pericardial friction rub or other signs of pericardial effusion. The most common murmur associated with ARF is mitral regurgitation followed by aortic insufficiency. First-degree heart block may be seen on the electrocardiogram, but it is neither specific nor prognostically important. There is no characteristic electrocardiogram pattern for ARF.

Diagnosis

Establishing a definitive diagnosis of rheumatic fever is important not only for acute management of disease manifestations, but also because of the potential need for antibiotic prophylaxis. In addition to the Jones criteria (Table 2), the diagnosis depends on establishing an antecedent streptococcal infection by laboratory tests; an

TABLE 1 SITES OF INVOLVEMENT OF RHEUMATIC DISEASES AND THE HEART

Disease	Aortic root	Pericardium	Myocardium	Endocardium	Coronary arteries	Conduction abnormality	Arrhythmias
Acute rheumatic fever	—	Pericarditis	Cardiomyopathy	Valvulitis, chronic valvular disease	—	+	—
Lyme disease	—	Pericarditis	Cardiomyopathy	—	—	Atrioventricular block	Atrial and ventricular tachyarrhythmias
Systemic lupus erythematosus	Aortitis (rare)	Pericarditis (tamponade, constriction)	Myocarditis (rare)	Libman–Sacks syndrome, thrombosis (antiphospholipid antibody syndrome)	Vasculitis, accelerated atherosclerotic disease, thrombosis (antiphospholipid antibody syndrome), embolic antiphospholipid antibody syndrome	Atrioventricular block (neonatal)	Ventricular
Rheumatoid arthritis	Granulomatous vasculitis	Pericarditis, constriction	Granulomatous myocarditis, interstitial myocarditis	Valvulitis	Vasculitis, accelerated atherosclerotic disease	+	—
Systemic sclerosis (scleroderma)	—	Pericarditis	Myocardial fibrosis, cor pulmonale	—	Intimal hyperplasia	+	Supra and ventricular
Dermatomyositis and polymyositis	—	—	Myocarditis	—	Vasculitis	+	+
Vasculitis	—	Pericarditis	Myocardial infarction	—	Vasculitis	+	+
Spondyloarthropathies (ankylosing spondylitis, Reiter's syndrome)	Aortitis	—	—	Aortic regurgitation	—	+	—
Polychondritis	Aortitis	Pericarditis (rare)	—	Aortic and mitral valvulitis	Vasculitis	+	+
Marfan syndrome	Dilatation, dissection	—	—	Mitral valve prolapse, aortic insufficiency	—	—	—
Ehlers–Danlos syndrome	Dilatation	—	Ventricular and atrial septal defects	Aortic insufficiency, mitral prolapse, tricuspid prolapse, bicuspid aortic valves, pulmonary regurgitation	—	—	—
Amyloidosis	—	Constrictive pericarditis	Restrictive cardiomyopathy	Valvular disease (tricuspid, mitral)	Intraarterial deposition	+	+

TABLE 2 JONES CRITERIA (REVISED) FOR DIAGNOSIS OF INITIAL ATTACK OF RHEUMATIC FEVER

Major manifestations
Carditis
Polyarthritis
Chorea
Erythrema marginatum
Subcutaneous nodules
Minor manifestations
Clinical
  Arthralgia
  Fever
Laboratory
  Elevated erythrocyte sedimentation rate
  C-reactive protein
  Leukocytosis
  Prolonged P-R interval
Supporting evidence of streptococcal infection
Increased titer of antistreptococcal antibodies
  (antistreptolysin-O or others)
Positive throat culture for group A *Streptococcus*

Adapted from Shulman *et al.* [1]; with permission.

develop 4 to 8 weeks after exposure to an infected tick, but they can occur as early as 4 days after the onset of the initial illness [4•]. Sometimes, they may predate the initial antibody response.

The most common cardiac abnormalities (Table 1) include atrioventricular block, myopericarditis, and left ventricular dysfunction, but cardiomyopathy and atrial and ventricular tachycardias have been reported [4•]. Almost all patients with atrioventricular conduction disturbances manifest first-degree block at some time during their course; high-grade block occurs in up to 50% of patients, and symptomatic complete heart block, in approximately 8% [4•]. The block is usually at or above the level of the atrioventricular node, predicting a benign prognosis, but more sinister conduction disturbances may occur. Temporary cardiac pacing is frequently needed by patients who have severe heart block with hemodynamic instability. Permanent pacemaker insertion is rarely indicated. The block generally resolves completely with antibiotic treatment, and the long-term prognosis is excellent (Table 4) [5].

elevated titer of at least one antibody on the antistreptolysin-O assay, anti-DNAse B, or antihyaluronidase test can be detected in approximately 95% of patients with ARF [2]. The rapid Streptozyme (Wampole Laboratories, Cranbury, NJ) slide test is not recommended because of its variable results.

Treatment

The current recommended treatment course is outlined in Table 3. All household members should have throat cultures taken, because reinfection may occur if the organism is not eradicated from the environment. Antiinflammatory medication is usually administered for arthritis, fever, and mild carditis, although it is not protective against the subsequent development of chronic rheumatic heart disease. Patients with severe carditis require prompt administration of corticosteroid therapy as an adjunct to their cardiac medications.

Secondary prophylaxis is recommended for patients who have had ARF (Table 3). Duration of prophylaxis remains controversial, but it can safely be discontinued if 1) the patient is older than 20 years of age; 2) the most recent attack occurred more than 5 years previously; 3) there was no carditis with the previous attack; and 4) there is no evidence of rheumatic heart disease [3]. The likelihood of the patient's exposure to children and the patient's reliability are considerations.

SYSTEMIC LUPUS ERYTHEMATOSUS

Cardiovascular involvement occurs in 29% to 66% of patients with systemic lupus erythematosus (SLE) (Table 1) [6]. Autopsy and even echocardiographic studies may document significant findings in the heart without clinically apparent disease.

Pericardial disease is the most common cardiac manifestation of SLE, documented at autopsy in approximately 80% of patients but seen as symptomatic disease in 8% to 50% of patients. It usually presents in association with SLE disease activity in other organs.

Patients with symptomatic pericarditis generally present with anterior or substernal chest pain that is characteristically pleuritic and relieved by leaning forward. The pain may be associated with dyspnea or arrhythmias. A pericardial friction rub may be heard on auscultation. A chest roentgenogram may reveal an enlarged cardiac silhouette. Transient electrocardiographic changes (ST-segment elevation and PR-interval depression) may be seen. Echocardiography may reveal pericardial effusions or pericardial thickening. Life-threatening complications of pericarditis include cardiac tamponade and

LYME DISEASE

Lyme disease, a systemic illness caused by the spirochete *Borrelia burgdorferi*, has cardiac manifestations in 4% to 10% of untreated patients. The cardiac complications usually

TABLE 3 TREATMENT RECOMMENDATIONS FOR ACUTE RHEUMATIC FEVER

Drug	Dosage
Acute treatment	
Penicillin	250 mg four times daily for 10 days
Erythromycin	250 mg four times daily for 10 days
Prophylaxis	
Penicillin G benzathine	1.2×10^6 U intramuscularly every 4 weeks
Penicillin V	250 mg orally twice daily
Sulfadiazine	0.5 g orally once daily
Erythromycin	250 mg orally twice daily

TABLE 4 ANTIBIOTIC THERAPY FOR LYME DISEASE

Stage-symptoms	Regimen*	Length, *d*
Early Lyme disease	Doxycycline, 100 mg b.i.d. or amoxicillin, 500 mg t.i.d. or erythromycin, 250 mg q.i.d.	10–21
Neurologic symptoms		
Bell's palsy only	Doxycycline, 100 mg b.i.d. or amoxicillin, 500 mg t.i.d.	21
Meningitis, encephalitis	Penicillin G, 20 million U/d IV or ceftriaxone, 2 g/d	14–21
Radiculoneuropathy		
Lyme carditis		
Mild (first-degree AV block, normal left ventricular function)	Doxycycline, 100 mg b.i.d.	30
Moderate to severe (high degree AV block)	Penicillin G, 20 million U/d IV or ceftriaxone, 2 q/d IV May require temporary pacemaker	14–21
Lyme arthritis	Doxycycline, 100 mg b.i.d. or amoxicillin, 500 mg q.i.d. plus probenecid, 500 mg q.i.d. or penicillin G, 20 million U/d IV or ceftriaxone, 2 g/d IV	30
Pregnancy		
Early-localized	Amoxicillin, 500 mg t.i.d.	21
Late-disseminated	Penicillin G, 20 million U/d IV or ceftriaxone 2 g/d IV	14–21

*Failures occur with all regimens.
AV—atrioventricular; b.i.d.—twice per day; IV—intravenous; q.i.d.—four times per day; t.i.d.—three times per day.

constriction, but both are rare. Pericardial fluid is usually exudative with high protein and normal to low glucose levels compared with serum.

Symptomatic pericarditis can often be successfully treated with nonsteroidal antiinflammatory drugs such as indomethacin, 50 mg three times daily, and, occasionally, oral corticosteroids at low dosages (15 to 30 mg/d). Hemodynamically compromising effusions require pericardial aspiration and high-dose intravenous corticosteroids.

Myocardial involvement in SLE should be categorized as primary or secondary. Primary myocarditis is rare, occurring clinically in 2.1% to 14% of patients with SLE. Patients present with unexplained tachycardia, congestive heart failure (rarely), ventricular arrhythmias, conduction defects, electrocardiogram abnormalities (including ST-T wave changes), and cardiomegaly without evidence of valvular or pericardial disease. Endocardial biopsy specimens may confirm histologically the presence of myocarditis.

Secondary causes of myocardial dysfunction in SLE include systemic hypertension, valvular disease, pulmonary disease, coronary artery ischemia, drug toxicity, and amyloidosis. These secondary causes are often clinically more important than true lupus myocarditis.

Treatment of SLE patients with carditis includes distinguishing primary from secondary disorders and appropriately treating any secondary cardiac insult. Antiinflammatory and immunosuppressive therapy should be reserved for active lupus carditis.

Coronary artery involvement in SLE includes embolic events, thromboses [7], vasculitis, and premature atherosclerosis. The treatment of the SLE patient with acute myocardial ischemia initially should be similar to that of patients with atherosclerotic coronary artery disease. However, the etiology of the ischemia must be determined by arteriography because coronary arteritis must be treated with corticosteroids and immunosuppressant agents.

The most characteristic cardiac manifestation of SLE is nonbacterial verrucous endocarditis, so-called Libman-Sacks endocarditis, which occurs on the ventricular surface of the mitral valve. A similar lesion involving the aortic valve has also been described, as well as a necrotizing valvulitis secondary to vasculitis of the smaller vessels supplying the valve. Libman-Sacks lesions rarely produce significant valvular dysfunction. However, hemodynamically significant aortic and mitral insufficiency may occur. Valve replacements may be required, but the associated mortality has been as high as 25%. Rarely, lesional material of Libman-Sacks endocarditis may dislodge and embolize.

Conduction abnormalities and arrhythmias owing to SLE are not usually clinically significant and should be managed the same way as in patients without SLE. If acute conduction disease is suspected clinically to be secondary to myocarditis or arteritis, a short trial of corticosteroids should be initiated in the hemodynamically compromised patient [6].

The infants of mothers with SLE also may suffer cardiac disease, most commonly in the form of neonatal heart block. This syndrome in infants is referred to as permanent neonatal lupus and is associated with maternal anti–Ro (SSA) antibodies.

RHEUMATOID ARTHRITIS

Rheumatoid arthritis may involve all structures of the heart as the result of granulomatous proliferation or vasculitis

(Table 1) [8]. Echocardiography can detect pericarditis and valvular disease, whereas endocardial biopsies can diagnose myocardial involvement [9].

Pericarditis, the most common of the rheumatoid cardiac manifestations with an incidence of approximately 50% by autopsy studies, rarely causes impairment of left ventricular function. However, constrictive pericarditis or a large pericardial effusion may compromise cardiac output and require pericardial aspiration or pericardiectomy.

Pericardial effusions generally respond to administration of 30 to 40 mg/d of prednisone over a several-week period. Pericardiocentesis should be performed early if tamponade is suspected or if there is a question of septic or suppurative pericarditis. In cases of constrictive pericarditis, pericardiectomy is the only effective therapy.

The myocardium may be affected by granulomatous inflammation, interstitial myocarditis, and coronary artery vasculitis. Cardiac conduction abnormalities, including complete heart block, may develop as a result of rheumatoid nodules. The heart block tends to occur in patients with severe, erosive, nodular-forming disease and is generally permanent. Coronary arteritis and amyloidosis are less common causes of heart block.

Arteritis in the rheumatoid patient may affect the coronary arteries and aorta, resulting in myocardial infarction, dilatation of the aortic root, and aortic valvular insufficiency, respectively.

Endocardial involvement is generally a result of granulomatous inflammation that may affect all four valves. Aortic valvular insufficiency is well documented. Mitral and tricuspid disease so severe as to cause symptoms is very rare.

SCLERODERMA

Systemic sclerosis (scleroderma) is a generalized disorder of connective tissue characterized by fibrosis and vascular obliteration. Cardiac involvement (Table 1) may be primary or secondary to involvement of other organ systems and, together with renal disease, is the leading cause of early death [10]. Cardiac disease in systemic sclerosis may also be secondary to other organ system involvement, such as malignant hypertension, uremia, and cor pulmonale as a result of severe pulmonary hypertension or severe interstitial lung disease.

Pericardial disease, although common at autopsy, is not often recognized clinically. Pericardial involvement presents most commonly as an indolent chronic pericardial effusion of variable size in an asymptomatic patient or in one who may have nonspecific findings such as chest pain, dyspnea, and cardiomegaly or symptoms of congestive heart failure. Chronic pericardial effusions may be a premonitory indicator of the development of renal failure within 6 months. Less commonly, pericardial disease may occur as an acute inflammatory process with dyspnea, chest pain, fever, and pericardial friction rub.

Asymptomatic pericardial disease usually does not predict a poor clinical course in contrast to symptomatic involvement.

Pericardial tamponade may occur but is thought to be uncommon. Constrictive and restrictive pericarditis have been reported but appear to be extremely rare.

Involvement of the myocardium, specifically focal myocardial fibrosis, has been found in autopsied scleroderma patients, but clinically evident disease occurs much less frequently. Vasospasm of the coronary microvasculature may be the primary etiology [11]. In patients with the CREST (calcinosis, Raynaud's disease, esophageal dysfunction, sclerodactyly, telangiectasia) variant of scleroderma, resting right ventricular function is abnormal more commonly than in generalized scleroderma (systemic sclerosis) and is usually secondary to pulmonary vascular disease.

Conduction and electrocardiogram abnormalities in systemic sclerosis are common and diverse. The electrocardiogram is normal in approximately 50% of patients. Only 10% of patients had electrocardiogram infarct patterns, most commonly in the septal region. Low-voltage and nonspecific ST segment abnormalities are the most common electrocardiogram disturbances. Ventricular conduction abnormalities occur in approximately 2% to 5% of systemic sclerosis patients. Infarcts and conduction disease also are thought to be caused by diffuse myocardial fibrosis. These abnormalities may lead to complete heart block or asystole. Thus, myocardial fibrosis and thallium perfusion abnormalities are common in patients with systemic sclerosis, but global left ventricular function is usually maintained. Ventricular arrhythmias are the primary cause of sudden death in up to 60% of patients.

Diagnosis

Because of the frequency of subclinical cardiac involvement and the high cardiac mortality in patients with systemic sclerosis, baseline cardiac evaluation should be performed in all newly diagnosed patients, including ambulatory 24-hour electrocardiogram monitoring, electrocardiograms, and radionucleotide imaging (thallium perfusion scans). If patients have symptoms suggestive of coronary artery disease, cardiac catheterization should be considered to evaluate for coexistent atherosclerosis.

Treatment

Treatment of cardiac manifestations of systemic sclerosis and CREST remains somewhat empiric but should be directed at the specific symptoms or problems. Angiotensin-converting enzyme inhibitors or calcium channel blockers should be used to manage hypertension. Angina resulting from coronary vasospasm may respond to calcium channel blockers. Angina secondary to coronary artery disease should be treated as it is for non–systemic sclerosis patients. Symptomatic pericardial effusions usually respond to nonsteroidal antiinflammatory agents, but corticosteroids are occasionally required. Drugs that can exacerbate underlying conduction disturbances should be avoided. Because of a possible increased mortality associated with use of antiarrhythmic agents, systemic sclerosis patients so treated should be monitored closely with repeated ambulatory electrocardiograms.

Polymyositis and Dermatomyositis

Cardiac abnormalities in polymyositis and dermatomyositis (Table 1) have been identified in as many as 40% of patients, perhaps more commonly in dermatomyositis. Only approximately 15% of patients have symptomatic cardiac involvement. Some have suggested that cardiac disease is an important prognostic factor in polymyositis and dermatomyositis [12].

The electrocardiogram is abnormal in 25% to 100% of patients. The most common abnormalities are nonspecific ST-T wave changes, atrioventricular block, and axis deviation. Rarely, complete heart block requiring permanent pacemaker implantation may occur. Abnormal Q waves resembling myocardial infarction may occur without underlying coronary artery disease. Arrhythmias occur less frequently.

Congestive heart failure may occur either as a result of the disease or secondary to hypertension associated with long-term corticosteroid therapy. Myocarditis has been found at autopsy in some patients with histories of congestive heart failure as well as in patients who have not had congestive heart failure prior to death. Myocardial fibrosis has not been a common histologic finding.

Studies of coronary arteries have shown vasculitis, arteritis obliterans, and angiographically normal vessels despite ischemic changes on the electrocardiogram. Coexistent atherosclerotic disease also may be found.

The diagnostic evaluation of patients with polymyositis and dermatomyositis should include a baseline electrocardiogram, creatine phosphokinase with MB fraction, and echocardiogram. It is not clear if 24-hour ambulatory electrocardiogram monitoring should be performed as a screening study in all newly diagnosed patients or only those with symptoms of rhythm disturbances. Persistent elevation of creatine phosphokinase-MB despite normal skeletal muscle strength may indicate ongoing myocarditis and should prompt further noninvasive testing such as thallium perfusion scanning.

There are no controlled trials that specifically evaluate treatment of cardiac disease in polymyositis and dermatomyositis. High-dose prednisone (60 to 80 mg/d) is usually required for at least 6 weeks at diagnosis, with tapering as indicated by clinical examination and muscle enzyme testing. Management of congestive heart failure, in addition to the conventional measures, may also require use of high-dose corticosteroids.

Vasculitis

The vasculitides are a group of disorders in which inflammation and necrosis of blood vessel walls result in organ system abnormalities caused by thrombosis and hemorrhage. Several forms of necrotizing systemic vasculitis may involve the heart. Kawasaki syndrome, which causes giant coronary artery aneurysms, occurs in children. Polyarteritis nodosa, Wegener's granulomatosis, and the Churg-Strauss syndrome may affect the heart and are discussed herein. Cardiac involvement in these disorders requires no special treatment.

Wegener's Granulomatosis

This relatively rare form of vasculitis shows cardiac involvement (Table 1) in up to 30% of untreated patients but in only 10% to 15% of those treated with cytotoxic agents. Coronary arteritis leading to myocardial infarction and pericarditis are the most common cardiac complications. Pericarditis often is symptomatic and may lead to tamponade. Any portion of the heart may be involved, leading to congestive heart failure, heart block, or arrhythmias, but these complications are much less common [13•].

Polyarteritis

Polyarteritis is a necrotizing vasculitis involving small and medium-sized muscular arteries. Cardiac involvement (Table 1) is observed in nearly 60% of patients in autopsy series but is often clinically silent. Congestive heart failure, pericarditis, myocardial infarction, and conduction abnormalities are the most common manifestations. Congestive heart failure may be caused by hypertension, which is seen in greater than 50% of patients, or by coronary insufficiency.

Churg-Strauss Syndrome

Also called allergic granulomatous angiitis, Churg-Strauss syndrome usually occurs in patients with a history of asthma or allergic rhinitis. The heart is a primary target organ (Table 1). Cardiac granulomas are commonly found at autopsy [13•]. Widespread myocardial damage may result from vasculitis affecting the coronary vessels. Cardiac disease may present as acute pericarditis, constrictive pericarditis, congestive heart failure, or myocardial infarction and accounts for approximately 50% of deaths of patients with Churg-Strauss syndrome. Electrocardiograms are abnormal in at least 50% of patients. Careful cardiovascular evaluation should be done early in patients with suspected Churg-Strauss syndrome because delayed treatment can lead to myocardial infarction and intractable congestive heart failure [13•].

Spondyloarthropathies

The seronegative spondyloarthropathies are a group of disorders that include ankylosing spondylitis, Reiter's syndrome or reactive arthritis, psoriatic arthritis, and the arthritis of inflammatory bowel disease (ulcerative colitis and regional enteritis, or Crohn's disease).

Cardiac involvement (Table 1) occurs in approximately 5% of individuals with ankylosing spondylitis, generally in patients with longstanding disease [14]. Inflammation of the aortic valve and root and of the atrioventricular node may cause aortic regurgitation and conduction abnormalities that may also occur in patients with Reiter's syndrome. Aortic valve fibrosis and thickening may be appreciated by echocardiography. Fibrosis extending to the interventricular system may cause complete heart block or milder forms of atrioventricular conduction abnormalities in 5% to 10% of men with ankylosing spondylitis. HLA-B27 has also been associated with isolated aortic regurgitation and with aortic regurgitation associated with severe conduction abnormalities. Subtle abnormalities of diastolic function have been found frequently in patients with ankylosing spondylitis.

Heart block and aortitis have been reported in up to 10% of individuals with severe, longstanding Reiter's syndrome. Conduction defects, such as P-R interval prolongation, second-degree block with Wenckebach's phenomenon, and complete heart block, may occur early in Reiter's syndrome [15].

Relapsing Polychondritis

Polychondritis is an episodic disorder of cartilage associated with inflammatory arthritis, aortitis, and inflammation of the aortic and mitral valves. It affects predominately middle-aged, white individuals, although cardiac involvement is more common in men.

Cardiac involvement (Table 1) occurs in 20% to 40% of patients and is the second most common cause of death, beyond respiratory tract involvement. Abnormalities include aortic insufficiency and mitral insufficiency and, less commonly, pericarditis, abnormal electrocardiograms, paroxysmal atrial tachycardia, cardiac ischemia, and the conduction abnormalities, including complete heart block [16].

Because cardiac involvement may be asymptomatic, some authors suggest baseline electrocardiograms, chest roentgenograms, and echocardiograms in all patients with relapsing polychondritis. If valvular disease is detected, the echocardiogram can be useful for follow-up.

Corticosteroids have been the mainstay of therapy, but immunosuppressives also have been used for organ-threatening, corticosteroid-resistant disease activity. Successful valvuloplasty and valve replacements have been reported, but valve dehiscence may occur as a result of persistent inflammation [17].

Connective Tissue Disease, Including Marfan Syndrome and Ehlers-Danlos Syndrome

Cardiovascular abnormalities associated with Marfan syndrome (Table 1) include aneurysmal dilatation of the ascending aorta, aortic valve insufficiency, coarctation of the aorta, mitral valve prolapse, mitral annulus calcification with mitral regurgitation, atrial and ventricular septal defects, tetralogy of Fallot, patent ductus arteriosus, and pulmonary artery aneurysms. Aneurysmal dilatation of the ascending aorta with rupture and aortic regurgitation are the causes of the shortened lifespan of 32 years in patients with Marfan syndrome. Annual echocardiographic monitoring is recommended until the aorta exceeds 50% of normal for body surface area, at which time echocardiographic monitoring should be done every 6 months. Management of aortic dilatation in Marfan syndrome includes β-blockade, specifically propranolol, and avoidance of vigorous activity. Pregnancy appears to be safe if aortic dilatation is not present. Surgical intervention with aortic grafting repair has proved beneficial when aortic dilatation reaches 6 cm [18].

Cardiovascular abnormalities in patients with Ehlers-Danlos syndrome (Table 1) include large artery aneurysms (the most serious manifestation of the syndrome), atrial septic defects, aortic valve insufficiency, ventricular papillary muscle dysfunction, dextrocardia, and conduction abnormalities. In patients with type IV Ehlers-Danlos syndrome, the so-called "vascular" or "ecchymotic" type, death generally occurs within the first two decades of life because of rupture of major arteries and gastrointestinal bleeding. Tetralogy of Fallot, peripheral pulmonary stenosis, bifid pulmonary artery, and dextrocardia also have been reported [19].

Mitral valve prolapse is a fairly common cardiac manifestation of both Marfan syndrome and Ehlers-Danlos syndrome. Therefore, patients with mitral valve prolapse should be evaluated clinically for these diseases.

Amyloidosis

The heart is a common site of amyloid deposition in both systemic and localized forms of amyloidosis (Table 5). Cardiac involvement is universally present in primary and myeloma-associated amyloidosis and is a major cause of death [20]. Amyloid also frequently affects the hearts of individuals with familial-hereditary amyloidosis but rarely occurs in those with secondary amyloidosis.

The primary manifestations of amyloid heart disease are cardiomegaly and low-output congestive heart failure. Cardiac

TABLE 5 COMPARISONS OF CARDIAC AMYLOIDOSIS IN PRIMARY AMYLOID VERSUS SENILE CARDIAC AMYLOID		
	Heart in primary amyloid ($n = 21$)	**Senile cardiac amyloid ($n = 26$)**
Cardiac amyloid deposits	Higher grade deposits, perifiber and mixed, frequent vascular involvement	Lower grade deposits, predominantly nodular distribution pattern, infrequent vascular involvement
Mean age of patients, y	57.6	83
Male-to-female ratio	1.6:1	5.5:1
Congestive heart failure, %	76	35
Pseudoinfarction electrocardiogram findings, %	45	Uncommon
Sudden death, %	33	19

Data from Smith *et al.* [20]; with permission.

amyloidosis also may present as constrictive pericarditis, restrictive cardiomyopathy, cardiac conduction disorders, and arrhythmias and may simulate ischemic heart disease with typical or atypical angina and "pseudoinfarct" electrocardiogram findings [20]. The diagnosis of amyloid heart disease should be considered in elderly individuals with heart disease of unknown etiology, particularly in those without atherosclerosis and valvular heart disease, and in patients in their fifth and sixth decades of life who have multisystem disease consistent with systemic amyloidosis and have the previously mentioned cardiac presentations.

Intractable heart failure may be the first manifestation and the cause of death in systemic amyloidosis. Amyloid is deposited diffusely in the myocardium but also may involve the pericardium, endocardium, and heart valves. The atrioventricular valves are more commonly involved than the pulmonary and aortic valves [20]. Murmurs are present occasionally.

Pericardial effusions are rare, but signs of constrictive pericarditis or restrictive myocardiopathy may develop. Pericardial involvement tends to occur in patients with high-grade amyloid deposits [20]. The demonstration of left ventricular diastolic pressures greater than those on the right helps to distinguish restrictive cardiomyopathy from constrictive pericarditis.

Ischemic heart disease secondary to amyloid deposition in intramyocardial arteries occurs in less than 2% of patients. Electrocardiograms may reveal the pattern of anteroseptal infarction in the absence of evidence of infarction at autopsy.

Amyloid deposits in the sinus node or fibrosis of the conduction system may cause rhythm disturbances in both patients with primary amyloid and senile cardiac amyloid [20]. Amyloid-induced neuropathy resulting in orthostatic hypotension may also cause dizziness, light-headedness, or syncope in the patient with amyloid heart disease.

Various invasive and noninvasive procedures are used to evaluate for cardiac amyloidosis. Echocardiograms may reveal thick-walled ventricles with normal or reduced-sized cavities. Left ventricular diastolic abnormalities are detectable by echocardiography even prior to development of clinically apparent amyloid heart disease. Ejection fractions may be normal despite significant heart failure, reflecting impaired cardiac relaxation (impaired diastolic function). Two-dimensional echocardiograms may reveal "granular sparkling." Diffuse uptake of 99m pyrophosphate may reflect the severity of myocardial Tc2 amyloid infiltration. Endomyocardial biopsy is the only definitive means of detecting amyloid deposits in the heart [20].

The median survival after diagnosis of primary or multiple myeloma-associated amyloid is approximately 12 months, with median survival of only 6 months from the onset of congestive heart failure in those with cardiac involvement. Of patients with primary amyloid, cardiac disease is reported to be the cause of death in 30% to 50% and is probably underreported [20]. The three variables of congestive heart failure, amount of weight loss, and presence of monoclonal light chains in urine predict poor outcome.

Although there is no specific therapy for amyloidosis, treatment of a predisposing disease may be useful. Alkylating agents have been used to treat primary amyloidosis, but they do not reverse the disease. Colchicine prevents acute febrile attacks in familial Mediterranean fever and retards amyloid deposition and further renal function deterioration in these individuals. Colchicine also may prolong survival in patients with primary amyloid.

Congestive heart failure secondary to amyloid heart disease should be treated with salt restriction and judicious use of diuretics. Hypovolemia should be avoided because ventricular filling may be compromised secondary to of ventricular wall stiffening. Postural hypotension also may result from volume depletion secondary to decreased fluid intake or protein–osmotic diuresis, adrenal insufficiency, autonomic neuropathy, and low-output cardiac failure. Mineralocorticoids, elastic stockings, treatment of malabsorption, and fluid supplementation are supportive therapies. Great care should be used when treating with digitalis because of the risk of conduction abnormalities and arrhythmias in patients with cardiac amyloid.

REFERENCES AND RECOMMENDED READING

Recently published papers of particular interest have been highlighted as

- Of interest
- Of outstanding interest

1. Shulman ST, Kaplan EL, Bisno AL, *et al.*: Jones criteria (revised) for guidance in the diagnosis of rheumatic fever. *Circulation* 1984, 69:203A–208A.

2. Gaasch WH: Guidelines for the diagnosis of rheumatic fever. *JAMA* 1992, 268:2069–2073.

3. Berrios X, del Campo E, Guzman B, *et al.*: Discontinuing rheumatic fever prophylaxis in selected adolescents and young adults. *Ann Intern Med* 1993, 118:401–406.

4.• Nagi KS, Joshi R, Thakur, RF: Cardiac manifestations of Lyme disease: a review. *Canadian J Cardiol* 1996, 12:503–506.

5. Sigal LH: Early disseminated Lyme disease: cardiac manifestations. *Amer J Med* 1995, 98:25S–29S.

6. De Inocencio J, Lovell DJ: Cardiac function in systemic lupus erythematosus. *J Rheumatol* 1994, 21:2147–2156.

7. Hojnik M, George J, Ziporen L, *et al.*: Heart valve involvement (Libman-Sacks endocarditis) in the antiphospholipid syndrome. *Circulation* 1996, 93:1579–1587.

8. Harris ED Jr: Clinical features of rheumatoid arthritis. In *Textbook of Rheumatology*, edn 4. Edited by Kelly WN, Harris ED Jr, Ruddy S, Sledge CB. Philadelphia: WB Saunders; 1993:898–900.

9. Carrao S, Salli L, Arnone S, *et al.*: Cardiac involvement in rheumatoid arthritis: evidence of silent heart disease. *Eur Heart J* 1995, 16:253–256.

10. Follansbee WP, Zerbe TR, Medsger TA, Jr: Cardiac and skeletal muscle disease in systemic sclerosis (scleroderma): A high risk association. *Am Heart J* 1993, 125:194–203.

11. Steen VD, Follansbee WP, Conte CG, *et al.*: Thallium perfusion defects predict subsequent cardiac dysfunction in patients with systemic sclerosis. *Arthritis Rheum* 1996, 39:677–681.

12. Hochberg MC, Feldman D, Stevens MB: Adult onset polymyositis/dermatomyositis: an analysis of clinical and laboratory features and survival in 76 patients with a review of the literature. *Semin Arthritis Rheum* 1986, 15:168–178.

13.• Goodfield NE, Bhandari S, Plant WD, *et al.*: Cardiac involvement in Wegener's granulomatosis. *Br Heart J* 1995, 73:110–115.

14. Arnett FC: Seronegative spondyloarthropathies. *Bull Rheum Dis* 1987, 37:1–12.

15. Dier T, Rosencrance JG, Chillag SA: Cardiac conduction manifestations of Reiter's syndrome. *South Med J* 1991, 84:799–800.

16. Bowness P, Hawley IC, Morris T, *et al.*: Complete heart block and severe aortic incompetence in relapsing polychondritis: clinicopathologic findings. *Arthritis Rheum* 1991, 34:97–100.

17. Lan-Lazdunski L, Hvass U, Paillole C, *et al.*: Cardiac valve replacement in relapsing polychondritis. A review. *J Heart Valve Dis* 1995, 4:277–235.

18. Gott VL, Pyeritz RE, Magovern GJ, *et al.*: Surgical treatment of aneurysms of the ascending aorta in the Marfan syndrome: results of composite-graft repair in 50 patients. *N Engl J Med* 1986, 314:1070–1074.

19. Leier CV, Call TD, Fulkerson PK, *et al.*: The spectrum of cardiac defects in the Ehlers-Danlos syndrome. *Ann Intern Med* 1980, 92:171–178.

20. Smith JT, Kyle RA, Lie JT: Clinical significance of histopathologic patterns of cardiac amyloidosis. *Mayo Clin Proc* 1984, 59:574–555.

SELECT BIBLIOGRAPHY

Askari AD, Huetter TL: Cardiac abnormalities in polymyositis/dermatomyositis. *Semin Arthritis Rheum* 1982, 12:208–219.

Bergfeldt L: HLA-B27 associated rheumatic diseases with severe cardiac bradyarrhythmias. *Am J Med* 1983, 75:210–215.

Buyon JP: Neonatal lupus syndromes. *Curr Opin Rheumatol* 1994, 6:523–529.

Dubrey S, Mendes L, Skinner M, *et al.*: Resolution of heart failure in patients with AL amyloidosis. *Ann Intern Med* 1996, 125:482–484.

Evans J: Lyme disease. *Curr Opin Rheumatol* 1994, 6:415–422.

Feldman T: Rheumatic heart disease. *Curr Opin Cardiol* 1996, 11:126–130.

Galve E, Ordi J, Barquinero J, *et al.*: Valvular heart disease in the primary antiphospholipid syndrome. *Ann Intern Med* 1992, 16:293–298.

Grant SCD, Levy RD, Venning MC, *et al.*: Wegener's granulomatosis and the heart. *Br Heart J* 1994, 71:82–86.

Khamashta MA, Hughes GRU: Antiphospholipid antibodies and valve disease in patients with systemic lupus erythematosus [letter]. *J Am Coll Cardiol* 1993, 22:1269–1270.

Narang R, Chopra P, Wasir HS: Cardiac amyloidosis presenting as ischemic heart disease. A case report and review of literature. *Cardiology* 1993, 82:294–300.

O'Neill TW, King G, Graham IM, *et al.*: Echocardiographic abnormalities in ankylosing spondylitis. *Ann Rheum Dis* 1992, 51:652–654.

Renaldini E, Spandrio S, Cerudelli B, *et al.*: Cardiac involvement in Churg-Strauss syndrome: A follow-up of three cases. *Eur Heart J* 1993, 14:1712–1716.

Roldan CA, Crawford M: Reply [letter]. *J Am Coll Cardiol* 1993, 22:1269–1270.

Steers AC, Grodzicki RL, Kornblatt AN, *et al.*: The spirochete etiology of Lyme disease. *N Engl J Med* 1983, 308:733–740.

Veasy LG, Wiedmeier SE, Orsmond GS, *et al.*: Resurgence of acute rheumatic fever in the intermountain area of the United States. *N Engl J Med* 1987, 316:421–426.

The Aging Heart 44
J. V. Nixon

Key Points
- Morphologic, physiologic, and cellular changes in the cardiovascular system are associated with the normal aging process.
- The prevalence of cardiovascular disease processes, including chronic ischemic heart disease, acute myocardial infarction, hypertension, arrhythmias, and valvular heart disease, changes with age.
- Medical therapy should be focused on cardiovascular risk factor modification as well as preservation of cardiac preload, heart rate, and contractility.
- The value of surgical or interventional therapy must be assessed for age.

Clinical assessment of the older cardiovascular patient must incorporate a series of unique variables. Aging is accompanied by changes in the cardiovascular system [1]. Furthermore, lifestyle impacts the extent and rate of these cardiovascular changes. Thus, in the general aging population, the assessment of changes in cardiovascular function must encompass changes in lifestyle and disease prevalence as well as alterations caused by aging [2•].

CHANGES IN CARDIAC ANATOMY AND PHYSIOLOGY

Aging is associated with a gradual increase in cardiac weight, principally in left ventricular mass and wall thickness [3] (Table 1). Aortic root dilatation and left atrial enlargement have been demonstrated. Importantly, left ventricular volumes remain unchanged. Furthermore, there is an age-related decline in vascular endothelial function [4]. Experimental studies have shown that an increase in collagen-tissue laydown with a diffuse development of fibrous tissue as well as an increase in myocardial cell size are associated with the age-related cardiac hypertrophy [5] (Fig. 1). These data generally agree with morphologic and biopsy studies in older patients [6]. In addition, several experimental studies have documented the myocardial cellular changes associated with aging (Table 2).

Details of functional changes in the aging cardiovasculature of humans are limited by the suitability of the population selected, the lifestyle of such a study population, and the utility of noninvasive diagnostic technologies with specific self-imposed limitations. Nevertheless, systolic function is maintained both at rest and during exercise [7] (Fig. 2). The response of heart rate to exercise is attenuated in the elderly. Thus, during exercise, the older heart compensates for the attenuated heart-rate response by increasing end-diastolic and stroke volumes to preserve cardiac output [7]. The increased left ventricular wall mass serves to maintain a normal wall stress in the presence of increased left ventricular volumes during exercise. When exercise responses of older men are compared with those of women, both sexes show parallel declines in peak exercise performance with age despite an overall higher exercise capacity in men. Only men show an age-related decrease in cardiac volumes at rest and exercise; cardiac index and ejection fraction declined equally with age in both sexes [8]. Also,

TABLE 1 AGE-RELATED CHANGES IN CARDIAC ANATOMY

Experimental studies

Myocardial hypertrophy
Individual cellular enlargement
Increased collagen
Increased fibrous tissue

Human studies

Increased left ventricular mass
Increased interventricular septal and posterior left ventricular wall thickness
Left atrial enlargement
Aortic root dilatation

TABLE 2 AGE-RELATED CHANGES IN CARDIAC PHYSIOLOGY

Experimental studies

Prolonged calcium transient
Prolonged transmembrane potential
Prolonged contraction duration
Prolonged relaxation
Increased resting and dynamic stiffness
Diminished responses to digitalis glycosides, norepinephrine, and isoproterenol

Human studies

Increased left ventricular wall mass
Increased left ventricular stroke volume during exercise
Decreased diastolic stiffness
Decreased diastolic filling

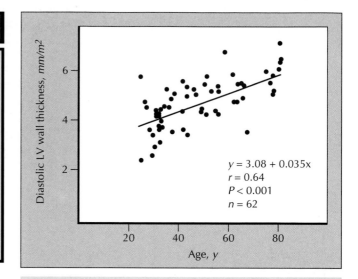

FIGURE 1 Linear regression plot showing the relation between increased age and increased diastolic left ventricular (LV) wall thickness in male participants in the Baltimore Longitudinal Aging Population. (*From* Gerstenblith *et al.* [3]; with permission.)

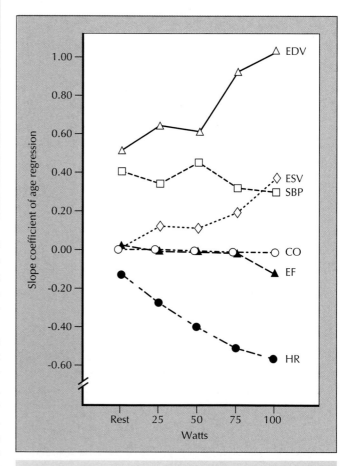

FIGURE 2 The slopes of the regression functions of age for end-diastolic volume (EDV), end-systolic volume (ESV), systolic blood pressure (SBP), cardiac output (CO), ejection fraction (EF), and heart rate (HR) at rest and increasing incremental workloads from 25 to 100 W during dynamic exercise in the Baltimore Longitudinal Aging Population. (*From* Rodeheffer *et al.* [7]; with permission.)

the attenuated chronotropic and inotropic responses and the cardiac dilatation associated with dynamic exercise in the elderly is due to the age-related blunting of β-adrenergic responsiveness [9]. Furthermore, this increasing stiffness with age does not appear to be slowed or reversed by dynamic training programs or by prolonged endurance training [10–12].

Although the altered diastolic function or compliance clearly shown in experimental studies is difficult to document accurately in humans by noninvasive methods, several noninvasive parameters of diastolic filling have consistently been shown to be altered with age [10]. Both Doppler echocardiographic and radionuclide techniques show the reduction in early rapid diastolic filling and the increased dependence on atrial contraction seen with aging (Figs. 3, 4, and 5). These findings reflect the increased stiffness associated with the morphologic changes of the aging heart.

AGING AND CARDIOVASCULAR DISEASE

Table 3 summarizes the changes that occur in the cardiovascular system with aging. Any treatment algorithm in an older cardiovascular patient has many branches. In the older patient, prevalence of the disease process and any unique forms of presentation must be considered. The value of surgical or interventional therapy must be assessed for age. Furthermore, medical therapy is directed at the preservation of cardiac preload, heart rate, and contractility, emphasizing controlled afterload reduction as an option.

CHRONIC ISCHEMIC HEART DISEASE

Prevalence

The prevalence of atherosclerotic heart disease increases significantly with age; more than 50% of people older than 65 years of age die from the effects of coronary artery disease

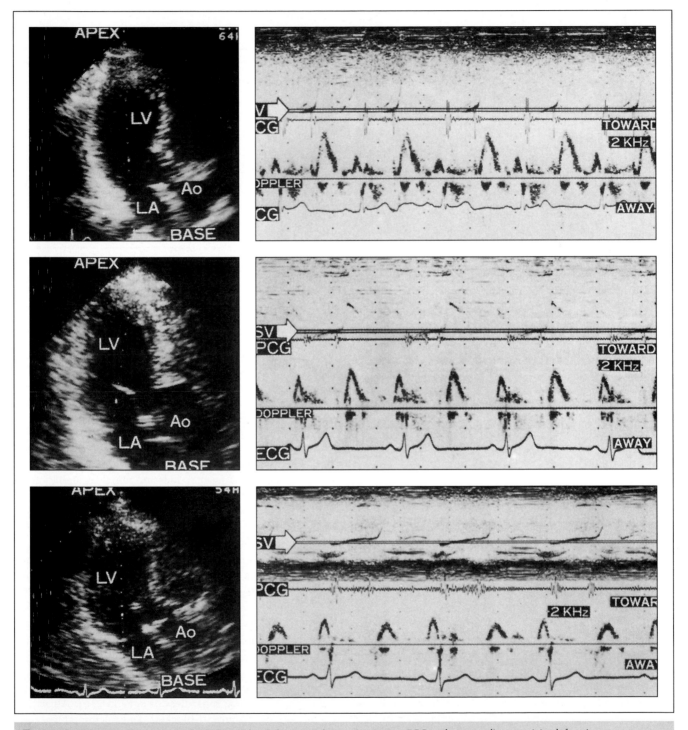

FIGURE 3 Changes in Doppler echocardiographic left ventricular (LV) diastolic filling patterns in normal subjects. **Top**, A 26-year-old man. **Middle**, A 48-year-old man. **Lower**, A 59-year-old man.

Ao—aorta; ECG—electrocardiogram; LA—left atrium; PCE—phonocardiogram; SV—sample volume. (*From* Miyatake *et al.* [37]; with permission.)

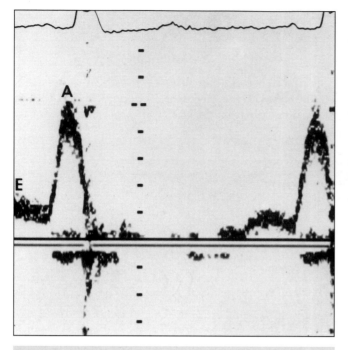

FIGURE 4 Doppler echocardiographic left ventricular diastolic filling pattern in an elderly patient with hypertension showing slow deceleration of the E wave, prolonged deceleration time, prominent A wave, and altered E:A ratio. (*From* Shah and Pai [38]; with permission.)

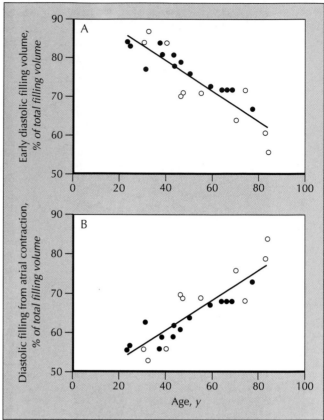

FIGURE 5 The relative contribution of early diastolic filling (**A**) and atrial contraction (**B**) to left ventricular filling as assessed by Doppler echocardiography in healthy men (*closed circles*) and women (*open circles*) ranging from 20 to 80 years of age. (*From* Lakatta [39]; with permission.)

TABLE 3 PHYSIOLOGIC IMPLICATIONS OF AGE-RELATED CHANGES IN CARDIOVASCULAR SYSTEM

Central effects

Preload	Attenuated
Contractility	Not attenuated
Heart rate	Attenuated at all levels of exercise
Afterload	Not attenuated

Peripheral effects

Decreased vascular distensibility

Decreased β-adrenergic responsiveness

[2••]. Furthermore, the prevalence of diagnosed coronary disease in this age group is only 30% to 50% of the prevalence of significant disease found at autopsy.

Thus, the recommendation of categories of therapeutic agents such as calcium channel–blocking agents, angiotensin-converting enzyme inhibitors, and α-adrenergic blocking agents occurs for the management of such common cardiovascular diseases in the older patient as ischemic heart disease, congestive heart failure, and hypertension (Table 4).

Diagnosis

Because of an age-related, altered lifestyle, including a decline in physical activity, presenting symptoms are often different than with younger patients. As a manifestation of systolic or diastolic dysfunction, dyspnea is a more prominent symptom than pain, which is usually a manifestation of physical exertion. Also, silent myocardial ischemia is more prevalent in older patients [13]. Added heart sounds and mitral regurgitation are normal variants related to age. Exercise stress testing may be of limited value in older patients because of their altered physical capability and the increased incidence of resting ST-segment electrocardiogram abnormalities. Thus, stress-imaging techniques, both stress echocardiography and stress thallium perfusion, and in particular pharmacologic stress-imaging technology, may be more productive in older patients [14].

Therapy

Appropriate management of risk factors, particularly hypertension therapy and smoking cessation, applies at all ages [2••]. Recent data show the benefits of lipid-lowering agents in hypercholesterolemic patients and estrogen therapy in postmenopausal women, regardless of age [15•,16]. All antiischemic agents, nitrates, β-blockers, and calcium antagonists are effective in older patients. Therapy is more favorably directed at afterload reduction, however, which is effectively performed by dihydropyridine calcium antagonists. Concomitant consideration of the higher prevalence of silent ischemia in these patients suggests the selection of controlled or

Clinical variables	Diuretic	α-blocker	ACE inhibitor	β-blocker	Calcium antagonist
Volume depletion	+	–	–	–	–
Suppression of heart rate	–	–	–	+	±
Suppression of cardiac output	–	–	–	+	±
Regression of LVH	–	+	+	±	+
Suppression of VEA	–	–	–	+	+
Preservation of renal function	+	–	+	–	+
Regression of atherosclerosis	–	±	–	±	+
Improved lipid profile	–	±	±	±	±
Effective with low PRA	+	+	–	–	+

+—variable associated with this class of drug; - —variable not associated with this class of drug; ±—variable associated with this class of drug in some cases, but not in others; ACE—angiotensin-converting enzyme; LVH—left ventricular hypertrophy; PRA—plasma renin activity; VEA—ventricular ectopic activity.
From Nixon [26]; with permission.

TABLE 5 RESULTS OF CORONARY ANGIOPLASTY IN THE ELDERLY

	Older (> 65 y)*	Younger (< 65 y)†
Total series		
Primary success	98 (81%)	412 (80%)
Mean CSA stenosis	92 → 35	87 → 15
Gradient, *mm Hg*	41 → 8	57 → 15
Last 200 cases	43	157
Primary success	40 (93%)	142 (90%)
Major complications		
Emergency CABG	5 (4.1%)	24 (4.7%)
MI (Q wave)	3 (2.5%)	15 (2.9%)
Death	1 (0.8%)	0

*n=121.
†n=518.
CABG—coronary artery bypass surgery; CSA—cross-sectional area; MI—myocardial infarction.
From Raisner *et al.* [17]; with permission.

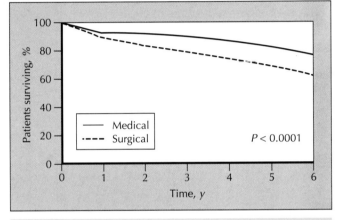

FIGURE 6 Cumulative 6-year survival in surgical and medical groups among 1491 patients 65 years of age or older from the Coronary Artery Surgery Study (CASS) registry. Survival is adjusted for left ventricular wall motion, congestive heart failure, number of diseased vessels, and associated medical diseases, and age at angiography. (*From* Gersch *et al.* [18]; with permission.)

sustained-release preparations or those with a prolonged intrinsic half-life to maintain constant therapeutic plasma levels. Percutaneous transluminal coronary angioplasty is a therapeutic option in older patients in whom low mortality rates persist regardless of age [17] (Table 5). Data from the Coronary Artery Surgery Study (CASS) show increased intra-operative mortality and morbidity rates in older patients after bypass surgery, yet long-term survival and pain relief are compatible with results in younger patients (Fig. 6) [18].

ACUTE MYOCARDIAL INFARCTION

Prevalence

The increased prevalence of coronary atherosclerosis was discussed in the previous section.

Diagnosis

The diagnostic methods used in younger patients are equally accurate in older patients. Presenting symptoms may be altered by age. Older patients with acute myocardial infarction may present more often with dyspnea or arrhythmias rather than chest pain (Table 6).

Therapy

Mortality and morbidity rates are higher in older patients [2••]. These higher rates may be age-related, caused by the higher prevalence of ischemic heart disease, or they may be caused by the greater frequency of concomitant diseases, particularly hypertension. Results vary among trials of throm-bolytic therapies in older patients with acute myocardial infarction, although recent data show lower mortality rates in the treated groups. Contraindications to thrombolytic therapy

TABLE 6 PRESENTING SYMPTOMS OF ACUTE MYOCARDIAL INFARCTION IN ELDERLY PATIENTS

	Patients, %		
Symptoms	**65–74 y**	**75–84 y**	**> 85 y**
Chest pain	78	60	38
Dyspnea	41	44	43
Sweating	34	23	14
Syncope	3	18	18
Confusion	3	8	19
Stroke	2	7	7

From Reeder and Gersch [40]; with permission.

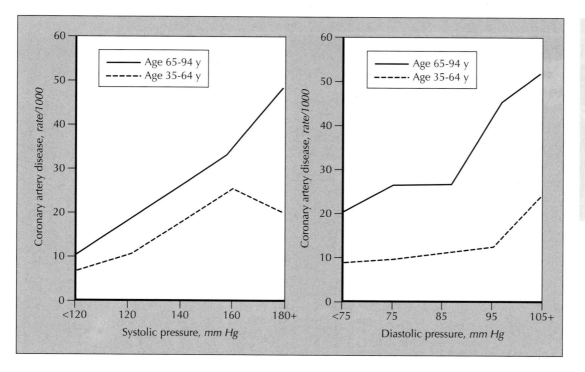

FIGURE 7
Biennial rate of coronary artery disease according to blood pressure and relation to age for men in the Framingham Study. (*From* Levy *et al.* [41]; with permission.)

increase with age. Secondary prophylactic therapy with β-blockers, angiotensin-converting enzyme inhibitors, and lipid-lowering agents are equally effective in older and younger patients who have had myocardial infarction [15•,19,20].

HYPERTENSION

Prevalence

Although prevalence of both systolic and diastolic hypertension in the elderly is not as high as previously thought,the third Natioinal Health and Nutrition Examination reported an incidence of hypertension of 54% in patients 65 to 74 years old [21, 22]. Antihypertensive therapy significantly reduces mortality and morbidity in patients over the age of 65 years [23]. Systolic and diastolic hypertension remain significant independent cardiovascular risk factors for both mortality and morbidity (Fig. 7) [24]. Furthermore, the prevalence of associated left ventricular hypertrophy

compounds substantially the cardiovascular risk [25]. Identification of pseudohypertension in this age group also significantly reduces the frequency of the diagnosis of hypertension [26] (Fig. 8).

Diagnosis

Recent data provide suitable endpoints above or below which the mortality and morbidity risk of the disease significantly increases. Recently, the Systolic Hypertension in the Elderly Program (SHEP) showed that morbidity rates are reduced when patients older than 60 years with isolated systolic hypertension above 160 mm Hg are treated with diuretics [27] (Fig. 9). Also, Cruickshank and coworkers [28] report increased coronary events when diastolic pressures are lowered below a J point of 85 to 90 mm Hg (Fig. 10).

Therapy

As stated above, effective management of hypertension improves survival and decreases cardiovascular morbidity in the

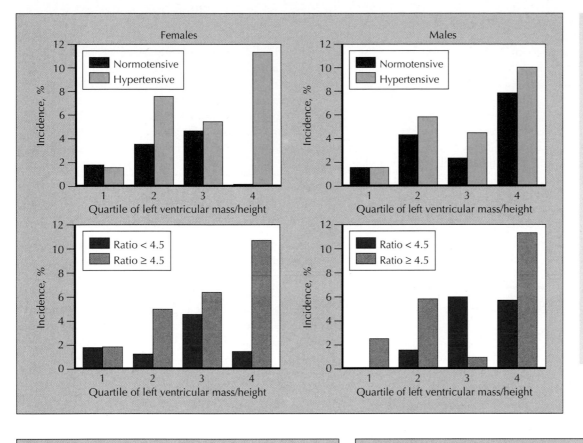

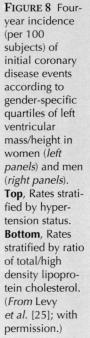

FIGURE 8 Four-year incidence (per 100 subjects) of initial coronary disease events according to gender-specific quartiles of left ventricular mass/height in women (*left panels*) and men (*right panels*). **Top**, Rates stratified by hypertension status. **Bottom**, Rates stratified by ratio of total/high density lipoprotein cholesterol. (*From* Levy *et al.* [25]; with permission.)

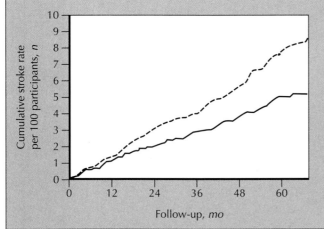

FIGURE 9 Cumulative fatal plus nonfatal stroke rate per 100 participants in the active treatment (*solid line*) and placebo (*broken line*) groups during the Systolic Hypertension in the Elderly Program (SHEP). (*From* SHEP Cooperative Research Group [27]; with permission.)

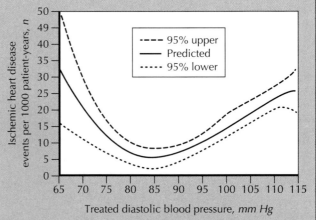

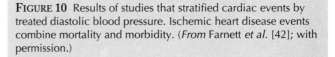

FIGURE 10 Results of studies that stratified cardiac events by treated diastolic blood pressure. Ischemic heart disease events combine mortality and morbidity. (*From* Farnett *et al.* [42]; with permission.)

elderly [23]. Recommended nonpharmacologic modalities include dietary modifications, weight loss, consistent exercise, sodium restrictions, and reduction in alcohol consumption [29]. Pharmacologic therapy may be more favorably directed in the older patient by maintaining cardiac preload, heart rate, and contractility, and by emphasizing the suitability of after-load reduction. Also, both contraindications to and the adverse effects of all medications are more frequent in older patients. Furthermore, certain therapies are better suited to the older patient. Diuretics effectively reduce morbidity rates in older

patients with systolic hypertension [25]. Their less desirable characteristics include their primary physiologic effect on cardiac preload and their potential for precipitating hypokalemic arrhythmias, particularly in the presence of left ventricular hypertrophy [26].

The negative inotropic and chronotropic effects of β-blockers reduce their suitability in older patients, as does their tendency to suppress conduction system activity. Nevertheless, β-blockers are the optimal form of secondary prophylaxis after myocardial infarction in all age groups [19]. Also, the incidence of postural hypotension after application of primary vasodilators is higher in the elderly [26].

The dose response to an angiotensin-converting enzyme inhibitor may be lower in an older patient, because plasma renin activity levels are attenuated with age [26]. The incidence of adverse effects, such as coughing, and contraindications are higher in older patients. Nevertheless, recent studies show these compounds to be effective secondary agents in older patients with mild hypertension [29]. Calcium antagonists, particularly dihydropyridenes, are the vasodilator of choice in patients with low renin activity. These compounds effectively induce regression of left ventricular hypertrophy. Furthermore, calcium antagonists may suppress ventricular arrhythmias in patients with left ventricular hypertrophy, improve abnormal diastolic function, and potentially regress atherosclerotic plaques [26, 29] (Table 4).

ARRHYTHMIAS

Prevalence

Arrhythmias occur with greater frequency in older cardiovascular patients because of their increased prevalence of coronary artery disease and hypertension; however, this increased prevalence of arrhythmias does not appear to be associated with increased mortality or morbidity [2••]. Also, bradyarrhythmias may occur with greater frequency in older patients because of the increased prevalence of nodal and conduction system disease [2••]. Atrial fibrillation is the most common supraventricular arrhythmia in patients over the age of 65 years [30]. It may precipitate or worsen congestive heart failure or ischemia and is associated with an increased incidence of stroke [2••, 16].

Diagnosis

Arrhythmias, particularly tachyarrhythmias, may have more profound hemodynamic manifestations in older patients because of age-related diastolic dysfunction, requiring a sustained diastolic filling period and a significant atrial contraction.

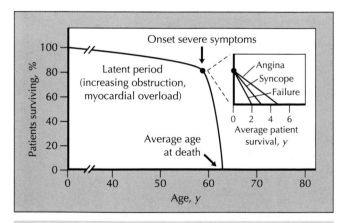

FIGURE 11 The natural history of aortic stenosis. (*From* Ross and Braunwald [43]; with permission.)

Therapy

As with other forms of cardiovascular therapy, the frequency of contraindications to and the adverse effects of antiarrhythmic drugs are greater in an older population. Sequential pacing is useful in older patients [2••]. Effective management of atrial fibrillation includes anticoagulation (if not contraindicated) and maintenance of normal sinus rhythm, if possible, with the consideration of flecainide, sotalol, or amiodarone [2••, 16].

VALVULAR DISEASE

Prevalence

As previously discussed, added heart sounds and systolic murmurs such as mitral regurgitation are normal variant findings in an elderly population. The cause and prevalence of valvular pathology in the elderly relates primarily to degenerative disease. Senile degeneration and calcification of the aortic valve renders aortic stenosis a disease of the sixth, seventh, and eighth decades [31] (Fig. 11). Although aortic regurgitation may result from a congenitally bicuspid valve, it is mainly a condition of middle rather than old age [32]. The diminishing incidence of rheumatic heart disease has resulted in a reducing prevalence of mitral stenosis among the older population. The prevalence of coexisting coronary artery disease is higher in this age population, which may impact both diagnosis and management.

Diagnosis

The clinical characteristics of different valvular diseases may be altered or suppressed by the presence of age-related characteristics that are normal variants. The clinical suspicion of coexistent valvular pathology in an older patient warrants careful assessment by Doppler echocardiography, which is capable of accurately quantifying valvular stenosis and estimating valvular regurgitation [33].

Therapy

In general, surgical intervention in the management of valvular heart disease is only affected by an increased intraoperative surgical risk and any concomitant age-related conditions such as coronary artery disease [2••,32]. The outcome after valve replacement for aortic stenosis and mitral stenosis does not appear to be impacted by age [32] (Fig. 12). Balloon aortic valvuloplasty is a therapeutic option in older patients with significant aortic stenosis; however, restenosis rates of up to 80% within 2 years leave questions of therapeutic efficacy [34]. Balloon mitral valvuloplasty appears to be a therapeutic option for a younger mitral stenosis patient as confirmed by experience and limitations imposed by a preoperative echocardiographic scoring system [32,33]. Clinical indications for valvular replacement in aortic regurgitation and mitral regurgitation also do not appear to be affected by age [32]; however, the same reservations regarding age-related concomitant diseases do apply.

Cardiology for the Primary Care Physician

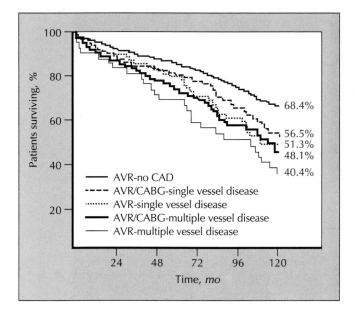

FIGURE 12 Late survival for patients undergoing isolated aortic valve replacement (AVR) and AVR plus coronary artery bypass grafting (CABG), grouped according to no coronary artery disease (CAD), single-vessel CAD, and multiple-vessel CAD. (*From* Lytle *et al.* [44]; with permission.)

Figure legend (within plot):
- AVR-no CAD
- AVR/CABG-single vessel disease
- AVR-single vessel disease
- AVR/CABG-multiple vessel disease
- AVR-multiple vessel disease

68.4%
56.5%
51.3%
48.1%
40.4%

CONGESTIVE HEART FAILURE

Prevalence

The prevalence of congestive heart failure as a manifestation of end-stage ischemic, hypertensive, or valvular heart disease is as high as two million patients in the United States, with an additional 400,000 being diagnosed each year [2••, 16]. Mortality is 50% within 5 years of the diagnosis [35]. Although the mortality associated with coronary disease and stroke has diminished in the last 20 years, it has continued to increase with congestive heart failure.

Diagnosis

When a patient is evaluated for congestive heart failure, it is necessary to determine whether the predominant component is systolic or diastolic dysfunction [2••, 16]. This differential diagnosis is optimally made by echocardiography. Predominant diastolic dysfunction with a normal ejection fraction is usually associated with hypertension and often occurs in conjunction with left ventricular hypertrophy. Systolic dysfunction with a depressed ejection fraction is often associated with ischemic heart disease or hypertension.

Management

A critical part of the management of congestive heart failure is management of the principal etiology. In addition, diastolic dysfunction and regression of increased left ventricular mass is optimally treated with long-acting calcium channel blocking agents or angiotensin-converting enzyme inhibitors [36]. Systolic dysfunction usually necessitates the use of several modalities: *eg*, the decreased neurohormonal activation and ventricular remodeling produced by an angiotensin-converting enzyme inhibitor, a diuretic, and digoxin.

DRUG USE IN THE OLDER PATIENT

Aging may influence the cardiovascular response to any drug, including any cardiovascular drug. The aging process also affects other organ systems, including the kidney and the liver, both of which are significantly involved in the metabolism and excretion of drugs. Because cardiovascular disease and the administration of cardiovascular agents is more prevalent in the elderly, drug heterogeneity of response, absorption rates, drug interactions, and associated system morbidity become important considerations in the appropriate therapeutic management of these older patients.

REFERENCES AND RECOMMENDED READING

Recently published papers of particular interest have been highlighted as:

• Of interest

•• Of outstanding interest

1. Nixon JV: Effects of aging on the heart. *Choices Cardiol* 1993, 7:119–120.

2.• Lakatta EG, Gerstenblith G, Weisfeldt ML: The aging heart: structure, function and disease. In *Heart Disease*, edn 5. Edited by Braunwald E. Philadelphia: WB Saunders; 1997:1687–1703.

3. Gerstenblith G, Fredrickson J, Yin FCP, *et al.*: Echocardiographic assessment of a normal adult aging population. *Circulation* 1977, 56:273.

4. Celemajer DS, Sorensen KE, Spiegelhalter DJ, *et al.*: Aging is associated with endothelial function in healthy men years before the age-related decline in women. *J Am Coll Cardiol* 1994, 24:471–476.

5. Lakatta EG: Alterations in the cardiovascular system that occur with advancing age. *Fed Proc* 1979, 38:163.

6. Unverforth DV, Fetter JK, Unverforth BJ, *et al.*: Human myocardial histologic characteristics in congestive heart failure. *Circulation* 1983, 68:1194.

7. Rodeheffer RJ, Gerstenblith G, Becker LC, *et al.*: Exercise cardiac output Is maintained with advancing age in healthy human subjects: cardiac dilatation and increased stroke volumes compensate for diminished heart rate. *Circulation* 1984, 69:203.

8. Fleg JL, O'Connor F, Gerstenblith G, *et al.*: Impact of age on the cardiovascular response to upright exercise in healthy men and women. *J Appl Physiol* 1995, 78:890–900.

9. Fleg JL, Schulman S, O'Connor F, *et al.*: Effects of acute beta-adrenergic receptor blockage on age-associated changes in cardiovascular performance during dynamic exercise. *Circulation* 1994, 90:2333–2341.

10. Nixon JV, Burns CA: Cardiac effects of aging and diastolic dysfunction in the elderly. In *Heart Failure and Left Ventricular Diastolic Dysfunction*, edn 1. Edited by Gaasch WH, LeWinter M. Philadelphia: Lea & Febiger; 1994:427–435.

11. Fleg JL, Shapiro EP, O'Connor F, *et al.*: Left ventricular filling performance in older male athletes. *JAMA* 1995, 273:1371–1375.

12. Tran UL, Arrowood JA, Nixon JV: Effects of long-term dynamic conditioning on cardiac function in the older human heart. *J Invest Med* 1995, 43:299.

13. Miller PF, Sheps DS, Bragdon EE, *et al.*: Aging and pain perception in ischemic heart disease. *Am Heart J* 1990, 120:22.

14. Lam JYT, Chaitman BR, Glaenzer M: Safety and diagnostic accuracy of dipyridamole-thallium imaging in the elderly. *J Am Coll Cardiol* 1988, 11:585.

15.• Scandinavian Simvastatin Survival Study Group: Randomized trial of cholesterol lowering in 4444 patients with coronary artery disease: the Scandinavian Simvastatin Survival Study (4S) *Lancet* 1994, 344:1383.

16. Stampfer MJ, Colditz GA, Willett WC, *et al.*: Postmenopausal estrogen therapy and cardiovascular disease: ten year follow-up from the Nurses' Health Study. *N Engl J Med* 1991, 325:756.

17. Raisner AE, Hust RG, Lewis JM, *et al.*: Transluminal coronary angioplasty in the elderly. *Am J Cardiol* 1986, 57:29.

18. Gersch BJ, Krenmal RA, Schaff HV, *et al.*: Comparison of coronary artery bypass surgery and medical therapy in patients 65 years of age or older. *N Engl J Med* 1985, 313:217.

19. Norwegian Multicenter Study Group: Timolol-induced reduction in mortality and reinfarction in patients surviving acute myocardial infarction. *N Engl J Med* 1981, 304:801.

20. Pfeffer MA, Braunwald E, Moye LA, *et al.*: Effect of captopril on mortality and morbidity in patients with left ventricular dysfunction after myocardial infarction. *N Engl J Med* 1992, 327:669.

21. Hypertension Detection and Follow-up Program Cooperative Group: Five year findings of the Hypertension Detection and Follow-Up Program. Mortality by race, sex, and age. *JAMA* 1979, 242:2572.

22. Joint National Committee on Detection, Evaluation and Treatment of High Blood Pressure: The fifth report of the Joint National Committee on Detection, Evaluation and Treatment of High Blood Pressure. *Arch Intern Med* 1993, 153:154.

23 Insura JT, Sacks HS, Lau TS, *et al.*: Drug treatment of hypertension in the elderly. *Ann Intern Med* 1994, 121:355.

24. Kannel WB, Gordon T, Schwartz MJ: Systolic versus diastolic blood pressure and risk for coronary heart disease: the Framingham Study. *Am J Cardiol* 1971, 27:335.

25. Levy D, Garrison RJ, Savage DD, *et al.*: Left ventricular mass and incidence of coronary heart disease in an elderly cohort. *Ann Intern Med* 1989, 110:101.

26. Nixon JV: Treating hypertension in the elderly: a physiological basis for selections of therapy. *Cardiol Elderly* 1993, 1:441–446.

27. SHEP Cooperative Research Group: Prevention of stroke by antihypertensive drug treatment in older persons with isolated systolic hypertension: final results in the systolic hypertension in the elderly program (SHEP). *JAMA* 1991, 265:3255.

28. Cruickshank JM, Thorp JM, Zacharias FJ: Benefits and potential harm of lowering high blood pressure. *Lancet* 1987, i:581.

29. Applegate WB: Hypertension in elderly patients. *Ann Intern Med* 1989, 110:901.

30. Furberg CD, Psaty BM, Manolio TA, *et al.*: Prevalence of atrial fibrillation in elderly subjects (the Cardiovascular health Study). *Am J Cardiol* 1994, 74:236.

31. Carabello BA: Timing of surgery in mitral and aortic stenosis. *Cardiovasc Clin* 1991, 9:229.

32. Braunwald E: Valvular heart disease. In *Heart Disease*, edn 4. Edited by Braunwald E. Philadelphia: WB Saunders; 1992:1007.

33. Feigenbaum H: Echocardiography. In *Heart Disease*, edn 4. Edited by Braunwald E. Philadelphia: WB Saunders; 1992:81.

34. Safian RD, Kentz RE, Berman AD: Aortic valvuloplasty. *Cardiovasc Clin* 1991, 9:289.

35. Massie BM, Conway M: Survival of patients with congestive heart failure: past, present and future prospects. *Circulation* 1987, 756:IV–11.

36. Schulman SP, Weiss JL, Becker LC, *et al.*: The effects of antihypertensive therapy on left ventricular mass in elderly hypertensive patients. *N Engl J Med* 1990, 322:1350.

37. Miyatake K, Okamoto M, Kinoshiter N, *et al.*: Augmentation of atrial contribution to left ventricular inflow with aging as assessed by intracardiac Doppler flowmetry. *Am J Cardiol* 1984, 53:586.

38. Shah PM, Pai RG: Diastolic heart failure. *Curr Probl Cardiol* 1992, 12:821.

39. Lakatta EG: The aging heart. *Ann Intern Med* 1990, 113:456.

40. Reeder GS, Gersch BJ: Acute myocardial infarction. In *Stein's Internal Medicine*. Edited by Stein JH. St. Louis: Mosby–Year Book; 1993.

41. Levy D, Wilson PWF, Anderson KM, *et al.*: Stratifying the patient at risk from coronary disease: new insights from the Framingham Study. *Am Heart J* 1990, 119:712.

42. Farnett L, Mulrow CD, Linn WD, *et al.*: The J-curve phenomenon and the treatment of hypertension: is there a point beyond which pressure reduction is dangerous? *JAMA* 1991, 265:489.

43. Ross J Jr, Braunwald E: Aortic stenosis. *Circulation* 1968, 38(suppl 5):61.

44. Lytle BW, Cosgrove DM, Gill CC, *et al.*: Aortic valve replacement combined with myocardial revascularization: late results and determinants of risk for 471 in-hospital survivors. *J Thorac Cardiovasc Surg* 1988, 95:402.

SELECT BIBLIOGRAPHY

Wenger NK: Cardiovascular disease in the elderly. In *Current Problems in Cardiology*. Edited by O'Rourke RA. St. Louis: Mosby–Year Book; 1992:10.

Pregnancy and the Heart 45

Brad S. Burlew
Howard R. Horn
Jay M. Sullivan

Key Points
- Pregnancy imposes a hemodynamic burden on the cardiovascular system.
- Severe valvular stenotic lesions are poorly tolerated; regurgitant lesions have better outcomes.
- Mitral valve prolapse is rarely a problem.
- Anticoagulation worsens the outcome during pregnancy.
- Pulmonary hypertension is associated with a very poor outcome.
- With careful medical care and appropriate hemodynamic monitoring, most patients with cardiac disease can be safely carried through pregnancy and delivery.

Pregnancy is a condition that places temporary but significant hemodynamic stresses on the woman with underlying cardiac disease. The risk of complications from these stresses depends on the nature of the maternal cardiac abnormality; ranging from negligible risk with mitral valve prolapse to a very high likelihood of maternal and fetal death in patients with advanced pulmonary hypertension. Skillful management of the gravid patient with cardiac disease depends on an understanding of the normal clinical findings associated with the gravid state, the recognition of cardiac disease in the pregnant woman, and an understanding of the likely response of a specific disorder to the hemodynamic changes.

Fortunately, the prevalence of heart disease in the reproductive female population is fairly low (between 0.4% and 4.1%) [1,2]. Worldwide, rheumatic heart disease accounts for up to 90% of the cardiac disorders seen in pregnant women. Mitral stenosis is the most common lesion, occurring in approximately 90% of women with rheumatic heart disease. In the United States, Canada, and Western Europe, rheumatic heart disease now accounts for a diminishing portion (approximately 45% to 75%) of all cases of heart disease [2–4]. Congenital heart disease accounts for much of the remainder, with patients with surgically corrected congenital heart disease and those with prosthetic valves forming a relatively new category of pregnant women with heart disorders.

SIGNS AND SYMPTOMS ASSOCIATED WITH PREGNANCY

The signs and symptoms of pregnancy are a consequence of the normal physiologic changes that occur. These changes include an increase in maternal total blood volume, which reaches maximal values of 50% above baseline (nongravid) values. Plasma volume increases more than the red blood cell mass, which increases by only approximately 10%, resulting in a relative hemodilution [1]. This accounts for the physiologic anemia of pregnancy (Fig. 1).

Resting cardiac output also increases during pregnancy approximately 40% to 50% above that of the nongravid state (Fig. 2) [5]. Increased cardiac output is initially mediated through an increased stroke volume; the stroke volume then

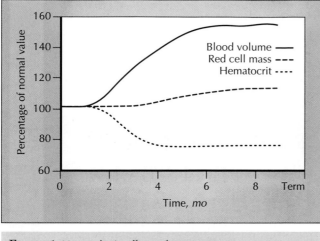

FIGURE 1 Hematologic effects of pregnancy.

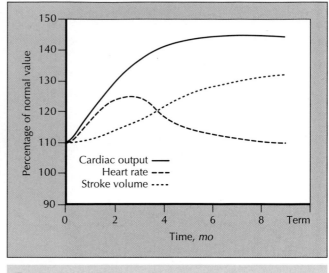

FIGURE 2 Hemodynamic effects of pregnancy.

returns toward the normal range while the heart rate progressively increases. The gravid uterus occasionally compresses the inferior vena cava in the recumbent and standing positions, reducing venous return and cardiac output (Fig. 3) [6,7].

As pregnancy progresses, variations occur in cardiac output, stroke volume, and regional perfusion patterns. As the uterus enlarges, alterations occur in venous return to the central circulation as well. These changes are associated with the development of symptoms and signs that may mimic heart disease. For example, exertional dyspnea normally occurs in over 50% of pregnant women. Orthopnea, paroxysmal nocturnal dyspnea, dizziness, and easy fatigability are quite common. Syncope and presyncope may occur in the normal gravid woman, presumably caused by compression of the inferior vena cava by the uterus. Patients also may experience chest discomfort, mimicking angina pectoris.

On physical examination, normal patients may have prominent neck veins, inspiratory rales, ventricular (S_3) gallops, cardiomegaly, and peripheral edema. Murmurs, particularly systolic flow murmurs with an intensity of up to grade 2 (out of 6), are often heard (Fig. 4). Although diastolic murmurs are unusual in pregnancy, a diastolic murmur over the pulmonic area similar to the Graham Steell murmur is sometimes heard. This murmur, which is believed to be related to a physiologic dilatation of the pulmonary artery, vanishes soon after delivery [1]. A diastolic flow murmur arising from the tricuspid valve is occasionally heard; it likewise disappears after delivery. Venous sounds such as venous hums and mammary souffles also can be heard [8].

ACQUIRED VALVULAR HEART DISEASE

Worldwide, mitral stenosis is the most frequently observed acquired valvular lesion in reproductive women. It also poses one of the most substantial risks to the survival of the mother and the fetus. Depending on the degree of stenosis, a pressure gradient develops across the valve, resulting in elevated pressures in the left atrium and the pulmonary

veins. Factors that increase the left atrial pressure are those that increase the diastolic mitral valvular flow rate through an increase in cardiac output or heart rate (which diminishes the duration of diastole, increasing the diastolic transvalvular gradient).

Because of the normal physiologic increases in cardiac output during pregnancy and delivery, left atrial pressures tend to be more severely elevated in the gravid state as the diastolic flow across the stenotic mitral valve increases. The elevation in left atrial pressure can result in pulmonary edema and hypoxemia. Clinically, patients develop dyspnea, tachypnea, orthop-

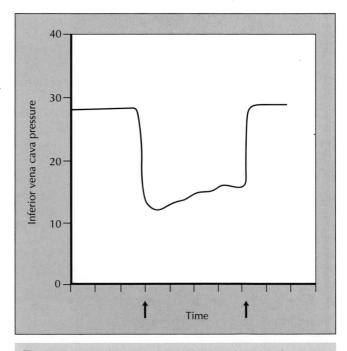

FIGURE 3 Hemodynamic effect of the gravid uterus. The uterus is lifted between the *arrows*. (*From* Kerr [6]; with permission.)

Cardiology for the Primary Care Physician

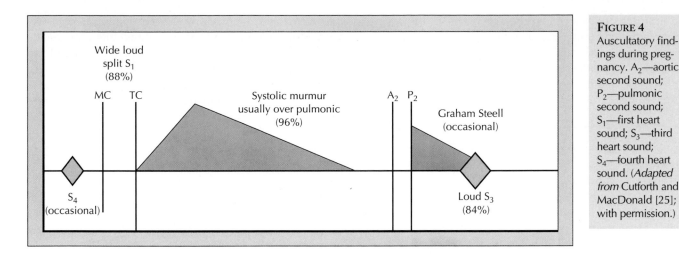

Figure 4
Auscultatory findings during pregnancy. A_2—aortic second sound; P_2—pulmonic second sound; S_1—first heart sound; S_3—third heart sound; S_4—fourth heart sound. (*Adapted from* Cutforth and MacDonald [25]; with permission.)

nea, and paroxysmal nocturnal dyspnea, which are also symptoms often experienced by the normal gravid woman. Frank pulmonary edema and hemoptysis can occur in the third trimester and in the immediate postpartum period. Even patients who appear to be doing well can decompensate suddenly with the onset of rapid atrial tachycardia. Symptomatic tachycardias therefore must be treated promptly and effectively with digoxin and perhaps β-blockade, because pulmonary edema frequently ensues. Patients with refractory symptomatic atrial fibrillation should have cardioversion. Infection and even mild hyperthyroidism also need to be treated promptly in this setting, because these disorders can similarly trigger tachycardia and subsequent pulmonary edema. At parturition, monitoring of the patient's volume status with a pulmonary artery catheter is recommended [1,9,10].

Aortic stenosis appears to affect pregnancy adversely, with a 17% overall maternal mortality rate [11]. Patients with severe aortic stenosis are preload dependent with a fixed stroke volume. Any increase in cardiac output is mediated through an increase in heart rate. Medications that decrease heart rate or preload should be avoided if possible. Vasodilators should also be avoided. If critical stenosis is diagnosed before pregnancy, surgical correction should be recommended.

Mitral and aortic valvular insufficiency are typically well tolerated in the gravid patient. The severity of valvular regurgitation may actually decrease during pregnancy because of the physiologic decrease in peripheral vascular resistance. Patients generally respond well to conservative therapy if they become symptomatic.

Mitral valve prolapse unassociated with other cardiovascular abnormalities does not increase maternal or fetal risk [12]. The use of prophylactic antibiotics in this setting remains controversial.

PROSTHETIC VALVES

Hemodynamically, patients with prosthetic valves tend to fare quite well throughout pregnancy, although the spontaneous abortion rate in patients receiving anticoagulant therapy is approximately 50% [13]. A dominant concern in these patients is the teratogenesis associated with warfarin therapy.

Warfarin exposure at 6 to 9 weeks of gestation carries an 8% incidence of warfarin embryopathy [14]. Although heparin does not cross the placenta, prolonged intravenous therapy is associated with maternal complications, including development of heparin-induced osteopenia. In view of these issues, widely followed recommendations for anticoagulation during pregnancy consist of the administration of intravenous heparin during the first trimester and use of oral warfarin therapy during the second and third trimesters [15]. During the last weeks of pregnancy, intravenous heparin is again administered, because late exposure to warfarin is clearly associated with increased peripartum hemorrhage.

Although this protocol was designed to minimize risk to the fetus and the mother, the use of intravenous heparin does not appear to result in a significantly better outcome [16]. Because of this, pregnancy in patients requiring systemic anticoagulation is probably best avoided. Management of the anticoagulated pregnant patient with a prosthetic valve is probably best accomplished in consultation with a cardiologist or another physician familiar with this problem.

PERIPARTUM CARDIOMYOPATHY

Peripartum cardiomyopathy is a disease of unknown etiology associated with development of congestive heart failure during the final month of pregnancy or during the 5 months after delivery. This disorder occurs initially in people who have not previously had heart disease and in whom other explanations for congestive failure are not apparent. It is more common among blacks, is more likely to occur in a woman of 30 years of age or older, who is pregnant with twins or who has toxemia, and is more likely to occur during a third or subsequent pregnancy. If the patient has ever acquired peripartum cardiomyopathy, it is likely to return in subsequent pregnancies, particularly if the patient had persistent postpartum cardiomegaly. Hypertension, myocarditis, and dietary factors may play roles in the development of peripartum cardiomyopathy [17•,18].

Standard therapy with digoxin and diuretics is usually sufficient. If needed, hydralazine and nitrates also can be used, because no studies have demonstrated the induction of teratogenesis in humans with the use of these agents. Prepartum use of angiotensin-converting enzyme inhibitors is strictly contraindicated during pregnancy because of their association with neonatal craniofacial deformities, renal failure, and death. However, postpartum use of angiotensin-converting enzyme inhibitors is appropriate, although breast-feeding should be strongly discouraged.

MYOCARDIAL INFARCTION

Fortunately, ischemic heart disease during pregnancy is quite uncommon, undoubtedly because women of reproductive age are at extremely low risk for its development. In view of the current US trend toward bearing children later in life, myocardial infarction among pregnant women will probably be seen more frequently in the future. The present frequency of myocardial infarction in pregnancy is very low, with an incidence of only approximately 10,000 pregnancies [19••]; the overall maternal mortality rate in this population is approximately 21%.

Current management recommendations include bedrest, aspirin, heparin, intravenous nitroglycerine, and beta blockade. There are anecdotal reports of successful preterm percutaneous transluminal coronary angioplasty (PTCA) and stent deployment, although routine use of interventional techniques has not yet been extensively studied. Similarly, there are a number of reports of thrombolytic therapy in the gravid female, usually for pulmonary embolism. There does not appear to be any teratogenic effect of thrombolytic agents, although experience with their use in acute myocardial infarction is limited. It was previously recommended that oxytocin not be used in patients with ischemic heart disease. Currently, however, synthetic oxytocin, which does not contain arginine vasopressin, is available; in appropriate doses, it is unlikely to increase coronary vasoconstriction. With the intravenous bolus administration of 5 to 12 U, oxytocin does produce a 30% decrease in mean arterial pressure and a 50% increase in cardiac output among healthy patients undergoing tocolysis. These hemodynamic effects can be avoided by the administration of oxytocin as a dilute solution [20]. Synthetic oxytocin has been used successfully in pregnant patients after myocardial infarction.

SELECTED DEVELOPMENTAL ABNORMALITIES

Primary pulmonary hypertension is associated with high fetal and maternal mortality rates. Generally, cardiac abnormalities associated with pulmonary hypertension (with or without right-to-left communication) are associated with a maternal mortality rate of approximately 50% [8]. Avoidance or interruption of pregnancy is indicated. Congenital heart disease in the pregnant woman usually poses some hazard to the mother. These patients are best treated in conjunction with a specialist familiar with these abnormalities. Genetic counseling also may be appropriate.

Other developmental abnormalities include Marfan syndrome and hypertrophic cardiomyopathy. With its connective tissue abnormality, Marfan syndrome is associated with a high incidence of aneurysmal dilatation of the aortic root. In one study [21], dissection or rupture of the aortic root occurred in 50% of affected pregnant women, although in our experience the frequency of these events is much lower. Serial echocardiography has been recommended to monitor the progression of dilatation or the development of dissection of the aortic root. The risk of sudden death is believed to be proportional to the diameter of the aortic root [21]. Nonetheless, undetected dissections have occurred despite close echocardiographic monitoring; the availability of endoscopic echocardiography may improve sensitivity in this regard. Meticulous control of blood pressure with β-blockade is an approach we have used for this condition.

Hypertrophic obstructive cardiomyopathy is usually associated with uneventful pregnancies. The outflow obstruction is dynamic and dependent on factors such as blood pressure and ventricular preload, both of which should be maintained if possible. During pregnancy, patients should be encouraged to lie preferentially in the lateral decubitus positions. This maneuver relieves inferior vena caval obstruction, preserving ventricular preload. Because of the likelihood of marked worsening of the dynamic outflow obstruction, β-sympathomimetic tocolytic agents are strictly contraindicated in this disorder. Regional anesthesia, with its risk of hypotension, should also be avoided [22].

CONCLUSIONS

With careful medical care and appropriate hemodynamic monitoring, most patients with cardiac disease can be safely carried through pregnancy and delivery [23]. Unfortunately, termination of the pregnancy is still sometimes indicated. In patients with severe congestive failure, termination should be considered during early pregnancy, because continuation of the pregnancy is likely to result in an unacceptable outcome for both the mother and fetus. Similarly, therapeutic abortion should be considered in patients with primary or secondary pulmonary hypertension (with or without right-to-left communications) and in those with cyanotic congenital heart disease. These clinical conditions can be associated with maternal mortality rates in excess of 50%. Termination of the pregnancy during the first or second trimester presents a more favorable risk to the patient [24].

KEY REFERENCES

Recently published papers of outstanding interest, as identified in *References and Recommended Reading*, have been annotated.

•• Roth A, Elkayam U: Acute myocardial infarction associated with pregnancy. *Ann Intern Med* 1996, 125:751–762.
Excellent, comprehensive review of the epidemiology, course, diagnosis, prognosis, and treatment of acute myocardial infarction during pregnancy.

REFERENCES AND RECOMMENDED READING

Recently published papers of particular interest have been highlighted as:
- Of interest
- •• Of outstanding interest

1. Conradsson T, Werkö L: Management of heart disease in pregnancy. *Prog Cardiovasc Dis* 1974, 16:407–419.

2. McFaul PB, Dornan JC, Lamki H, Boyle D: Pregnancy complicated by maternal heart disease: a review of 519 women. *Br J Obstet Gynaecol* 1988, 95:861–867.

3. Szekely P, Snaith L: *Heart Disease and Pregnancy.* London: Churchill Livingstone; 1974:53.

4. Shime J, Mocarski EJM, Hastings D, *et al.*: Congenital heart disease in pregnancy: short and long term implications. *Am J Obstet Gynecol* 1987, 156:313–322.

5. Robson SC, Hunter S, Boys RJ, Dunlop W: Serial study of factors influencing changes in cardiac output during pregnancy. *Am J Physiol* 1989, 256:H1060–H1065.

6. Kerr MG: The mechanical effects of the gravid uterus in late pregnancy. *J Obstet Gynaecol Br Comm* 1965, 72:513–529.

7. Metcalf J, Ueland K: Maternal cardiovascular adjustment to pregnancy. *Prog Cardiovasc Dis* 1974, 16:363–374.

8. McAnulty JH, Metcalfe J, Ueland K: General guidelines in the management of cardiac disease. *Clin Obstet Gynecol* 1981, 24:773–789.

9. Lang RM, Borow KM: Pregnancy and heart disease. *Clin Perinatol* 1985, 12:551–569.

10. Ueland K, Hansen JM: Maternal cardiovascular dynamics II: posture and uterine contractions. *Am J Obstet Gynecol* 1969, 103:1–7.

11. Arias F, Pineda J: Aortic stenosis and pregnancy. *J Reprod Med* 1978, 20:229–232.

12. Tang LCH, Chan SYW, Wong VCW, Ma H: Pregnancy in patients with mitral valve prolapse. *Int J Gynaecol Obstet* 1985, 23:217–221.

13. Vitali E, Donnatelli F, Quaini E, *et al.*: Pregnancy in patients with mechanical prosthetic heart valves. *J Cardiovasc Surg* 1986, 27:221–227.

14. Pauli RM, Hall JG, Wilson KM: Risks of anticoagulation during pregnancy. *Am Heart J* 1980, 100:761–762.

15. Hirsch J, Cade JF, O'Sullivan EF: Clinical experience with anti-coagulation therapy during pregnancy. *BMJ* 1970, 1:270–275.

16. Hall JG, Pauli RM, Wilson KM: Maternal and fetal sequelae of anticoagulation during pregnancy. *Am J Med* 1980, 68:122–140.

17.• Lampert MB, Lang RM: Peripartum cardiomyopathy. *Am J Heart J* 1995, 130:960–970.

18. O'Connell JB, Costanzo-Nordin MR, Subramanian R, *et al.*: Peripartum cardiomyopathy: clinical, hemodynamic, histologic and prognostic characteristics. *J Am Coll Cardiol* 1986, 8:52–56.

19.•• Roth A, Elkayam U: Acute myocardial infarction associated with pregnancy. *Ann Intern Med* 1996, 125:751–762.

20. Weis FR, Markello R, Mo B, Bochiecho P: Cardiovascular effects of oxytocin. *Obstet Gynecol* 1975, 46:211–214.

21. Pyeritz RE: Maternal and fetal complications of pregnancy in the Marfan syndrome. *Am J Med* 1981, 71:784–790.

22. Shah DM, Sunderji SG: Hypertrophic cardiomyopathy and pregnancy: report of a maternal mortality and review of literature. *Obstet Gynecol Surv* 1985, 40:444–448.

23. Whittemore R, Hobbins JC, Engle MA: Pregnancy and its outcome on women with and without surgical treatment of congenital heart disease. *Am J Cardiol* 1982, 50:641–651.

24. Elkayam U, Gleicher N: Cardiac problems in pregnancy. *JAMA* 1984, 251:2838–2839.

25. Cutforth R, MacDonald CB: Heart sounds and murmurs during pregnancy. *Am Heart J* 1966, 71:741–747.

The Transplanted Heart 46

Charles K. Moore
John B. O'Connell

Key Points

- Heart transplantation is now firmly established as a treatment option for some patients with end-stage heart disease.

- Five-year survival rates following heart transplantation in many centers now exceed 70%.

- Exercise testing with measurement of peak oxygen consumption is a useful adjunct in assessing the need for transplantation.

- The most common maintenance immunosuppression regimen following heart transplantation uses cyclosporine, azathioprine, and prednisone in combination.

- The leading cause of death beyond the first year after transplantation is accelerated coronary artery disease, a process believed to represent a form of "chronic rejection."

In the 1990s, heart transplantation plays a successful role in the treatment of advanced heart disease. Following its highly publicized beginnings in the late 1960s, the procedure suffered from relatively poor survival rates, limiting application of heart transplantation to just a few centers worldwide through the 1970s. Advancements such as the development of the transvenous endomyocardial biopsy, and especially the introduction of the immunosuppressant cyclosporine in 1981, dramatically improved success rates and led to rapid increases in the use of cardiac transplantation throughout the United States.

CURRENT RESULTS

Centers performing heart transplantation proliferated rapidly in the first half of the 1980s after the introduction of cyclosporine (Fig. 1*A*) [1]. Both the number of active centers and the total number of heart transplantations performed yearly (both worldwide and in the United States), however, have now leveled off (Fig. 1*B*) (United Network for Organ Sharing Scientific Registry, Unpublished data) [1]. Heart transplantation currently is strictly limited by the availability of donor hearts.

The dramatic improvement in survival after heart transplantation over the last 25 years is clearly evident in Figure 2 [2]. Many centers now achieve 1-year actuarial survival rates exceeding 90%. Five-year actuarial survival rates now surpass 70%, and individual heart transplant recipients have survived more than 20 years (United Network for Organ Sharing Scientific Registry, Unpublished data). Equally important, heart transplantation dramatically improves functional status. One year after transplant, 86% of recipients are in New York Heart Association (NYHA) class I [3], and 50% are employed full-time [4].

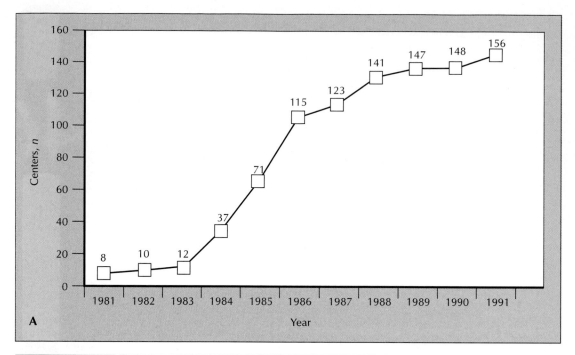

FIGURE 1
A, Number of heart transplant centers in the United States by year. (*From* O'Connell and coworkers [1]; with permission.)
B, Number of heart transplants performed in the United States by year. (*From* O'Connell *et al.* [1] and United Network for Organ Sharing Scientific Registry [Unpublished data]; with permission.)

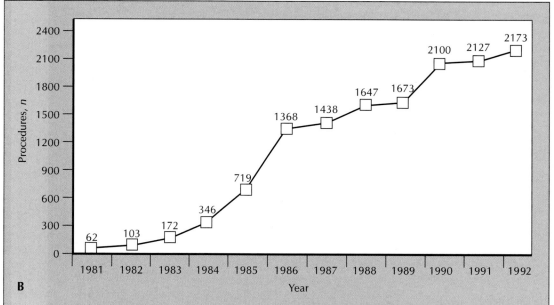

FIGURE 2 Actuarial survival associated with heart transplantation during three successive periods. (*From* Kriett and Kaye [2]; with permission.)

RECIPIENT SELECTION

The improvement in survival rates after heart transplantation combined with an increasing prevalence of congestive heart failure has led to a marked increase in the number of patients likely to benefit from transplantation. Unfortunately, the supply of donor hearts has stagnated in recent years (as noted previously). As a result, the number of patients awaiting transplantation continues to escalate (Fig. 3). In 1991, more than 800 patients died awaiting heart transplantation. Over 300 patients are added to the waiting list each month, and only 150 receive transplants (Fig. 3). While efforts to expand the number of donor organs continue, the importance of selecting patients most likely to benefit from transplantation is obvious.

Indications

Any cardiac condition associated with substantial morbidity and mortality not amenable to any other form of therapy may be an indication for heart transplantation. Dilated cardiomyopathy remains the most common indication, but severe coronary artery disease or "ischemic cardiomyopathy" is a close second (Fig. 4) [5]. Other possible indications are shown in Table 1. Although the causes of heart disease may vary, severe symptoms (NYHA functional class III to IV) or a poor expected 12-month survival should be present. In the last decade, 71% of heart transplant recipients have been in NYHA class IV and 25% in class III [3]. The determination of prognosis in patients with advanced heart disease is difficult at best, with numerous factors playing a role (Table 2). Poor left ventricular systolic function (low ejection fraction) alone is not sufficient for transplant candidacy, because usually only those patients with associated advanced symptoms of heart failure or life-threatening arrhythmias carry a 6- to 12-month mortality risk great enough to warrant immediate transplant consideration.

Exercise testing with measurement of oxygen consumption by expired gas analysis is a useful adjunct in assessing the need

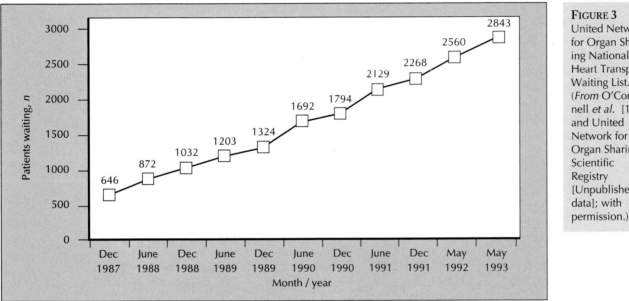

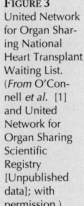

FIGURE 3 United Network for Organ Sharing National Heart Transplant Waiting List. (*From* O'Connell *et al.* [1] and United Network for Organ Sharing Scientific Registry [Unpublished data]; with permission.)

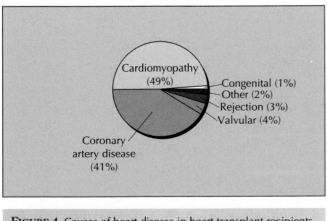

FIGURE 4 Causes of heart disease in heart transplant recipients. (*From* Kaye [5]; with permission.)

TABLE 1 CAUSES OF HEART DISEASE IN TRANSPLANT CANDIDATES

End-stage cardiomyopathy
  Idiopathic dilated
  Ischemic
  Infiltrative, restrictive (*eg*, amyloidosis, sarcoidosis)
  Valvular
  Hypertrophic
Myocarditis
Refractory angina, ischemia not amenable to surgery
  or angioplasty
Inoperable primary cardiac tumors
Refractory life-threatening arrhythmias not controllable
  with implantable cardioverter defibrillator
Uncorrectable congenital heart disease
Refractory heart transplant rejection

TABLE 2 ADVERSE PROGNOSTIC FACTORS IN HEART FAILURE
Low left ventricular ejection fraction
Advanced NYHA functional class
Presence of a ventricular S_3 gallop
Reduced serum sodium
Elevated plasma catecholamine levels
Increased pulmonary capillary wedge pressure
Reduced cardiac index
Low peak exercise oxygen consumption
Ventricular tachycardia
Antiarrhythmic drug use
NYHA—New York Heart Association.

for transplantation. Not only does it provide an objective confirmation of the subjective determination of NYHA functional class, peak exercise oxygen consumption (pVO_2) has also been shown to predict 12-month survival in patients with severe left ventricular systolic dysfunction and resultant congestive heart failure [6].

Contraindications

Although a transplant candidate's present level of symptoms and cardiovascular prognosis are critical to the selection process, expected morbidity and mortality *after* heart transplantation must also be addressed. Patients with end-stage heart disease and irreversible, uncontrollable, or untreatable comorbid conditions are not suitable candidates for transplantation (Table 3). Coexisting medical problems independently affect posttransplantation morbidity and mortality adversely, or they may do so in combination with the toxicity of immunosuppressive drugs.

As experience with heart transplantation has grown, the number of absolute contraindications has decreased. Some

patients with diabetes mellitus now routinely undergo transplantation and appear to have similar morbidity and mortality rates to patients without diabetes in the first year after transplantation [7]. The upper age limit has steadily increased to the degree that most transplantation programs now consider selecting patients up to 65 years of age (or even older in highly selected patients).

The Selection Process

Patients with NYHA class III or IV symptoms caused by heart disease not amenable to other treatment modalities and without absolute contraindication should be referred to a heart transplant center for consideration. Such patients will undergo an extensive evaluation directed at identifying and assessing all of the factors noted previously (Table 4). A committee of physicians and other health-care personnel generally makes a decision on each candidate. Some patients will be found to be unacceptable because of one or more contraindications, whereas others may have transplantation deferred because of symptoms of insufficient severity or a relatively favorable prognosis (Fig. 5). Those patients deemed acceptable and in imminent need of transplantation will be actively "listed" on a computerized, nationwide waiting list. Organs are allocated based on severity of illness, blood group, body size, and finally, time on the waiting list. Severity of illness is generally limited to two categories (Table 5). Waiting time for a suitable donor heart ranges from as little as 1 day to 1 year or more, with a median of approximately 6 months [8].

MANAGEMENT

At the time of transplantation, the recipient trades advanced heart disease for another significant problem—suppression of the immune system to prevent rejection of the donor heart. Despite introduction of more specific immunosuppressive agents such as cyclosporine, the toxic potential of the modern immunosuppressive regimen remains formidable, and optimal

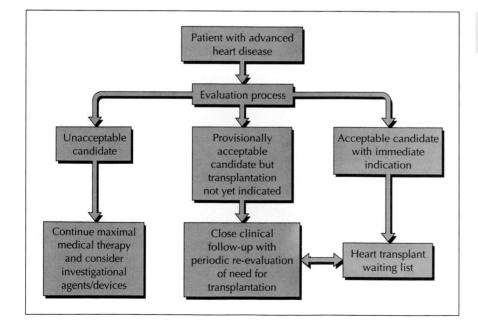

FIGURE 5 Outcomes of referral for heart transplantation.

TABLE 5 HEART TRANSPLANT RECIPIENT STATUS CRITERIA

Status 1

Patients requiring cardiac or pulmonary assistance with one or more of the following devices:
    Total artificial heart
    Left and/or right ventricular assist systems
    Intraaortic balloon pump
    Ventilator
Or, patients meeting both of the following criteria:
    In an intensive care unit
    Requires inotropic agents to maintain adequate cardiac output
Or, patients less than 6 months old

Status 2

All other waiting patients who do not meet Status 1 criteria

From United Network for Organ Sharing Scientific Registry [Unpublished data]

TABLE 4 MEDICAL EVALUATION BEFORE CARDIAC TRANSPLANTATION

History and physical (complete)

Hematologic profile

Complete blood count, chemistries, BUN, Cr, ALT, AST, ALP, GGT, total and direct bilirubin, prothrombin time, partial thromboplastin time

Stool occult blood testing

Serologic assays

Hepatitis A, B, C; syphilis; human immunodeficiency virus; cytomegalovirus; Epstein-Barr virus; *Toxoplasma gondii*; varicella

Histocompatibility testing

Blood type and antibody screen
Panel-reactive antibody screen
HLA typing

Urine profile

Urinalysis
Creatinine clearance (24-h collection)

Radiologic testing

Chest radiography
Radionuclide ventriculography
Abdominal ultrasonography
Carotid and peripheral Doppler studies*

Ventilatory testing

Complete pulmonary function studies
Exercise capacity testing (pVo_2)

Cardiologic evaluation

Electrocardiogram
Echocardiogram
Right heart catheterization
Left heart catheterization*
Coronary angiogram*
Endomyocardial biopsy*
Radionuclide ventriculogram*

Consultation

Social services
Dentistry
Psychiatry*

*As indicated.
ALP—alkaline phosphatase; ALT—alanine aminotransferase; AST—aspartate aminotransferase; BUN—blood urea nitrogen; Cr—creatinine; GGT—gamma-glutamyl transferase; HLA—human lymphocyte antigen.
From Olinde *et al.* [19]; with permission.

posttransplantation care requires constant vigilance for potential complications.

Normal Allograft Physiology

The surgical technique of orthotopic heart transplantation is simplified by anastomosing a residual cuff of the recipient's right and left atrial tissue to the donor atria rather than separately anastomosing two venae cava and four pulmonary veins (Fig. 6). As a result, two sinus nodes are present postoperatively. Atrial activity from the recipient sinus node can often be seen on the electrocardiogram dissociated from the sinus rhythm of the donor heart. This recipient atrial activity is electrically isolated from the donor heart by the suture line.

Another unique feature of the donor heart is denervation. All transplanted hearts remain denervated for at least 1 year and are partially denervated thereafter. Without the normally dominant inhibitory parasympathetic influence, resting heart rate in the transplant recipient frequently exceeds 90 bpm. Denervation also modifies the response of the donor heart to exercise. Without direct sympathetic innervation, the tachycardic response to exercise depends on circulating catecholamines, an

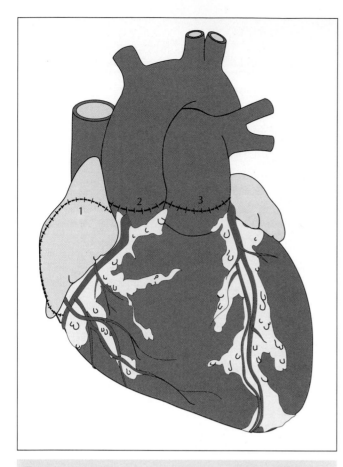

FIGURE 6 Anterior view after orthotopic heart transplantation demonstrates right atrial (1), aortic (2), and pulmonary arterial (3) suture lines. The left atrial suture line is hidden behind the heart in this view.

polyclonal and monoclonal antilymphocyte antibody preparations are available (*eg*, antithymocyte globulin and muromonab-CD3).

Maintenance Immunosuppression

The majority of heart transplant centers now practice "triple therapy" maintenance immunosuppressive therapy, using cyclosporine, azathioprine, and corticosteroids. Use of several agents allows a total level of immunosuppression sufficient to keep rejection at bay yet avoid significant toxicity from any single agent (Fig. 8). Each immunosuppressant carries a unique toxicity profile (Table 7). Morbidity secondary to chronic corticosteroid administration can be especially problematic, prompting many programs to wean steroid doses gradually to a minimal level or even discontinue therapy with these agents entirely in some patients.

In addition to the intrinsic toxicity of immunosuppressive drugs, significant interactions with other commonly prescribed medications pose a real threat to the heart transplant recipient. The metabolism of cyclosporine in particular can be dramatically affected, leading to either elevated blood levels and toxicity (*eg*, renal failure) or decreased blood levels and transplant rejection (Table 8). Other drugs to be used only with caution include nonsteroidal antiinflammatory drugs, which exacerbate nephrotoxicity from cyclosporine, and allopurinol, which dramatically impairs metabolism of azathioprine, therefore requiring a three- or fourfold dose reduction. Recipients are routinely advised to contact the heart transplant center before starting therapy with *any* new drugs.

Infections

Suppression of the immune system to prevent rejection also enhances susceptibility of the transplant recipient to a variety of infectious agents. Before cyclosporine was available, infections accounted for over 50% of all deaths in heart transplant recipients [10]. With cyclosporine-based immunosuppressive

inherently slower mechanism. Thus, transplant recipients require a longer warm-up and cool-down phase during exercise. Despite these differences in physiology, heart transplant recipients are generally capable of achieving normal exercise tolerance; some even participate in competitive athletics.

Rejection

The incidence of acute allograft rejection and death resulting from transplant rejection is greatest early after transplantation and diminishes gradually with time (Fig. 7) [9]. The transvenous right ventricular endomyocardial biopsy technique allows unprecedented surveillance for rejection on a repetitive outpatient basis. Consequently, most episodes of acute rejection are diagnosed before significant symptoms develop or the systolic function of the allograft decreases. Signs and symptoms that may suggest acute allograft rejection are shown in Table 6. Suspicion of acute rejection is a medical emergency and warrants immediate consultation with the transplant center. Treatment options for acute rejection are numerous, but "pulse" therapy with intravenous methylprednisolone (*eg*, 1 g of methylprednisolone intravenously four times a day for 3 days) or oral prednisone remains the most common therapy for episodes of sufficient severity to warrant a significant augmentation in immunosuppressive treatment. For more severe or corticosteroid-resistant rejection episodes, potent

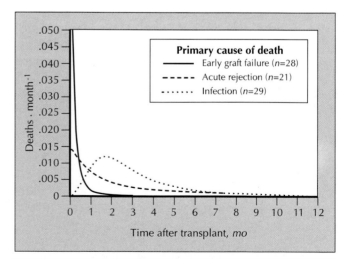

FIGURE 7 Risk of death from early graft failure, acute rejection, and infection for 914 patients in the Transplant Cardiologists Research Database. (*From* Bourge *et al.* [9]; with permission.)

TABLE 6 SIGNS AND SYMPTOMS OF ACUTE CARDIAC ALLOGRAFT REJECTION*

Signs	Symptoms
Relative hypotension	Dyspnea
Elevated jugular venous pressure	Fatigue
Ventricular S_3 gallop	Orthopnea
Rales	
Peripheral edema	
Low-grade fever	
Arrhythmias	

*Rejection commonly occurs without any signs or symptoms however.

TABLE 7 SIDE EFFECTS AND TOXICITY OF IMMUNOSUPPRESSANTS

Corticosteroids	Cyclosporine
Cushing's syndrome	Hypertension
Osteoporosis	Renal insufficiency
Myopathy	Hirsutism
Cataracts	Tremor
Peptic ulcer disease	Gingival hyperplasia
Impaired wound healing	Elevated LFT results
Hyperlipidemia	Seizures
Glucose intolerance	Headache
Hypertension	Hypomagnesemia
Osteonecrosis	Photosensitivity
Emotional lability	Paresthesias
Acne	

Azathioprine
Leukopenia
Anemia
Thrombocytopenia
Pancreatitis
Nausea
Elevated LFT results

LFT—liver function test.

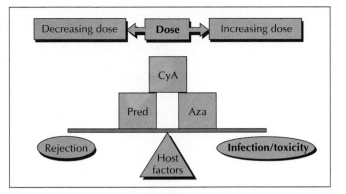

FIGURE 8 Adjusting the doses of immunosuppressive drugs requires a balance between insufficient (leading to rejection) and excessive (resulting in infection or toxicity) immunosuppression. Aza—azathioprine); CyA—cyclosporine; Pred—prednisone.

TABLE 8 COMMON DRUG INTERACTIONS WITH CYCLOSPORINE

Increases cyclosporine blood levels
Erythromycin
Ketoconazole
Fluconazole
Itraconazole
Diltiazem
Verapamil
Nicardipine
Metoclopramide

Decreases cyclosporine blood levels
Carbamazepine
Phenobarbital
Phenytoin
Rifampin

regimens, the infectious mortality rate is now less than 15% [11]. Deaths from infection peak at 1 to 3 months after transplantation, with a steady decline thereafter [2].

Bacterial pathogens account for the majority of severe infections, but viral, fungal, and protozoal agents each play an important role (Fig. 9) [12]. The single most common severe infection is bacterial pneumonia (usually resulting from *Pneumococcus* infection in outpatients) [12].

The majority of serious viral illnesses that arise after heart transplantation are caused by cytomegalovirus [12], which is commonly associated with asymptomatic infection but can also result in life-threatening pneumonitis, hepatitis, or enteri-

tis. "Cytomegalovirus syndrome" is a mononucleosis-like illness with fever, fatigue, and leukopenia. Patients who are seronegative before transplantation and then receive a heart from a seropositive donor are at highest risk for cytomegalovirus disease. Most programs use prophylactic therapy with intravenous ganciclovir, high-dose oral acyclovir, hyperimmune intravenous immunoglobulin, or some combination for at-risk patients during the first 3 to 4 months after transplantation (when the incidence of cytomegalovirus infection is greatest).

Infection with *Pneumocystis carinii* accounts for most protozoal infections and almost always induces pneumonitis [12]. The incidence of *Pneumocystis* infections seems to vary by location, but many programs administer oral trimethoprim-sulfamethoxazole prophylaxis during the first 9 to 12 months after transplantation and at other times when patients are heavily immunosuppressed.

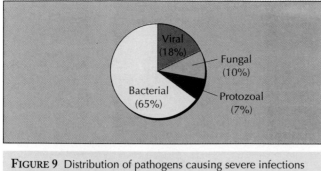

FIGURE 9 Distribution of pathogens causing severe infections in heart transplant recipients. (*From* Dummer [12•]; with permission.)

Accelerated Coronary Artery Disease

The donor heart is susceptible to a process involving accelerated intimal proliferation throughout the coronary vessels that can lead to myocardial ischemia and even infarction. The most widely accepted hypothesis proposes that the vasculature of the donor heart stimulates an immune response that culminates in myointimal thickening. As a result, this process has also been labeled *chronic rejection*. Coronary angiography has shown that this vascular abnormality can be seen in approximately 25% of recipients by 2 years after transplantation (Fig. 10) [13]; beyond the first year after transplantation, it is the leading cause of death [14]. Because of denervation of the donor heart, most patients with advanced allograft vasculopathy do not experience angina but may present with signs and symptoms of congestive heart failure. Because of the limited sensitivity and specificity of noninvasive studies in this population, most transplant programs perform yearly coronary angiography to screen for this process. At present, treatment options are limited, because the diffuse coronary lesions are rarely amenable to coronary artery bypass surgery or percutaneous transluminal coronary angioplasty. There is evidence, however, that lowering serum total and LDL cholesterol

levels with a statin drug, *eg*, pravastatin, decreases rejection and the associated coronary artery disease [15]. Some patients may be candidates for repeat transplantation.

Other Complications

A myriad of other complications may strike the heart transplant recipient (Table 9) [14]. Arterial hypertension is particularly common, with over 90% of patients receiving immunosuppressive maintenance "triple-therapy" requiring antihypertensive therapy by 6 months [16]. Corticosteroids, and especially cyclosporine, have been implicated as causative agents. Hemodynamic studies have shown elevated systemic vascular resistance with normal cardiac output [16]. Calcium channel blockers are very effective therapeutically, as are many other agents.

An increased incidence of malignancy is a well-recognized complication of chronic immunosuppression. Lymphoproliferative disorders can be especially lethal and may occur either early or late after transplantation. Therefore, regular assessment of transplant recipients should include careful examination for lymphadenopathy. Heavy immunosuppression, particularly with potent antilymphocyte-antibody preparations, is associated with an increased incidence of lymphoproliferative disease [17]. Some of these malignancies will respond to a reduction in immunosuppressive therapy alone [18]. Skin cancers are also a major problem, especially in patients who have had excessive exposure to the sun. Squamous cell carcinomas predominate and can be life-threatening if not detected early and aggressively treated.

ROLE OF THE GENERALIST

Despite a relatively favorable expected quality of life and survival after heart transplantation, regular and thorough general medical care is critical in minimizing complications. Most transplant programs encourage continued participation by the patient's primary-care provider, especially when the frequency of visits to the transplant center for biopsies dimin-

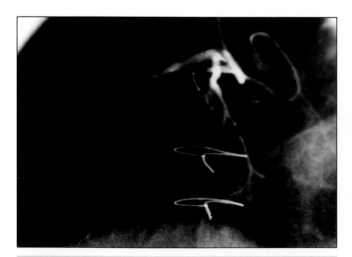

FIGURE 10 Angiography of the left coronary artery of a transplanted heart with accelerated coronary artery disease demonstrates rapid tapering of the lumen with loss of small distal vessels.

TABLE 9 COMPLICATIONS FOLLOWING HEART TRANSPLANTATION
Acute rejection
Infection
Accelerated coronary artery disease
Systemic hypertension
Malignancy
Chronic renal insufficiency
Gout
Hyperlipidemia
Osteoporosis
Osteonecrosis
Obesity
Glucose intolerance

ishes. Close communication between the primary-care physician and the transplant team allows many problems to be appropriately handled close to the patient's home, obviating travel to the sometimes distant transplant center.

REFERENCES

1. O'Connell J, Gunnar R, Evans R, *et al.*: Task Force 1: Organization of heart transplantation in the US. *J Am Coll Cardiol* 1993, 22:8–14.

2. Kriett J, Kaye M: The Registry of the International Society for Heart and Lung Transplantation: Eighth Official Report—1991. *J Heart Lung Transplant* 1991, 10:491–498.

3. Kaye M: The Registry of the International Society for Heart and Lung Transplantation: Tenth Official Report—1993. *J Heart Lung Transplant* 1993, 12:541–548.

4. Young J, Winters W, Bourge R, *et al.*: Task Force 4: Function of the heart transplant recipient. *J Am Coll Cardiol* 1993, 22:31–41.

5. Kaye M: The Registry of the International Society for Heart and Lung Transplantation: Ninth Official Report—1992. *J Heart Lung Transplant* 1992, 11:599–606.

6. Mancini D, Eisen H, Kussmaul W, *et al.*: Value of peak exercise oxygen consumption for optimal timing of cardiac transplantation in ambulatory patients with heart failure. *Circulation* 1991, 83:778–786.

7. Ladowski J, Kormos R, Uretsky B, *et al.*: Heart transplantation in diabetic recipients. *Transplantation* 1990, 49:303–305.

8. United Network of Organ Sharing: *Annual Report of the U.S. Scientific Registry for Organ Transplantation and the Organ Procurement and Transplantation Network.* Publication number ES-1, D-12. Rockville, MD: US Department of Health and Human Services; 1990.

9. Bourge R, Naftel D, Costanzo-Nordin M, *et al.*: Pretransplantation risk factors for death after heart transplantation: a multiinstitutional study. *J Heart Lung Transplant* 1993, 12:549–562.

10. Pennock J, Oyer P, Reitz B, *et al.*: Cardiac transplantation in perspective for the future. *J Thorac Cardiovasc Surg* 1982, 83:168–177.

11. Hofflin J, Potasmon I, Baldwin J, *et al.*: Infectious complications in heart transplant recipients receiving cyclosporine and corticosteroids. *Ann Intern Med* 1987, 106:209–216.

12. Dummer J: Infectious complications of transplantation. *Cardiovasc Clin* 1990, 20:163–178.

13. Olivari M, Homans D, Wilson R, *et al.*: Coronary artery disease in cardiac transplant patients receiving triple-drug immunosuppressive therapy. *Circulation* 1989, 80:111–115.

14. Miller L: Long-term complications of cardiac transplantation. *Prog Cardiovasc Dis* 1991, 33:229–282.

15. Kobashigawa JA, Katznelson S, Laks H, *et al.:* Effect of provastatin on outcomes after cardiac transplantation. *N Engl J Med* 1995, 333:621–627.

16. Olivari M, Antolick A, Ring W: Arterial hypertension in heart transplant recipients treated with triple-drug immunosuppressive therapy. *J Heart Transplant* 1989, 8:34–39.

17. Swinnen L, Costanzo-Nordin M, Fisher S, *et al.*: Increased incidence of lymphoproliferative disorder after immunosuppression with the monoclonal antibody OKT3 in cardiac transplant recipients. *N Engl J Med* 1990, 323:1723–1728.

18. Penn I: Cancers after cyclosporine therapy. *Transplant Proc* 1988, 20:276–279.

19. Olinde KD, Moore CK, O'Connell JB: The selection of recipients for cardiac transplantation. *Develop Cardiol* 1993, 3:1–12.

SELECT BIBLIOGRAPHY

Blum A, Aravot D: Heart transplantation—an update. *Clin Cardiol* 1996, 19:930–938.

Costanzo MR, Augustine S, Bourge R, *et al.*: Selection and treatment of candidates for heart transplantation. *Circulation* 1995, 92:3593–3612.

Miller L, Naftel D, Bourge R, *et al.*: Infection after heart transplantation: a multiinstitutional study. *J Heart Lung Transplant* 1994, 13:381–383.

Olson L, Rodeheffer R: Management of patients after cardiac transplantation. *Mayo Clin Proc* 1992, 67:775–784.

Stevenson L: Advanced congestive heart failure. Inpatient treatment and selection for cardiac transplantation. *Postgrad Med* 1993, 94:97–112.

Young J: Cardiac allograft arteriopathy: an ischemic burden of a different sort. *Am J Cardiol* 1992, 70:9F–13F.

Index

Page numbers followed by a *t* or *f* indicate tables or figures, respectively.

Color Plates

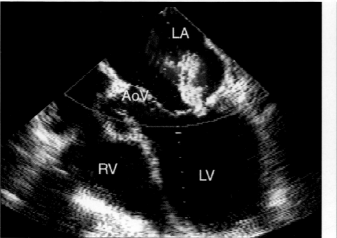

Chapter 4, Figure 6, p. 34

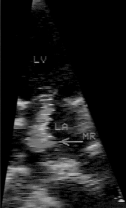

Chapter 6, Figure 3B, p. 53

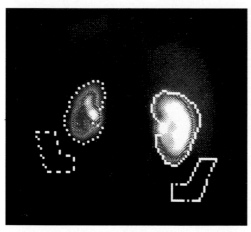

Chapter 16, Figure 5, p. 140

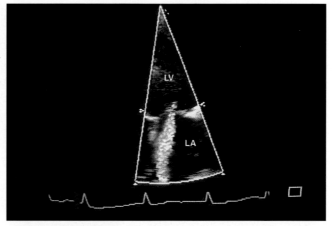

Chapter 21, Figure 3, p. 185

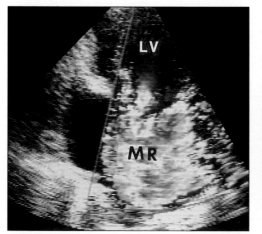

Chapter 22, Figure 11, p. 193

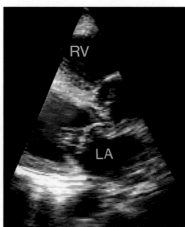

Chapter 23, Figure 8B, p. 204

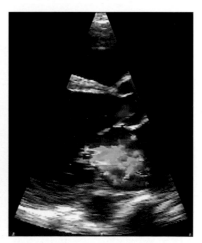

Chapter 26, Figure 4C, p. 223

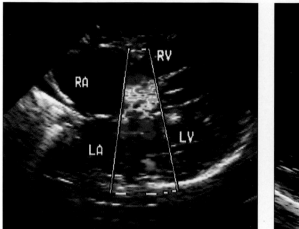

Chapter 31, Figure 2, p. 269

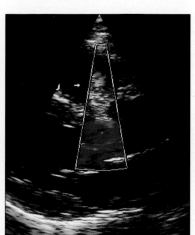

Chapter 31, Figure 3, p. 271

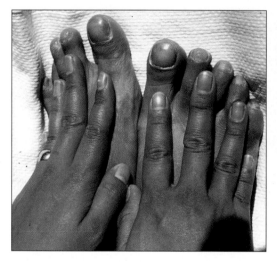

Chapter 31, Figure 4, p. 272

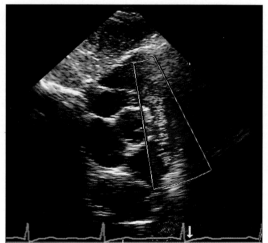

Chapter 31, Figure 5, p. 272

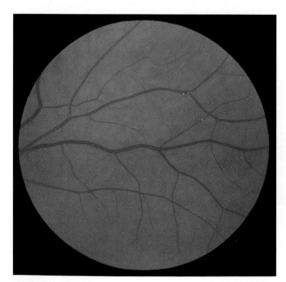

Chapter 38, Figure 2, p. 332